T0316404

TECHNOPATHOGENOLOGY

Guillermo Miguel Eguiazu & Alberto Motta

TECHNOPATHOGENOLOGY

TECHNOLOGY AND NON-EVIDENT RISKS – A CONTRIBUTION TO PREVENTION

PETER LANG

Bern · Berlin · Bruxelles · Frankfurt am Main · New York · Oxford · Wien

Bibliographic information published by die Deutsche Nationalbibliothek
Die Deutsche Nationalbibliothek lists this publication in the Deutsche National-
bibliografie; detailed bibliographic data is available on the Internet
at ‹http://dnb.d-nb.de›.

British Library Cataloguing-in-Publication Data:
A catalogue record for this book is available from The British Library, Great Britain

Library of Congress Cataloging-in-Publication Data

Eguiazu, Guillermo M.
Technopathogenology : technology and non-evident risks : a contribution to
prevention / Guillermo Miguel Eguiazu & Alberto Motta.
p. ; cm.
Includes bibliographical references.
ISBN 978-3-03-430612-6
I. Motta, Alberto. II. Title.
(DNLM: 1. Environmental Exposure–adverse effects. 2. Technology.
3. Hazardous Substances–adverse effects. 4. Hazardous Substances.
5. Risk Assessment. 6. Risk Management. QT 140)

614.4–dc23

2012004459

The text was originally written in Spanish and translated for this publication
by Lucila Cordone.
The translation was meticulously revised and corrected by the authors in
collaboration with Prof. Armin Tenner. The authors guarantee that the text at
hand corresponds to the original Spanish version.

Cover design: Didier Studer, Peter Lang AG

ISBN 978-3-0343-0612-6

© Peter Lang AG, International Academic Publishers, Bern 2012
Hochfeldstrasse 32, CH-3012 Bern, Switzerland
info@peterlang.com, www.peterlang.com

Printed in Hungary

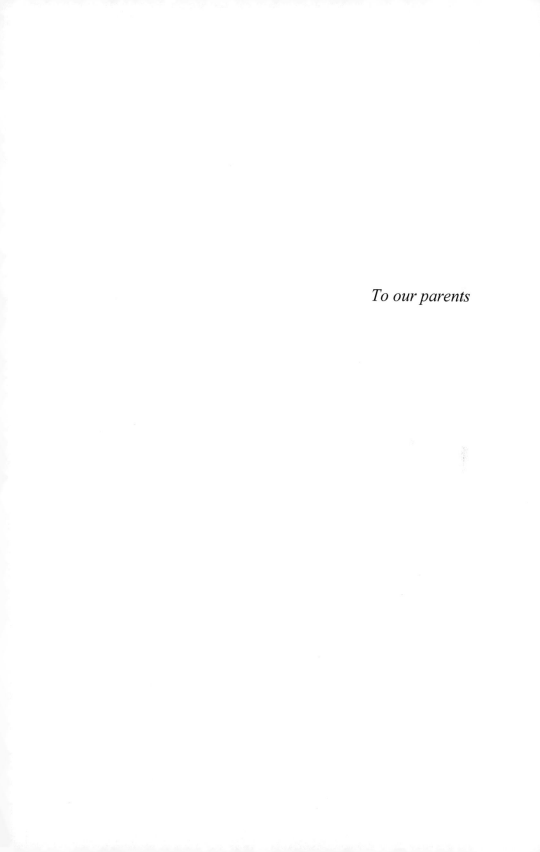

To our parents

Acknowledgements

This book could not have been possible had it not been for the recognition, trust and committment of three honourable persons who supported our work.

Should our discipline contribute to protect human beings from non-evident technological risk, it will not be our credit alone but their's too. These persons are:

- Professor Dr. Heinrich Beck, who, through his work and personal charisma has given us the intellectual thrust needed to understand the essence of Technique in our object of study. We thank him for his encouragement and support, for his commitment in the dissemination of our work and for his devotion in the evaluation of the manuscript. (*)

- Dr. Günter Emde, founder and first director of the INESPE project, for his moral support, but especially for the continuous material support given through the years to A. Motta after he was expelled from the University due to the whistleblower nature of our work. Had it not been for Dr. Emde's integrity and generosity we wouldn't have been able to carry out this work.

- Professor Dr. Armin Tenner, member and former Chairman of the INES network, for his moral support, for encouraging us to write this book, for his dedication during the writing process and meticulous revision and correction of the translation of the chapters and especially, for financing its publication.

We would also like to thank:

- Katrin Forrer, for her excellent disposition and unconditional and essential support in the text typesetting.

- Peter Lang AG, for trusting in our work.

- Marta Taborda de Eguiazu, for her kind support in the writing of this book.

- Andrés Guillermo Eguiazu, for his good disposition and computer technical support.

- Bolsa de Comercio de Rosario, whose uninterrupted and unselfish support since 1976 allowed us to be the first to detect aflatoxins in local corn.

(*) Prof. Beck's report on our work is included in the Annex.

Preface

We could define science as a kind of adventure. Like a cave explorer, or a deep sea diver, who enters unknown territories driven by curiosity and the need to discover something new, a scientist also dives into the unknown territories of science, into that *ontic* universe where there is so much yet to discover, driven by a feeling that there is something out there and by the desire to discover it.

However, just like an explorer, who must face the obstacles posted by the places he or she dives in, a scientist entering new fields of knowledge might also face many obstacles, and keep going forward *in spite of* such obstacles. These obstacles include not only those inherent to the field of knowledge to be explored, but also those generated by colleagues and people within the field.

We are saying this because we ourselves have found unexpected obstacles while exploring this new field of knowledge of technology we call Technopathogenology, many of such obstacles coming as a result of the ethical commitment we assumed in the unconditional search for knowledge.

These obstacles made Dr. Günter Emde, founder and leader of INESPE, the project for Ethical Engagement of INES (International Network of Engineers and Scientists for Global Responsibility), regard us as ethical objectors within the scientific field – a figure that, while common in private business, seemed unconceivable in science.

In 2005, Prof. Armin Tenner – former chairman of INES – reaching a good understanding of our research encouraged us to write a book dealing with the foundations of our proposal for a new discipline. His request was materialized in the present book.

Our proposal is based on our personal search and experience. We do not intend to be conclusive, but to leave it open for other researchers to continue its development.

We are neither philosophers nor epistemologists, so the aspects related to these disciplines might be treated rather rudimentarily. We neither intend to impose a new epistemological doctrine. We are just two technologists who have noticed a phenomenon, an event or simply something that happens which was absent from our academic education. We are technologists who value our first hand knowledge in technology, thanks to which we are well aware of the cost, in terms of effort and money, of developing any new technique; a cost that makes it especially difficult to abandon or recall a technique which was found too late to pose a risk on health. We have simply detected an imperfection in the way technology is developed, wishing with all our hearts that this proposal contributes to detect and correct this imperfection with enough time in advance to prevent technopathogenic risk to human health and to help the industries involved avoid economic loss.

Delving into our research, we discovered a surprising world of voids in science and technology. The significance of some of these voids supports our proposal for the creation of a new science, Technopathogenology, for their study.

The risks of technique are well known. Science makes enormous efforts to prevent them. We consider that the discipline we propose can help accomplish such task and join the group of disciplines developed in the risk prevention field.

This book is the result of the compilation of lectures grouped in three areas: The phenomenon, its disciplinary void, and the proposal for a discipline for its study. These subjects form the first three chapters of the book. Other lectures are included in Chapter 4 as complementary reading matters. They were part of a course on Environmental Technopathogeny we created in 1988 and offered until 2002 to disseminate the fundamentals of Technopathogenology among graduate and undergraduate students.

The authors

Table of Contents

CHAPTER III – Technopathogenology – The science and its method

CHAPTER IV – Technopathogenology and its impact on society

ANNEX

Introduction

'The LORD God then took the man and settled him in the Garden of Eden, to cultivate and care for it'

Genesis 2, 15

According to the general proceedings of the advancement of knowledge, the problems, phenomena or events described in this book are framed within disciplines. When only one discipline is not enough to solve a given problem, many disciplines are used in what we call a *multidiscipline*. But when all the disciplines at hand cannot break the problem apart to reassemble it like a puzzle we talk about a *transdiscipline*, thus leading to the creation of a new discipline. In other words, the nature of the problem leads to the development of a transdiscipline, i.e., a language which can be understood by all the parties who are trying to solve it. The answers are not broken apart any longer but connected. This means that when a new phenomenon presents itself or is detected, what can happen is that after making the effort of framing it, the problem – which is relatively new or not very much studied – cannot be completely clarified by the existing disciplines, thus leaving still a *void in the residual knowledge*. If such phenomenon is important enough so that it needs further clarifying *in spite of*, a new discipline must be sketched out – that is to say, a new way of clarifying the phenomenon must be created. This must be the last resource, when there's no possible solution through previous methods. Finally, the void in knowledge and the void in a methodology to study it – which denounces a phenomenon not very much clarified yet – allows to draft out a specific science.

Every search begins with a question. If whoever asks it is not satisfied with the first answer, a new question may arise, and then another and another, making the subject to be successively re-studied or re-investigated (research, recherche, ricerca). Such is the beginning of research itself. Every research is a continuous search, an *endless search* (Popper, 1973) or an *unconditional search for knowledge* (Westerholm, 1999). This search that begins with the question can be clarified through experimental means, but can be also be pursued intellectually, leaving aside experimental means which would only lead to a dead end in spite of the formal beauty of the task. The search is then carried out with the *whole person*, metaphorically speaking, with a *common sense method* in which every tool that the researcher has is eclectically accepted. In some cases, his or her experimental tools may not be the most important to clarify the problem and in other cases they may be crucial. Therefore, each tool is adjusted to each question.

We will observe how a new phenomenon was found while trying to develop an in-depth answer to a question. A problem which *should not be but actually was there* and it had negative consequences to human health. A problem we call Technopathogeny. A problem whose disciplinary void allows for the creation of a new discipline for its study: Technopathogenology. We are saying that it should not have been there because within the positivist conception of science, the Technique that emerges spontaneously from the accumulation of positive knowledge should be as perfect as the science it originated from.

We will try to frame this new discipline within the framework provided by the generally accepted epistemological criteria.

The aim of science is to learn more about a problem, and we all agree on that. But there are different types of problems. Some problems are so complex that it could take a whole life to approach them correctly. The so-called environmental problem is one of them.

Our approach on the subject led us to abandon dozens of possible *solutions* to the problem and to dive, once again, into a new uncertainty. A problem can be solved superficially, making us feel satisfied. But we can also feel unsatisfied, so we start delving into the problem through a different question or a different approach that takes us away from the comfort and *settlement* of an established science. We all know that in an established science it is easy to get papers published just by having the formal requirements, financial aid, promotions, etc. On the other hand, the new approach, enormously risky and uncomfortable, pushes the investigators into an unknown field where, given that it is not *settled*, it is hard to obtain financial aid, promotions, etc. Our story is that of an endless search in an *unsettled* area. It is the result, like we said before, of an unconditional search for knowledge in reply to honest questions such as: How can I know more? What is the actual problem? If I carry on this way, will I know more about the problem?

These questions, which seem so simple, were always the ones we wanted to answer and when we managed, somehow, to answer them, we had to ask ourselves the question again and review what we had done. It is in this way that we have continuously searched for a new result that allowed us to re-focus or re-ask ourselves questions about the problem. We know that there are both simple and complex problems. We also know that some answers are completely satisfying, but others are not satisfactory at all. Our way was to be always unsatisfied with the answers to the problem and to search for more profound solutions. Our work is the result of a succession of dead-ends which lead to the search of new alternatives. What we describe in this book is the result of a search which was sometimes like making our way in the dark of a labyrinth.

We finally arrived to the conclusion that a new science was required to provide the means to prevent this new phenomenon, Technopathogeny.

However, the fact that this phenomenon emerges within the knowledge that will originate a new Technique does not mean that every single technological object will have an undetermined and unknown side which can cause a Technopathogeny. We would fall in a kind of immobility that would stop any type of technological change. This will always exist. The sciences that determine the technological progress are empirical sciences, and, in Goblot's words (Goblot, 1943):

> Every knowledge that lies within an empirical verification always has a part of speculation and approximation which can be very much reduced, but never eliminated

The origin of a Technopathogeny can lie within that part which cannot be eliminated. The aim of Technopathogenology is to provide the means to make any technological change or advancement safe and not random and to gradually and progressively reduce its risks. We aim for technological changes whose search and accomplishments in terms of benefits for human beings do not drift apart from the responsibility assigned to humans ever since their creation, as the Bible passage above cited prays. A change that does not *spoil* the environment or affect fellow humans, many of whom many times are not the direct beneficiaries of the works created by the Technical Man.

It was a principle of the ancient Greeks to execute all their tasks according to clear, certain and funded rules (Goblot, 1943). Similarly, the aim of Technopathogenology is to contribute to the establishment of a series of *canons* that technology should respect, so that the generated change does not lead to adverse effects of late manifestation in human health.

Technopathogenology also contributes to the control or prevention *a posteriori* of technological risks, but this aim is also pursued by other disciplines such as Risk Evaluation, Technological Evaluation, etc. However, the most important and substantial goal is to achieve a control *a priori* of such risk. An *a priori* control means the early recognition of indicators or signs that indicate that a technique is being developed with potential mistakes or flaws which are hazardous to human health. Chapter III includes the proposals and developed criteria of Technopathogenology on the subject.

Upon this book being in the correction stage, we were informed of the seminar *Other science, other technologies are possible* organised by INES and WFSW (World Federation of Scientific Workers) (May-June 2007) (INES, 2007). We feel that the title of this seminar is the best way to express in our Introduction that "a science that contributes to the development of technology without risks is possible".

CHAPTER I

Technopathogeny – The Phenomenon

'From the price of progress to the priceless progress'

I. The discovery of a phenomenon still undescribed

More than three decades ago we began our research having as *leitmotiv* the protection of human health from non-evident and non-acceptable technological risk. This beginning led to learning about a new phenomenon. Upon realising its relevance, magnitude and scope, in 1984 we created a specific program: Programa de Investigación Calidad Biológica y Biopatológica del Entorno Humano (PROCABIE) (Biological and Biopathological Quality of Human Environment Research Program) (Eguiazu & Motta, 1991). This program was originally called Programa de Investigación de la Calidad Biológica y Ecotoxicológica del Entorno Humano (Biological and Ecotoxicological Quality of Human Environment Research Program) since the concept of *biopathological* – which we would later use and whose fundamentals we will explain when we refer to the characteristics of neoplastic disease – was still not understood. The concept of biopathological is more precise and goes beyond the idea of ecotoxicological, which is, in turn, related to Ecology.

The scientific fundamentals of the program were outlined in 1985, at the 12th Argentine Symposium on Mycology (San Luis, Argentina, October 9th to 12th). They were presented in a paper which dealt with the origin and prophylaxis of mycotoxins and their connection with the technological modification of primeval grain. These fundamentals were later consolidated in 1988 in the International Congress of Toxicology (Buenos Aires, April 11th to 15th) in a paper dealing with non-evident and non-acceptable risk of pesticides.

As we advanced in the understanding of the problem, we started focusing on a phenomenon requiring special attention – a phenomenon we called *Technopathogeny* (first called as *Technogeny*).

We realized that the disciplinary, multidisciplinary and interdisciplinary approach from traditional sciences was insufficient. Therefore a radically different approach was required.

Any single phenomenon which is approached from different disciplines will be studied through different points of view and the results or conclusions will differ accordingly. For example, we could take a plant species which one researcher wants to study from the medical point of view and another researcher from a taxonomic point of view. Each researcher will answer different questions about the same plant species.

That is why we say that we need a different approach to study Technopathogeny. This new approach implies a change of paradigm, which, in some cases, as we have said before, can be described as *transdisciplinary*. This means that in order to study this phenomenon, we should not resort to a group of disciplines, but rather contemplate the question by liberating it from the existing disciplines: *the construction of knowledge around the problem as such.*

This transdisciplinary approach is particularly necessary when we refer to the phenomenon of unexpected side effects in Technique, especially regarding those which are negative to human health.

So far, we have discussed non-evident and non-acceptable risk: Technopathogeny. We add to that the need to create a new discipline to study it: *Technopathogenology.*

Below we will focus on explaining why Technopathogeny is a phenomenon and why is Technopathogenology necessary to study it.

The existence of so many disciplines gave rise to the following question: which are the concurrent elements within the framework of logic to allow for the discussion of the need of a new science?

Because we are technologists and, therefore, not specialized in epistemology, we consulted specialists in this field of philosophy about the conditions that the study of a field of knowledge must have in order to justify the need of a new science or discipline for its study. We could not obtain clear information.

At first, we tried to study the problem of aflatoxins – which we later defined as a Technopathogeny and which will be described in detail in Chapter II – by framing it within some of the existing disciplines and establishing a framework for this new phenomenon. We started out with a multidisciplinary criterion since we could not anticipate at the time the framing difficulties we would encounter. We found that none of the disciplines around us – Mycology, Ecology, and Grain Handling, among others – could provide for the outlines for the right prophylaxis.

The opportunity of having to later evaluate the problem of pesticides, along with the findings on aflatoxins, allowed us to find a common thread. This allowed us to consolidate the existence of a problem linked to Technique, a problem that, having such a dimension could be framed as a new phenomenon: Technopathogeny.

Later, once the phenomenon was explained, a new question arose: could this phenomenon be framed within the various existing disciplines for its study (Medicine, Toxicology, Epidemiology, etc.)? We also found that, just like with aflatoxins, only some of the aspects of this phenomenon could be studied by each of these disciplines, but not like a particular object of study.

The evidence of this new phenomenon and the finding of a disciplinary void for its study allowed us to propose the need of a specific discipline: Technopathogenology. It may seem a hard path, but as any project entailing difficulties but propelled by great aims, it shouldn't discourage anyone willing to tackle it. Besides, it is a way to accept the challenge of striving for a *priceless progress,* the motto we chose for this first chapter. The opposite would be to accept the easy and comfortable position of accepting the apparently unavoidable price for every innovation in modern Technology.

If we say that in order to study Technopathogeny we need a new discipline, let's now consider which are the required conditions for a phenomenon that justify the creation of a specific science for its study.

II. Epistemological criteria for the creation of a science

As in any factual science, apart from the need of the actual existence of a phenomenon, Technopathogenology must rely on a series of theories. Also, considering this definition of science (Colacilli de Muro, 1978). "Science is a complex human enterprise which, through trustworthy methods, can be applied to obtain bodies of formulated knowledge", we also see that in order to be able to speak of a new science the methodological rigor as well as the results (the obtained bodies of knowledge) are of utmost importance.

To sum it up, and without intending to delve ourselves into philosophical discussions regarding whether the criteria is correct or not, if we can find a logical concatenation among the elements which make up the epistemological group: *Phenomenon, Theories, Methodologies, Results,* we can then assert that Technopathogenology is a new science.

III. Epistemological group in Technopathogenology

We will refer to such elements in order to be able to justify our thesis on the need of the creation of a new science called Technopathogenology.

We will then start with the first element required to arrive to the description of a new science: *The Phenomenon.*

IV. The phenomenon

In order to justify why we can refer to Technopathogeny as a new phenomenon, we will begin by dealing with the subject that triggered our first investigations: aflatoxins – toxins which are part of the broader mycotoxins family.

To do so, we will refer to an ancient activity of humankind to obtain food: agriculture and livestock production – the area of Technology we specialized in.

Agriculture and livestock production, which is the combination of the ancient *agriculture* or mechanical art of agriculture and some aspects of the *venatio*, or mechanical art of hunting and handling and exploitation of animals, had a very slow evolution at first, coexisting with a human species that was evolving in parallel. The chronological time and the innovation rate grew at a very slow pace, vegetative, synchronic. The adaptation of Man to innovation did not require processes which were painful to him and innovation did not entail prospective unexpected risk to humans.

Inventions were gradually refined and improved human condition by permitting to feed more population with less human work.

This idyllic situation was maintained until the 20th century. During that century, the efficiency in production reached unthought-of limits, thanks to the development of the classical genetic selection first and of genetic engineering later. In addition, the intensive use of chemicals in agriculture managed, through Liebig's Law, the scientific application of fertilization laws and, since the discovery of the first pesticides, the control of microbial plagues in plants and animals. Both achievements resulted in an enormous increase in production. Nowadays improvements are more radical. They entail the exchange of specific genes from different species, a feat that would have never been achieved through classical methods.

The discovery of DDT was hailed as a success of human spirit in the war against pests. However, more realistic voices which recommended its careful use were ignored (Cottam, 1946).

Nowadays, a combination between biological and chemical innovation is used. On the one hand, genes are incorporated to species in order to improve certain yield characteristics and, on the other, plants are adapted to survive in an environment with high doses of pesticides. Some pests have become more resistant to a given pesticide after various generations of contact with the active principle, thus needing increasingly higher doses in order to be eliminated. It is therefore more economical to modify the plant in order to make it more resistant to pesticides (transgenic soy, for example) than to create a new pesticide. The resistance of species to agrochemicals also proves how short lived the technologist's *eureka!* can be. Sooner or later nature manages to muffle it by resorting to its own laws.

Production systems for meat, milk, etc. have been designed with the aid of several chemical coadjuvants – such as antibiotics, beta blockers, anabolic steroids or animal protein concentrates (questionably used on strictly herbivores) – to enhance considerably the turnout of the produce. The amount of meat is considerably increased depending less on the size of the land and more on resources such as food or chemical coadjuvants.

During storage, a series of measures are resorted to, including the use of pesticides in grains, sprouting inhibitors in tubers, liquid fungicides in fruits or others, such as controlled gas.

Finally, the product reaches the consumer – raw in the case of fruits, vegetables and meat, and processed in the case of cereal, dairy products, etc.

Many chemical products are used in the production process of food and only a few of them are known to be completely innocuous. In certain situations, for purely economic reasons, the unethical criterion of hiding toxicological evidence of the chemical product is resorted to so as to favor the company instead of the consumer. Many companies seem to choose this motto: *The lack or small quantity of evidence of health risks equals to No Risk at all.*

As an example, we will see the case of the different criteria used while considering the toxicological results of an active ingredient used as fungicide, from a company's perspective and from scientific organisms perspective.

Following economic rather that nutritional guidelines for its production process, the food product – now on the consumer's table ready to be ingested – has suffered a series of transformations. These transformations begin in its production, in the countryside. They continue with post-harvest storage and handling, industrial processing and final conservation by cold chain until the product is finally consumed.

Paradoxically, the excess of production can do little to help the hungry, since they have no wealth to buy the food they need. This last aspect is closely related to the problem of vernacular agricultural models, their biodiversity and autonomy of external resources – aspects which are clearly dodged in modern agriculture.

Some alarm signals begin to sound, all having unexpected side effects as a common element. Those signals present themselves as questions regarding the hidden error or defect that had not been contemplated earlier in the successful model until its belated manifestation. This belated manifestation, maybe after decades of work, usually occurs without those enthusiastically applying the model suspecting it.

Having described this situation referred to the production of food and the risk it entails to human beings – the object of study chosen not for its technopathogenic relevance but because of our agronomic background – we initiate the reflections on the phenomenon.

The Technopathogenic phenomenon: Its detection

The principle leading to the detection of this phenomenon was the coming to our knowledge of the 1972 Stockholm Conference recommendations on the need to prevent the damaging effects coming from the various environmental contaminants which humans are exposed to. These recommendations motivated us to start a line of research following the aim above described. Given our specialization in agronomy, we chose, among all the contaminants related to food production, one that had been discovered in England barely a decade before and which was considered of utmost importance: mycotoxins – a subject which had not been dealt with yet in our field. From this family of fungus related substances we chose one of them: aflatoxins – a potent carcinogenic considered a non-evident risk to human health.

After working for many years on mycotoxins, after many years of *rambling* from discipline to discipline as we will explain in next chapter, we could refer to the problem of mycotoxins as deeply connected to technology, in this case, to grain production. For this reason, and because the damages to health associated with these contaminants manifest themselves not only as acute intoxication but also as a long term condition, we could first refer to it as a Technopathogeny. Technopathogeny refers to long term damage, a type of risk we were especially interested in at the time since it is caused inadvertently. As we will see in next chapter, the risk implied by these contaminants motivated us to extend the question on the risk to other contaminants in particular and to Technique in general. We found that the Technopathogeny phenomenon manifested itself in the most diverse technologies.

Due to the relevance this phenomenon has for humans, we considered that in order to achieve the above cited aims it was necessary to create a specific program, thus giving birth to PROCABIE in 1984. The disciplinary field we then thought of including in our studies was Anthropoecology. After only a year of work within this framework, we came across a problem that, since it went beyond the environment, it did not fit the field of Ecology, as we will see later on. By the end of 1985 we started referring to the problem as Technopathogeny – which we called at first Technogeny. Below we list some of our lectures, courses and papers on the subject from those early years of research:

Table 1:   Events and Publications where the concept of Technopathogeny was presented

Year	Event – Publication
1985	*"Las Micotoxinas desde una perspectiva antropo-ecológica"* (Mycotoxins from an antropo-ecological perspective) – 12th Argentine Symposium on Mycology (San Luis, October 9th to 12th) – Oral Presentation. (Eguiazu, 1985)
1987	*"Pesticidas y Profilaxis del Error Tecnológico"* (Pesticides and Prophylaxis of the Technological Error) (Eguiazu, 1987a)
1987	*"Las Micotoxinas desde una perspectiva antropo-ecológica" (Mycotoxins from an antropo-ecological perspective)* (Eguiazu, 1987b)
1988	*"Plaguicidas y Error Tecnogénico"* (Pesticides and Technogenic Error) (Eguiazu, 1988).
1988	First Theoretical-Practical Course on Environmental Technogenic – (October-December) – Fac. De Ciencias Agrarias – Universidad Nacional de Rosario – Rosario – Rep. Argentina (Tecnogenia Ambiental).
1989	"2nd National Seminar on University and Environment" (Paraná, Entre Ríos, October 25th to 27th) Argentina. (Motta & Eguiazu, 1989) (Eguiazu, 1991).
1991	*"Programa de Investigación de la Calidad Biológica y Ecotoxicológica del Entorno Humano"* (Biological and ecotoxicological quality of human environment research program). (Eguiazu & Motta, 1991). *Tecnogenología – Una respuesta a la necesidad de prevenir los efectos nocivos ocultos en la Técnica"* (Technogenology: an answer to the need to prevent technique's hidden side effects) (Eguiazu, 1991).

V.   Technopathogeny and Technique

Our starting point was agriculture and livestock production and, within this field, food production specifically. We have seen that the production of food entails the application of Techniques. The fact that such Techniques can bring about certain risks leads to the following question:

Why can we say that Technique causes non-evident and non-acceptable risk?

More generally, we could say that in their constant search for goods to satisfy their needs, humans adapt and create objects transforming matter and energy by means of procedures or Techniques developed from bodies of knowledge or Technologies. Here we should distinguish the term *Technique* from the term *Technology*. Although they are sometimes used as synonyms in everyday language, in fact they are not so. For the purpose of this book, we can make the following distinction:

Technique: refers to the group of processes used to achieve a specific aim, either goods or services.

Technology: is the group of necessary bodies of knowledge for the development or creation of a Technique.

One given good, service or goal – whatever might be called – can be achieved by means of different Techniques. For example, in medicine, certain illnesses required invasive techniques or procedures that needed a long recovery period. A series of new technologies – development of new materials like optical fiber and more profound knowledge of light physics – allowed for the development of a new technique: laparoscopy, which causes much less pain on the patient and reduces significantly the recovery time.

The need for faster change determines the existence of missing elements or voids which can cause flaws in the Technique developed. These flaws, in turn, can generate factors which can be harmful to human health and can cause the non-evident risks we have referred to before. This is why we can call these factors *Technopathogenous*.

Every Technique has *Positive Aspects* – the ones its creator was looking for in the first place. Such aspects must exist within the technological object to comply with the aim or aims for which the object was conceived, that is to say, to satisfy the needs of the people it was created for. For example: to cure a disease, to fight a plague, to color food, to transmit a signal, etc. This way an immediate problem can be successfully solved. But there can also be *Negative Aspects*. The Technician is aware of such negative aspects (or at least, like we will see later on, of some of the negative aspects), and that is why certain levels of risk and the consequent safety precautions are established for the Technique in particular.

Regarding the negative aspects of the Technique and the risks it entails, it is interesting to see a comparison made by scientists between catastrophes produced by natural and technological causes, in both cases referring to catastrophes producing 100 or more cases of acute deaths (Gassen, 1988):

Table 2: Frequency of catastrophe with 100 cases or more of acute death, based on natural and technological disasters

Technical Causes	Can happen once every:
Air crash (with occupants death)	2 years
Big fire	7 years
Explosion	16 years
Dam break	25 years
Air crash (with death of people on land)	100 years
Nuclear reactor accident	100,000 years
Natural disasters	**Can happen once every:**
Tornadoes or hurricanes	5 years
Earthquakes	20 years
Meteorite Impact	100,000 years

Interestingly enough, scientists gave the same probability of occurrence to a nuclear accident and a meteorite impact producing the same amount of deaths (over 100, not including long term deaths). Chernobyl proved them wrong. This supports the idea that the gestational process of any technology based on a nuclear phenomenon must be reconsidered.

This leads us to another reflection. In spite of all the safety precautions taken, accidents do take place in munitions and explosives warehouses – whether spontaneous or sabotage related. However, a modern nuclear reactor is not considered as risky as an explosives warehouse. Something in the nature of nuclear technology is not quite right if a nuclear reactor used for peaceful aims poses the same risk as a warfare facility. Even though the aim of the nuclear reactor is purely peaceful, it engenders the same risk as a warfare facility.

Later on we will observe this technological activity, the generation of energy, through two different techniques – fossil fuel and nuclear fuel – and we will analyze their differences concerning technogenic risk. We will see that the differences are quite clear.

Let's now think of another type of accident that can occur in any industry working with microorganisms. Let's first think of an accident that produces the liberation of natural pathogens in a medical or pharmaceutical laboratory. Lacking the highly controlled conditions it had in the laboratory, it will most likely either die or eventually disappear (having no selective advantage). That is to say, the pathogen might infect the immediate operators and nearby population, but having no selective advantages over the rest of the organisms in the environment, it will most probably not be able to spread significantly.

Let's now consider an accident in which some organism with synthetic genome is liberated. In the best of cases, it will not spread significantly but will be naturally controlled by balancing with the medium. But we should consider the possibility that a modification in its genetic information could give the organism selective advantages thus making it more dangerous to Humans. If it is a new pathogen, it could affect them. If it is an organism that was developed with economic aims, it could alter the balance between species. Thus, a genetically engineered vegetable or fruit could pose a threat to other existing vegetables or fruits due to its capacity to compete and spread without control (von Weizsäcker, 1986).

We will get back to this point when we refer to risks of genetically modified organisms.

These negative aspects produce an imbalance between the *necessary harmony between humans and their human environment.* Below we will explain what we understand by human environment and why we speak of a necessary harmony.

VI.   Characteristics of the human / human environment harmony

1) Human Environment

Used alone, the term Environment is commonly related to Ecology or easily linked to Ecology. In this context, the alterations in the environment caused by Technique are also defined as Environmental Unbalance. The affected beings would include animals, plants and, of course, Humans.

In relation to the causes of cancer and the Environment it is interesting to refer to the following concept of the National Cancer Institute (NCI-NIH, 2003), that say:

> Several factors both inside and outside the body contribute to the development of cancer. In this context, scientists refer to everything outside the body that interacts with humans as the *Environment*.

29

About environment it is mentioned that "unfortunately, the statements were sometimes repeated with *environment* used to mean only air, water, and soil pollution" (Congress of the United States/Office of the Technology Assessment, 1981).

In order to avoid misinterpretations we prefer to use the concept of *Human Environment* because it is much more precise. Apart from the environmental components – soil, air, and water – it also refers to everything that enters in contact with Humans and their exposed surfaces, including the digestive system, the respiratory system and the skin. It therefore includes the substances which are ingested with food (additives, contaminants and substances drunk or inhaled). It also includes natural or medical radiation, exposure in the workplace, medication and other aspects, apart from factors present on the soil, air and water (Congress of the United States/Office of the Technology Assessment, 1981) (U.S. DHHS-PHS, 2002). We are especially interested in the risks that affect human beings. Such risks arise from elements originated in natural science but they are also caused by human actions or errors, therefore we distance ourselves from the narrow minded biologicist mechanism which excludes from this concept everything that is essentially human. These aspects can be only taken into account accepting human environment in its broader sense.

2) Harmony

We speak of harmony because the relationship between humans and the components of their human environment is characterized by three conditions: a) Finiteness; b) Fragility; c) Supratemporality (Eguiazu, 1985).

a) The finiteness indicates that the proportion and correspondence between Humans and the components of their human environment that make life possible is limited.

b) Fragility indicates that the proportion and correspondence can be easily altered. For example, Technique can determine a bigger proportion of carcinogenic substances in the human environment. This can exceed the capacity of the organism to counteract or repair the damage these substances produce, therefore causing more cases of neoplasia in the population inhabiting the area.

c) Supratemporality indicates that Technique can alter the proportion and correspondence between Humans and the components of their

Human Environment so significantly that not only Humans living today can be harmed but also humans living in the future. This is the case of areas contaminated with radioactivity, areas contaminated with substances having high physicochemical stability, etc. In the case of substances having high physicochemical stability, it will mean a long persistence of such substances in the human environment, representing an increase in risk for people who might be exposed as well as their descendants. Such substances include the chlorinated pesticides which, even in regions where they have been prohibited, residues continue to be detected after many years.

3) Necessary

We say it is Necessary because Humans require certain amount and correspondence among the elements of their human environment, without which life for them is either very difficult or impossible. If some of the air components are above the normal level, for example, they can be a cause of death. Certain amount of pesticide residue can cause intoxication. For some carcinogenic substances, like we will observe later on, its mere presence in the human environment is enough to pose a high risk of carcinogenesis, regardless of proportion. Only the complete absence of such substances in the human environment will make it completely safe.

VII. Technology's approach to maintain the balance

We have said that technicians are aware that technique can have negative aspects. But we have also said that they are aware of only some of them. And here is the reason why: Negative aspects can be *evident* or *non evident*. *Evident aspects* are, for example, acute toxicity risk (in the short term) for a given substance, electrocution risk, loss of limb risk, etc. These are risks the technician is aware of. *Non evident negative aspects*, on the other hand, are those which manifest themselves after many years or even generations, like in the case of carcinogenic substances, for example. In general, technicians are not aware of such negative aspects.

Humans correct or prevent the imbalance in harmony that a negative aspect causes or may cause, provided such imbalance is evident and obvious. In the case of pesticides, for example, the technician performs a series of trials to measure how toxic the product is using the Median Lethal Dose (LD50) as reference. This value is applied to acute or single dose toxicity, and means that this dose of the product can kill 50% of the animals exposed to the trial. The lower the DL50 value, the higher the toxicity of the product. This value indicates the Technician which is the proportion of pesticide residue that humans can ingest without it posing a risk to their health. With that information, he calculates the Acceptable Daily Intake (ADI) value.

Knowing the physicochemical properties of the pesticide, for example, the technician can estimate the level of degradation of the product. He or she can then know when is the last possible pre-harvest time to apply the product in a crop so that the pesticide's proportion of active ingredient is within the levels of innocuousness when harvested.

However, this is not the case with Non Evident Negative Aspects. They remain hidden within the Technique, in built or adapted objects, only coming to light in the long term.

Among the Non evident Negative Aspects we find, for example, the carcinogenicity of a substance.

Apart from satisfying consumers' needs, goods are produced within a business framework which also aims for an efficient production which increases profit or benefits. Like we said before, this can lead to a hasty application of knowledge that is still full of voids, thus posing unnoticed risks on health.

Pathogen are those "influences or elements that originate or favor the development of diseases" (Diccionario Enciclopédico Ilustrado de la Lengua Española). As we have said before, we have proposed to define those influences or elements coming from Technique that originate or favor the development of diseases as *Technopathogen*. Technopathogenology studies those non evident risks. Similarly, following the term *Iatrogenic* – a disease inadvertently caused by a physician – we coined the neologism *Technogenic*. Later, with the aim of making the meaning more explicit, we coined the term *Technopathogeny:*

> The diseases or harm to health either physical or psychic caused to human beings, not occurring immediately after but after many years or generations as a conse-

quence of exposure to non evident aspects generated by Technique or Technopathogens that are present in the Human Environment, produced by hidden immanent Errors or Flaws.

We have used the terms *immanent* and *hidden* – which we will detail later on – to refer to the damage Technique causes inadvertently to health, significant errors in the conception and construction of a Technique which were unnoticed by the technologist during the developmental stage.

This is clearly different from evident damage or possible damage caused by technology, which lie within human risk or error management, such as an oil spill.

Technopathogenesis is a group of successive stages or processes that lead to make evident the phenomenon of the Technopathogeny.

To sum up, we have coined the following neologisms: Technopathogeny; Technopathogenesis; Technopathogenic. From all these terms the concept of *Technogenology* or *Technopathogenology* is derived.

VIII. Technopathogeny: Analyzing its defining terms

This object of study deserves a thorough explanation on each of its parts (Eguiazu, 1992,1998) (Eguiazu & Motta, 1991).

First and foremost, we would like to state that our object of study, Technopathogeny, is in no way related to *Good or Bad Praxis* – which are terms used to define a different phenomenon in technological activities, including medicine. In this case, it is not the nature of the technological tool what is in question, but the expertise of the technician who uses it.

In a case of bad praxis what would be questioned is not the nature of the medicine or crop treatment technique, but the decision of the technician whether to apply it or not. If there is a negative effect, it will be due to the technician's lack of knowledge or expertise.

Bad praxis is a consequence of a technician's error or lack of expertise. Technopathogeny, however, comes from a flaw or error within the technological object. An example of this would be the collateral effects of a medicine or a pesticide, which will be manifested notwithstanding the technician's proficiency.

Having defined the three concepts (Human Environment, Harmony and Need), let's now define the other terms present in the definition of Technopathogeny.

Negative consequences to human health

By negative consequences to human health we refer to the concrete manifestation of the Technopathogeny phenomenon, i.e., illnesses or conditions which are harmful to human health, either somatically or psychically, and which do not manifest themselves immediately after exposure but after many years or generations.

It is clear that there is no such thing as a Technique without unexpected results or collateral effects, which can either be positive, neutral or negative. We will focus on those negative effects that appear after the application of a certain technology, which are relevant enough so as to be taken as objects of study in scientific research. We are then narrowing down the field of study to the negative effects on human health such as negative or unwanted collateral effects caused by the technological object. We are also interested in damages to the ecosystem or other living creatures but always in connection to the risk entailed on humans (Eguiazu, 1991), or when such damages can be taken as indicators of a potential technopathogenic risk.

In relation to Technopathogeny, cancer can be taken as a paradigmatic case. A 60% to 90% of cases of cancer or neoplasia are thought to be caused by agents on the human environment (Congress of United States/Office of Technology Assessment, 1981).

For the purpose of this book, we would like to define:

Neoplasia: The process through which a tumor is formed and grows (U.S. DHHS-PHS-NTP, 1985).

Neoplasm: Any new and abnormal cell growth which can be benign or malignant (U.S. DHHS-PHS-NTP, 1985).

Cancer: A malignant tumor characterized by the proliferation of abnormal cells (carcinoma o sarcoma) (NIOSH, 1979).

Carcinoma: New growth of a malignant tumor (NIOSH, 1979).

Sarcoma: Malignant neoplasm deriving from connective tissue (U.S. DHHS-PHS-NTP, 1985).

34

Neoplasia, then, refers to the development of a tumor, whilst cancer refers to the development of a malignant tumor.

However, the US National Toxicology Program (NTP) Toxicology and Carcinogenesis research report (US DHHS-PHS-NIH-NTP, 2001) used to establish the level of carcinogenesis evidence needed to consider an agent as presenting *Clear Evidence of Carcinogenic Activity*, when:

> It is demonstrated by studies that are interpreted as showing a dose-related (i) increase in malignant neoplasms, (ii) increase in a combination of malignant and benign neoplasms, or (iii) marked increase of benign neoplasms if there is an indication from this of other studies of the ability of such tumors to progress to malignancy.

In the level of evidence needed to consider an agent as presenting *Some evidence of carcinogenic activity*, the report (US DHHS-PHS-NIH-NTP, 2001) indicates:

> It is demonstrated by studies that are interpreted as showing a chemical-related increase incidence of neoplasms (malignant, benign, or combined) in which the strength of the response is less than that required for clear evidence.

Also, for an agent to be *Listed as reasonably anticipated to be a human carcinogen,* in point (b) the NTP (U.S. DHHS-PHS-NTP, 2002), indicates:

> There is sufficient evidence of carcinogenicity in experimental studies with animals, which indicates an increase of malignant tumors incidence or a combination of benign and malignant tumors.

Table 8 references expand on this criterion.

The International Agency for Research on Cancer defines Chemical Carcinogenesis (IARC, 1983a), as:

> The induction by chemicals of neoplasms that are not usually observed, the early induction by chemicals of neoplasms that are commonly observed, and/or the induction by chemicals of more neoplasms that are usually found-although fundamentally different mechanisms may be involved in these three situations. Etymologically, the term *carcinogenesis*, means the induction of cancer, that is, of malignant neoplasms; however, the commonly accepted meaning is the induction of various types of neoplasms or of a combination of malignant and benign tumors. In the monographs, the words *tumor* and *neoplasms*, are used interchangeably. (In scientific literature the terms *tumorigen, oncogen,* and *blastomogen,* have all been used synonymously with *carcinogen*, although occasionally *tumorigen* has been used specifically to denote a substance that induces benign tumours).

That is to say, it refers to neoplasms, not limiting chemical carcinogenesis to malignant tumors.

In relation to Technopathogenology, what is relevant is to know whether this factor can, among others, develop a tumor. It is not relevant whether it is benign or malignant since, as we have seen, a benign tumor can evolve into a malignant tumor.

Some quotes on cancer of technopathogenological relevance are:

"American statistics state that one every four Americans will have cancer and one every five will die of this malignancy" (U.S. DHHS-PHS-NTP, 1985).

Some of the agents causing cancer are: occupational exposure to unknown etiological elements, medicines, pesticides, food additives, cosmetics, natural substances, solvents, inks, pigments, etc. (U.S. DHHS-PHS-NTP, 1985).

About 200 diseases can be considered as a type of cancer. Cancer epidemiology and experimental carcinogenesis have established that the carcinogenic process is *multifactor* in causation and *multistage* in its development (Congress of United States-Office of Technology Assessment, 1981). Cancer develops through different stages: *initiation, promotion* and *progression* (U.S. DHHS-PHS, 1984). More general terms for the two first stages are *early* and *late* events (Congress of United States-Office of Technology Assessment, 1981).

The substances capable of initiating and promoting a cancer process are known as *complete carcinogens*. They function both as *initiators* and *promoters* (Congress of United States-Office of Technology Assessment, 1981). There are certain substances or more generally agents, called *initiators* that can only initiate a cancer process. "The initiator is a chemical that permanently alters a cell or group of cells and, in the case of carcinogens, it is tumor-producing" (U.S. DHHS-PHS-NTP, 2002). According to another definition (Congress of United States-Office of Technology Assessment, 1981), an initiator is:

An external stimulus or agent that produces a cell that is *latently premalignant.* An initiation event, or more generally *early event*, may be a mutational change in the cell's genetic material, but the change is unexpressed, and it causes no detectable change in the cell's growth pattern. The change is considered to be irreversible.

"Initiated cells may lie quiescent if they are not *turned on* by a *promoter* and cancer may never develop if sufficient exposures to promoter do not occur" (Congress of United States-Office of Technology Assessment, 1981).

We have said that the initiation is defined as mutational change. It is mentioned (U.S. DHHS-PHS, 1984) that:

> There is indeed sufficient evidence to believe that the process of carcinogenesis – initiation in particular – results from mutational changes occurring in somatic cells. But mutation is used in the broad sense as a change in DNA or chromosome structure that is inheritable at the somatic level. It may include specific changes in DNA sequence, i.e., point mutations (based substitution, frame shift), deletions, insertions, gene rearrangement and gene amplification as well as gross chromosomal changes, i.e. translocations, aneuploidy, etc.

Initiation is considered irreversible (Congress of United States-Office of Technology Assessment, 1981) (U.S. DHHS-PHS-NTP, 2002). Also, it is mentioned (Weinstein, 1982) that:

> There is also considerable evidence that the successive stages in carcinogenesis may involve qualitatively different events that can be enhanced or inhibited by quite different types of environmental and host factors, and that the early stages (at least) are often reversible.

While other substances, or more generally: agents, called *promoters* can only promote the cancer process. "Promoter is a chemical that, although not carcinogenic itself, serves to dramatically potentiate the effect of a low dose of a carcinogen" (U.S. DHHS-PHS-NTP, 2002). Another definition (Congress of United States/Office of Technology Assessment, 1981) describes promoter as:

> An influence or agent causing an initiated cell to produce a tumor. Promotion events, or more generally, *late events*, can occur only in initiated cells, and are somewhat reversible. Discontinuation of exposure to a promoter, if exposure has not yet caused a tumor, may prevent the appearance of a tumor.

"Promoters convert only initiated cells to tumor cells and have not lasting effects on non initiated cells" (Congress of United States-Office of Technology Assessment, 1981). If the organism has no initiated cells, promoter substances will have no effect whatsoever.

When we analyze technopathogenic risk associated to electromagnetic fields, we will see that they can only promote the development of tumors – that is to say, cancer can only develop if there is one or various initiated cells. This does not mean, however, that electromagnetic fields are harmless. We should bear in mind the enormous amount of substances of daily use produced by humans and the action of contaminants which determine that some of those substances which humans might have been exposed to may have left a mark, an initiation process through which promotional factors can favor the development of a tumor.

About the classification of carcinogens as initiators and promoters, it is also said (U.S. DHHS-PHS, 1984) that:

> The classification of carcinogens as initiators and promoters does not seem justified in an absolute sense, since a carcinogen could act as an initiating agent in one tissue and as promoter in another. For example, urethane is carcinogenic for mice lungs but not for the skin, which goes to say that urethane has only got an initiating activity in the skin.

It is very important to explain that the development of cancer also depends on *host factors* (U.S. DHHS-PHS-NTP, 1985).

> Host factors are attributes of human organisms associated with individual differences in the risk of developing a specified cancer. A host factor may be associated with reduced risk of a cancer, not only with increased risk. Examples of host factors are: immunological and endocrine functions, nutritional status, genetic constitution, age and sex.

To sum up, we understand by *initiator* the external stimulus or agent generating a cell called latently premalignant, an initiation event or more commonly known as an *early event*. It can be a mutational change in the genetic material of a cell, but the change is not expressed and it does not provoke noticeable changes in the growing patterns of the cell. What we understand as *promoter* is the influence or agent that causes that an initiating cell originates a tumor. The promotional events or more commonly known as *late events* can only occur in an initiated cell and they can be reversible. If the exposure to the promoting agent is discontinued or interrupted, and if exposure hasn't caused the apparition of the tumor yet, such apparition could be prevented (Congress of United States-Office of Technology Assessment, 1981).

Other interesting properties are *synergism* and *co-carcinogenesis*.

"Synergism is the aspect of two agents interacting to produce an effect greater than the sum of the agents' individual effects" (U.S. DHHS-PHS-NTP, 2002).

An example of this is cigarette consumption and exposure to asbestos. The incidence of cancer on people exposed to both factors is higher than the incidence of cancer exposed only to cigarette smoking or only to asbestos (Congress of United States-Office of Technology Assessment, 1981).

Cocarcinogenic is "an agent that is not carcinogenic itself, but enhances the activity of another agent that is carcinogenic" (U.S. DHHS-PHS-NTP, 2002).

These characteristics of neoplastic diseases and of factors causing them imply that even if the carcinogenic property of a technopathogen is discovered, it is very difficult to prevent their risk. Even if there is legislation forbidding its usage – if it is used in a technique – or making a compulsory analysis and control if it is a contaminant – if the person has already been exposed, he or she might end up getting the disease. This example further supports the notion that a correct or anticipated prophylaxis in technological design would be the logical road towards successful prevention.

The wide variety of etiological agents shows us that adverse effects in technique do not circumscribe to a specific group in society. On the contrary, every single person can be exposed to causal agents.

Considering the labor environment, a report prepared by the International Labor Organization, states that "at least 7 out of 10 diseases and injuries related to work (included in a list conceived by the National Institute for Occupational Safety and Health (NIOSH) of the United States) are originated totally or partially by exposure to hazardous substances" (ILO, 1987). "Many diseases which are probably not caused by labor environment exposure can be worsened by it" (ILO, 1987).

When we defined Technopathogeny, we talked about psychological as well as physical damage. It is easy to identify a Technopathogeny in somatic manifestations such as neoplastic diseases. It is easy to understand a Technopathogeny at the reproductive and gestational level, as well as the aetiology of other conditions such as diabetes, neurological, etc. These technopathogenies of somatic manifestation can also cause psychic damage such as, for example, neurological conditions that can cause damage at the psychological, psychiatric or behavioral level (Anger, 1993).

Technopathogenies associated to psychic damage, loss of intelligence, mental retardation and speech skills diminishing were found in children whose mothers had been exposed to ionizing radiation in Chernobyl during their gestational period. The peak of these conditions is significant over nine months after the incident (Schmitz-Feuerhake, 2006).

This description enables us to see clearly the negative consequences on human health associated with Technopathogeny.

As we have mentioned before, we were inspired on the term Iatrogenesis to define this phenomenon. Even though Medicine is a Technique in itself, it uses other techniques for the treatment of the most diverse diseases and even there are different techniques to treat one single condition, so it is interesting to analyze the big differences between Technopathogeny and Iatrogenesis (Eguiazu, 1991). From a logical point of view, Iatrogenesis, because medicine is a technique, is also a Technopathogeny. In table 3, we will find the answer.

Factors generated by Technique or Technopathogenous agents

Chemical substances, physical factors, biological factors and cultural and psychological factors are factors that can be generated by technique or technopatogenous agents that can originate or favour a Technopathogeny.

Table 3:   Differences between Iatrogenesis and Technopathogeny

Technopathogeny	Iatrogenesis
Technological origin	Medical origin
Maximum spatial dimension	Minimum spatial dimension
The recipient is usually not someone who profits from the technique causing the technopathogeny.	The recipient is who receives the medicine or his or her immediate descendants (for example, through the placenta)
The risk and benefit does not necessarily affect the same person	The risk and benefit do affect the same person or immediate descendants, users of the medical technique
The cause-effect relationship is complex and hard to prove.	The cause-effect relationship is relatively simple.
Multifactorial	One cause – one effect
Effects of sub-chronic doses during relatively long periods of time	Relatively high doses during relatively short periods of time

Chemical factors

Include these substances:
- natural
- synthetic
- of usage
- contaminants

Physical factors

Include:
- Electric fields
- Magnetic fields
- Microwaves
- Radiofrequencies
- Radiation
- UV light
- etc.

Biological factors

Include:
- Organic dust
- Transgenic products

Cultural or psychological Factors:

If we consider, like we briefly will later on, that apart from the intervention of technique in the fields of Physics, Chemistry and Biology, humans can also intervene in the cultural field through Psychotechnique and Sociotechnique, we should not underestimate these techniques as generators of cultural and psychological factors that can cause Technopathogeny.

As we have said before, technopathogens can be evident or non-evident. An evident technopathogen could be heat generated or toxic vapor emanated by a technique in particular which can harm the people exposed if they are not adequately protected. Like we have said before, Technopathogenology is interested in non-evident risk.

Technopathogens can, in turn, cause a Technopathogeny directly or indirectly. They do it directly when a technopathogen causes the damage without needing modification. They do it indirectly when the technopathogen requires a previous transformation. For example, some substances need to be metabolized in the organism in order to have a carcinogenic effect. Other substances require a prior chemical reaction with another substance in order to have a carcinogenic effect – like we will see later on with Nitroso compounds.

Technique

Taking the most abstract definition, and regardless the obvious redundancy, we can talk about *theory in movement*. This means *the knowledge with which an invention with a determined and concrete aim is carried out*. What we state here is that this usage of so-called scientific knowledge is deeply imperfect. Due to its inevitable methodological reductionism, the so-called scientific knowledge of reality is fragile It is so fragile that a theory can only be asked to be falsifiable but nothing else (Popper, 1973). For this work's specific purpose what we understand by *falsify, forge, forgery, falsifier* is the possible demonstration of falseness of a hypothesis, theory, etc.

When making *Techne* (Art – Technique) based on this incomplete knowledge – and considering that this *Techne* is further distanced from the ancient empirics or rudimentary way of generating knowledge to become what we now know as Techno-logy – *we do not know what will come up along with the expected.* In some cases, for personal, economic, etc. reasons even the possibility of *something* coming up along with the expected can be denied. This statement seems rather exaggerated, given the fact that our culture has a blind faith in science, technology and the technologist's work. Everything seems to be under perfect control and we find it very hard to distance ourselves from this *blind faith* in Science and Technology. However, if we distance ourselves from the dogma of believing that scientific work is perfect, or that there is a unique method to achieve perfect knowledge or that science is almost perfect, the logical conclusion is that it is highly likely to find collaterality along with the expected.

Human Environment

Even though we have already referred to this term, we would like to insist that the reason why we prefer this concept is because it is more closely linked to humans, whereas environment is more related to ecology.

The idea of human environment is more precise, since apart from including the environment components – soil, air, water – it also includes whatever is related to humans, to whatever is in contact with their exposed surfaces (digestive system, respiratory system and skin). It therefore includes substances which are ingested with food, such as additives, contaminants, drunk and inhaled substances. Natural and/or medical radiation, exposure on the workplace, medicines and other aspects; elements present in the soil, air and water are also included.

Error or Flaw

In a broader sense what we are dealing with here is the technical object, which could be as diverse as a machine, a chemical substance, or even something immaterial, like a psychological method. When we speak of error or flaw, we are referring to the manifestation produced in the *Techne's* kinetics, an unwanted effect, unexpected when applied. We say that the error or flaw lies within the technical object because it is independent from the use of technique – the error lies within the nature of the technique.

To illustrate this concept, we could use the example of the architect. If an architect designs a beam conceived with an error or miscalculation by which it ends up being built with less iron or concrete than it should have, the beam could collapse. Therefore, the error or misconception lies within the plan long before the beam is actually made. Should the beam be constructed, it would, metaphorically speaking, cause a Technopathogeny – in this case, a spectacular collapse of the structure. If we took this to the technological field, the plan would represent the paper or article published. Even if there is a flaw in the paper, nothing will happen if the proposal is not materialized or if the object is finished but it is never applied. That is to say, in the light of current knowledge, as long as the hidden flaws lie within the theory – they *remain static* – they will be harmless. But if the theory *starts moving*, they will become harmful. That is, if it becomes *kinetic*. We are saying in the light of current knowledge, because the aim of the science we are proposing is to detect such hidden flaws very early in the process, even in the gestational period of the technical object, so as to avoid this discovery when applying the technique.

Immanent

We should stop at such a serious term to specify that we refer to the most common definition, that is what is *indwelling, inherent*, and not to the philosophical concept. As we have stated in previous works and in the introduction, this is based on the basic characteristics of modern technological-scientific work, i.e.:

a) Speeding up of the process of discovery-development-application.

b) Increasing preponderance of nuclear phenomena (atomic and cellular nucleus).

c) Scientist, technologist and system manager's ethical misdemeanors.

Within a system that blindly trusts the *method,* this turns the possibility of imperfect knowledge inception into a reality. The apparent safety of a paper that passes all the evaluations does not guarantee the exclusion of technopathogenies in the kinetic application of the knowledge contained in it. According to Prof. Heinrich Beck, "the lack of verification of an existent does not mean the verification of a non-existent" (Beck, 2000).

We could then say that due to the characteristics of scientific knowledge, the construction of a new technological object within knowledge's current status that does not find an *existent risk* cannot predict the impossibility of a Technopathogeny or risk that was considered non-existent.

Hidden

We say that it is *hidden* because this error or flaw which is relevant in terms of Technopathogenology must not be evident or known before its application, for in that case we would be dealing with a problem of bad praxis due to the lack of ability or expertise of the technician. There are several examples coming from different technologies, ranging from engineering to healing professions.

Every Technique has its own known risks that must be handled by the technician after a more or less exact evaluation of risks and benefits, but those are not our subject of study. We are neither referring to those techniques released in the market with a clear knowledge of the risks implied but which are not revealed to the technician or the population. This would be a clear case of lack of ethics.

By referring to hidden, we mean a flaw whose existence went unnoticed by the Scientific and Technique safety system. A hidden flaw or error causing a Technopathogeny is manifested in spite of having applied all the regular Science and Technique safety systems. This error or flaw manifests itself during the usage of the technique in spite of having applied the relevant regulatory trials.

IX. The increase in complexity of Technique comes along with the increase of risk

As we have stated before, Technique entails non-evident risks to health; Technique's development and increasing complexity also cause an increase in non-evident risks. The problem is that Technique is not interested in such situation and it will always profit from knowledge, be it truthful or not, provided the desired benefit is obtained. Rather than aiming at the search for knowledge, technology aims at the search for benefit.

Unfortunately, this state of things is neither as simple nor as positive as modern Technique presents it. Unlike what happened in ancient times, where simple and macroscopic changes were made to objects of nature and neither technicians nor their community suffered a significant risk, modern Technique does affect technicians and their community. The great voids or gaps in the knowledge that is used for the development of new processes determine that certain unexpected situations can occur, which in some cases are irreparable and cause an enormous amount of harm.

This is evidently so: how much could the ancient man ignore about the pointed stick he used for ploughing that might pose a risk on him and his community? The stick might be weak and eventually break and hurt the ploughman, but no more than that. Even in more modern cases, for example, the case of the steam boiler, whether fed by wood, coal, or any other combustion fuel. How many people could be harmed by an accident caused by the voids or gaps in the knowledge used for the construction of the boiler? If the construction presented flaws regarding the resistance of materials, an explosion could affect the people nearby. The inadequate combustion and lack of ventilation could also be harmful to workers, causing acute intoxication due to the inhaling of carbon monoxide or chronic intoxication due to the inhaling of products of incomplete combustion

If we compare the boiler to a nuclear reactor – the modern boiler – the voids or gaps in the knowledge used in its construction and operations might result in an unexpected accident. This would be hazardous not only to the people directly exposed (workers) but also to the community surrounding the plant and even communities far from it. The other difference between both techniques (steam boiler and nuclear reactor) is the lasting effect. The effect of a fossil combustion boiler explosion is limited to the time of the actual explosion, but the nuclear reactor explosion will cause a long term damage which will remain for centuries (Eguiazu, 1994) (Motta, 1994).

Table 4 summarizes this comparison (Eguiazu, 1991).

Table 4:   Comparison between a primitive boiler and a modern nuclear reactor

Primitive boiler explosion	Modern nuclear incident
Limited	Very difficult to limit
Damage caused only by heat or pressure	Apart from the damage caused by heat or pressure, there would be ionizing radiation and liberation of radioactive nuclei
Low probability of mutagenicity, carcinogenicity, teratogenicity and fetal damage.	High probability of mutagenicity, carcinogenicity, teratogenicity and fetal damage.
No long-term consequences. Spatially restricted	Long-term consequences No spatial restriction

The overt technological differences between a wood-fed boiler and a nuclear power plant are an example of the evolution of Ancient Technique to Modern Technique.

In order to analyze this evolution process and the growing complexity of Technique – which is closely linked to or responsible for the Phenomenon that is our object of study – it is interesting to revise the definition of Technique in ancient times. In the Antiquity, Technique was more closely related to Art, that is, the ability or skill to develop any activity. They separated intellectual activities or Liberal Arts from manual activities or Mechanical Arts (Beck, 1979a), as can be observed in the following table.

Table 5:   Ancient classifications of the Arts, whether manual or intellectual

Liberal Arts		Mechanical Arts
Arts that don't modify the matter		Arts that modify the matter, an approximate conception to the modern idea of Technique
Grammar Dialectics Rhetoric	Trivium (Logics)	Agriculture Venatio Navigatio Texture
Geometry Arithmetic Astronomy Music	Quadrivium (Mathematics)	Armatoria Medicine Spectaculum

If we analyze this ancient classification, we will notice that Liberal Arts scarcely modified matter, or not at all. These were intellectual arts. It was only manifested through verbal or written expression and it was never made into concrete tangible objects.

Mechanical Arts, on the other hand, did modify matter either by hand or through the use of machines (*mechane*) – what is curious is to see spectaculum included in this group.

The Greek word *mechane* means machine. It is interesting to see that the transformations of matter, whether it is animate or inanimate, are usually carried out with the help of machines – objects we could also define as the product or result of modification of matter. These machines go from basic designs such as wedges (present in scalpels, ploughs or axes) to more complex designs in modern machines.

Chemical and nuclear modifications are not mentioned yet, neither those derived from genetic engineering, since in those times only the more evident modifications of a physical or mechanical nature were taken into account.

The seven mechanical arts described before roughly represent the totality of the *industry* in the Ancient world. All the activities derived from them. For example: the food industry derived from *agriculture* and *venatio*; the chemical industry derived from *texture*, since the art of *weaving* included everything related to color dyes; and the pharmaceutical industry derived from *medicine*.

This way, mechanical arts in Antiquity represented the application of knowledge at the time to develop techniques and to apply them systematically through industry (Beck, 1979a).

Every Mechanical Art can be related to some industrial activity in Antiquity. Similarly, they can also be roughly related to current industrial activities. Some of them can be related with particularly contaminant modern industries (Jerneloew, 1989), as can be observed in table 6 (Eguiazu, 1991).

Table 7 (Eguiazu, 1991) describes other differences between ancient and modern techniques. These differences explain not only the short-term deterioration processes but also the manifestation of technopathogenies.

In addition to the case of a nuclear reactor mentioned before, we could mention other examples that are a direct consequence of this trend in technological changes.

Table 6:   Relationship between Modern Industries and Antique Mechanical Arts

Modern Industrial Sector	Ancient Mechanical Art Related
Cement	Armaturia (art of warfare that included the building of fortifications).
Textile	Texture
Tannin	Venatio (leather tanning)
Aluminium	Armaturia, Navigatio
Slaughterhouses	Venatio (which included, apart from the hunting, everything related to slaughter and meat products conservation)
Breweries – Distilleries	Agriculture (which included not only farming but also the derived processes of agriculture and livestock products)
Steelwork	Armaturia – Navigatio – others
Pulp and Paper	Others
Fertilizers	Agriculture

48

Table 7:   Differences between antique and modern Mechanical Arts

Antique	Modern
Modification of matter taking the physical and observable as a starting point.	Modification of matter taking the nuclear – atomic or cellular – as a starting point.
Rudimentary chemical modifications – extraction and concentration.	Deep chemical modifications – synthesis and dispersion.
Low modification efficiency. Low energy phenomena.	High modification efficiency. High energy phenomena.
Relatively low and reversible action on the ecosystem.	High and frequently irreversible action on the ecosystem.
The slow reequilibrium natural processes are enough to protect the ecosystem. Respect for evolution.	The slow reequilibrium natural processes are insufficient. Manipulation of evolution.
Scattered and unfocused economy. Craftsmanship.	High economic pressure. Great volume of products. Mass production of products
Limited mutagenic, carcinogenic, teratogenic or fetal damage effects.	High mutagenic, carcinogenic, teratogenic or fetal damage effects.
High occurrence of observable negative effects and low occurrence of hidden negative effects.	Low occurrence of observable negative effects and high occurrence of hidden negative effects.
Short term, temporarily limited modifications	Long term, temporarily non-limited non-observable modifications
Future humans relatively not submitted to risk	Future humans submitted to high risk

For instance, the use of pesticides in food production, which, due to its high stability and resistance to degradation, will remain in the environment for many years representing a risk to the people exposed.

Another case, also related to Chemical Industry, is constituted by the various substances which are incorporated day by day to the long list of chemicals. Every year, 200 or more of the 1.000 new substances are placed in the market in quantities of more than one ton and used in many different ways. But most of them are not studied in reference to their possible adverse effects (ILO, 1987).

For some substances, after many years of usage, a carcinogenic effect is detected through experiments or epidemiology. Table 8 clearly shows this.

Although many substances are listed in this table, we have only included some of the ones whose carcinogenic risk is known, probable or possible. There is a large number of substances with very little or no data at all. Going back to Prof. Beck's reflection, the fact that the existence of risk to humans cannot be verified does not mean it can be disallowed.

The list includes information from the International Agency for Research on Cancer: *IARC Monographs on the Evaluation of Carcinogenic Risks to Humans,* and the U.S. Department of Health and Human Services, Public Health Services, National Toxicology Program: *10th Report on Carcinogens – 2002..*

The table may include substances whose use has already been prohibited. Due to their carcinogenic risk, many substances already have legislation controlling their use, but it is impossible to know whether the criterion for such control is the same for all countries. For example, the dye Ponceau 3R was forbidden in some countries but only after many years of usage. The United States approved its usage as a food additive in 1906, and on the basis of animal toxicity studies, banned it as such in 1960. However, the usage was permitted for external usage in medicines and cosmetics until 1966 when it was completely forbidden (IARC, 1975a).

Similarly, 4-Dimethylaminoazobenzene (or *para*-Dimethylaminoazobenzene), a possibly carcinogenic substance, had been permitted in the United States as a food additive in 1918, but was forbidden six months later after detecting that it produced dermatitis in workers exposed to it (IARC, 1975a).

The fact that some substances have been banned in some countries does not mean that they are not in use in other countries.

The aim of naming substances which were eventually retrieved from the market (like the above cited Ponceau 3R) is to show how technology exposed humans to a substance whose risk was discovered much later.

In the case of cancer, for example, even if a substance is retrieved from the market, a person who was exposed to it for a determined amount of time can still be affected.

Another interesting case is benzene, a carcinogenic substance which can present risk not only due to its direct usage but also due to its residual presence in distilled solvents or fuels.

The case of Chloramphenicol, an antibiotic, and Ethylene Oxide a substance used in the chemical industry are also worth mentioning here. Both substances were originally listed in a category of carcinogenic risk, but later, based on new evidence, they were listed in another category of greater carcinogenic risk. In 1987 the first substance was classified by IARC as possibly carcinogenic to humans (IARC, 1987b), and in 1990 as probably carcinogenic to humans (IARC, 1990b). The second substance was classified for the NTP in 1985 as Reasonably Anticipated to be human carcinogens, and in 2000 as Known to be human carcinogen (U.S. DHHS-PHS-NTP, 2002).

About the evaluation criteria it is also worth mentioning what happened with the 3-Chloro-2-methylpropene. In 1995, the International Agency for Research on Cancer did not find enough carcinogenic evidence (inadequate evidence in humans and limited evidence in experimental animals), and it was therefore considered *not classifiable as to its carcinogenicity to humans* (Group 3) (IARC, 1995). But in 1989, the National Toxicological Program classified this substance as *reasonably anticipated as to be carcinogenic in humans*, maintaining this category in the 11th Annual Report on Carcinogens (2004) (US. DHHS-PHS-NTP, 2004).

There are substances which are considered carcinogenic because they are metabolized into a carcinogenic substance. For example, Direct Black 38, Direct Blue 6, and Direct Brown 95 (three dyes not enclosed in the table) are considered as carcinogenic to humans because they are metabolized to Benzidine which is a human carcinogen (IARC, 2010)

Table References

Column "A" indicates the chemical name of the substance. Due to the existence of various synonyms and for some, even several commercial names, the Chemical Abstract Services (CAS) register number was also included.

Column "B" indicates the use/uses of each substance. This list is not complete; it is a mere example to show the reader the various ways in which humans can be exposed to a substance in particular.

Column "C" indicates the carcinogenic risk or the evidence of carcinogenicity.

We will consider categories proposed by the International Agency for Research on Cancer (IARC) (IARC, 1987b) and categories proposed by the National Toxicology Program (NTP) (U.S DHHS-PHS-NTP, 2002). Below we quote only the criteria taken for each category related with a real or potential risk to humans. The abbreviations in brackets and bold type are the ones included in column C.

IARC Categories

For the evaluation, *human carcinogenicity data* and *experimental carcinogenicity data* are used.

a) *Human carcinogenicity data*:
The evidence relevant to carcinogenicity from studies in humans is classified into one of the following categories:
Sufficient evidence of carcinogenicity: The working group considers that a causal relationship has been established between exposure to the agent and human cancer. That is, a positive relationship has been observed between exposure to the agent and cancer in studies in which chance, bias and confounding could be ruled out with reasonable confidence.
Limited evidence of carcinogenicity: A positive association has been observed between exposure to the agent and cancer for which a causal interpretation is considered by the Working Group to be credible, but chance, bias or confounding could not be ruled out with reasonable confidence.
Inadequate evidence of carcinogenicity: The available studies are of insufficient quality consistency or statistical power to permit a conclusion regarding the presence or absence of a causal association.

b) *Experimental carcinogenicity data*
Sufficient evidence of carcinogenicity (**S.E.A**): The Working Group considers that a causal relationship has been established between the agent and an increase incidence of malignant neoplasms or of an appropriate combination of benign and malignant neoplasms in (a) two or more species of animals (b) in two or more independent studies in one species carried out at different times or in different laboratories or under different protocols.
Exceptionally, a single study in one species might be considered to provide sufficient evidence of carcinogenicity when malignant neoplasms occur to an unusual degree with regard to incidence, site, type of tumor or age at onset.
In the absence of adequate data on humans, it is biologically plausible and prudent to regard agents for which there is *sufficient evidence* of carcinogenicity in experimental animals as if they presented a carcinogenic risk to humans.
Limited evidence of carcinogenicity (**L.E.A.**):The data suggest a carcinogenic effect but are limited for making a definitive evaluation because (a) the evidence of carcinogenicity is restricted to a single experiment; or (b) there are unresolved questions regarding the adequacy of the design, conduct or interpretation of the study; or (c) the agent increases the incidence only of benign neoplasms or lesions of uncertain neoplastic potential, or of certain neoplasms which may occur spontaneously in high incidences in certain strains.

IARC Overall evaluation

The agents with real or potential risk for humans are classified in four groups (IARC, 1987b). The abbreviations in brackets and bold type are the ones included in column C.

Group 1 – The agent is carcinogenic to humans (**C.H.**)
This category is used only when there is *sufficient evidence* of carcinogenicity in humans.

Group 2
This category includes agents for which, at one extreme, the degree of evidence of carcinogenicity in humans is almost sufficient, as well as agents for which, at the other extreme, there are no human data but for which there is experimental evidence of carcinogenicity. Agents are assigned to either 2A (probably carcinogenic) or 2B (possibly carcinogenic) on the basis of epidemiological, experimental and other relevant data.

Group 2A – The agent is probably carcinogenic to humans (**Pr.C.H.**)
This category is used when there is *limited evidence* of carcinogenicity in humans and *sufficient evidence* of carcinogenicity in experimental animals. Exceptionally, an agent may be classified into this category solely on the basis of *limited evidence* of carcinogenicity in humans or of *sufficient evidence* of carcinogenicity in experimental animals strengthened by supporting evidence from other relevant data.

Group 2B – The agent is possibly carcinogenic to humans (**Ps.C.H.**)
This category is generally used for agents for which there is *limited evidence* in humans in the absence of *sufficient evidence* in experimental animals. It may also be used when there is *inadequate evidence* of carcinogenicity in humans or when human data are nonexistent but there is *sufficient evidence* of carcinogenicity in experimental animals. In some instances, an agent for which there is *inadequate evidence* or no data in humans but *limited evidence* of carcinogenicity in experimental animals together with supporting evidence from other relevant data may be placed in this group.

NTP Categories

The agents with real or potential risk for humans are classified in two groups (U.S DHHS-PHS-NTP, 2002). The abbreviations in brackets and bold type are the ones included in column C.

Known to be human carcinogen (**K.H.C.**)
There is sufficient evidence of carcinogenicity from studies in humans, which indicates a causal relationship between exposure to the agent, substance, or mixture, and human cancer.

Reasonably Anticipated to be human carcinogens (**R.H.C.**)

a) There is limited evidence of carcinogenicity from studies in humans, which indicates that a causal interpretation is credible, but that alternative explanations, such as chance, bias, or confounding factors, could not adequately be excluded.

b) There is sufficient evidence of carcinogenicity from studies in experimental animals, which indicate there is an increased incidence of malignant and/or a combination of malignant and benign tumors (1) in multiple species or at multiple tissues sites, or (2) by multiple routs of exposure, or (3) to an unusual degree with regard to incidence, site of type of tumor, or age at onset.

c) There is less than sufficient evidence of carcinogenicity in humans or laboratory animals; however, the agent, substance, or mixture belong to a well-defined, structurally related class of substance whose members are listed in a previous Report on Carcinogens as either known to be a human carcinogen or reasonably anticipated to be a human carcinogens, or there is convincing relevant information that the agent acts through mechanisms indicating it would likely cause cancer in humans.

NTP Remarks

Conclusions regarding carcinogenicity in humans or experimental animals are based on scientific judgment, with consideration given to all relevant information. Relevant information includes, but there is not limited to, dose response, rout of exposure, chemical structure, metabolism, pharmacokinetics, sensitive subpopulations, genetic effects, or other data relating to mechanisms of action of factors that may be unique to a given substance. For example, there may be substances for which there is evidence of carcinogenicity in laboratory animals, but there are compelling data indicating that the agent acts through mechanisms which do not operate in humans and would therefore not reasonably be anticipated to cause cancer in humans.

Column "D" lists the year in which the substance was discovered, synthesized for the first time or the year of the bibliographical reference where such data is cited from.

Column "E" lists the year in which the substance started to be produced commercially or the chemical effect discovered: Antibiotic, Antioxidant, etc.

Column "F" indicates the year in which IARC evaluated the substance, or re-evaluated it or indicated the risk, or evaluated its carcinogenicity.

The order in which the categories are placed in the column "C", correspond to the order in which the underlining year in the column "F" is placed. For example, 1,1-Dimethylhydrazine, was enclosed as R.H.C. (Reasonably Anticipated to be human carcinogens) in the Annual Report on Carcinogens in 1985, and enclosed in the IARC report as Ps.C.H. (possibly carcinogenic to humans) in 1987.

54

Table 8:   List of 100 chemicals of carcinogenic risk for man

A – Chemical	B – Use	C	D	E	F
1,1-Dimethyl-hydrazine CAS N° 57-14-7	High-energy propellant for liquid-fuelled rockets. Plant growth regulator. In photography.	R.H.C. Ps.C.H.	1956	1961	1974 1985 1987
1,2-Dichloroethane CAS N° 107-06-2	Chemical Industry: production of diverse substances. Various solvent applications. Fumigant for grain, upholstery and carpets. Lead scavenger. It is a major ingredient of many petrol antiknock mixtures. Paint. Varnish. Finish removers. Component of metal degreasing formulations. In soaps. Wetting and penetrating agents. Etc.	R.H.C. Ps.C.H.	1795	1922	1979 1981 1999
1,3-Butadiene CAS N° 106-99-0	Chemical Industry: Production of synthetic rubbers; polymers, etc.	Ps.C.H. R.H.C. Pr.C.H. K.H.C.	1890	1930s	1985 1987 1989 1999 2000
1,3-Propane Sultone CAS N° 1120-71-4	Chemical industry: Synthesis of diverse substances.	Ps.C.H. Ps.C.H.		1963	1974 1987 1999
1,4-Dioxane CAS N° 123-91-1	Solvent in: Lacquers, paints, varnishes, paints and varnish removers. Wetting and dispersing agent in textile products; dye baths; printing compositions; cleaning and detergent preparations; cements; cosmetics; deodorants; fumigants; emulsions and polishing preparations; stabilizer for chlorinated solvents.	R.H.C. Ps.C.H.		1951	1976 1981 1999
2,3-Dibromo-1-propanol CAS N° 96-13-9	Production of flame retardants, insecticides and pharmaceuticals. Was used in the production of flame retardants, insecticides and pharmaceuticals. Was used in the production of TRIS-BP, a flame re-	R.H.C.			2002

A – Chemical	B – Use	C	D	E	F
2,3-Dibromo-1-propanol (cont.)	tardant used in children's clothing and other products.				
2,4,6-Trichloro-phenol CAS N° 88-06-2	Wood preservative. Glue preservative. Insecticide ingredient, bactericide and anti-mildew treatment for textiles. Used to prepare fungicides.	R.H.C. Ps.C.H.	1836	1950	1979 1983 1987
2,4-Diamino-anisole Sulphate CAS N° 39156-41-7	Cosmetics: Component of oxidizing permanent hair- and fur-dye formulations. In the synthesis of C.I. Basic Brown 2 used to dye furs, acrylic fibbers, cotton, wool, nylon, polyester, and leather and suede and is an ingredient of shoe polishes.	R.H.C. Ps.C.H.	1913	1933	1978 1983 1987
2,4-Diamino-toluene CAS N° 95-80-7	Chemical Industry: Synthesis of diverse substances. Production of dyes for textile, leather, and furs and in hair-dye formulations.	R.H.C. Ps.C.H.	1861	1920	1978 1981 1987
2-Naphtylamine CAS N° 91-59-8	Chemical Industry.	K.H.C. C.H.		1920	1974 1980 1987
3,3'-Dichloro-benzidine CAS N° 91-94-1	Chemical Industry: Organic pigments.	R.H.C. Ps.C.H.	1900	1932	1982 1981 1987
3-Chloro-2-methyl-propene CAS N° 563-47-3	Used as an insecticide and fumigant and as intermediate in the production of plastics, pharmaceuticals and other organic chemicals. In the production of Carbofuran, an insecticide. In the production of herbicides. Used: as a textile additive, as a perfume additive. Was used as fumigant in: grains, tobacco, and soil.	R.H.C.			1989 1995
4-Chloro-o-phenyl-enediamine CAS N° 95-83-0	Cosmetic: Was used as a dye intermediate in a hair-dye component.	R.H.C. Ps.C.H.	1876	1941-1943	1982 1985 1987

A – Chemical	B – Use	C	D	E	F
4-Dimethyl-aminoazobenzene CAS N° 60-11-7	Coloring polishes and other wax products, polystyrene, petrol, soap, as an indicator of dyers and colorists, and for the determination of free hydrochloric acid in gastric juice.	R.H.C. Ps.C.H.	1876	1914	1975 1981 1987
Acetaldehyde CAS N° 75-07-0	Chemical Industry: intermediate in the manufacture of acetic acid and in the synthesis of various other substances. Other use: In the silvering of mirrors; in the leather tanning; as a denaturant alcohol; in fuel mixtures; as a hardener for gelatine fibers; in glue and casein products; as a preservative of fish and fruits; in the paper industry; as a synthetic flavoring agents; in the manufacture of cosmetics, aniline dyes, plastics, and synthetic rubber.	R.H.C. Ps.C.H.	1774	1968	1985 1991 1999
Acrylamide CAS N° 79-06-1	Chemical Industry: Chemical intermediate in the production and synthesis of polacrylamides. The principle end use of Acrylamide is in water-soluble polymers used as additives for water treatment, enhanced oil recovery, flocculants, papermaking aids, thickeners, soil conditioning agents, sewage and waste treatment, ore processing, and permanent-press fabrics. Is also used in the synthesis of dyes, in copolymers for contact lenses, and the construction of dam foundations, tunnels, and sewers. Polyacrylamides are used in the treating municipal drinking water and waste water. The polymers are also used to remove suspended solids from industri-	Ps.C.H. R.H.C.	1893	1954	1986 1987 1991

A – Chemical	B – Use	C	D	E	F
Acrylamide (cont.)	al waste water before discharge, reuse or disposal. Other uses: Oil-drilling processes; pulp and paper industry; incorporated to cement to slow the dehydration; in foundry operations; in cosmetic and soaps preparations; in dental fixtures; hair grooming preparations; preshave lotions; explosives; binders in adhesives and adhesives tapes; etc.				
Acrylonitrile CAS N° 107-13-1	Principal uses: Acrylic fibers, acrylonitrile-butadiene-styrene (ABS) resins, adiponitrile, nitrile rubbers, elastomers, and styrene-acrylonitrile (SAN) resins. In the past was used as a fumigant with carbon tetrachloride, and in pesticide formulations.	R.H.C. Ps.C.H.	1893	1960	1981 1999
Adriamicyn CAS N° 23214-92-8	Cytotoxic antibiotic. Drug: Used in the treatment of neoplastics diseases: acute lymphoblastic leukemia, estrogenic sarcomas, and other.	R.H.C. Pr.C.H.	1967		1976 1985 1987
Asbestos CAS N° 1332-21-4	Most Asbestos is used in the construction industry. Over 3000 uses have been identified. Important uses include: asbestos cement sheets and pipes, insulation materials, taping compounds and floor and ceiling tiles. Friction materials: clutch facings and brakes for cars, lorries, railways carriages, and airplanes. Braking materials are widely used in the industry for machinery. In insulation materials. Sprayed asbestos materials are used for decorative and acoustic purposes, as well as for the fireproofing of structural elements in buildings. In paper	K.H.C. C.H.		1880	1977 1980 1987

A – Chemical	B – Use	C	D	E	F
Asbestos (cont.)	maché materials used by school children and fireproof clothing and gloves to filler for plastics.				
Azacitidine CAS N° 320-67-2	Drug: Is a cytostatic agent. It has been used principally in the treatment of leukemia. It has also been tested for use in the treatment of a variety of solid tumors.	Pr.C.H. R.H.C.	1970		<u>1990</u> <u>1998</u>
Azathioprina CAS N° 446-86-6	Drug: Immunosuppressive agent used, usually in combination with a corticosteroid, to prevent rejection following renal homotransplantations. It is also used following the transplantation of other organs. Other uses are in the in the treatment of a variety of presumed autoimmune diseases.	K.H.C. C.H.	1962	1970	1981 <u>1985</u> <u>1987</u>
Benzene CAS N° 71-43-2	Chemical Industry: Synthesis of diverse substances. In the past, benzene was used widely as a solvent, but the amounts used now for this purpose are believed to be relatively small and decreasing. While its use as a gasoline additive has been largely reduced in the U.S., benzene continue to be used in the U.S. and more extensively in many countries for the production of commercial gasoline.	K.H.C. C.H.	1825 1833		<u>1980</u> 1982 <u>1987</u>
Benzidine CAS N° 92-87-5	Chemical Industry: Dyes. Other uses: Rubber Industry; adhesives; plastics; in analytical chemistry as reactive; etc.	K.H.C. C.H.	1845	1880	1982 <u>1980</u> <u>1987</u>
Bleomycin CAS N° 11056-06-7	Drug: Antineoplastic agent.	Ps.C.H.	1965	1969	1981 <u>1987</u>
Bromodichloromethane CAS N° 75-27-4	Chemical Industry: in organic synthesis. It has also been used to separate mineral and salt, as a flame retardant, and fire ex-	Ps.C.H. R.H.C.			<u>1991</u> <u>1991</u>

59

A – Chemical	B – Use	C	D	E	F
Bromodichlorome-thane (cont.)	tinguishers. Currently used on-ly as a standard in the analysis of drinking-water.				
Butylated hydrox-yanisole CAS N° 25013-16-5	Antioxidant in fat-contain foods and edible fats and oils. Food additive in butter, lard, meats, cereals, baked goods, sweet and beer. Used in vege-table oils, potato crisp, snacks foods, nuts, dehydrated pota-toes and flavoring materials. In Cosmetics: as a preservative and antioxidant in cosmetics formulations. BHA is used as a preservative and antioxidant in pharmaceut-icals preparations containing fats and oils. Antioxidants are used to delay the deterioration of food flavors and odors and substantially in-crease the self life of many foods. Since 1947, it has been added to edible fats and fat-containing foods for its antioxi-dant properties; it prevents food from becoming rancid and de-veloping objectionable odors.	R.H.C.		1947	1986 <u>1991</u>
Carbon Tetra-chloride CAS N° 56-23-5	Chemical Industry: Synthesis of chlorinated organic com-pounds. In solvents. Agricul-tural fumigant. Pesticide. It is also used as a vermidical agent in human medicine. Solvent in the production of semiconduc-tors, in the processing of fats, oil and rubber. In laboratory applications.	R.H.C. Ps.C.H.	1839	1907	1979 <u>1981</u> <u>1987</u> 1999
Catechol CAS N° 120-80-9	In polymerization inhibitors and antioxidants. In electro sensitive copying papers. In the synthesis of pharmaceuti-cals and pesticides. In photo-graphy and in rubber com-	Ps.C.H.	1839	1920	1977 <u>1999</u>

A – Chemical	B – Use	C	D	E	F
Catecol (cont.)	pounding aids. As starting material for insecticides, for perfumes and drugs. As an antiseptic; in photography; dyestuffs; special inks; anti-oxidants and light stabilizers; and in organic synthesis.				
Chlorambucil CAS N° 305-03-3	Drug: Used in human medicine as an antineoplastic agent.	K.H.C. C.H.	1953	1957	1981 1981 1987
Chloramphenicol CAS N° 56-75-7	Antibiotic. Used for the treatment of *Salmonella* infections, and many other infectious diseases. In veterinary medicine as a broad-spectrum antibiotic treatment (purpose that might result in the presence of residues in food for human consumption)	R.H.C. Ps.C.H. Pr.C.H. R.H.C	1947	1948	1976 1980 1987 1990 2002
Chlorendic acid CAS N° 115-28-6	Chemical Industry: chemical intermediate in the manufacture of unsaturated polyester resins. Used: to impart flame resistance to polyurethane foams; in composites for flame retardant building and transport materials; as anti-corrosion equipment. In the textile industry: as a flame retardant treatment of wool fabrics. Other uses: As an extreme pressure lubricant.	R.H.C. Ps.C.H.			1989 1990
Chlornaphazine CAS N° 494-03-1	Drug: Chemotherapeutic agent for the treatment of leukemia	C.H.		1964	1974 1987
Chloroform CAS N° 67-66-3	It was first used as anesthetic. Chemical Industry: Production of fluorocarbon for use in refrigerants. Miscellaneous uses: Drugs; cosmetics (including tooth-pastes); solvent; grain fumigant; intermediate in	R.H.C. Ps.C.H.	1831	1903	1979 1981 1987

A – Chemical	B – Use	C	D	E	F
Chloroform (cont.)	preparations of dyes, drugs and pesticides.				
Chloroprene CAS N° 126-99-8	It is used almost exclusively in the production of specialized elastomers, known as polych-loroprene. It is also used to produce polychloroprene latex. Rubber of vulcanized po-lychloroprene include electric-al insulating and sheathing materials, hoses, conveyor belts, flexible bellows, trans-mission belts, sealing mate-rials, diving suits and other protective suits. Adhesive grades of polychloroprene are used mainly in the footwear industry. Polychloroprene la-tex has been used for dipped goods (balloons, gloves), latex foam, fiber binders, adhesives and rug backing.	Ps.C.H. R.H.C.		1932	1999 2000
Chlorozotocin CAS N° 54749-90-5	Drug. It is a cytostatic agent. It can be used in the treatment of cancers of the stomach, large bowel, pancreas and lung, melanoma and multiple myeloma.	Pr.C.H. R.H.C.	1975		1990 1998
CI Acid Orange 3 CAS N° 6373-74-6	Cosmetic: In semi permanent hair coloring products. In the industry it is also used to dye textiles.	I.E.H. L.E.A.	1911	1920s	1993
CI Acid Red 114 CAS N° 6459-94-5	It is used to dye wool, silk, jute and leather.	Ps.C.H.		1900s	1993
CI Basic Red 9 Monohydrochlo-ride CAS N° 569-61-9	It has been used extensively as textile dyes. Current use of tri-alylmethane dyes is mainly for non textile purposes. They are used in the prepara-tion of organic pigments for printing inks and in printing. They are also used: extensively in high-speed photoduplicating	R.H.C. Ps.C.H.	1850s		1989 1993

A – Chemical	B – Use	C	D	E	F
CI Basic Red 9 Monohydrochloride (cont.)	and photo imaging systems. In tinting automobile antifreeze solutions and toilet sanitary preparations. In the manufacture of carbon paper, in ink and typewriter ribbons and in jet printing for high-speed computer printers. To color other substrates such as: leather, fur, anodized aluminium, glass, waxes, polishes, soaps, plastics, drugs, and cosmetics. They are also used extensively as microbial stains.				
Ciclosporin CAS N° 79217-60-0	Drug. It is an agent immuno-supresor. It is extensively in the prevention and treatment of graft-*versus*-host in bone marrow transplantation, and for the prevention of rejection of kidney, heart and liver transplants. It has also been tested for the therapy of a large variety of other diseases in which immunological factors may have a pathogenesis role: diabetes mellitus; chronic active hepatitis, etc.	C.H.	1976		1990
Cisplatin CAS N° 15663-27-1	Drug: Used in human medicine for the treatment of a variety of malignancies usually in combinations of other agents.	Pr.C.H. R.H.C.	1840s		1981 1987 1989
Citrus Red N° 2 CAS N° 6358-53-8	In the US, this color is permitted only for coloring the skins of oranges that are not intended or used for processing.	Ps.C.H.	1940	1960	1975 1987
Creosotes CAS N° 8007-45-2 (Coal-tars General)	In the US, it is used almost exclusively in wood preservation. In the US, it is registered for use as animal or bird repellent, animal dip, miticide, fungicide, herbicide and insecticide, in limited quantities it is used only three of these applications: as	K.H.C. Pr.C.H.		1917	1980 1987

A – Chemical	B – Use	C	D	E	F
Creosotes (cont.)	an animal or bird repellent, as an insecticide and as an animal dip. It is also used as a feedstock for the production of carbon blacks.				
Cyclophosphamide CAS N° 6055-19-2 (Anhyrous 50-18-0)	Drug: Used in human medicine as an antineoplastic agent in a variety applications.	K.H.C. C.H.	1958	1962	1980 1981 1987
D&C Red N° 9 CAS N° 5160-02-1	It is used in some countries in the cosmetic and drug industry in such applications as a lipstick colorant, mouthwashes, dentifrices and drugs. It is widely used in printing inks. It has been used extensively in letter press and offset inks and also in gravure inks. It is used in water- and solvent-based flexography inks. It also finds substantial use in coated papers and crayons. Other uses: in polystyrene and rubber, in tin printing and baking enamels.	L.E.A. I.E.H.	1903		1993
Dacarbazine CAS N° 4342-03-4	Drug: Used in human medicine as an antineoplastic agent in the treatment of diseases such as malignant melanomas, and other.	R.H.C. Ps.C.H.	1962		1981 1985 1987
Dantron (1,8-Dihydroxi-anthraquinone) CAS N° 117-10-2	It has been widely used since the beginning of the 20´century as a laxative, and as an intermediate for dyes.	Ps.C.H. R.H.C.	1981		1990 1998
Daunomycin CAS N° 20830-81-3	Drug. Used in the treatment of acute leukemia and solid tumors.	Ps.C.H.	1960s	1965	1976 1987
Dichloromethane CAS N° 75-09-2	Solvent in paint strippers. Extraction solvent for spices and beer hops and for decaffeination of coffee. Solvent: in textile industry, in	Ps.C.H. R.H.C.	1840	1934	1979 1987 1989 1999

A – Chemical	B – Use	C	D	E	F
Dichloromethane (cont.)	the manufacture of photographic film, for vapor degreasing of metal parts. Component of low-pressure refrigerants, in air-conditioning installations. In the manufacture of polycarbonate plastics, photo resists coating, insecticides and herbicides. Grain fumigation; oil dewaxing; in inks and adhesives. In the pharmaceutical industry: solvent for the manufacture of steroids, vitamins, antibiotics, for the coating of tablets. Paint removers; aerosol propellants.				
Diepoxybutane CAS N° 1464-53-5	It has been used in the curing of polymers, for cross-linking textile fibers and in the prevention of microbial spoilage. It is also used in polymer, paper and textile treatment and as chemical intermediate.	R.H.C. Ps.C.H.	1884		1976 1983 1987
Diethyl Sulphate CAS N° 64-67-5	Chemical Industry. Mutagenic agent to produce a new variety of barley.	R.H.C. Pr.C.H.		1920	1974 1985 1987
Diethylstilboestrol CAS N° 56-53-1 (No steroidal estrogens)	In human medicine, it is used for the treatment of symptom arising during the climateric and following ovariectomy, and other treatments. It is used as an emergency contraceptive. It is used for chemotherapy of advanced carcinoma of the breast. In Veterinary medicine, it is used in replacement therapy for underdeveloped females, to induce heath in anoestrus, to prevent conception in mismated bitches, and other	K.H.C. C.H.	1938	1941	1979 1980 1987

A – Chemical	B – Use	C	D	E	F
Diethylstilboestrol (cont.)	treatments. It was used as a growth promoter in poultry and in beef cattle.				
Dimethylcarbamoyl chloride CAS N° 79-44-7	The only known use is a chemical intermediate in the production of drugs and pesticides.	R.H.C. Pr.C.H.	1879	1958	1976 <u>1981</u> <u>1987</u>
Dimethyl Sulphate CAS N° 77-78-1	Chemical industry	R.H.C. Pr.C.H.		1920	1974 <u>1981</u> <u>1987</u>
d-Limonene CAS N° 5989-27-5	It has been used widely as flavor and fragrance additives in perfume, soap, food and beverages. It has been used in non-alcoholic beverages; ice crams and ices; sweets; baked goods; gelatines and puddings; and chewing gum. In the Chemical Industry: in the synthesis of *l*-Carvone. In terpene resins manufacture as a wetting and dispersing agent. In the synthesis of tackifying resins for adhesives. It has been used as a solvent, cleaner and odor. It has been used to dissolve retained cholesterol gallstones postoperatively. In insect control. In treatment of breast cancer and other tumors, and chemoprevention trials are under considerations.	I.E.H. S.E.A.		1941-42	1993 <u>1999</u>
Epichlorohydrin CAS N° 106-89-8	It has been used to crosslink starch in food and industrial uses. It is a major raw material for epoxy and phenoxy resins, and is used in the manufacture of glycerine, in curing propylene-based rubbers, as a solvent for cellulose esters and ethers, and in resins with high wet-strength for the paper industry.	R.H.C. Pr.C.H.	1854	1937	1976 <u>1985</u> <u>1987</u> 1999

66

A – Chemical	B – Use	C	D	E	F
Erionite CAS N° 66733-21-9	It is used as a noble metal-impregnated catalyst in a hydrocarbon cracking process. It is used for house-building materials. It has been investigated for use to increase soil fertility and to control odors in livestock production.	C.H. K.H.C	1898	1954	1987 1994
Ethylene Dibromide CAS N° 106-93-4	The major uses are as lead scavenger in tetraalkyl lead petrol and antiknock preparations. It is also used as a soil and grain fumigant. As an intermediate in the synthesis of dyes and pharmaceuticals and as solvent for resins, gum, and waxes	R.H.C. Pr.C.H.	1826	1923	1977 1981 1987
Ethylene Oxide CAS N° 75-21-8	Chemical Industry: Chemical intermediate. Production of non-ionic surfactants used in a variety of household and industrial products as low-foam detergents. Fumigant and sterilizing in a variety of applications. Fumigate products such as: bread, cocoa, desiccated coconut, dried egg powder, fish, flour, dried fruits, meat, spices, dehydrated vegetables and walnut meats, clothing, furs, leather and textiles, cosmetics and drugs, cigarette tobacco, dental, medical, pharmaceutical and other scientific equipment and supplies including disposable and reusable medical items: packaging materials; paper and books; railway passenger- and freight cars and buses; motor oil; and other products including: experimental animals, beehives, bone meal, furniture, museum artefacts, and soils. Sterilization of spices.	R.H.C. Pr.C.H. K.H.C.	1859	1920	1985 1985 1987 2000

A – Chemical	B – Use	C	D	E	F
Etoposide CAS N° 33419-42-0	It is one of the most widely used cytotoxic drugs and has strong antitumor activity in cases of small-cell lung cancer, testicular cancer, lymphomas and a variety of childhood malignancies.	Pr.C.H.	1963	1999	2000
Formaldehyde CAS N° 50-00-0	Plastics and resins manufacture. Urea-formaldehyde resins – phenolic resins; polyacetal resins; and melamine resins. Production of diverse substances. Additional minor use: agriculture, concrete and plaster; cosmetics (foot antiperspirants); deodorant in rooms; disinfectants and fumigants; embalming; histopathology; leather. In Medicine: Treatment of athlete's foot; sterilizing. Metal industry: corrosion inhibitor. Paper industry; photography. Rubber industry: biocide in latex rubber. Solvents. Textile Industry; wood preservative. Veterinary medicine: as antiseptic and fumigant for the control of tympani, diarrhea, mastitis, pneumonia, and internal bleeding.	R.H.C. Pr.C.H.	1859	1900s	1981 1982 1987
HC Blue N° 1 CAS N° 2784-94-3	Cosmetic: It was used exclusively as a dye semi-permanent hair coloring products.	Ps.C.H.		1960s	1993
Hexamethylphosphoramide CAS N° 680-31-9	It is used as a solvent for polymers, as a selective solvent for gases, as a polymerization catalyst, as a stabilizer against thermal degradation in polystyrene, as an additive to polyvinyl and polyoleofins resins	R.H.C. Ps.C.H.	1903		1977 1985 1987

A – Chemical	B – Use	C	D	E	F
Hexamethylphos-phoramide (cont.)	to protect against degradation to ultra violet light. It has been tested as chemosterilant for insects. As an antistatic agent, as a flame retardant, and de-icing additive for jet fuels				
Hydrazine CAS N° 302-01-2	Chemical Industry: Manufacture of diverse substances; agricultural pesticides; water treatment; antioxidants; pharmaceuticals; photography; xerography; dyes; explosives; high-energy fuels; rocket propellants.	R.H.C. Ps.C.H.	1887	1907 1940	1974 1983 1999
Melphalan CAS N° 148-82-3	It is used in human medicine for the treatment of various malignant diseases, especially for multiple malignant myeloma, malignant melanomas and adenocarcinomas of the ovary.	K.H.C. C.H.	1954	1975	1975 1980 1987
Methyleugenol CAS N° 93-15-2	It is used as a flavoring agent in jellies, bake goods, non-alcoholic beverages, chewing gum, candy, pudding, relish, and ice creams. It has been used as an anesthetic in rodents. It also is used as an insect attractant in combination with insecticides. It has been used as an agent in sunscreens.	R.H.C.			2002
Methylthiouracil CAS N° 56-04-2	Drug: Treatment of hyperthyroidism.	Ps.C.H.		1940s	2001
Metronidazole CAS N° 443-48-1	Drug: It is effective on oral administration in infections due to *Entamoeba histolytica, Trichomonas vaginalis,* and *Giardia lamblia.* It has been evaluated for use in the treatment of alcoholism. Its use in the treatment of acne rosaceous has been suggested.	R.H.C. Ps.C.H.	1960	1963	1977 1985 1987

A – Chemical	B – Use	C	D	E	F
Mitomycin C CAS N° 50-07-7	Antibiotic. Used in the treatment of advances carcinomas.	Ps.C.H.		1959	1976 1987
Myleran CAS N° 55-98-1	Drug: Chemotherapeutic agent for the treatment of some form of leukemia (chronic myelocytic leukemia).	K.H.C. C.H.		1954	1974 1985 1987
Nafenopin CAS N° 3771-19-5	It has been studied for use in the treatment of hypercholesterolemia or hypertriglyceridemia.	Ps.C.H.	1963		1980 1987
Nitrilotriacetic Acid CAS N° 139-13-9	Numerous commercial applications: as a metal ion chelator, including principally its use in cleaning products, industrial water treatment, textile preparations and metal finishing. Used in pulp and paper industry; in rubber processing; in photographic products, in the electrochemical industry; in the tanning of leather; and in cosmetics. As the trisodium salt, in detergent systems as a chelating agent and a laundry detergent builder.	R.H.C. Ps.C.H.	1862	1930s	1983 1990
ortho-Toluidine CAS N° 95-53-4	Chemical Industry: Synthesis of a variety of dyes. Used an intermediate for rubber chemical, pharmaceuticals and pesticides.	R.H.C. Ps.C.H.	1844	1880	1982 1983 1987
para-Aminoazo- benzene CAS N° 60-09-3	Used as a dye for lacquers, varnishes, wax products, oil stain and styrene resins. Intermediate in the production of acid yellow, diazo dyes and indulines.	Ps.C.H.	1861	1924	1975 1987
para-Cresidine CAS N° 120-71-8	Used almost exclusively as a dye intermediate. Intermediate to produce azo dyes and pigments, such as Direct Orange 72, Direct Violet 9, and other, used in the textile industry.	R.H.C. Ps.C.H.		1926	1981 1982 1987

70

A – Chemical	B – Use	C	D	E	F
para-Dichloro-benzene CAS N° 106-46-7 (1,4-Dichloro-benzene)	Space deodorant. Insecticide: Smooth control. Germicide/disinfectant. Soil fumigant – Insecticide for fruit borers and ants. Animal repellent. Chemical Industry: chemical intermediate for dyes, insecti-cides, pharmaceuticals, and other organic chemicals. In the production of plastics used in the electrical and electronic industries.	Ps.C.H R.H.C.	1850 1905	1909	1982 1987 1989
Phenacetin CAS N° 62-44-2	In human medicine, it is used as analgesic and antipyretic drugs. It is used alone, or in combination with aspirin and caffeine. In Veterinary medicine it is used as an analgesic and anti-pyretic agent. It is also used as a stabilizer for hydrogen peroxide in hair bleaching preparations.	R.H.C. Pr.C.H.	1887	1925	1977 1980 1980 1987
Phenazopyridine Hydrochloride CAS N° 136-40-3	It is used as an analgesic and antiseptic in the management of genitourinary-tract infections.	R.H.C. Ps.C.H.	1914	1944	1980 1981 1987
Phenobarbital CAS N° 50-06-6	In long-acting barbiturates used in human medicine as hypnotic, sedatives and in the treatment of epilepsy. In Veterinary medicine it is used as sedative and anticon-vulsant.	Ps.C.H.	1911	1925	1977 1987
Phenolphthalein CAS N° 77-09-8	It is a stimulant laxative which has been used for the treatment of constipation and for the bowel evacuation be-fore investigational proce-dures or surgery. In an alco-holic solution is also used as a visual indicator in titrations of mineral and organic acids and most alkalis.	R.H.C. Ps.C.H.		1902	2000 2000

A – Chemical	B – Use	C	D	E	F
Phenytoin CAS N° 57-41-0	It is used largely in the treatment of grand mal and psychomotor seizures. It is used as a cardiac depressant (anti-arrhythmic). It has been used in the treatment of corea or Parkinson's syndrome. Its use has been investigated for the treatment of trigeminal neuralgia, migraine, polyneuritis of pregnancy, acute alcoholism, and certain psychoses. In veterinary medicine it is used to control epileptiform convulsions in dogs.	R.H.C. Ps.C.H.	1911	1946	1977 1980 1987
Polybrominated Biphenyls	As flame retardants for synthetic fibers and molded thermoplastic parts. The Hexabromobiphenyls was incorporated into ABS (Acrylontrile/butadiene/styrene) plastics, coatings and lacquers, and polyurethane foam. Used in light-sensitive compositions to act as color activators. As wood preservative, and electrical insulation. Radio and television parts, thermostats, shavers and hand-tool housings. Used in typewriters, calculators, microfilm readers, and business machine housings. Miscellaneous small automotive parts, e.g., electrical wire connectors, switch connectors, speaker grills.	R.H.C. Ps.C.H.	1964	1970	1986 1985 1987
Polychlorinated Biphenyls	Used in numerous industrial products prior to 1972. Where emissions into the environment are not probable, are used: in heat transfer, hydrau-	R.H.C. Pr.C.H.	1867	1929	1978 1981 1987

A – Chemical	B – Use	C	D	E	F
Polychlorinated Biphenyls (cont.)	lic fluids and lubricants. Used in transformers cooling liquid. Where the emission into the environment is more probable since it is not controlled, are used: plasticizers, surface coatings, inks, adhesives, pesticide extenders and for micro encapsulation of dyes for carbonless duplicating paper. In insecticide and bactericide formulations. To insulate electric wires and cables in the mining and ship-building industries. In immersion oil for micro-scopes.				
Ponceau 3R CAS N° 3564-09-8	Has been used to dye wool. Has been permitted in US as food colors (removed in 1960). Was permitted in externally applied drugs and cosmetics. The DFG, reported that this substance was approved for use as general food coloring in some countries.	Ps.C.H.	1878	1914	1975 1987
Ponceau MX CAS N° 3761-53-3	Used principally as a textile and leather dye. Used to color inks, paper, pigment, wood stains and in fruits (specifically in the United Kingdom), confectionary and meat products. Used in the United States in drugs and cosmetics, and cancelled in 1966. The DFG reported that the product was approved for food use in some countries.	Ps.C.H.	1878	1914	1975 1987
Potassium Bromate CAS N° 7758-01-2	Is used primarily as maturing agent for flour and as a dough conditioner. In fish-paste products. It is also a component of food for yeast and is used in the	Ps.C.H.			1986 1999

A – Chemical	B – Use	C	D	E	F
Potassium Bromate (cont.)	malting of beer. It may be used in the manufacture of cheese. Used as laboratory reagent and oxidizing agent. Other uses: In home permanent-wave neutralizing compounds. As a food additive. In explosives.				
Propylene Oxide CAS N° 75-56-9	Main use as chemical intermediate in the manufacture of diverse products. Fumigant, principally for sterilizing packages food products in fumigation chambers. Direct or indirect food additive: as an etherifying agent in the production of modified food starch; and a package fumigant for certain fruit products and as a fumigant for bulk quantities of several food products.	Pr.C.H. R.H.C.	1860	1925	1985 1987 1991
Propylthiouracil CAS N° 51-52-5	Drug: Treatment of hyperthyroidism.	R.H.C. Ps.C.H.		1940s	1985 1987
Silica Crystalline (Silica: CAS N° 7631-86-9) (Quartz: CAS N° 14808-60-7)	Silica sand has been used for many different purposes for many years; its principal use throughout history has been in the manufacture of glass. It is also used in the manufacture of ceramics. Other major use is in foundry castings. Another significant industrial application is incorporation into abrasives, such as sandpaper, grinding and polishing agents, and sandblasting materials. It is also used in hydraulic fracturing suspended in a fluid pumped into oil or gas wells. It is used as a raw material for the production of silicon and	Pr.C.H. R.H.C. K.H.C.			1987 1991 2000

A – Chemical	B – Use	C	D	E	F
Silica Crystalline (cont.)	ferrosilicon metals, the abrasive silicon carbide, activated silica, silica gel desiccants and sodium silicate and as a builder in detergents. It may also used in filtering. Finely ground sand (silica flour) has been used as filler in paints, rubber, paper, plastics, asphalt, scouring powders, cement, and other products. Quartz Crystals: are used in jewellery and electronic applications.				
Sodium saccharin CAS N° 128-44-9	Sweetness without adding calories. In: beverages, foods, cosmetics, and pharmaceuticals.	I.E.H. S.E.A.	1878	1900	1999
Styrene CAS N° 100-42-5	It is one of the most important monomers worldwide, and its polymers and copolymers are used in an increasing wide range of applications. The major uses for styrene are in plastics, latex paints, and coatings, synthetic rubbers, polyesters and styrene-alkyl coatings. The broad spectrum of uses includes constructions, packaging, automotive, and household goods. Polystyrene resins are used extensively in the fabrication of plastic packaging, disposable beverage tumblers, toys, and other molded goods. Expandable polystyrene beads are used for disposable cups, containers and packaging as well as for insulation. Packaging is the single largest use in which styrene-containing resins, particularly foams, are used as fillers and cushioning.	Ps.C.H.	1831	1925	1979 1987 1994

A – Chemical	B – Use	C	D	E	F
Styrene (cont.)	Construction applications include pipes, fittings, tanks, lighting fixtures, and corrosion-resistant products. Household goods include synthetic marble, flooring, disposable tableware and molded furnishings. Transport applications range from tires to reinforced plastics and automobile body putty.				
Styrene Oxide CAS N° 96-09-3	Chemical Industry: Reactive plasticizer or diluents in epoxy resins. Approved for US FDA for use as a cross-linking agent for epoxy resins in coatings for containers intended for repeated use in contact with alcoholic beverages containing up to 8% of ethanol by volume.	S.E.A. R.H.C.	1905	1974	1985 2002
Testosterone CAS N° 58-22-0 (Androgenic Anabolics Steroids)	It is used in human medicine for the treatment of a variety of conditions in both men and women. It is used in Veterinary medicine, in dogs and horses.	Pr.C.H	1935	1939	1979 1987
Tetrachloro-ethylene CAS N° 127-18-4	Textile industry: dry-cleaning. Industrial metal cleaning: degreasing of metal. Chemical intermediate: synthesis of Fluorocarbons. Drug against hookworms and some nematodes.	Ps.C.H. R.H.C.	1821	1925	1979 1987 1989
Thiotepa (Tris(1-aziridinyl)-phosphina sulphyde) CAS N° 52-24-4	Drug. It is a cytostatic agent. It has been used in the treatment of lymphoma and a variety of solid tumors, such as those of breast and ovary. It has also been used in cases of urinary bladder malignancies, meningeal carcinomatosis and various soft-tissue tumors.	R.H.C. C.H. K.H.C.	1954		1981 1990 1998

A – Chemical	B – Use	C	D	E	F
Toluene Diisocyanate CAS N° 584-84-9	Mainly in the production of Polyurethane foams. Polyurethane coatings and elastomers. Flexible Polyurethane foams are used in furniture and bedding industry. In carpet underlay. In automotive seating and padding. Rigid Polyuretane foams are primarily used as insulation. This foam is used in household refrigerators and in board or laminate form for residential sheathing or commercial roofing. This foam is also used as insulation for truck trailers, railroad freight cars and cargo containers. Polyurethane coating are used as floor finishes, wood finishes and paints. They are also used as wood and concrete sealants and floor finishes. Aircraft, truck and passenger-car coatings are often comprised of these prepolymer systems. Elastomers are used in applications requiring strength, flexibility and shock-absorption, and are resistant to oil, solvent and ultraviolet radiation. They are also used in adhesive and sealant compounds, in automobile parts, shoe soles, roller skate wells, pod liners, blood bags. In oil fields and mines.	R.H.C. Ps.C.H.		1930s	1985 1985 1987
Treosulphan CAS N° 299-75-2	Drug: Used in human medicine as antineoplastic agent for the treatment of ovarian cancer.	C.H.	1961	1969	1981 1987
Trypan Blue CAS N° 72-57-1	Used for dyeing textiles, leather and paper, as a stain in biological investigations and as therapeutic agent in the treatment of sleeping sickness.	Ps.C.H.	1890	1921	1975 1987

A – Chemical	B – Use	C	D	E	F
Vinyl Bromide CAS N° 593-60-2	Chemical Industry: intermediate in organic synthesis, and in the manufacture of polymers, copolymers, flame retardants, pharmaceuticals and fumigants. Vinyl bromide-Vinyl chloride copolymers are used for preparation films, for laminating fibers and as rubbers substitutes. It is also used in leather and fabricated metal products.	Pr.C.H. R.H.C.	1835	1968	1979 1985 1987 2002
Vinyl Chloride CAS N° 75-01-4	Chemical Industry: It is used for the production of vinyl chloride resins. The largest use for resins is in the production of plastic piping and conduit. Other important uses are in floor covering; in consumer's goods; in electrical applications; and in transport applications. Vinyl chloride has been used as a refrigerant, as an extraction solvent, for heat-sensitive materials. Limited quantities were used in the US as an aerosol propellant (banned in 1974). In self-pressurized household containers, and as ingredient of drug and cosmetic products.	K.H.C. C.H.	1835	1920s	1979 1980 1987
Zidovudine (AZT) CAS N° 30516-87-1	It was originally synthesized as possible anti-cancer agent, but was found to be ineffective. In 1985, was found to be active against HIV-1.	Ps.C.H.	1960s	1985	2000

Bibliography for table 8

1,1-Dimethylhydrazine (IARC, 1974; IARC, 1987b; US DHHS-PHS-NTP, 2002), *1,2-Dichloroethane* (IARC, 1979b; IARC, 1999b; US DHHS-PHS-NTP, 2002), *1,3-Butadiene* (IARC, 1985d; IARC, 1987b;

IARC, 1999a; US DHHS-PHS-NTP, 2002), *1,3-Propane Sultone* (IARC, 1974; IARC, 1987b; IARC, 1999c), *1,4-Dioxane* (IARC, 1976b; IARC, 1999b; US DHHS-PHS-NTP, 2002), *2,3-Dibromo-1-propanol* (US DHHS-PHS-NTP, 2002), *2,4,6-Trichlorophenol* (IARC, 1979b; IARC, 1987b; US DHHS-PHS-NTP, 2002), *2,4-Diaminoanisole Sulfate* (IARC, 1978a; IARC, 1987b; US DHHS-PHS-NTP, 2002), *2,4-Diaminotoluene* (IARC, 1978a; IARC, 1987b; US DHHS-PHS-NTP, 2002), *2-Naphtylamine* (IARC, 1974; IARC, 1987b), *3,3'-Dichlorobenzidine* (IARC, 1982b; IARC, 1987b; US DHHS-PHS-NTP, 2002), *3-Chloro-2-methylpropene* (IARC, 1995; US DHHS-PHS-NTP, 2002), *4-Chloro-o-phenylenediamine* (IARC, 1982a; IARC, 1987b; US DHHS-PHS-NTP, 2002), *4-Dimethylaminoazobenzene* (IARC, 1975a; IARC, 1987b; US DHHS-PHS-NTP, 2002), *Acetaldehyde* (IARC, 1985b; IARC, 1999b; US DHHS-PHS-NTP, 2002), *Acrylamide* (IARC, 1985d; IARC, 1987b; US DHHS-PHS-NTP, 2002), *Acrylonitrile* (IARC, 1999a; US DHHS-PHS-NTP, 2002), *Adriamicyn* (IARC, 1976a; IARC, 1987b; US DHHS-PHS-NTP, 2002), *Asbestos* (IARC, 1977b; IARC, 1987b), *Azacitidine* (IARC, 1990b; US DHHS-PHS-NTP, 2002), *Azathioprina* (IARC, 1981; IARC, 1987b; US DHHS-PHS-NTP, 2002), *Benzene* (IARC, 1982b; IARC, 1987b; US DHHS-PHS-NTP, 2002), *Benzidine* (IARC, 1982b; IARC, 1987b; US DHHS-PHS-NTP, 2002), *Bleomycin* (IARC, 1981; IARC, 1987b), *Bromodichloromethane* (IARC, 1991; US DHHS-PHS-NTP, 2002), *Butylated hydroxyanisole* (IACR, 1986a; US DHHS-PHS-NTP, 2002), *Carbon Tetrachloride* (IARC, 1979b; IARC, 1987b; IARC, 1999b; US DHHS-PHS-NTP, 2002), *Catechol* (IARC, 1977c; IARC, 1999b), *Chlorambucil* (IARC, 1981; IARC, 1987b; US DHHS-PHS-NTP, 2002), *Chloramphenicol* (IARC, 1976a; IARC, 1987b; IARC, 1990b; US DHHS-PHS-NTP, 2002), *Chlorendic acid* (IARC, 1990a; US DHHS-PHS-NTP, 2002), *Chlornaphazine* (IARC, 1974; IARC, 1987b; US DHHS-PHS-NTP, 2002), *Chloroform* (IARC, 1979b; IARC, 1987b; US DHHS-PHS-NTP, 2002), *Chloroprene* (IARC, 1999a; US DHHS-PHS-NTP, 2002), *Chlorozotocine* (IARC, 1990b; US DHHS-PHS-NTP, 2002), *CI Acid Orange 3* (IARC, 1993b), *CI Acid Red 114* (IARC, 1993b), *CI Basic Red 9* (IARC, 1993b; US DHHS-PHS-NTP, 2002), *Ciclosporin* (IARC, 1990b), *Cisplatin* (IARC, 1981; IARC, 1987b; US DHHS-PHS-NTP, 2002), *Citrus Red N° 2* (IARC, 1975a; IARC, 1987b), *Creosotes* (IARC, 1985a; IARC, 1987b; US DHHS-PHS-NTP, 2002), *Cyclophosphamide* (IARC, 1981; IARC, 1987b; US DHHS-PHS-NTP,

2002), *D&C Red N° 9* (IARC, 1993b), *Dacarbazine* (IARC, 1981; IARC, 1987b; US DHHS-PHS-NTP, 2002), *Dantron* (IARC, 1990b; US DHHS-PHS-NTP, 2002), *Daunomycin* (IARC, 1976a; IARC, 1987b), *Dichloromethane* (IARC, 1979b; IARC, 1987b; IARC, 1999a; US DHHS-PHS-NTP, 2002), *Diepoxybutane* (IARC, 1976b; IARC, 1987b; US DHHS-PHS-NTP, 2002), *Diethyl Sulphate* (IARC, 1974; IARC, 1987b; US DHHS-PHS-NTP, 2002), *Diethylstilboestrol* (IARC, 1979c; IARC, 1987b; US DHHS-PHS-NTP, 2002), *Dimethyl Sulphate* (IARC, 1974; IARC, 1987b; US DHHS-PHS-NTP, 2002), *Dimethylcarbamoyl chloride* (IARC, 1976c; IARC, 1987b; US DHHS-PHS-NTP, 2002), *d-Limonene* (IARC, 1993a; IARC, 1999d), *Epichlorohydrin* (IARC, 1976b; IARC, 1987b; IARC, 1999b; US DHHS-PHS-NTP, 2002), *Erionite* (IARC, 1987a; IARC, 1987b; US DHHS-PHS-NTP, 2002), *Ethylene Dibromide* (IARC, 1977c, IARC, 1987b; US DHHS-PHS-NTP, 2002), *Ethylene Oxide* (IARC, 1985b; IARC, 1987b; US DHHS-PHS-NTP, 2002), *Etoposide* (IARC, 2000a), *Formaldehyde* (IARC, 1982b; IARC, 1987b; US DHHS-PHS-NTP, 2002), *HC Blue N° 1* (IARC, 1993b), *Hexamethylphosphoramide* (IARC, 1977c; IARC, 1987b; US DHHS-PHS-NTP, 2002), *Hydrazine* (IARC, 1974; IARC, 1999c; US DHHS-PHS-NTP, 2002), *Melphalan* (IARC, 1975b; IARC, 1987b; US DHHS-PHS-NTP, 2002), *Methyleugenol* (US DHHS-PHS-NTP, 2002), *Methylthiouracil* (IARC, 2000b), *Metronidazole* (IARC, 1977a; IARC, 1987b; US DHHS-PHS-NTP, 2002), *Mitomycin C* (IARC, 1976a; IARC, 1987b), *Myleran* (IARC, 1974; IARC, 1987b; US DHHS-PHS-NTP, 2002), *Nafenopin* (IARC, 1980; IARC, 1987b), *Nitrilotriacetic Acid* (IARC, 1990a; US DHHS-PHS-NTP, 2002), *ortho-Toluidine* (IARC, 1982a; IARC, 1987b; US DHHS-PHS-NTP, 2002), *para-Aminoazobenzene* (IARC, 1975a; IARC, 1987b), *para-Cresidine* (IARC, 1982a; IARC, 1987b; US DHHS-PHS-NTP, 2002), *para-Dichlorobenzene* (IARC, 1982b; IARC, 1987b; US DHHS-PHS-NTP, 2002), *Phenacetin* (IARC, 1977a; IARC, 1980; IARC, 1987b; US DHHS-PHS-NTP, 2002), *Phenazopyridine Hydrochloride* (IARC, 1980; IARC, 1987b; US DHHS-PHS-NTP, 2002), *Phenobarbital* (IARC, 1977a; IARC, 1987b), *Phenolphthalein* (IARC, 2000a; US DHHS-PHS-NTP, 2002), *Phenytoin* (IARC, 1977a; IARC, 1987b; US DHHS-PHS-NTP, 2002), *Polybrominated Biphenyls* (IARC, 1986b; IARC, 1987b; US DHHS-PHS-NTP, 2002), *Polychlorinated Biphenyls* (IARC, 1978c; IARC, 1987b; US DHHS-PHS-NTP, 2002), *Ponceau 3R* (IARC, 1975a; IARC, 1987b), *Ponceau MX*

(IARC, 1975a; IARC, 1987b), *Potassium Bromate* (IARC, 1986a; IARC, 1999d), *Propylene Oxide* (IARC, 1985b; IARC, 1987b; US DHHS-PHS-NTP, 2002), *Propylthiouracil* (IARC, 1987b; US DHHS-PHS-NTP, 2002), *Silica Cristaline, Silica, Quartz* (IARC, 1987a; IARC, 1987b; US DHHS-PHS-NTP, 2002), *Sodium Saccharin* (IARC, 1999d), *Styrene* (IARC, 1979a; IARC, 1987b; IARC, 1994), *Styrene Oxide* (IARC, 1985b, IARC, 1987b; US DHHS-PHS-NTP, 2002), *Testosterone* (IARC, 1979c; IARC, 1987b), *Tetrachloroethylene* (IARC, 1979b; IARC, 1987b; US DHHS-PHS-NTP, 2002), *Thiotepa* (IARC, 1990b; US DHHS-PHS-NTP, 2002), *Toluene Diisocyanate* (IARC, 1985d; IARC, 1987b; US DHHS-PHS-NTP, 2002), *Treosulphan* (IARC, 1981; IARC, 1987b), *Trypan Blue* (IARC, 1975a; IARC, 1987b), *Vinyl Bromide* (IARC, 1979a; IARC, 1985d, IARC, 1987b; US DHHS-PHS-NTP, 2002), *Vinyl Chloride* (IARC, 1979a; IARC, 1987b; US DHHS-PHS-NTP, 2002), *Zidovudine* (IARC, 2000a).

Another interesting point of technopathogenic relevance is the time span between Discovery-Development-Application. As the following table shows, the time span between one and the other is progressively short-ened (Eguiazu, 1991).

Table 9: Evolution of the time span between discovery and the development / application of a technique exemplified through several techniques Source: Gassen, 1988

Discovery	Time until its commercial application (years)
Photography	112
Electrical Motor	65
Telephone	56
Radio	35
X- ray tube	18
Television	12
Atomic reactor	10
Atomic bomb	6
Genetic Engineering	2

Finally, the Technician is aware of the risks implied but economic, cultural, etc. pressures lead him to justify such risks. He uses fallacious concepts (Motta, 1994), such as:

a) The Price of Progress: Progress, modernization and development will always entail paying a price. But, as we've seen before, the price is not always paid by the one who benefits from the technique. The other question is: who decides who must pay or not pay the price?

b) Air and water are great dilutants: The substances eliminated in the air, through chimneys, for example, or dumped into the river, will not be harmful because they will be diluted to innocuous levels.

c) We must accept certain level of contamination in food: Otherwise pests would prevent humans from using food raw materials. Pests would devour all the existing crops.

d) Future techniques will solve the problems: Future science will eventually solve the current technical flaws and the damage they cause.

e) The techniques posing risks to developed countries do not necessarily affect developing countries. At the same time, they must tolerate more risk than developed countries until they achieve development (Frank, 1980-1983).

Regarding point "b", a study published in 1990 in the former Soviet Union indicated that the volume of water necessary to dilute the effluents coming from all the country's waterways had surpassed the volume or annual discharge of all the country's rivers combined (Loukjanenko, 1990).

Point "d" would lead us to accept certain techniques even though they can cause cancer, because future medicine will discover a cure for this disease.

The point "e" concept was ruled out in the 1960's. The advancements in contamination studies allowed us to get to know the causes more thoroughly and thus conclude that contamination does affect all the countries whether they are industrialized or not (FAO, 1982).

To sum up

The problem with modern Technique is that when a new technique is developed to create new objects, what is being sought for is the positive aspect, that is, the characteristics required to accomplish the aims for which it was conceived. Developers are also aware that there will be certain negative aspects – for example, the risk of acute toxicity in a substance – so they take the relevant measures to prevent the associated risk.

As we have described before, negative aspects can be divided in two groups: Evident and Non-evident.

For instance, if we take a pesticide, the evident negative aspect is its risk to cause acute toxicity, that is, intoxication in the short term. Modern technique can estimate this risk and establish preventive measures. Non-evident negative aspects can be, for example, carcinogenic risk. Non-toxic substances can be carcinogenic or have any other long-term effect. This characteristic is measurable, but it takes a long time to do so and it has a high economic cost. At the same time, the only preventive measure could turn out to be to avoid using the substance altogether, which is something impossible to accept for the technician due to the economic investment involved.

Having analyzed the characteristics of modern technique – the above mentioned, among others, the attitude of scientists, technicians and corporations, the *non-observable negative aspects* – and motivated by the work of Prof. Heinrich Beck on the relationship between Technique and Culture (Beck, 1979a), we came to see the existence of this new phenomenon we have defined as Technopathogeny.

Prof. Heinrich Beck has a wide philosophical background including several works on Technique, a subject he has been exploring for many years. Apart from his cited works, we include some others for those interested in further exploring the subject from the point of view of Philosophy (Beck, 1969, 1972, 1974, 1977, 1979b, 1981, 1982, 1984, 1986, 1987).

X.   Technopathogeny: The first three approaches

At this stage we can present the first three theses or approaches used in the clarification of the phenomenon:

I. Technopathogeny is defined as the damage caused to health in humans which is not immediately manifested but after many years or generations, as a consequence of factors caused by technique, product of immanent and hidden errors or flaws within it.

II. Technopathogeny will be a phenomenon whose intensity will be in crescendo for the following reasons:
1. The nature of the new mechanical arts is qualitatively different from the nature of ancient mechanical arts because they are increasingly based on nuclear phenomena (atomic and cellular nucleus).
2. The increasingly shortened process of Discovery-Development-Application makes prevention of damage more difficult.
3. The skimp soundness of the fundamentals of classical science anticipates imperfect use of knowledge.
4. Ethical mishaps in people involved in the creation of knowledge process, in the development of techniques and in their commercial application.
5. There is no science that allows for the study of Technopathogeny as a unique phenomenon.

III. We postulate the need for the development of a science – Technopathogenology – that allows for the study of Technopathogeny as an object of study on its own.

XI.   Technopathogeny: Its causes – The fourth approach

As the only rational beings on Earth, humans have always been driven by an unexplainable and unlimited need for change (maybe defined by

84

the terms: Progress, Evolution, Modernization, etc.). This has led humans to use the knowledge with which they developed arts or techniques to modify elements or objects from nature and create new objects. By *cultural objects* we understand objects which humans have built or have invented; by *culturized objects*, objects which humans have adapted from nature (Colacilli de Muro, 1978), for example, by domesticating animals as cattle or by selecting a determined plant to grow it – cereals, oleaginous plants, fruits, etc.

At first, the modifications, adaptations and alterations of objects were rudimentary, simple and macroscopic. As we have said before, this barely posed any risk on the Technician or on the community. That was the case of the wedged stick.

With time, science has evolved and diversified in the most diverse areas of knowledge – whether abstract or concrete – and each area, in turn, has become more and more specific and isolated from the rest. Knowledge has become atomized and a holistic view of reality has been lost.

These advances have allowed technicians to move from simple, rudimentary changes to more profound, complex and microscopic ones. One example is chemical synthesis. Other examples are the penetration in the atomic nucleus (nuclear energy) and in the cellular nucleus (genetic engineering) which have allowed us to define them as *nuclear phenomena* (Eguiazu, 1991).

When compared to ancient techniques, modern techniques imply bigger observable risks as well as long term non-observable risks. In addition, among all the disciplines and sub disciplines that have been developed, we haven't found one which successfully focuses on studying this problem of modern technique: *the non-evident negative effects on human health.*

We have thus arrived to a point in which we see there is a specific problem and, as it will be explained in the following chapter, there is no adequate discipline for its study. But there are still certain doubts about the phenomenon. How did it originate?

If Technopathogeny is a concrete problem which is harmful to human health caused by a factor generated by a defect in a technique, the question is: which are the causes that allow for these hidden effects that provoke technopathogenies to appear? When we speak of Technique we are also referring to concrete elements. Every technique generates – directly or indirectly – physical, chemical or biological elements. In order to develop a technique, therefore, these bodies of knowledge we call technologies are required. It is rather obvious that if a technique has a defect it is probably due to the fact that insufficient or erroneous elements were used during its development.

The urgent need of adaptation or invention of new objects and the need to develop new techniques for that purpose increase the pressure on scientists to generate more knowledge. As we have said before, Technologies is the group of necessary bodies of knowledge needed for the development or creation of a Technique.

This pressure leads to hastily consider many bodies of knowledge as complete. They may be flawed bodies of knowledge or technologies and as such, they are not completely truthful. These technologies are used to develop new techniques (equipments, devices, substances, seeds, etc.) which, being ill conceived from their inception, can be defined as *Technological Freaks*. We are using the term *Freak* without any apocalyptical undertone, relying on its definition in Spanish language as "work wrongly conceived and wrongly carried" (Diccionario Enciclopédico Ilustrado de la Lengua Española),

The existence of these Technological Freaks, which lay at the very origin of Technopathogeny, lead to a study (Motta, 1994) which was based on a question arising from the following reasoning: The only way to get to know an object completely, in a truthful manner, is to know all the truth about it, i.e., to know everything about the object. If the object presents a flaw, it means that the technician who developed it did not know the object completely, or ignored part of it. For example, the case of the laboratory that elaborated a new medicine and both the laboratory and the physician ignored that apart from the known pharmacological properties, the medicine was teratogenic. The medicine in question had unknown or ill-known aspects. The question is therefore: which are the attitudes regarding the truth that can lead to the lack of knowledge or ill knowledge of the factors that lead to the manifestation of negative non-evident effects?

The Ancient Greeks followed the principle of "Executing all their tasks according to clear, certain and well-funded rules" (Goblot, 1943).

To them, "Every flaw or defect is a consequence of ignorance or an error".

"The Greeks considered that every single good could be reached from the truth as a starting point" (Goblot, 1943).

Ignorance and error are two attitudes regarding truth. (Colacilli de Muro, 1978) Now, are they also the only ones connected to the manifestation of a Technopathogeny?

In the study above mentioned that question was analyzed (Motta, 1994). Some factors causing technopathogenies were studied to establish that the role of knowledge in itself was at the root of the problem. The study demonstrated that not only Ignorance and Error can cause a Technopathogeny, but also other attitudes could.

Apart from Ignorance and Error, Certainty, Doubt, Opinion and even Mendacity are attitudes regarding truth and can therefore be responsible for gaps or voids in the bodies of knowledge used in the future to develop possibly flawed new techniques that carry the germ of Technopathogeny.

We will analyze each of these attitudes regarding truth and we will see that each of them can be responsible for a Technopathogeny.

XII. Attitudes regarding truth and its consequences on Technique

Certainty

"Is defined as the attitude according to which a determined result of knowledge is unconditionally accepted" (Colacilli de Muro, 1978).

In every case, Certainty provides an effective security over which it adheres to, but in no case whatsoever can certainty guarantee that correctness, validity, truth, authenticity or their opposites have been effectively obtained.

Certainty is produced by evidence.

Let's take the case of a substance that is evaluated to determine whether it is or not carcinogenic. The studies are carried out on experimental animals (usually rats and mice). If the trial provides enough evidence of carcinogenicity on experimental animals, then it can be anticipated that it will also be carcinogenic to humans (IARC, 1983) (U.S. DHHS-PHS, 1984).

On the other hand, if the results are negative, the substance will not be considered carcinogenic to humans.

The carcinogenicity trials or evaluation of trials carried out by prestigious organisms are strict enough to estimate that if the results are negative, the substance will be innocuous to humans. This is based on a more or less approximate extrapolation that infers the possible effect on humans using experimental animals.

So far we do not know of any case that indicates the contrary. The certainty of such trials has been established because in some cases, for certain substances, the experimental evidence on animals preceded the epidemiological evidence in humans as, for example, with Aflatoxins and Diethylstilboestrol. This shows that the results obtained in the long term trials conducted on experimental animals could be used to predict similar effects on humans. They should also be considered in the implementation of Public Health measures for the primary prevention of cancer (U.S. DHHS-PHS, 1984).

Even when there are certain substances for which there is only animal evidence regarding its carcinogenic effect (whether positive or negative), there are substances for which there is accumulated evidence to consider them Carcinogenic to humans. An example of this are the substances included in the Annual Report on Carcinogens (USA) under the title *Substances or group of substances, occupational exposures associated with technological processes and medical treatments that are known to be carcinogenic.* In this group of substances there is evidence that indicates that there is a cause-effect relationship between exposure and development of cancer (U.S. DHHS-PHS-NTP, 1985). That necessarily has to mean that humans inadvertently ended up being the objects of experimentation.

Experimental trials on animals do not guarantee that the whole truth about a substance regarding its carcinogenic effect is known. This could only be so if humans were used on trials, which is, of course, not ethically possible. However, in some cases this *experimentum crucis* has been carried out contradicting all the rules of ethics. As we have seen before, only in accidental cases or due to inadvertent exposure is this value obtained. If a trial on experimental animals shows that there is not enough evidence that a specific substance is carcinogenic to humans, but then it ends up being carcinogenic to humans, we would consider this a case of

Technopathogeny (even though in this case, as we will detail later on, this Technopathogeny will be motivated by an Error).

Uncertainty

"Uncertainty is the lack of certainty produced by the lack of evidence" (Colacilli de Muro, 1978).

As it has already been mentioned, the toxicology trials for the study of carcinogenicity of a substance uses different species of animals, specially rats and mice of both sexes that for two years are strictly controlled so that the results – either positive or negative – can be attributed to the substance investigated (U.S. DHHS-PHS-NIH-NTP, 1992a).

According to the results obtained in such trials, the substances are classified in three levels regarding their Carcinogenic Activity: *Enough Evidence, Limited Evidence* and *No Evidence* (U.S. DHHS-PHS-NIH-NTP, 1992a). These three levels are established when, upon the general evaluation of a substance or agent, the results of various trials are considered. A trial in particular can provide several levels of evidence like *Clear Evidence, Some Evidence, Contradictory Evidence* or *No Evidence* (U.S. DHHS-PHS-NIH-NTP, 1992a).

Following the aforementioned definition of Certainty, we can only say that the substance will be innocuous to humans if the trial results on experimental animals indicate that there is No Evidence of Carcinogenic Activity.

A substance for which there is limited evidence or some evidence or contradictory evidence of carcinogenic activity cannot be considered a carcinogen to humans, but at the same time cannot be considered not to be a carcinogen. The same will happen if the results indicate, for example, *Clear Evidence* of carcinogenic activity on one of the species used on the trial, or on one of the sexes used of both species, giving contradictory or inadequate evidence to the other species or the other sex to establish a conclusion.

Therefore, if there are not enough studies to classify the risk of carcinogenicity of a substance on humans and such substance ends up being harmful, the origin of the Technopathogeny will be Uncertainty.

As it was the case with uncertainty, "Doubt is also produced by the lack of evidence" (Colacilli de Muro, 1978). But, unlike Uncertainty, Doubt implies a decision on how to take the results of the trials.

This is the attitude usually adopted by corporations. As it was said before, certain substances are used without having carried out the necessary studies to determine their innocuousness or lack of innocuousness in humans.

In this case, the companies commercializing such substances or products bluntly state that the substance or product is innocuous for humans since *there hasn't been any study so far demonstrating the long term or short term harmful side effects*. We could define this attitude as the companies giving themselves *the benefit of the doubt*. But the technopathogenological criterion is to apply the old juridical concept *in dubio pro reo* (the doubt in favor of the defendant) and, considering the consumer as the defendant, say: *the doubt in favor of the consumer*.

If a substance or technique used this way turns out to be harmful to humans, this would be a case of a Technopathogeny caused by Doubt.

It is interesting to mention here the case of an agrochemical company which, within the framework of its safety, health and environmental policy, published a document which included several products they commercialized including safety data (Rohm & Hass, 1986). In the page containing safety data on a product with the active ingredient Maneb (a fungicide), regarding the possibility of tumor development or birth defects, it indicates and stresses that:

> According to the trials on animals and on human experience THERE IS NO EVI-DENCE that the commercial product containing Maneb active ingredient can cause tumors or birth defects.

This report was elaborated in 1986. The IRPTC Datum Profile of Maneb prepared by the United Nations Environment Program International Register of Potentially Toxic Chemical transcribes the report elaborated by IARC in 1976 (IRPTC, 1987h), which states:

> Maneb has been tested on mice and rats through oral administration and subcutaneous injection. Oral administration produced an increase in lung tumors in one line of mice, but no effects were observed in other three lines. The studies in rats cannot

be evaluated due to the small number of surviving animals. No evaluation of the carcinogenicity of this compound can be realized.

We have seen that based on scientific evidence, the International Agency for Research on Cancer classifies substances in different groups. In table 8, we have mentioned three groups: Group 1, Group 2a and Group 2b. We have also mentioned Group 3: agents which do not fall into any other group. These are non-classifiable agents regarding carcinogenicity on humans due to the limited evidence on humans, or the limited or inadequate experimental evidence on animals. Then we also mentioned Group 4: This category is used for agents for which there is *evidence suggesting lack of carcinogenicity* in humans together with *evidence suggesting lack of carcinogenicity* in experimental animals. In some circumstances, this group can also include agents for which there is *inadequate evidence* or no data of carcinogenicity in humans but there is *evidence suggesting lack of carcinogenicity* in experimental animals, consistently and strongly supported by a broad range of other relevant data (IARC, 1987b).

In the case of Maneb, the evidence on animals is limited and therefore, as the IARC report indicates, the substance is not classifiable regarding its risk of carcinogenicity in humans, which goes to say it would belong to Group 3. It could by no means be included in Group 4, which could consider the substance – Maneb, in this case – innocuous to humans.

The company report provides a false certainty. Instead of saying There is No Evidence, it should say that the evidence is limited, inadequate or insufficient – as it is the actual case.

As we have said before, the doubt favored the company.

Opinion

"Opinion is defined as the conscious attitude that gives provisional acceptance before any trial regarding correctness, validity, truth, authenticity and their opposites" (Colacilli de Muro, 1978).

Let's take the case of chemical products. We have selected them to explain technopathogenies or possible technopathogenies that can occur due to faults regarding truth or due to voids in knowledge. In the case of these products, Opinion, i.e., its use for their development or application, can be the most important cause of a Technopathogeny.

Having been demonstrated that there are substances which can cause neoplasias in humans, each new substance must prove its innocuousness. But the innocuousness can only be determined if there is enough evidence supporting it.

It is believed that developed countries are currently using maybe more than 100,000 substances for everyday products. Only a few hundreds have been analyzed for their carcinogenesis risk. Of a yet smaller number there is enough data to determine whether they are carcinogenic or potentially carcinogenic to humans.

The lack of proof for the thousands remaining substances – substances for which there is not even limited or insufficient evidence – makes it only possible to guess (maybe from the study of its physico-chemical properties or molecular structure) that a determined substance will not be carcinogenic. In many cases the substance is used not baring in mind such possibility.

This is the case with pesticide substances (see table 12), which were used for many years until it was discovered that they presented carcinogenic risks to humans.

Ignorance

"Ignorance is defined as the lack of a determined knowledge" (Colacilli de Muro, 1978). Even though it can be manifested through error, they are not synonyms. If a person is affected by cancer for having been exposed to a substance in particular, it is impossible to say that it was due to ignorance that this person suffered or suffers such disease. Evidently, having discovered that there are substances which are carcinogenic, only an adequate study can prove whether a new substance poses a risk or not. In other words, if a person has cancer because of exposure to a carcinogenic substance, he or she may have not known the carcinogenic effect the substance had, but health authorities should have been aware of it.

We can include as examples of technopathogenies caused due to Ignorance those techniques associated to the use or apparition of determined substances. This is the case of the Aflatoxins. Aflatoxins were discovered in England in 1960 when heavy mortality was experienced among young turkeys which had been fed with food contaminated with them.

It was later discovered that they were a powerful carcinogen to humans, when several cases were detected in different communities.

Aflatoxins are naturally occurring mycotoxins that are produced by many species of Aspergillus, a fungus. Until 1960, among the fungi that were known to be toxic were the ones belonging to the Basidiomycota family (which includes the most common poisonous fungi) and the claviceps purpurea – whose toxic components, alkaloids, were isolated in 1875. Fungi also were responsible for the alimentary toxic aleukia that occurred in Russia during the 1940s, caused by the consumption of molded grains, especially millet, which had remained in the fields. In spite of this situation, there was no apparent interest on researchers to get to know the possible consequences on health that these fungi represented in less dramatic conditions (FAO, 1982). This is the reason why until 1960 it was not known that microscopic fungi (deuteromycetes), from the mould group, could generate carcinogenic substances. Since many species of moulds are pests of several grains that are part of human diet, humans could easily be inadvertently exposed to such substances. Therefore, the cases of cancer caused by exposure to any of such substances were cases of Technopathogeny due to Ignorance.

The discovery of Aflatoxins marked the beginning of several studies that resulted in the discovery of other substances produced by other species of fungi which can also be harmful to humans, causing cancer and other diseases (FAO, 1982).

Another case that can be included as Technopathogeny due to Ignorance is the case of Thalidomide. Even though the relevant short term and long term toxicology tests were said to be performed, its use proved it to be a potent teratogen. In this case, the factibility of the extrapolation of its effect on experimental animals to humans was erroneously inferred.

Another Technopathogeny due to Ignorance is the case of the incidence of diabetes in children whose parents ingested smoked food not long before conception. This food-processing technique is associated to the contamination with N-Nitrosamines, which were the cause of such cases of diabetes (Helgason, 1984). Due to its importance and because they are probably the cause of other technopathogenies, we will refer to these substances later on.

Other cases of technopathogenies due to Ignorance include: the incidence of leukemia in infants whose parents had been exposed to radiations for working in nuclear plants (Gardener, 1991); veterinary medicines that are harmful to humans and whose residues accumulate in the animal's organs or systems (FAO, 1985); chlorinated pesticides used in the protection of pastures which, ingested by cattle, led to the apparition of residues in meat thus harming consumers – a process called *carrying over.*

Even though so far we have presented it just as a hypothesis, another case of Technopathogeny connected to Ignorance is the one caused by a technique which is associated to the apparition of Aflatoxins. We have found that this substance is connected with the techniques which are used in the production of grains. One of such techniques is the use of plant enhancers, which aim at obtaining bigger yields. Certain characteristics are selected, for example, to obtain a bigger yield in the volume of the grain or a larger quantity of one of its components, oil, for example. One of our hypothesis is that due to aiming at such objectives – the search for genetic characteristics that lead to a bigger yield – the genetic selection determines that genes which naturally provided the grain with resistance to the attack of biological agents producing mycotoxins, are lost and become absent in the grain. This would favor the exposure of such grains to the contamination with Aflatoxins. We will expand on this hypothesis in Chapter II (Eguiazu, 1985) (Eguiazu & Motta, 1986) (Motta & Eguiazu, 1991a).

We could think that technicians ignored that selecting certain genetic characteristics resulted in the genetic erosion of others.

Error

As we have said before, there is an interrelationship between some of the attitudes regarding truth. Therefore, Certainty, Doubt or Opinion can occur due to Error. Even Ignorance can be manifested through Error and Error is applied on what is ignored. However, while Ignorance is the absence of certain knowledge in particular, the "Error is an unconscious attitude – just like Ignorance – accepting as true what is false and as false what is true and so on" (Colacilli de Muro, 1978).

Even though Ignorance is manifested through Error, you cannot commit an error for something that you ignore.

Ignorance implies that a knowledge in particular is not known, whilst Error implies that the knowledge is known, but, as it what said before, what is ignored is that such knowledge is false instead of true or true instead of false.

The Error is fortuitous, it appeals to chance. If knowledge is considered true, and it is indeed true, we are in the presence of a Correct fact.

Regarding the trials on carcinogenicity, for the extrapolation of the results on experimental animals to humans to provide a possible way to obtain true conclusions, such criterion must be fully applicable, in which case, the choice of such trials will have proven Correct.

Actually, a possible example of Error due to Ignorance could indeed be the extrapolation to humans of the results obtained on animals. When we described Certainty we said that if the toxicology tests of a substance in particular render negative results, such substance can be deemed not carcinogenic to humans. However, such results only produce Certainty, and this is why when there is enough evidence on experimental animals, some evaluators use the term *reasonably* in their prediction of carcinogenic risk (IARC, 1983).

The same term should be applied when trials render negative results.

It is not ignored that substances can be carcinogenic. Therefore, if the toxicology trials on experimental animals lead to think that a substance in particular has negative carcinogenic effects, but it unexpectedly causes cancer in humans, we would be in the presence of a Technopathogeny caused by Error, i.e., for accepting as truth that the conclusions of the extrapolation to humans of the results obtained on experimental animals for that substance were applicable to humans.

In the aforementioned case of the Thalidomide, the Error of extrapolating results of animal trials to humans led to Thalidomide causing teratogenicity – an example of Ignorance in the technique of toxicology evaluation.

Other cases of Error can be motivated by Insecurity, Doubt and Opinion.

Evidently, if we accept the criterion of believing a substance to be innocuous to humans because at the time there is limited evidence of carcinogenity on experimental animals (Doubt or Uncertainty), or because no study has been carried out and the non-risk conclusion was based on the substance's chemical structure, and the substance ends up being harmful to humans, the Error lies in having adopted such criterion.

In order to clearly differentiate Error from Ignorance and the Technopathogenies generated by them, we resort, once again, to the example of the incidence of diabetes in children whose parents had eaten smoked meat contaminated with N-Nitrosamines not long before conception. If the incidence of diabetes had occurred in spite of the fact that until that moment there was sufficient evidence that the consumption of smoked meat did not produce any effect on descendants, this would be a case of Technopathogeny caused by Error – for regarding as true a statement that turned out to be false.

However, the incidence of diabetes was caused because until then it was not known that the consumption of smoked meat not long before conception could have such effect. This is a case where the Technopathogeny was caused by Ignorance.

Another case of Error is caused by one of the concepts used by modern technique as justification, which we included in the list of fallacious concepts. In this case, the old criteria that air and water are great dilutants. As we have seen, the study published in 1990 by the former Soviet Union indicated that the volume of water necessary to dilute the effluents coming from all the country's waterways had surpassed the volume or annual discharge of all the rivers in the country (Loukjanenko, 1990).

Another case of Error is the Paracelsus' (1493-1541) concept. Regarding toxic substances, he believed that *Dosis sola facta venenum* (The dose makes the poison). This universally accepted concept no longer applies to all the substances that can be harmful to health. Nowadays, some hypotheses support the idea that there is a cumulative effect of the damage produced even by very small doses of carcinogenic substances (Preussmann, 1976, 1980). Let's not forget that the level of toxicity of a substance is based on the LD50 parameter. To exemplify this and with reference to the lack of relationship between the LD50 and the carcinogenic risk of a substance, we must remember that the value of ADI (Acceptable Daily Intake) in the United States of America does not apply to carcinogenic food additives or pesticides. The Food Additive Amendment to the Federal Food, Drug, and Cosmetic Act states (U.S. DHHS-PHS-FDA, 1998), which says:

> No additive shall be deemed to be safe if it is found, after tests which are appropriate for the evaluation of the safety of food additives, to induce cancer in man or animal...

Finally, another example of Error was to consider that contamination only affected industrialized countries (FAO, 1982).

This attitude can also cause a Technopathogeny. "It is a conscious and deliberate attitude which takes as false what is in fact true and as true what is in fact false" (Colacilli de Muro, 1978). It is an outrageous attitude.

This is the case of people commercializing or advertising chemical products or substances to be used by consumers or in a Technique – for example, a pesticide active principle – who, maybe under pressure by economic or market interests, either indicate that the product is not harmful or hide its adverse effects when there is enough evidence indicating the contrary. In this case, the persons commercializing the product can justify their attitude underrating the risk. They know the substance can have a carcinogenic risk on the person/s exposed to it. However, they *consider*, without any support whatsoever, that the substance in question will not produce a harmful level of exposure for users, or that there will be no residues left in the final products since they will degrade before the product reaches the consumer. It is worth quoting here an important toxicologist (Korte, 1998), who said that:

> Developing countries should not worry about the use of substances which can represent a risk when such substances are used in the production of food. If such substances weren't used, pests would devour all the crops and the problem generated would be much more serious than the one that is trying to be avoided. In addition, the annual average temperature is much higher in developing countries than in developed countries, which might lead us to expect that the degradation of these products once they are applied is fast enough so as to avoid constituting a risk.

We would like to stress the fact that consumers or users in general are not aware of the risks implied by the exposure to certain products (PNUMA, 1985b).

There are people occupationally exposed to complex chemical products of unknown composition – maybe due to the fact that the manufacturing company ascribes to commercial secrecy, which makes it impossible to estimate the risk implied. In this case, the protection of the consumer or user's health will depend on the veracity or mendacity of the person offering the product or Technique.

In these cases we can see that lying can also cause a Technopathogeny.

Within Mendacity we can also include the negligent attitude of some producers who use a technique knowing it can pose a risk on humans –

for example, applying a pesticide that can affect the crop's final product. If this application is done at a time too close to harvest – knowing that there will not be enough time to allow the product to degrade to an innocuous level to consumers – the producer would have incurred in the ethical fault we are describing here. We refer to this attitude as Mendacity because the producer hands over a product saying it is innocuous knowing that in fact it is not.

Accumulation of effects

It is important to bear in mind that the aforementioned attitudes were described as a direct or ultimate cause determining the manifestation of a Technopathogeny.

However, as it was seen in previous examples, an attitude regarding the truth that is the ultimate or direct cause of a Technopathogeny can, in turn, have been motivated or caused by another attitude regarding the truth, and such attitude, in turn, by another.

This is so because there are various stages involved in the development of any Technique – from obtaining the necessary knowledge to the final development. In the development of any given Technique, there are always other techniques involved. This is why what might be considered an error in an intermediate technique can end up being of technopathogenic relevance in the final product.

To clarify this idea, we could go back to the example of the person thinking that a substance is innocuous when in fact there are no sufficient tests proving the opposite.

Another example we could go back to is the one referred to toxicology trials to determine the carcinogenicity of a substance. When producing a substance, different techniques can be applied: Synthesis techniques, purification techniques, etc., as well as toxicology techniques to determine the risk on health. As we have seen, a flaw in these intermediate techniques – or even in the ones evaluating the innocuousness of a product – can be transferred to the technique or final product. If – in spite of the trials resulting to be negative in terms of the risk posed on humans – the substance ends up being harmful, what happened is that a lack of knowledge due to ignorance in the bodies of knowledge used for the development of toxicology techniques led to an error in the technique/s they were applied to. We are referring here to a toxicological trial which was either badly projected or that used erroneous tools, due to which the risk analysis on such substance rendered an erroneous result as well as an erroneous conclusion that was adopted as truth: the substance has no effect on human health. This is what happened with certain pesticides, which were used thinking they were innocuous only to discover later that they presented a carcinogenic risk.

To sum up: The flaw in the Technique to control pests (a pesticide with carcinogenic collateral effects) is motivated by a flaw in an intermediate technique: the toxicology technique. Interestingly, this defect in the toxicology technique does not pose a risk on the toxicology technician. For example, some substances are mutagenic due to the action of their metabolic products and not due to the action of the substance itself. Therefore, in order to be able to extrapolate the result with more certainty in humans, it is important to activate the substance metabolically so that it shows its carcinogenic potential. If the substance is not metabolically activated, the trial result will be negative despite its potential carcinogenic risk. However, such substance does not pose a technopathogenic risk on the toxicology technician. Due to the safety measures adopted in laboratories, he or she will not be exposed to the substance being evaluated – unlike the users or consumers of the product where the substance can be present as residue.

That is to say, there was an error in the application of the result of the toxicological technique. Such error, in turn, determined a flaw in the final technique by using a carcinogenic substance. Knowing any substance could be carcinogenic, the risk was considered negative for the substance in question. The direct cause of the Technopathogeny was an error caused by the lack of knowledge in the development of the toxicological technique. This determined a flaw which, even though it did not pose a risk on the lab technician, it did render erroneous results in the evaluation of substances thus posing a Technopathogeny risk for users or consumers exposed to it.

We have used a similar example in the evaluation of innocuousness of aflatoxins. Since the analysis technique was badly conceived, as we will describe later on, giving false positive or false negative results gives the final product an uncertainty or a false certainty.

In other cases the substance used as part of a technique might not entail a technopathogenic risk, i.e. the final technique will not entail technopathogenic risks. Nevertheless, the techniques used in the elaboration process of such substance may originate intermediate substances or derived sub products which do pose a technopathogenic risk on humans. In this case, the final technique using such innocuous substance does not entail a pathogenic risk, but the intermediate techniques applied in its elaboration do.

We can then see that the Greeks were right. It has been demonstrated that there are technopathogenies (they call them flaws or defects) that can be associated not only to ignorance or error but also to other attitudes.

This means that even at the level of knowledge, voids or flaws must be detected so as to avoid applying the erroneous knowledge in the development of a Technique that can cause a Technopathogeny. Technopathogenology would act like an architect detecting the errors in a plan drawn by somebody else. If the construction was carried out, it would have structural flaws which could cause its collapse (Motta, 1994).

Apart from preventing the harmful effect on people, Technopathogenology can also save money to companies.

Interestingly, it was also shown that the two attitudes quoted from the Greeks – Ignorance and Error – are the only ones which could be accepted as ethical in the manifestation of a Technopathogeny. We will further comment on this in Chapter III when we deal with Technopathogenology Methodology to prevent technopathogenies.

Having progressed in the analysis, we can draw up a fourth thesis or approach:

> VI. The immanent and hidden flaws in a Technique that can produce the generation of factors (Technopathogens) which can be harmful to humans in the long term (Technopathogeny) are a consequence of either lack of truth or the existence of a void in the bodies of knowledge used for its development.

XIII. The ethical attitude that causes the phenomenon: The fifth approach

We have seen that Techniques are developed so as to produce objects to satisfy needs. Goods are produced within a business framework. Companies are constantly developing or applying new techniques and new goods from the bodies of knowledge generated by their own researchers as well as by others, thus obtaining an economic benefit. Such benefit is considered retribution to business risk (Motta & Eguiazu, 2005).

We have also seen that scientists are under a lot of pressure to generate knowledge. In the State scientific community (State because of working in government organizations) this is known as "publish or perish", (Chargaff, 1989) (Eguiazu, 1991). Couldn't we think, then, that private companies' researchers are under a lot more pressure? The competition among companies also leads to an increase in pressure. When the research is carried out in a State environment everything can be circumscribed to a report or a subsidy and nothing is expected in return. However, when research is carried out in a private company, there is great pressure of return because of the invested capital.

We have seen that the nature of the process: Generation of knowledge – Development – Application increasingly shortens the time span between each of these stages. There is indeed a marked *acceleration* of the process.

We have observed in the attitudes above mentioned an eagerness to develop new Techniques (products, goods, processes) and the necessary knowledge to achieve such Techniques.

According to the dictionary definition, what we understand by *eager* is: "Impatiently desirous of something" (Standard Encyclopedic Dictionary).

Since to get to the fourth approach we have resorted to Ancient Greeks, in order to get to the fifth approach, we will also resort to ancient wisdom. In 1 Tm 6,10 we can read in the Bible (in one Spanish version) (San Pablo): "Porque la raíz de todos los males es el afán de dinero..." (literal translation: Because the root of every evil is the eagerness for money...) and in one English version (Paul – First letter to Timothy):

> Indeed the love of money is the root of every evil. Because of this greed, some have wandered away from the faith, bringing on themselves affliction of every kind.

According to the English version, the root of all evils is not money itself or the need to look for money, but *love* and therefore, greed to obtain money. We can briefly reflect about this last term: *greed*, which refers to attitudes such as *avid, fervent, and vehement*. According to the dictionary definition, *vehement* means: *arising of marked by impetuosity of feeling or passion*, that is, *to act on sudden impulse and without forethought*. A synonym of *vehement* is the worth *eager*, which coincides with the Bible Spanish version.

Whatever the Bible version is, we can say that the root of all evils is not money itself or the need to obtain money, but the *eagerness* to obtain money. Well, why are we saying this?

Companies aim for economic benefits, that is to say, to make money with the production of goods. They are eager to produce new goods. But technological knowledge created by other scientists or by technologists of the own company is need for the production of these goods. All the generated knowledge may be imperfect, but if knowledge was generated with eagerness it is highly likely to find a void in the bodies of knowledge used for the development of new goods. This hasty generation of new technologies my result in faulty goods.

For example, due to inter-company competition, or for a faster return of an inversion, many goods can enter the market without being, using Jorge Luis Borges' words, *fully invented*[1]. We are referring to goods produced suddenly and without the forethought duty. As we have mentioned before, in order to achieve this rapid production of goods there is also an eager impulse to generate technological knowledge. In the Chapter III, we will go back to the concept of *patience*. Considering that when we speak of Technopathogeny we refer to something being *harmful* to health, we could then merge both concepts and apply them to technological developments to conclude that (Motta & Eguiazu, 2005): "The eager or hasty generation of new Technologies is the root of all Technopathogenies".

We thus arrive to the fifth approach:

V. The voids in knowledge that are responsible for Technopathogenies are a consequence of the hasty generation or of the eager attitude for obtaining such knowledge.

---

1   Jorge Luis Borges (1899-1986) was a famous Argentine writer. The quoted expression was frequently used by him, when he jokingly justified his fear for the elevator saying that he preferred using the stairs because, unlike the elevator, he considered them "fully invented".

XIV. Flaws by action and flaws by omission

Some Techniques that entail Technopathogenic risk such as Mycotoxins, Pesticides, Nuclear Reactors, etc., can be grouped as Techniques with *Flaws by Action* – that is to say, flaws generating technopathogens (physical, chemical or biological) linked to carcinogenic, mutagenic or toxic effects. But we also find *Flaws by Omission* that causes Technopathogenies (Eguiazu & Motta, 2001a). Flaws by *Omission* include substances which remove positive aspects or create negative conditions of development due to the removal of characteristics that prevent the development of such negative aspects, for example, Techniques whose application imply the production of food with less vitamins which are essential for the protection of human health. As we will see in Chapter IV, both kinds of flaws led us to establish new criterion of quality.

A Technopathogeny by action, for instance, can be exemplified by the apparition of aflatoxins and the increasing risk of primary liver cancer, or the non-Hodgkin's lymphoma in workers exposed to 2,4D, or the higher incidence of leukemia in people exposed to electromagnetic fields. As examples of Technopathogeny by omission, we find the apparition of Beriberi due to white rice polishing (loss of vitamin B), or the absence of healthy elements that constitute the biological quality of food – such as vitamins, minerals, antioxidants, etc. – which favor the apparition of diseases, among them neoplasias, since many of such elements are defined as *chemopreventive* agents.

Either by action or by omission, 70 to 90% of neoplasias originate in the human environment (Congress of the United States-Office of the Technology Assessment, 1981) either due to the presence of destructive factors or due to the absence of protective factors (vitamins, minerals, antioxidants, etc.). We call these factors *destructive* and not exclusively technopathogenic since there are factors which are not necessarily associated with Technique which are also connected to the development of neoplasias (for example, UV solar light, areas with high natural radiation, radioactive gas emissions, etc.).

XV. Vector system to exemplify the risks within Technique

To complement the extensive explanation about Technique and its evident and non-evident or technopathogenic risks we will illustrate it with a vector system analysis.

In Physical Mechanics, the result of two concurrent forces is another force that can easily be obtained by applying the Parallelogram Rule, represented in the Figure 1.

One of the definitions of vector, applied to biology or medicine is: "A carrier of pathogenic microorganisms from one host to another" (Standard Encyclopedic Dictionary). We can then apply such concept to Technique and call the objects produced by it as *Technological Vectors*, defined as: *Technique which carry a technopathogen or technological germ of a chronic disease.*

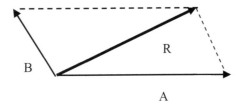

Figure 1:   Parallelogram Law to obtain R from two forces: A and B

The concept of *Vector* is also interesting, since factors generated by Technique that are harmful to humans are forces that, when applied to the organism, are harmful. Similarly, we call forces to the resources the technicians apply on a technological object so as to alter or diminish the forces that could be harmful.

Let us begin this analysis with a Technique that has no negative aspects.

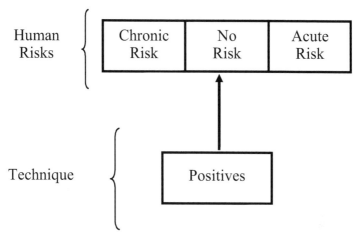

Figure 2:   Human-Technique Relationship for a Technique that has no negative effects

The Technique transmits its positive effects on humans, satisfying the needs for which it was conceived.

Let us now observe Techniques which have negative aspects – excluding, for clarifying purposes the positive vector. The short term chronic risks are indicated in the dotted line since they are not manifested in the short term. The opposite criterion is applied to long-term acute risks.

Let us begin with a Technique which has Evident Negative Effects, for example, a high toxicity pesticide. Figure 3.

In this case the technician is aware of the damage that the substance can cause, which is indicated in the chart by Vector "A" directed to the acute risk area (for example poisoning if this were a highly toxic product). The technician applies a concurrent force that can be the resultant of several forces, which is indicated by vector "B", in order to make the resultant, indicated by Vector "C" (in this case the negative effects of the substance) reach the *No Risk* zone.

For example, by establishing usage doses, special formulations, limits to the application time, safety measures for the applicator, etc., in such a way that the levels of the substance that can reach humans are innocuous enough.

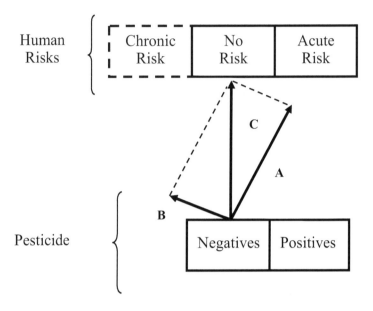

Figure 3:   Human-Technique Relationship for a Technique that has evident negative effects

Now we will discuss two technological products with a non-evident negative effect. The first case will be a medicine with a technopathogenic environmental factor (Thalidomide, for example) and the second case, a grain whose biopathological quality is altered by an unknown technopathogen (a kind of mycotoxin, aflatoxins). We will refer to this in the past since for a long time aflatoxins were unknown. Biopathological Quality – which we will develop later on – includes elements which are harmful to humans in the long-term.

Let us analyze the case of Thalidomide, a medicine.

In this case, the technician, who is aware of the risks that a substance can entail, performs the relevant trials and estimates that the substance – in this case, a medicine – poses *no risk* if taken in recommended doses.

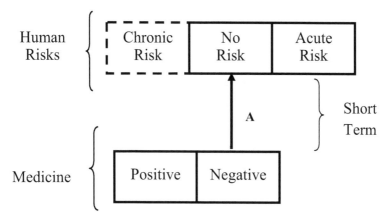

Figure 4: Short-Term Human/Technique relationship for a Technique that has a known factor (substance) causing a non-evident negative effect

Let us observe the grain with a bad biopathological quality due to the presence of aflatoxins. In this case, the bad biopathological quality determined by the presence of the xenobiotic with the non-evident negative effect is indicated with the dotted line since the factor with such negative effect was unknown.

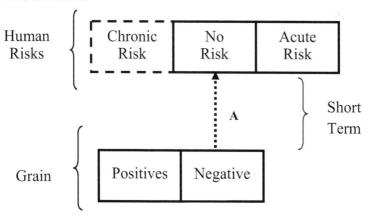

Figure 5: Short-Term Human/Technique relationship for a Technique that has a unknown factor (substance) causing a non-evident negative effect

Until it manifested its acute toxicological effects on young turkeys, aflatoxins were unknown. Surely enough, some people had already eaten food contaminated with this mycotoxin, but due to the low levels of concentration it did not cause acute intoxication or death. That is to say, the presence of this mycotoxin did not impoverish the biopathological quality in such a way that would lead to the apparition of acute or chronic effects.

In the short term, neither Thalidomide (in the correct doses) nor aflatoxins (in very low concentrations) implied risk.

Now let us observe what happened in the long-term. Let us analyze first the case of Thalidomide. Figure 6.

In this case, not only had the studies indicated that Thalidomide was innocuous in the short term (with the recommended doses), but it also indicated it was innocuous in the long-term. That is why, even in the long term, Vector "A" is directed towards the No Risk area. Technologists had estimated that there was no future risk.

But a flaw in the Technique, in this case, the Toxicology Technique (indicated by the small lower concurrent vector) determines that even if in the short term the resulting risk factor - in this case, the teratogenic power of the medicine - is driven towards the No Risk Area, in the long term it is driven towards the Chronic Risk. In the case of Thalidomide, even though the mother did not suffer the consequences, the foetus did.

Now let us analyze first the case of Aflatoxin. Figure 7.

In the case of aflatoxins, unlike Thalidomide, they were unknown substances. That is why both Vector "A", representing to the mycotoxins in general, and the resultant "R", representing aflatoxins in particular, are represented through dotted lines. As we have said before, until 1960 the existence of mycotoxins generated by moulds was unknown. The vector is therefore directed towards the No Risk area since until then no cases of acute intoxications in humans had been described.

Unlike Thalidomide – which was caused by a defect in the toxicological evaluation technique – we could think of two reasons why the presence of aflatoxins affected the grain's biopathological quality. The first reason could be that the genetic improvement technique in the grain led to a loss of biopathological quality that caused a weakening of the grain's genome. This provoked the loss of the genes that inhibit the development of parasite fungi in the grain. (This hypothesis will be further explored in Chapter II).

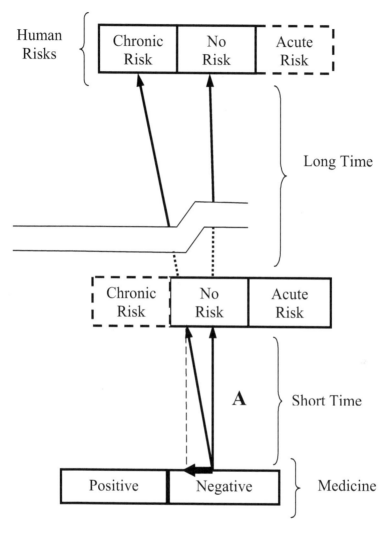

Figure 6: Long-term Human/Technique relationship for a Technique that has a known factor (substance) causing a non-evident negative effects

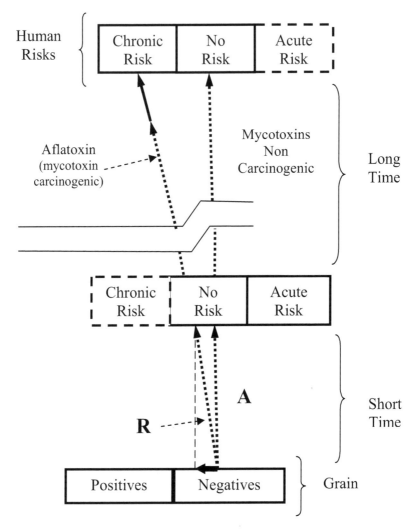

Figure 7: Long-term Human/Technique relationship for a Technique that has an unknown factor (substance) causing a non-evident negative effects

The second reason is related to the flaws in grain handling and manipulation.

Now, regarding the first reason, it is obvious that this weakening would not only allow for the development of aflatoxins generating *Aspergillus* strains but also for the development of non aflatoxins generating *Aspergillus* strains, as well as other fungi not producing carcinogenic metabolites. These moulds are of ubiquitous nature (they are present on the soil) and, therefore, grains can carry their pathogens – which can produce other metabolites that can indeed cause acute intoxication if its concentration allows for it.

In Figure 7 we see that Vector "A" is not directed towards the Acute Risk area in the short term, but towards the No-Risk area. In the case of carcinogenic mycotoxins this would indicate that, in small doses, they do not imply a risk in the short term. In the case of non-carcinogenic mycotoxins, also in small doses, this would indicate that they do not imply a risk either in the short or in the long term, so, in the long term, Vector "A" continues to the No Risk Area. Even with the existence of supporting data, the hypothesis of the weakening effect is still a hypothesis. The lower small concurrent vector representing the technique's flaw is used to illustrate such hypothesis: that the weakening of a genome can determine the possibility first, of an attack or allow for an increase in fungi attacks – some of which could produce substances which could eventually cause neoplasias in the long term (aflatoxin B1, for example), and second, the possibility of synthesis of such substances. These cases are represented by the resulting vector. This way we falsify the argument of the technicians that produce grains, which says that *even though the grains that went under genetic enhancement based on commercial parameters can be sensitive to the attack of fungi, they will not represent a risk to consumers since they will not reach a risk level.* Regarding the techniques of grain manipulation, this argument is also falsified below.

Being the genetic weakening effect still a hypothesis, some could also say that grains which do not go under human genetic selection can also develop fungi generating carcinogenic toxins and that there have always been people getting cancer because of these substances, and that humans have not become extinct for this reason (Frank, 1980-1983). In this case, Vector "A" would initially have an inclination that, in the long term, would be directed towards the chronic risk area. However, the idea that even in ancient times people caught cancer for eating contaminated grain is merely an opinion. Reality shows us that cases of cancer caused by aflatoxins were detected on the second half of the twentieth century – when modern production techniques were applied.

The small inferior concurrent vector could also illustrate the second reason for the apparition of mycotoxins. This vector illustrates the flaws in grain handling, manipulation and storage techniques that may favour the development of fungi – which is of high relevance for the carcinogenic toxins generators. In this case, the flaws would make the small concurrent vector change the direction of the resulting vector towards the chronic risk area. The resulting vector illustrates the case where the flaws in the handling, manipulation and storage techniques allow for the apparition of carcinogenic mycotoxins (it would have no effect whatsoever in the generation of a technopathogenic process if it only allowed for the apparition of other toxins with no long term risk). In this case, for a short term risk to exist, the flaws in the handling, manipulation and storage techniques should be of such significance that the damage produced by moulds in grains would be evident. An example of this is what happened in Siberia during the Second World War with the alimentary toxic aleukia caused by the consumption of grain contaminated with toxins associated with *Fusarium* fungi (IARC, 1993a). Even though the grains were clearly molded, the extreme hunger led people to consume it instead of disposing of it (Eguiazu, 1985).

Given that aflatoxins were only known when their toxicological effect was manifested, the resulting vector is only fully traced at the tip.

Even though, unlike Thalidomide, aflatoxins are natural substances, we consider that the flaws in the genetic selection, in the post-harvest handling, and in the industrialization allowed this substance to become of technopathogenic relevance by modifying the biopathological quality of food at such extent that it could pose a risk on health.

We will further analyze the flaws in grain handling and manipulation techniques in Chapter II when we deal with mycotoxins and the hypothesis of post harvest grain handling, and in Chapter IV, when we deal with the new criteria on quality.

The simple nature of charts has clearly illustrated the Technopathogenies caused by the presence of two substances (aflatoxins and Thalidomide) in two technological products: a medicine and a grain. As we have mentioned before, there are different techniques involved in the production of a desired object (a medicine, in this case) or in the generation of an undesired object in food (mycotoxins).

In addition, and before ending this chapter, another important aspect to consider in Technopathogeny – and that we will further explore in Chapter II when we refer to some characteristics of neoplasias – is that a Technopathogeny can be engendered by a combination of different objects (either physical, chemical and/or biological) produced by different techniques. Following the vector system analysis we see that the favorable or unfavorable resultant to human health is the combination of negative factors to health neutralized by biological quality factors (vitamins, antioxidants, etc). Metaphorically speaking, the final effect on health would be the *resultant* of all this *vector calculation* of positive and negative vectors.

XVI. Conclusion

We believe we have made a case for the classification of a group of negative and non evident effects related to technique as a new phenomenon. We call such phenomenon Technopathogeny. We consider that it has an identity and a magnitude or scope (i.e., sufficient singularity) to call for the creation of a new discipline.

This phenomenon makes up the particular field of study of Technopathogenology.

We can sum up the basic concepts on the phenomenon of Technopathogenology in the following theses:

I. Technopathogeny is defined as the damage caused to health in humans which is not immediately manifested but after many years or generations, as a consequence of factors caused by technique, product of immanent and hidden errors or flaws within it.

II. Technopathogeny will be a phenomenon whose intensity will be in crescendo for the following reasons:
1. The nature of the new mechanical arts is qualitatively different from the nature of ancient mechanical arts because they are increasingly based on nuclear phenomena (atomic and cellular nucleus).
2. The increasingly shortened process of Discovery-Development-Application makes prevention of damage more difficult.
3. The skimp soundness of the fundamentals of classical science anticipates imperfect use of knowledge.
4. Ethical mishaps in people involved in the creation of knowledge process, in the development of techniques and in their commercial application.
5. There is no science that allows for the study of Technopathogeny as a unique phenomenon.

III. We postulate the need for the development of a science – Technopathogenology – that allows for the study of Technopathogeny as an object of study on its own.

VI. The immanent and hidden flaws in a Technique that can produce the generation of factors (Technopathogens) which can be harmful to humans in the long term (Technopathogeny) are a consequence of either lack of truth or the existence of a void in the bodies of knowledge used for its development.

V. The voids in knowledge that are responsible for Technopathogenies are a consequence of the hasty generation or of the eager attitude for obtaining such knowledge.

CHAPTER II

Technopathogeny – Its disciplinary orphanage and a framing proposal

'Every phenomenon needs its own disciplinary home'

I.   Introduction

We have presented a phenomenon or object of study with a disciplinary void. Being this phenomenon the field of study of this new science, the first requirement to consider Technopathogenology as such is established. We must then provide the other three elements of the epistemological group (i.e.: Theories, Methodology and Results) in order to be able to speak of the need of creating a new science.

In the previous chapter we have observed how by studying two problems associated with technology – mycotoxins and pesticides – we became aware within a year of work of the existence of a phenomenon which was unknown to us upon the creation of PROCABIE in 1984 (formerly INCABIE) (Eguiazu & Motta, 1991). Even though we tried to fit our studies within the environmental sciences framework, more precisely within Anthropo-ecology, we realized that the technopathogeny phenomenon did not adequately fit within this framework. What we mean by this is that we were constantly forced to apply impoverishing reductionisms to the real object of study. Studying something so much reduced and impoverished all but shaded the original phenomenon.

In this Chapter we will focus on developing the hypotheses and theories presented which actually support the existence of this *disciplinary void* and led to the laying down of Technopathogenology which, as every science, as the French philosopher Goblot said, "had experience as its starting point" (Goblot, 1943). We will show how, in the philosopher's words, "having accumulated certain amount of empirical rules and induction truths before being in condition of systematizing them rationally," we were able to finally postulate this new science at the end of 1989.

We will now focus on what is perhaps the most daunting task of this work, which is trying to support the answer to the question: Why is it that in the world of science it is necessary to speak of a new science to study the phenomenon of Technopathogeny?

To illustrate this, we would like to quote Goblot once again:

> ...the beginning of every science or every part of science reminds us of a weaver weaving a tangled skein: he takes a thread, the first that comes up, and follows the thread in both directions to the point in which they are lost in the tangled mess. He takes another thread, and yet another. Sometimes, we pull two of such threads enough so as to discover that they are but one: a great discovery. Finally, we get to the end of a thread, that is to say, a logic beginning.

He continues saying that:

> ...the comparison is not that accurate. What we are trying to untangle is not a unique thread, but a ramified thread, like tree branches....From the moment the human spirit finds the end of a thread, it can follow it in opposite directions: science becomes deductive. But it is only threads that the spirit finds at the beginning, and might have to untangle many threads before getting to a beginning.

We indeed had to untangle many *threads* – hypotheses and theories – before arriving to the beginning of Technopathogenology. We had to resist many times to the temptation of taking the wrong thread from the tangled skein, which we had to discard since it led us to a new reduction and impoverishing consideration of the phenomenon. As the philosopher says, we had to untangle many threads, discard many alternatives before arriving to the beginning or foundation of Technopathogenology.

Paraphrasing part of the title of the philosopher's work, we can say that we took the real as our starting point – our experience – to arrive to the intelligible: the understanding of a phenomenon still undescribed.

II. The need of a new discipline: Basic concepts

If we could resort to Environmental Sciences, Ecology, Medicine, Workplace Health, etc. to study Technopathogeny, we would clearly be studying the phenomenon of technopathogenic risk from a multidisciplinary framework and not through a transdiscipline as we are proposing, with all the risks presented by such approach, as we will see later.

We will first describe our attempt to study technopathogeny within prior existent disciplines.

Among other examples we have used as analogies to support our proposal of creating a new disciplinary field, we will use the example also applied by Viktor Frankl (Frankl, 1988) (which he calls Dimensional Ontology) to the study of such a complex phenomenon as human psyche. Based on geometric solids projections, Frankl shows that a phenomenon can be seen differently depending on the projection chosen to see it. Similarly, depending on the projection chosen to see the technopathogenic problem, it can be perceived as belonging to the field of medicine or to the environmental sciences, for example. The problem is that they are just projections. The object is an entity in itself, and due to its complexity it is far bigger than the partial reductions produced by its projections in different disciplines.

Frankl makes a comparison with the projection of geometrical solids. We can easily mistake the nature of the solid if only a partial projection is analyzed – at a later stage, we will further analyze this interesting analogy.

As we already know, the usual procedure in scientific investigation is to state a hypothesis, usually rather constrained – which, in the case of the young scientist, is usually provided by his or her director.

The scientist must then investigate the history of the problem or hypothesis (Introduction), then pose a question and describe the methodology as well as the material and intellectual tools he or she will use to work it out (Materials and Methodology).

Later he or she will proceed to describe the experimental results obtained (Results) and then compare such results with the results obtained by other authors and confront them (Discussion). Finally, the scientist will arrive to the conclusions (Conclusion) where he or she will synthetically state what seems to be concluded from the observation or experiment.

The language employed is expected to be succinct, concise and accurate.

The whole experiment must be able to be repeated, and similar conclusions must be obtained after using the same starting point and the same methodology.

Usually, there is no doubt or discussion on which discipline the subject should be ascribed to. A half-open door to knowledge must be detected, and then everything must be elucidated empirically. But everything remains within the same well defined and consolidated discipline.

The success of the researcher's work will depend on his or her ability to plan the experiment, to tackle the phenomenon from an angle that allows him or her to arrive to deeper answers to the question posed. The success will also depend on the means that the researcher has for his or her work.

It is generally expected that the better the means or the more precise and sophisticated the devices are, the more successful the investigation will be. The phenomenon will be more and more encircled by papers which, like a puzzle, will contribute to clarify it.

III.   A science with ups and downs or the disciplinary orphanage

Scientists specialized in disciplines are so trained in a specific discipline that, in order to be effective, must ignore areas of knowledge other to the discipline they are focusing on.

This difficulty is allegedly solved through the Science and Technique system using a simple reasoning: a phenomenon which, due to its characteristics, calls for a new discipline or transdiscipline, must be forced to be studied through a multiple set of disciplines. Each discipline would take a part of the phenomenon, even those complex phenomena which do not perfectly fit in a consolidated discipline and at the end, putting together all the sub-evaluations, we can grasp the essence of the phenomenon.

This reasoning will not always necessarily work since in some cases, the phenomenon is not a jigsaw puzzle where each piece is a specific discipline and when all the pieces are finally put together the whole phenomenon could be grasped. The phenomenon as a whole, on the contrary, is hard to grasp using the *disciplinary puncher*. What remains on the surface – the punched area after each discipline has taken what belonged to it – is the part of the phenomenon that remains hidden or not taken into account which will not allow to recognize the phenomenon authentically even in the multidisciplinary framework. We will further analyze this and the jigsaw puzzle analogies when we refer to Technopathogenology as a science in Chapter III.

If we are speaking of a new science, before continuing with the topic of this chapter we must frame the science within the general framework of science classification.

Technopathogeny is a concrete phenomenon. We are speaking of Technique, Technopathogens and Health. We could therefore say that through what we have seen so far Technopathogenology is an Empirical Science.

Having proposed Technopathogenology, going back to the beginning of our work, we can ask ourselves: Which was the reasoning that we consciously or unconsciously followed to postulate this new science?

Reasoning can be: Deductive, inductive or by analogy (Fatone, 1969).

Having used a problem in particular as starting point (mycotoxins) in order to arrive to a universal statement – the postulation of a new science – the initial reasoning was inductive. Such induction was incomplete, following the principle that states that it must be so in order to constitute a progress in knowledge (Fatone, 1969).

Let us now look at the succession and concatenation of hypotheses and theories formulated that led to our conclusion.

IV. Hypotheses and theories that support the disciplinary void and the postulation of Technopathogenology as a science to study the phenomenon

The first two theories that we came upon as a result of our studies were on mycotoxins – the first *thread* we started pulling from this tangled skein that led us to propose Technopathogenology.

We could describe them as follows:

Theory I: Given their origin and the way they reach humans, the risk posed by mycotoxins to human health is a technological problem

Theory II: None of the existing disciplines can be efficient enough to prevent the risk they entail

The first theory states that even when mycotoxins are natural contaminants, because they appear in agricultural products and reach humans, they are caused by technology, since technology – either by action or omission – is part of the process.

In 1975, after talking to an expert in agricultural matters (Agriculturist Correa), and being ourselves interested in researching on subjects on human health protection from technological risks, we focused on researching on aflatoxins, which are mold generated carcinogenic substances.

Aflatoxins attack oleaginous plants and cereals and they concentrate mainly in corn.

Since corn is an essential raw material for Argentine industry out of which by-products and food are obtained for human use, we wanted to determine the levels of contamination with aflatoxins, since at the time there were no studies on the subject.

We started gathering international research data. As we have said in Chapter I, we were encouraged by the conclusions of the 1972 Stockholm Conference.

We quickly realized we were onto something important since aflatoxins not only attacked corn, a basic foodstuff, but were highly dangerous due to their high toxicity and, especially because they were a potent carcinogen, as shown by international research. Mold also develops spontaneously, since propagules (spores and mycelium), which are always present in grain, develop fast on fertile ground with favorable environmental conditions, allowing to generate the toxin rather quickly. In addition, contamination with aflatoxins proved to be difficult to determine. Without the proper complex analysis, contamination can go easily unnoticed.

Since mold can attack only under certain, always changing conditions, it is very difficult to produce preventing measures against these substances in agricultural products when the substratum is sensible.

By the time we started our research, aflatoxins had been found in different parts of the world. Scientists had discovered that aflatoxins could not only cause diseases in animals, but also that long term consumption in humans could cause liver cancer, as it was found in Africa and Thailand (Eguiazu, 1976).

All these facts convinced us that humans needed to be protected against this risk.

Thanks to the information we gathered from around the world, we were then able to publish a research paper on the subject, which was the first in this region, and it was awarded a prize (Eguiazu, 1976).

We then started our pilgrimage through different state departments with the hope of convincing authorities of the urgent need to protect consumers and, at the same time, trying to find financial support for our research.

Even though until then we had not yet arrived to any conclusion, we did have the information that the Argentine corn exported to European markets had been analyzed and tested positive for contamination with aflatoxins. In 1974, for example, Holland received Argentine corn and peanuts contaminated with aflatoxins (Eguiazu, 1976).

Considering this issue not only a health but also a commercial issue, we started analyzing corn in our region (Eguiazu, 1977, 1978a).

The results of regional tests showed that 4,9% of exporting quality corn was contaminated.

Considering the samples we analyzed were to be exported we then asked ourselves: if this corn, which is meant to be of high quality, is contaminated beyond what is considered tolerable, what can we expect of the corn meant for domestic consumption?

A comment by an expert on grain quality can cast some light on this: *If corn has a low degree of mold contamination, it will be exported, but if the mold contamination surpasses the limit to be exported to Europe, it will be used for domestic consumption.* This remark referred to the classification of corn grain due to its content of *verdín*[1] – a quality

---

1   This quality item includes molds of Genera *Aspergillus* and *Penicillum*. The action of these molds leaves green or blue-green stains in the embryo under the seed coat that can be observed in the intact grains or in broken grain. A related term is "blue-eye," but this term defines "a storage disease of corn caused by several species of *Penicillium*. These molds grow over the embryo but under the seed coat" (Kurtzman & Ciegler, 1970).

classification that includes fungi of the Genus *Aspergillus* and *Penicillum*, which can potentially produce mycotoxins, such as Aflatoxin.

This means that potentially contaminated corn is not exported, but consumed within the country. The fact that the toxic substance in question is harmful to humans encouraged us to further continue researching (Eguiazu, 1978b).

All this made us think that human action was more relevant than natural causes. What we wanted to consider was how humans, through technique, could change matter – in this case biologically organized, such as corn.

Mycotoxins and the question on prevention

Facts have shown that the study of mycotoxins were then and are now of high relevance to humans.

Then, the study could be tackled from different disciplines. But within our theoretical framework, the following question arose: could each of the existing disciplines or a combination of all of them be enough to achieve correct prevention? This triggered different hypotheses which we will develop below, each of them aiming at prevention. They were all falsified.

In connection with prevention of this issue, we formulated these hypotheses which allowed us to enunciate the theories above cited.

Question on prevention A – The search for an answer attempting to frame it within the existing disciplinary field

Hypothesis: Can prevention be achieved within a Biological Sciences framework?

Even though we are specialized in agricultural technology, the first attempt to frame our work within these disciplines failed because it was rejected by the Evaluation Board. One of the members, whose field of study was Plant Physiology, was first consulted as to whether the problem could be frameworked within his discipline. He rejected the proposal simply saying he did not consider the problem a physiological one.

Interestingly enough – as we will also see for Human Physiology – when the scholars of this discipline *realized* that this subject could help them get subsidies to their projects, they tried to include it in their discipline and frame it as a study problem they ridiculously called *Post-Harvest Physiology*, as we will see later.

We continued then with our attempt to frame our research within the framework of other Biological Sciences.

Hypothesis: Can prevention be achieved within an Ecological framework?

The first answer to this question was to frame our research within Ecology. Nevertheless, when we approached an ecologist to ask him whether we could include this study within his ecology program, he downgraded the scientific nature of this problem saying that:

> Contamination needs police control and punishment. If pollutant controls were improved, higher quality foodstuff, cleaner rivers and an unpolluted atmosphere could be obtained.

He used the example of the decontamination of the River Thames, which only required a series of regulations controlled by the police. According to this view, the presence of a carcinogen would only be a matter of control. Our question could not fit within the Ecological framework since, according to this expert, this problem was of low scientific relevance.

At a later stage, we will try to explain with more detail why this discipline which is apparently the most suitable to frame this problem, was not so. This explanation is based on the nature of the object of study.

Hypothesis: Can prevention be achieved within a Mycology framework?

Having failed at the attempt with Ecology, we passed on to try with this science.

Since the carcinogen is caused by mold (*Aspergillus flavus, Aspergillus parasiticus*) we continued our research in a Human Mycology program. Since this science was inscribed within the health field, it enabled a more suitable approach. Unlike Ecology, this science was interested in the carcinogen and, being this cancer caused by pathogen molds, it added an extra interest to this field of study. However, aflatoxins and the molds related to them were completely new as a scientific problem for Mycology and there was no experience on them at the time. Nevertheless, we initiated a research program on the carcinogen within this field. We encountered the first problem upon facing the core question: What is the role of natural substratum in the genesis of this contaminant? Why does it attack some grains and not others, even among the same species? This question did not particularly interest the directors of the course we worked on, since the course was more focused on the study of each mold in particular. The questions which lay outside this approach or interest were not considered. It focused on toxic and pathogenic fungus to humans. The fungi were cultivated in synthetic environments and their pathogenic action was determined. This permitted the isolation of the mold due to the previous experience with Aspergillus (especially due to the research on Aspergillus fumigatus infection – lung aspergilloma).

Even though we had advanced to a point in which the mold that produced aflatoxins could be isolated and cultivated in natural and artificial environments, this was not enough.

We have mentioned before our attempt to frame our proposal within the Plant Physiology framework. Interestingly enough, even though we did not try to frame our research within the Human Physiology framework, their exponents did include our proposal in their projects. Human Physiology is the part of Biology that studies human organs and the way they function (Diccionario Enciclopédico Ilustrado de la Lengua Española). Even though aflatoxins and their effect in physiology could be studied from the perspective of its pathological effect by a science or field of study we could call pathophysiology or physiopathology, this is not convincing either since here the causal relevance is still weaker than in Mycology. We will further analyze this topic in a specific reading we will include in the Annex, but first we would like to state that we believe that our project was only considered within the Human Physiology framework due to a reason of power within the system – to be the first or to obtain better financial support in research since physiologists conformed one of the most powerful lobbies in our field. The temptation of reducing any new question to this science may be hard to resist. This way the complex question – how to prevent food poisoning by mycotoxins – was reduced to a study of the toxins' effect in normal physiology.

Actually, it was further reduced to its effects on a perfusioned organ. This is what happened indeed. When we discovered aflatoxins in the region, experts in human physiology immediately asked for subsidies to apply them on rats' perfusioned livers so as to investigate their effect and dynamics on this organ. The scope is narrower than within mycology itself, even than within Biology. This path led to very profound questions but which further moved apart from our aim. The last few paragraphs, which we could describe as *very informal*, illustrate how some scientists would try to force framing a phenomenon within their discipline with a not strictly scientific motive.

As for the Human Physiology framework, we believe it is only useful for purely biochemical research with no relevance from the point of view of detection and prophylaxis.

To sum up, the questions on which other factors (including technological) could be used to explain the different aflatoxins attacks, on storage conditions and mainly on the relationship between grains and relative humidity could not be answered within the biological sciences proposed.

Having failed in the previous attempts, we went back to our origins: Technology.

Hypothesis: Can prevention be achieved within an Agronomic framework?

Since the products mentioned here as posing a risk on health were agricultural products, we considered framing prevention within an agronomic framework.

This hypothesis was analyzed from two points of view: Agricultural Chemistry and grain Post-harvest handling.

Hypothesis: Can prevention be achieved within an Agronomic framework? A: Agricultural Chemistry

We then tried to frame our question within this discipline. The main incoherence was that there was no room for a carcinogen as such – even less if it was generated by a mold, since this discipline was specifically interested in the old agricultural chemistry or in the analysis of foodstuffs, pesticides and fertilizers. A carcinogen raised the interest as a chemical substance that required control, but this interest decreased or disappeared when it was proved that the carcinogen was produced by a mold – which required a mycological methodology for its study.

The answer to this hypothesis was that at least within our university, we could not frame our project within this field of study.

Hypothesis: Can prevention be achieved within an Agronomic framework? B: Grain Post-Harvest Handling

In this discipline we pursued the question on storage technology.

Mycotoxins generating fungi are in general classified as storage fungi. It is obvious that proper storage contributes to decrease the incidence of biological damage due to fungi attack and subsequent mycotoxins formation. In Chapter IV we include a paper on the contribution of Technopathogenology to the adoption of new quality criterion – which includes the contribution of this science to grain post-harvest handling.

On the other hand, it was globally proved that these molds could attack grains prior to harvest, so a proper storage will only partially prevent this.

In addition, the nature of storage techniques determines great difficulty in preventing contamination with these substances. Molds require certain temperature and relative humidity conditions. If conditions are kept outside the values for molds to develop, this contamination can be avoided. However, storage techniques are quite diverse. Silos and other means of storage vary greatly in size and volume. For example, in a 2000 tonne silo, it is very difficult to control the temperature and relative humidity in the whole mass of grains. A small area could develop a risky micro environment by affecting, for example, a 0,5 ton of grain maybe due to humidity condensation or water leakage from outside. If conditions allow for the development of aflatoxicogenic fungi, this relatively small mass of grain will be contaminated with aflatoxins. Finally, when the silo is emptied, this mass of grain will get mixed with the rest and the whole content of the silo will be unsuitable for human consumption. The internationally accepted limit for the most toxic aflatoxin – Aflatoxin B1 – is 5 ppb (ppb stands for part per billion, which means, 1 milligram of a given substance per ton of product). We can see here that technological errors in storage techniques leading to mycotoxins contamination can be very difficult to solve and can be responsible for causing technopathogenies.

Hypothesis: Can prevention be achieved within an Analytical Chemistry framework?

If mycotoxins are relevant to humans for being, among other adverse effects, potential carcinogens, it was considered that through the analysis

126

in foodstuff products mycotoxins could be detected and this would avoid the product reaching the consumer.

Unlike certain products like fleshy fruit or dry fruits (nuts), which humans can consume directly, in general, agricultural products are used as raw materials to elaborate other foodstuffs. Here we want to make reference to the following: In Chapter I we have used the vector system to exemplify how grains whose biopathological quality was altered by aflatoxins caused a technopathogeny. When we referred to the errors in plant enhancement techniques as posing a technopathogenic risk, we said that some, rejecting our hypothesis, could say that since we are dealing with a natural contaminant, people could very well eat contaminated grains without the intervention of Technique. Those who support this theory say that there have always been people getting cancer because of this substance.

In order for this to happen, the person should have eaten the contaminated fruit directly. This is very unlikely, since fungi contaminated fruit can cause rejection. Apart from generating toxins, molds provoke organoleptic changes in the fruit: change of color, smell and especially flavor, which would cause immediate rejection. Just by seeing or tasting it, the consumer would reject the fruit.

However, industrialization and elaboration techniques can mask the contaminated raw material condition by adding additives and other ingredients used in the process. This is why industrialization techniques are also responsible for technopathogenies. Analytical Chemistry is therefore crucial to prevent the risk when the toxin is present in the raw material.

We wonder if the young turkeys that died because of feed elaborated with contaminated raw material would have actually eaten the molded grain contaminated with aflatoxins in its natural state. Had the industrialization process masked the organoleptic characteristics of the infected grain? Would the animals eat infected grain in its natural state?

These questions led us to initiate a series of international contacts to gather information on the analysis techniques used with these toxins. We then obtained information on analytical methods from Holland, USA (especially USDA) and Germany (Federal Research Centre for Nutrition). To begin our research we had to choose an area with intensive agricultural activity. We chose the fields near Rosario, Argentina, to look for the toxic substance in corn. This research – which was the first in the area confirming the existence of aflatoxins in corn – could be carried out thanks to the financial support of Bolsa de Comercio de Rosario (Rosario Stock Exchange) (Eguiazu, 1976, 1977, 1978a, 1978b).

In order to confirm the results, the tests were sent to the German Centre for Nutrition.

At the beginning of our research, part of our job was to study the most common analytical methods at the time: minicolumns.

But to identify contaminated corn lots, a quick previous inspection can be carried out by exposing the grains to ultraviolet light. A bright-green yellow fluorescence (BGYF) can be observed on the contaminated lots. This test might seem a great advantage since it would practically make the expensive chemical analysis unnecessary. However, this procedure might lead to an error hiding a technopathogenic risk, because the bright-green yellow fluorescence observed is not due to aflatoxins but due to another substance produced by the fungus: Kojic acid. Therefore, the presence of this acid would indicate a fungi attack, but not the amount of contamination with aflatoxins. We observed that lots with a low level of BGYF could be contaminated with high concentration of aflatoxins. The level of contamination with aflatoxins depends on the type of batch. What we also observed was that although observation with ultraviolet light might not necessarily indicate BGYF – which would lead to conclude that the sample was not affected by fungi – BGYF was observed in cracked grain. We can see here another error in the inspection technique. An uninformed grains producer can conclude that his or her lot was not contaminated with aflatoxins and therefore consider that such lot does not pose a risk on consumers.

Going back to analytical methods, when we studied commercial methods – specifically methods using minicolumns, which are very easy to use and very inexpensive – we discovered that these methods led to erroneous results (false negatives or false positives), a consequence of substances that have a fluorescence which looks exactly the same as the fluorescence produced by aflatoxins, the measuring device being incapable of distinguishing one from the other (Eguiazu, 1979). This is another technique error that can lead to a technopathogeny – an analytical method can lead to conclude that a product is innocuous when in fact it can pose a technopathogenic risk.

This fluorescence is produced by substances we could call deceptive because they fluoresce the same way aflatoxins do and are retained in the adsorbent just like aflatoxins.

128

This means some samples show positive results when they do not contain aflatoxins. How is it possible that in determining the existence of aflatoxins a great amount of samples can wrongly prove positive or negative? A corn lot wrongly believed to be contaminated will represent an unnecessary economic loss. But the most important risk here is that this technique can lead to believe that samples which are in fact infected are not contaminated and this can indeed be harmful to consumers.

All this happened because in order to avoid the problem of the *natural* fluorescence, the measuring device had to be calibrated to zero with an aflatoxins free sample. Corn has inherent substances which fluoresce just like aflatoxins which we call *natural* fluorescence. According to our study, the corn samples had a natural fluorescence oscillating between 2 to 12 ppb. If the sample taken for zero calibration had a high natural fluorescence and then low natural fluorescence samples were determined, there would be a 10 ppb gap of undetected aflatoxins. This means that if the device was calibrated to zero with a free of aflatoxins sample but with a natural fluorescence of 12 ppb, in another sample with 2 ppb natural fluorescence contaminated with 10 ppb of aflatoxins, the device will indicate zero.

This item, just like the previous one (the observation of bright-green yellow fluorescence) made us become aware of the big technical-analytical limitations existing at the time. We then asked ourselves, how can these techniques be improved in order to be more accurate?

We continued our research in Germany studying analytical methods. Our thesis director recommended focusing on a fast and simple technique (Frank, 1980-1983).

The task was to develop an analytical technique adapted to geographical areas with enormous limitations – typical of third world countries – where no existing sophisticated technique requiring complex elements or hard to get spare parts could be used. It had to be very inexpensive, simple and accurate. This seemed a problem impossible to solve. However, after working on it for a year we did find some solutions that allowed us to achieve our aim. As a result of our research we came across a new minicolumn technique, simple and inexpensive, which could be manufactured with minimal resources. This technique also helped us to solve the problems generated by the false positive of the technique we had originally used.

We also came across a substitute for aflatoxins: Blankophor (Eguiazu, 1983), a substance which could be absorbed in cellulose and used as a standard substitute. This substance, apart from having the same fluorescent properties as aflatoxins, was more stable and allowed us to use it more freely due to its lack of toxicity. This allowed us to prepare artificial standards with various concentrations to quantify the level of contamination of a sample, standards which had before to be prepared with pure toxin.

We also modified the cleaning methods of the mini columns so as to avoid interferences (Eguiazu & Frank, 1982, 1983).

The best achievement was a variation in the thin layer chromatography technique known as Self Activated Thin Layer Chamber-Plate (patented device) (Eguiazu, 1993). It is a very simple and inexpensive technique which completely excludes the false positives (Eguiazu, 2003).

Since this method only requires a minimum lab intervention, it can be used in the countryside or in small towns where there are no specialized laboratories. Grain lots can be quickly tested even in places where there are no complex laboratories. This method was considered another important contribution to protect consumers since identification of contaminated lots led to the prohibition of the distribution of such lots.

There are also kits prepared by laboratories, but they are expensive and cannot be manufactured by the interested parties.

In spite of the apparent success of the discovery of Blankophor P as a standard substitute and the Self Activated Thin Layer Chamber-Plate as a fast, simple and inexpensive method, there was still a question to be tackled: in order to answer our basic question, is it worth it to keep on researching on new low budget and high applicability analytical techniques which would allow us to publish many papers and patent devices? How does this contribute to the basic question on contamination? Or rather: Is this the heart of the problem? And here it was where we had to abandon this discipline, in spite of having many possibilities of developing a research career in it. The basic questions on why the contaminant appears and how can an efficient prevention be achieved could not be answered since Analytical Chemistry studies contamination once it has already happened but does not investigate its cause.

On the other hand, even though analytical scientists may develop techniques with very expensive equipment, every technique will always have a limited detection for any contaminant. No matter how precise analytical techniques might be, there will always be lots of contaminants which in spite of obtaining a negative result might have a low degree of contamination which is below the reading of the device. This is particularly true with mycotoxins. Regarding this, it is worth mentioning an interesting experiment carried out with samples considered aflatoxins-free, according to the result obtained with accurate techniques. To these samples very low concentration – 2 to 4 ppb – of aflatoxins were added. When the sample was extracted and analyzed with complex, sophisticated devices, highly accurate in detection, the results retrieved were negative. This indicates that small quantities are not detected, whether due to the nature of the extraction technique or of the measuring device. What happens if the digestive process removes the small quantities of contaminants from samples formally considered free of aflatoxins? Maybe the foodstuff is harmful to health?

It is important to reduce human exposure to contaminants as much as possible – the more precise the analytical techniques, the more contamination will be reduces. But, as we will see later, with carcinogenic substances zero tolerance is the best criterion. The fact that these substances cannot always be detected does not imply they do not pose a risk. Therefore, it is always better to prevent the contamination. As we will state later when we deal with Relative Humidity, prevention is far better than detection (Frank, 1980-1983).

The observations on inspection methods and analytical techniques made us think about how easily something contaminated can pass as uncontaminated. What failed here is something more basic: the substance should have never been there. What failed in technology that let it appear in the first place? Why was there no efficient prophylaxis?

We can conclude this hypothesis saying that: *Avoiding the mold is far better than detecting aflatoxins*, or, a more extreme version could be: *The worst prophylaxis is better than the best detection.*

Hypothesis: Can prevention be achieved within a Food Technology framework?

We continued our research in the German centre, but this time focused more on the causes for the appearance of the contaminant. This led to a series of questions.

The first question had to do with the weather conditions. The effect of several storage atmospheres was systematically studied. The air in contact with the grains was combined with different contents of water, nitrogen and carbon dioxide. This combination of gases varied from the most favorable to the least favorable for the development of mold. When exposing the grains to different atmospheres, differences were observed. However, strangely enough, unexplainable differences still appeared regarding the sensibility to mold attack and the generation of toxins even within the same grain species. Even though this basic question satisfactorily led to a doctoral thesis, the question on the origin of aflatoxins had not yet been fully answered – even less the question on causes and consequences of its contamination in humans. Here is where we came up with the question on the substratum: what is it that makes a given species, a given crop or even a given individual seed to generate the toxin in some cases but not in others in spite of having all the conditions for its development? The research had therefore to focus on storage; most importantly, on the basic technology or genetic selection criteria used during the genesis of the grain and during its storage.

Here we got to a crossroads: either we carry on looking for a suitable discipline to study the phenomenon or stop looking for one and specialize in any of the disciplines investigated so far. After researching on the relationship between environmental factors and the development of molds, we kept on exploring foodstuffs analysis at Landesuntersuchungsanstalt für Verbraucherschutz, Erlangen (Research Centre for Consumer Protection, Erlangen, Germany). There was always the difficulty that even though the analytical approach described the current state of a sample, it was somehow a one-dimensional phenomenon, equivalent to a straight line or a planar projection to describe something that required at least the dimension of volume and even other non-geometrical dimensions. Foodstuffs Science, Foodstuffs Chemistry and Foodstuffs Technology did not provide for the answer accurately enough. There was also an enormous amount of questions with a strong cultural or ethical component which were left unanswered. The disciplines we had explored did not answer the basic question on causes, effects and prophylaxis of food contamination, on its most profound aspects. There was the risk of specializing by quantitative apposition on the disciplines studied, leaving aside a more profound area. This more profound area could be merely delineated, but was not easy to fully grasp.

Hypothesis: Can prevention be achieved
within a Jurisprudence framework?

Following the ecologist's suggestion that the problem with contamination was a *police control* problem, we could think that a strict juridical structure could force those who apply the technologies to control contaminants and this could stop such contaminants from reaching consumers. Regarding mycotoxins in particular – although the case could also be considered for other contaminants – this was our experience:

After determining that the corn in our region could be dangerous to consumers due to its potential contamination, we made new attempts of convincing authorities that it was necessary to design mechanisms to avoid such contaminants from being consumed by population.

We then proceeded to develop a thorough bill dealing with detection and prophylaxis (Eguiazu, 1984d, 1990) based on the old German Law to control aflatoxins (Bundesministerium für Jugend, Familie und Gesundheit) (Eguiazu, 1990) which we sent to both chambers (Upper House and Lower House, in the Argentine Parliament). This would mean another contribution whose beneficiary would be the consumer. However, the bill was never treated and lost its parliamentary status.

That is to say, specifying that the degree of contamination in this country could signify great financial loss for some of the actors – the possible banning of the commercialization of such product in the domestic market – was the reason for not considering the bill. The fact that large quantities of corn originally destined for human consumption, if found contaminated, would have to end up as animal feed, thus lowering its price, or, more dramatically still, the complete financial loss this would signify if the product had to be destroyed, allowed us to see clearly the reason why the system was unwilling to unveil the facts.

The result is then that legislation, however efficient it might be, can only partially control a technopathogenic risk.

Question on prevention B – The search for an answer attempting to
frame it within the causes that originate these contaminants

Considering having studied all the existing disciplines to achieve prevention, we will analyze the causes that originate these contaminants.

We formulated the following hypotheses:

Hypothesis: Can intergranular relative humidity
be the prevention parameter?

As we have mentioned before, the development of microorganisms in grains depends on environmental factors. One of them is relative humidity or free water content, which is found above 70% of relative humidity. This is why we worked on this promising parameter to achieve prevention.

We continued with this subject using as starting point the results we had obtained in Germany (Eguiazu, 1983, 1984a, 1984b, 1984c, 1986) (Eguiazu & Frank, 1984) (Eguiazu & Grünewald, 1984). We used the intergranular relative humidity (that is, relative humidity in between grains) as an absolute parameter for prevention and we used it to investigate sunflower.

For this purpose, we developed a special container to which we could insert a hygrometer (Eguiazu & Motta, 1985).

We had arrived to the conclusion that the common practice of *Humidity* (water content in the grain) as a commercialization standard was not the most suitable. As we will see and explain at a later stage, samples containing a high content of oil were more prone to the attack and contamination of mycotoxins (Eguiazu & Motta, 1985) (Motta , 1985) (Motta & Eguiazu, 1991a).

The risks of using Humidity as a parameter for the commercialization and storage of grain were demonstrated also in corn (Motta & Eguiazu, 1993).

This is why we presented a proposal to apply a parameter of *Intergranular Relative Air Humidity* (IRAH), that is, the water contained in the air around the grain, to the commercialization and storage of all the grains (Motta & Eguiazu, 1991b).

Among the enormous number of techniques applied to the productive process of grain – from its genetic development until it reaches consumers – procedures we could call Commercialization Techniques are also applied. Here we can observe another case of technique flaw, in this case, the commercialization technique, which might be responsible for generating a technopathogeny.

The results of this research were presented in 1985, in an international conference on sunflower (Mar del Plata, Argentina) and were later published in an important international journal (Eguiazu & Motta, 1985). We also received an award for the parameter proposed to contribute to the prevention of contamination of grains with mycotoxins (Motta, 1985).

This research proved that Intergranular Relative Air Humidity (IRAH) and not the humidity of the grain – was the most suitable parameter for a proper prevention against molds and mycotoxins generation – among them, aflatoxins. This is how we support this hypothesis:

Humidity is a parameter that measures the amount of water that the grain has, whilst Relative Humidity measures the amount of water in the air surrounding the grain. The higher the Humidity Content, the higher the Relative Humidity will be. The exchange of water between the grain and the surrounding atmosphere is a dynamic process and it is produced until a balance is achieved. According to the level of water each of them has, the grain can either absorb atmosphere water or transfer water to it. Even if the Relative Humidity value is proportional to the Humidity Content we find the former to be more suitable, since the balance is influenced by different factors determining that for a given grain the same value of Humidity Content can retrieve different values of Relative Humidity. On the other hand, the development of molds is more determined by the Relative Humidity parameter since it indicates that the mold can or cannot have free water for it to gather and develop toxins (Eguiazu & Motta, 1985) (Motta, 1985). That is, the quantity of water in the substratum is not as relevant as the free water on its surface since the development of mold is essentially a superficial phenomenon. This superficial humidity is measured accurately taking into account the relative humidity of the intergranular air. The internationally accepted limit of Relative Humidity is of 70%.

The result of this research indicated an increasing risk of aflatoxins in highly modified grains with an elevated level of oil. The search for this characteristic was found to be related to a higher proneness to the attack of molds. However, having supported this hypothesis and proposed the usage of the IRAH parameter, as well as having developed a measuring device – which constitutes yet another contribution to decrease the contamination of grains with mycotoxins and therefore the risk on consumers – was not enough. This achievement did not satisfy our interest of finding a way for efficient prevention.

Going back to what is recommended in connection with prophylaxis, we can say that: *The worst prevention is better than the best detection.* Even though tackling the problem of prevention from the Agricultural

Sciences point of view contributes to decreasing the risk, it left many questions unanswered. To identical storage conditions, the questions were: Why is the attack and genesis of toxins so dissimilar? What is happening with the modification of the grain substratum? How does this highly modified grain differ from the original grain through which the ancestral species reproduced? We consider that postulating the use of IRAH parameter (instead of the Humidity Content parameter) was a landmark in the prevention of fungi development and mycotoxins contamination in stored grains. However, as we have mentioned before, grain post-harvest handling is a group of techniques (rather than a discipline) that includes the handling and final industrialization of grains. Basic questions are usually not of that much interest as practical answers to grain storage and transfer. Neither are the questions aiming at investigating new quality criteria for consumers of much interest as compared to new criteria on grain commerce and industrialization. One of the papers in Chapter IV deals with this subject in detail. This discipline also did not provide satisfactory answers to deceitful or adulteration practices which are very common in the market, which also implied an ethical element. Adulterations to the quality of products are known since immemorial times. What they have in common are the clear ethical mishaps which muddle transparency – crucial for a proper functioning of the market. The most common practice is to increase the mass of the product – thus producing less quality lots (even getting to the extreme process of adding water to them). Therefore, the post-handling process is a very limited discipline to tackle this problem in-depth.

Going back to the attempts to frame this problem within a disciplinary field, having us proven the relevance of environmental conditions in fungi and mycotoxins development and postulating the IRAH parameter, we could humorously suggest framing our study within the Climatology field. In fact, some Agricultural careers offer the specialization in Agricultural Climatology. But we could not disagree more in accepting such an impoverishing and reductionist proposal.

Post-harvest handling then did not help us answer our questions. It seemed that we had just to take the modified substratum the way it was and study the ways of conserving it the best possible way without considering the more profound modifications it had undergone. But then our initial question: *The causes and effects of contamination and its relevance on human beings,* could not be answered through this discipline.

We would clearly be digressing from the original question. It was also obvious that aflatoxins were just an example of the enormous quantity of natural contaminants that could be found in grains. Then the question we came up with was: Which of all those risky substances is it worth choosing and studying? Rather than trying to find an answer to such question, we considered it was more useful to try to find an answer to this other question: What is it that allows molds which can generate potentially risky substances to humans to be developed in grains?

We therefore formulated the following hypothesis:

Hypothesis: Is Technique the cause of loss of resistance
in cultivated species?

Having not found the centre or root of the problem to achieve an efficient prevention in any of the roads chosen, we asked ourselves: Why is it that mold is able to develop in certain substrates? With this question we started getting nearer to the root of the problem and we therefore started visualizing how to address efficient prevention.

The research carried out in Germany continued to be focused on the environmental factors conditioning the fungi development and mycotoxins generation.

Some results were obtained from experiments with sunflower. The first mycelium was observed on a sample of Argentine sunflowers exposed to humidity and controlled temperature (Eguiazu, 1983) (Eguiazu & Frank, 1984). This is an early stage of fungi development. Although the mycelium layer could be easily observed, it is too thin to produce detectable quantities of aflatoxins.

The apparition of the first visible mycelium in stored grains is important since it can predict risk at a low level of contamination. If it surpasses this level and starts an active fungi growth, it can reach the stage in which aflatoxins can appear. Just like plants which, in order to bear fruit they need to have reached a certain stage of development, fungi also need a certain stage of development in order to generate the toxin. It was also observed that a great amount of mold was developed below the seed cover, the pericarp. We removed the pericarp from the grain and we could observe the difference of speed with which atmosphere humidity was absorbed, that is, the re-hydration kinetics and the biological action of molds ending with the complete or partial degradation of grains (Eguiazu, 1983).

This kinetic phenomenon allowed us to evaluate and prevent the degree of damage through indirect indicators. After detecting the fungi attack through the first visible mycelium (a subjective visual parameter), we tried to detect the fungi with another indicator: the ergosterol analytic detection (an objective method). Even though this was an efficient method, it could not be used as general method to detect fungi activity of toxic molds since it is a fungi metabolic product not necessarily related to its toxic capacity. In addition, even though this parameter is an instrumental measurement, it was observed that the detection limit was higher to the limit observed in the first visible mycelium. That is to say, in order to determine ergosterol chemically, there needed to be a considerable fungi attack (Eguiazu, 1983).

Studies showed that products with a higher content of oil biodegraded faster, and this made us see clearly the important role of genetic selection. Modification on the original grain by *sifting* genes was causing this fast damage. We concluded then that genetic modification and, in a broader sense, the techniques to obtain new seeds were causing the loss of resistance.

Mankind manipulation played a more important role than the force of nature.

This makes sense and it is understandable. It is natural that seeds in their wild original state can be resown in order to perpetuate the species and that is why they must be resistant to fungi attack. Let us not forget that all the mycotoxins producing molds are reproduced in the soil and there are millions of their reproduction sources – spores or propagules – in every cubic centimeter of soil. Without resistance there is no budding and therefore no new plant, leading to the interruption of the life cycle of such species. This is why human modifications of technological nature are unnatural and attempt against the survival of the species unless they protect the resowing process and the resistance of the seed.

As we have mentioned when supporting the application of the IRAH parameter, seeds harvested with a high content of oil are much more prone to the attack of mycotoxins (Eguiazu & Motta, 1986).

Back in Argentina, we continued working on this aspect and developed a hypothesis we then called *Anthropo-ecologic Hypothesis* connected to the storage and resowing of seeds in relation to the spontane-

138

ous apparition of mycotoxins (Eguiazu, 1985). In the light of current knowledge we now could actually call this hypothesis *Technopathogenologic Hypothesis* (Eguiazu, 1999a) (Eguiazu & Motta, 2004a).

On the one hand, we focused in developing a commercial parameter that allowed for an early recognition of the storage conditions that would lead to a later damaging. On the other hand, as we have said before, we were interested in seeing whether the focus by genetics technicians in some commercial and industrial characteristics of grains was not detrimental to the resowing characteristics above described.

These aspects, among others, refer to the research of resistance against molds attack.

These papers were presented in 1985 in a mycology congress in Argentina and then published (Eguiazu, 1985) (Eguiazu & Motta, 1986) (Motta, 1985).

We realized that the molds attack issue was not simple at all, on the contrary, it got more and more complex.

We then decided to keep on working on the Anthropo-ecologic Hypothesis using this question as starting point: If a seed is placed in negative conditions for a determined amount of time, will this seed survive? If some grains survived, this would prove that they represent different genetic variations, that is, a wide genetic range where resistance genes are included. But if no seed survives, this would mean that the grains were so genetically modified that they lost their capacity of resistance. That is to say, they suffered a significant genetic erosion of the genes that would have ensured resistance in bad storage conditions and further fungi attack. We therefore performed a test we called *inverse anthropoecologic hypothesis*. In Karl Popper's words (Popper, 1973): "A risky hypothesis is important provided it is expressed in such a way that it allows for the experimental path of its own destruction." Including all the results in sunflower studies, we continued our research on corn. We exposed almost all the corn varieties grown in Argentina to extreme storage conditions: very high relative humidity (100%). We expected that some seeds survived this extreme condition since we refused to believe in our own hypothesis. Through these experiments we intended to prove our hypothesis false (Eguiazu, 2001).

But the hypothesis proved positive. The corn grains sown in Argentina we used in our trial do not have a natural resistance against this fungi attack. This proves the apparition of aflatoxins in Argentine exported grains, which can be continuously determined. Interestingly enough, every year since 1988 in the United States various conferences are held to discuss the protection of agricultural products against aflatoxins and which include several topics such as: plant protection and conventional hybridization, genetic manipulation, identification of fungi and aflatoxins' biosynthesis inhibitors, microbial ecology, and insect control. In recent years, thanks to the development of molecular biology sciences, there have been developments in fungal genomics, which is also included in strategies of control.

The last few congresses presented papers on the existence of proteins that could act as fungal inhibitors (Bressan *et al.*, 1995) (Chen *et al.*, 1997) (Molieux *et al.*, 2000) (Moore *et al.*, 1997) (Payne *et al.*, 2002).

This would further support our hypothesis, since we have to bear in mind that the synthesis of protein and other substances is regulated by DNA information. If certain genes for protein synthesis have gotten lost due to genetic selection, this means that certain proteins – including those that can inhibit fungi attack – will not be synthesized. This proves that the proneness of plants to fungi attack can be caused by this selection process.

Preliminary conclusion

The search for answers to the question on prevention attempting to properly frame the causes that originate these contaminants was the right approach. Having verified the last two hypotheses, especially the last one, we confirm our Theory I, which stated that technique was responsible for generating mycotoxins and transferring it to humans: *Given their origin and the way they reach humans, the risk of mycotoxins to human health is a technological problem* (technology/technique in the wider sense that is given is this book). Therefore, in order to obtain an efficient protection, research must be oriented towards that approach.

Along with the failed attempt to try to frame our research within an existing disciplinary frame (Theory II), both theories contributed significantly to support the existence of the Technopathogeny phenomenon and the need to create a new discipline: Technopathogenology.

We therefore formulated the following hypothesis:

*Hypothesis: Is it necessary then to frame the problem
within a new science in order to achieve prevention?*

There was no science where we could frame our question. It did not fit within the scientific structure of Science and Technology – therefore, it could not be classified as a scientific question. The evaluations were only interested in the aspects that linked this question with other branches or other existing disciplines. However, in the manner we presented the question, it could not be answered by any discipline.

Biological Sciences (Physiology, Mycology, Ecology) did not provide an answer to the essential problem of aflatoxins – they were just auxiliary tools that contributed to its resolution. The same thing happened with technological disciplines (Analytical Chemistry, Agronomy, Food Technology). Even after encountering such difficulties, if we still tried to frame our problem within those perspectives, we would find the following objections:

a) Every science or specialty would analyze the problem from its own perspective, unavoidably reducing it so as to make it fit within its framework. The vision of the problem would depend on the point of view. The study of this technopathogenic phenomenon cannot be fragmented.

In some cases, the loss of the sense of reality in the Science and Technology system is such that it sometimes prefers, rather unethically, to distort or impoverish the object of study rather than recognizing its own ignorance or limitations. The question is therefore reformulated so that the evaluation committee can frame it within the disciplines they know. Here lies a strong component of scientific pride mentioned by Eco (Ecco, 2000). An ignorant evaluator prefers to get away of this embarrassing situation denying the existence of what he or she does not know.

b) The study of the problem would lay outside the human environment (even when all its factors interact with human health) (Eguiazu & Motta, 2000).

Our experience allowed us to prove our hypothesis true.

Having confirmed the first two theories on mycotoxins and having detected in those theories a non-evident risk hard to detect and recognize, we came up with another hypothesis that led to a new theory:

Theory III: Being technological products, pesticides can also entail im-
manent and hidden risks

In this theory we state that non-evident technological risk could also manifest itself in the use of substances that humans themselves synthesize
to enhance production. Since they are elaborated by humans, it was expected that risks were either null or preventable.

The following hypotheses gave support to the above mentioned theory:

Hypothesis: If the non-evident technological risk of natural contami-
nants such as mycotoxins is a consequence of defects in one or various
Techniques applied to the production process, can such risk manifest it-
self in pesticides as well?

Hypothesis: Is the LD50 parameter applied to toxic substances a factor
that can achieve prevention of non-evident technological risk for the us-
er and/or consumer?

Humans are aware that substances developed to beat pests imply in many
ways that they are toxic and, therefore, can pose a risk on users or consumers.

Therefore, before a substance is used, there are several estimations on
the levels of innocuousness that must be obtained, so that the risk of toxicity is null or minimum – as we have seen with the vectors analogy, so
that the levels of pesticide reaching the user or consumer present no risk.

There are certain experiments that estimate a common value in
chemical substances (LD50 or Median Lethal Dose) which, as we have
already mentioned, indicates the level of concentration of a substance
that can cause death in 50% of the animals used in the experiment (generally rats) (IPCS, 2004). The higher the value, the lower the risk of toxicity of such substance. Therefore, the acute toxicity risk indicated by
LD50 is inversely proportionate to the indicated figure. In order to obtain
this value, it is determined whether the active principle is solid or liquid
and if exposure is oral or dermal.

To illustrate this, below we show the values indicated by the World
Health Organization.

Table 10:   Classification of dangerousness of pesticide active principles according to
            acute level of toxicity, type of exposure, and solid or liquid state (Source:
            IPCS, 2004)

Class		LD50 for the rat (mg/kg body weight)			
		Oral		Dermal	
		Solid	Liquid	Solid	Liquid
Ia	Extremely hazardous	5 or less	20 or less	10 or less	40 or less
Ib	Highly hazardous	5-50	20-200	10-100	40-400
II	Moderately hazardous	50-500	200-2000	100-1000	400-4000
III	Slightly hazardous	Over 500	Over 2000	Over 1000	Over 4000

The hypothesis falsification was easier than with mycotoxins. Comparing active principles used, the LD50 value and the carcinogenic risk, we were able to verify that some high value LD50 pesticides – that is, meant to be safe – did have a long term carcinogenic risk.

We can then say that both risks of toxicity – acute and chronic – are not necessarily related. That is to say, we cannot say that a highly toxic substance (low LD50 level) will be carcinogenic and that a low toxic substance (high LD50 level) will not be carcinogenic. On the other hand, as we have already mentioned, we have found that low toxicity substances (with LD50 values that classified them as innocuous) can indeed be carcinogenic (Eguiazu, 1988) (Eguiazu & Motta, 1991), as the following table shows:

Table 11:   Relationship between the toxicity shown by LD50 in six pesticides and the
            carcinogenic risk in each of them.

Active Pesticide Ingredient	LD50	Risk of Carcinogenesis
Alachlor	1200	High
Captafol	6000	High
Captan	9000	High
Amitrol	5000	High
Nitrofen	3000	High
Aldicarb	0.93	Low or Null

The LD50 is expressed in milligram of active principle per each kilogram of the animal. That is to say, a 70 kg person should eat 630 grams of captan active principle to have a risk of intoxication, whilst it would take almost ten times less of aldicarb (65.1) to run the same risk. However, aldicarb will not pose a carcinogenic risk in the long term (therefore, it will not pose a technopathogenic risk), whilst captan, although much less toxic, does present a carcinogenic risk and can therefore be responsible for a technopathogeny.

This hypothesis also showed that the carcinogenicity trial is not routinely applied on pesticides prior to their usage.

Many products were used for many years until a long term risk was proved as the following table shows (Motta, 1994). Column "A" indicates the date in which the substance was either mentioned for the first time, produced at large scale or produced commercially or sold for the first time. Column "B" indicates the date in which IARC mentions the substance was proved to be carcinogenic on experimental animals.

Table 12: Relationship between the date of discovery of eight pesticide active principles and the discovery or proof of carcinogenic risk.

Active Pesticide Ingredient	A	B
Amitrole	1954	1982
Aramite	1950	1982
Carbon tetrachloride	1907	1979
DDT	1939	1982
1,2-Dibromo-3-Chloropropane	1955	1979
Chlordecone	1966	1979
Nitrofen	1963	1983
Toxafene	1943	1979

Another example of Technopathogeny in pesticides is the case of hexachlorobenzene. This active principle is solid and of a very low level of toxicity (its dermal LD50 is of 10,000 mg/kg). By the values indicated in table 10 it is considered practically innocuous. However, the World Health Organization has included it in Group Ia, that is, *Extremely Dangerous,* since it was found to cause porphyrias in humans. In addition, its usage and production is highly restricted by the Stockholm Convention as it is considered a persistent organic contaminant (IPCS, 2004).

When we analyzed the question of prevention of the mycotoxins, attempting to frame it within the existing disciplinary field: Agronomy, Analytical Chemistry or Jurisprudence, etc., we concluded that the question could not be answered within the existing disciplinary field. Because pesticides as well as mycotoxins also carry along a non-evident technological risk, it was not necessary to investigate whether to achieve prevention its study had to be framed within the existing disciplinary field, because we could confirm what was already found in mycotoxins.

For example, regarding Analytical Chemistry, it is very interesting to mention the results of the studies carried out in the United States on fruits, vegetables and legumes (Mott & Snyder, 1987). In the case of lettuce, the authors mention the following data:

a) A third of the analyzed samples had residues of one or more pesticides.

b) Forty three pesticide active principles were detected in lettuce.

c) Out of the over 60 pesticide active principles used to grow lettuce, the lab methods usually employed by the Federal Government can only detect approximately 60%.

d) Active principles mentioned among the most frequently used presenting long term risk: mevinphos (Ia, L, 4D) (some evidence of mutagenicity); endosulphan (II, S, 80) (effects in the liver, kidneys and testicle atrophy in lab animals); permethrin (II, L, 500) (possible carcinogen in humans, reproductive toxicity); dimethoate (II, S, 150) (some evidence of carcinogenicity, birth defects, reproductive toxicity and mutagenic effects in lab animals); methomyl (Ib, S, 17) (effects in the kidneys, bladder and blood in lab animals; some evidence of mutagenicity).

The information in brackets describes: the active principle class according to its acute toxicity (as seen in table 10), its physical state: S (solid), L (liquid), and the LD_{50} value (expressed in milligrams of active principle per kilogram of body weight). These values are for oral exposure. Dermal exposure is indicated with letter "D" (IPCS, 2004). Even though the level of danger ranges from extremely dangerous to moderately dangerous, the concentration of residues will not be high enough so as to imply an acute risk. That is to say that alarm signals due to acute reasons are not produced or are so low that they can be attributed to other causes. That is why the chronic risks of these products are of higher relevance. Furthermore, it is important to consider that small quantities of various products add up to a larger, more significant quantity.

All this clearly shows the technopathogenic relevance of pesticides: the long-term effects, the presence of pesticides in foodstuffs and the impossibility of a reliable detection.

Having confirmed the Theory of Mycotoxins and Pesticides we went on to formulate the General Theory of Technologic Risks.

As we have said before, taking the medical term *Iatrogenesis* and the concepts developed by Prof. Beck on Culture and Technique, by induction from the problems on mycotoxins and pesticides, we were able to support the existence of a new phenomenon. Or rather, the need of framing the study of non-evident technological risks as a new phenomenon. We thus postulated the fourth theory:

Theory IV: The development and application of Techniques entail an immanent and hidden risk we call Technopathogeny

So far we have described our work on mycotoxins (detection and prophylaxis). Measures on protection and storage were achieved, and we further worked in the field of non-evident risks of pesticides.

We also proposed the theory of Technique being responsible for technopathogenic risks in these substances. That is to say, there was no biological or natural fatality but an utter human mistake – humans develop and choose wrong technologies, apply them systematically and recognize or not their mistakes.

However, we clearly saw that even if we managed to prevent the presence of these toxic substances in every product which could carry them, it would be only a small contribution to protection of consumers. Toxic substances are like a drop of water in the middle of the ocean if one considers the amount of toxic substances consumers are continuously exposed to. This is how, having two specific problems as starting point, through induction we formulated a general principle. Now, applying a deductive reasoning we tried to demonstrate that the phenomenon or problem of Technopathogeny is also found in other techniques. Using the Technopathogeny general principle we can demonstrate that this phenomenon is also manifested in other techniques.

Mycotoxins prove the existence of unknown technopathogens whose apparition is favored by Technique. Pesticides prove that products elaborated by the technical man can also become a technopathogen for having unknown non-evident effects the technician that developed them is responsible for. In both cases, mycotoxins and pesticides prove the existence of unexpected and unwanted collateral effects associated with a technique in particular.

146

We therefore came up with the most obvious and broad hypothesis: Were there other hidden and undiscovered contaminants? And mainly: Were there other techniques generating factors with a technopathogenic effect?

We thus formulated the following hypotheses:

Hypothesis: Which other carcinogenic substances – either hidden or semi-hidden – can affect human beings?

Mycotoxins and pesticides constitute only a portion of the vast amount of chemical substances.

In 1980, for example, the US Department of Health, Education and Welfare named 48,000 daily usage substances used during that year (US DHW-PHS, 1979). In that same year, an increase of 500 new substances each year was estimated. A 1981 report (US DHHS-PHS, 1980) indicated 60,000 daily usage substances with an increase of 700 to 1000 new substances each year. In 1985, 70,000 substances were already in use with an increase of 1000 new substances each year (ILO, 1987) (PNUMA, 1985b).

It is interesting to point out that daily usage substances only represent a 1% of the substances synthesized by Technical Chemistry. This means that only 1% of the substances find some kind of commercial application. For example, in 1985, the Chemical Abstract Service of the American Chemical Society had registered 7,000,000 substances. In this year, 420,000 new substances were being synthesized. As we have seen, only 70,000 substances were of daily usage and out of the 420,000 synthesized only 1000 were incorporated to the daily usage. In 1991, the Chemical Abstract Service registered 10,000,000 substances. By then, 600,000 new substances were synthesized every year and 100,000 substances were used in international commerce (PNUMA, 1991).

Since 1991, more than 100,000 different substances are of daily usage in the modern world. That same year, the Sixth Annual Report of Carcinogens (US DHHS-PHS-NTP, 1991) incorporated twenty-five substances or groups of substances, medical treatments and occupational exposures associated with technological processes known to be carcinogenic to humans because of evidence in humans that indicates a causal relationship between the exposure to such agents and cancer. It also included 148 substances or groups of substances and medical treatments which could reasonably be anticipated to be carcinogenic to humans because of a limited evidence of carcinogenicity in humans and enough evidence in experimental animals.

The high economic cost, time and complexity of the studies required to determine whether a substance is carcinogenic or not implies that only some of the substances can be tested and only after a strict selection. Serious trials use groups of rats and mice of both sexes for two years.

To illustrate the difficulties of the evaluation of the substances by carcinogenicity trials, in 1980, a trial capacity was estimated of 300 to 600 substances each year. As we have already mentioned, in that year 48,000 substances were commonly used, which means it would take 80 years for a thorough study. The conclusion is obvious considering the increase in the annual amount of substances.

This is why many of them are used with minimal data of the toxicology trials, as the table below indicates:

Table 13:   Toxicology data available to perform an evaluation on risk on human health (Source: Rall, 1990)

		Percentage with:			
		Health Hazard Assessment:		Toxicological Data:	
	Number	Complete	Partial	Minimal tox. data	Less than minimal data
Pesticides, ingredients	3300	10	24	2	64
Cosmetics, ingredients	3400	2	14	10	74
Drugs, ingredients	1800	18	18	3	61
Food additives	8600	5	14	1	80
Chemical in commerce	38000	0	11	11	78

As it is the case with pesticides, many substances with different uses – medicines, foodstuff additives, industrial chemical products, veterinary products – have also been found to be carcinogenic, and therefore, technopathogenic.

It is interesting to note that the number indicated in the daily usage substances – as table 13 shows – only considers the substances technicians have synthesized or elaborated for a specific purpose. This leads to the following question:

Hypothesis: What happens with substances
which are not produced by humans?

Apart from the risk entailed by the substances synthesized by humans, there are other substances generated by technicians as a consequence of the application of their techniques. There are an uncountable number of unwanted substances, some natural, some artificial, which are also responsible for health damages, including contaminants (mycotoxins, dioxins, products of incomplete combustion, etc.) as well as physical and biological factors.

In order to provide for the evaluation of the magnitude of the problem or risk entailed by these substances, we will briefly deal with some of the groups included in this hypothesis. Even though these substances are catalogued as contaminants, some of them have been elaborated with the intention of being used. Thus the paradox that certain substances elaborated with a certain positive aim can be considered contaminants if they appear in the wrong place.

Other Mycotoxins

As we have seen, the first hypotheses and theories that led to support the idea of the disciplinary void for the Technopathogeny phenomenon, referred to mycotoxins. Even though we referred to it as a general term, as we have also seen, we were particularly referring to a group of them: aflatoxins. In order to further analyze the problem they imply, we will only mention a few of these mold-generated substances. Among them, we will especially name those relevant to humans. Such substances were evaluated by IARC. Even though in some cases there is not enough experimental evidence to classify the certain substances in terms of its risk to humans, such risk should not be underestimated.

The following table indicates the toxin, the mold/s producing it, the products in which it was detected and the carcinogenic risk. Column "D" indicate: Adverse effects to Humans; Experimental Evidence for Carcinogenicity and/or Evaluation.

Table 14: Some mycotoxins and their risk on health.

Toxin	Fungi / Fungus Productors	Products in which was detected and/or Uses	(D)
Cyclochlorotine CAS N° 12663-46-6	*Penicillium islandicum*	Various grains, staple diet, barley, and prepared foodstuffs.	Carcinogenic in male mice.
Deoxynivalenol CAS N° 51481-10-8	*Fusarium graminearum* *Fusarium culmorum*	Wheat, corn, foods, oats, rice, flour, triticale, barley.	Inadequate evidence in humans. Inadequate evidence in experimental animals.
Fumonisins B1 CAS N° 116355-83-0	*Fusarium moniliforme* and some related species of *Fusaium*	Corn, corn products: corn meal, corn grits, corn feed, cornflakes.	Possibly carcinogenic to humans.
Fumonisins B2 CAS N° 116355-84-1	*Fusarium moniliforme* and some related species of *Fusaium*	Corn, cprm products: corn meal, corn grits, corn feed, cornflakes.	Possibly carcinogenic to humans.
Fusarenone X CAS N° 23255-69-8	*Fusarium nivale* and other species of *Fusarium*	Corn	Inadequate evidence in experimental animals.
Fusarin C CAS N° 79748-81-5	*Fusarium moniliforme* and several species of *Fusaium*	Corn	Possibly carcinogenic to humans.
Griseofulvin CAS N° 126-07-8	*Penicillum griseofulvum*	Antifungal antibiotic substance. It is used for the treatment and prophylaxis of human mycotic diseases. In Veterinary medicine is used for the treatment of ringworm.	Hepatocarcinogenic in mice. Possibly carcinogenic to humans.
Luteoskyrin CAS N° 21884-44-6	*Penicillum islandicum* *Mycelia sterilia*	Various grains, rice, barley.	Carcinogenic in mice.
Nivalenol CAS N° 23282-20-4	*Fusarium nivale* Other species of *Fusarium*	Wheat, corn, feed, cereals, barley, wheat flour.	Inadequate evidence in experimental animals.
Ochratoxin A CAS N° 303-47-9	*Aspergillus ochraceus,* and other species. *Penicil-*	Cereals, wheat, hay, grain, forage, peas beans, corn, barley,	Possibly carcinogenic to humans.

Toxin	Fungi / Fungus Productors	Products in which was detected and/or Uses	(D)
	lum sp.	cassava flour, feed, bran, flour, bread, breakfast cereals, cowpea, rice, copra, rye, oats, beans, peanut.	
Patulin CAS N° 149-29-1	*Penicillum expansum*	Apples, sweet apple cider	Sarcomas in rats.
Penicillic Acid CAS N° 90-65-3	*Penicillum puberulum* and other species of *Penicillum,* and species of *Aspergillus*	Corn; dried beans.	Sarcomas in mice and rats.
Sterigmatocystin CAS N° 10048-13-2	*Aspergillus versicolor*	Green coffee beans, wheat, salami.	Carcinogenic in rats and mice. Possibly carcinogenic to humans.
T-2 Toxin CAS N° 21259-20-1	*Fusarium sporotrichioides* and other species of *Fusarium*	Barley, feed, corn, grains, corn flour, oats, wheat, rice, sorghum, wheat flour, groundnuts.	"Alimentary toxic aleukia" in humans. Limited evidence in experimental animals for the carcinogenicity.
Zearalenone CAS N° 17924-92-4	*Fusarium graminearum,* and other species	Cereals, feeds, corn foods, wheat, barley, beer, malt. It is produced commercially as an intermediate in the preparation of Zeranol, which is used as a growth promoter in beef cattle, feedlot lambs, and suckling beef calves.	Inadequate evidence in humans. Limited evidence in experimental animals.

Bibliography Table 14:

Cyclochlorotine, Luteoskyrin, Patulin, Penicillic Acid (IARC, 1976a); *Griseofulvin, Sterigmatocystin*: (IARC, 1976a; 1987b); *Ochratoxin*: (IARC, 1976a; 1993a); *Deoxynivalenol, Fumonisins B1, Fumonisins B2,*

Fusarenone X, Fusarin C, Nivalenol, T-2 Toxin, Zearalenone: (IARC, 1993a)

As we can see, either advertently or inadvertently, Technique can lead to an uncountable amount of risks in relation to toxins. If zearalenone, for example, appears either spontaneously or by a weakening effect in the grain, it is already a risk. But if it (or its derivatives) is synthesized, produced industrially and used for its anabolic effect (better conversion or more efficient usage of the feed by the animal), the final residual effect that remains in the animal product can lead to a significant risk of higher Technopathogenic relevance. This proves that what poses the technological risk is not the substance itself but the circumstance of its technological use.

Polycyclic Aromatic Hydrocarbons

Polycyclic Aromatic Hydrocarbons or Polynuclear Aromatic Compounds are formed as a result of the incomplete combustion of organic compounds.

They occur ubiquitously in products of incomplete combustion and constitute a family which includes several substances. In a study on gas motor emissions more than 80 substances of this family were identified (IARC, 1989). The International Agency for Research on Cancer analyzed 42 substances (IARC, 1983). The following 15 substances were selected by the 10[th] Annual Report on Carcinogens (US DHHS-PHS-NTP, 2002) as substances which can be reasonably anticipated as carcinogens to humans.

Table 15: List of the 15 most common Polycyclic Aromatic Hydrocarbons which can be reasonably anticipated as carcinogens to humans.

	Name – CAS N°
1	Benz[a]anthracene CAS N° 56-55-3
2	Benzo[b]fluoranthene CAS N° 205-99-2
3	Benzo[j]fluoranthene CAS N° 205-82-3
4	Benzo[k]fluoranthene CAS N° 207-08-9
5	Benzo[a]pyrene CAS N° 50-32-8
6	Dibenz[a,h]acridine CAS N° 226-36-8
7	Dibenz[a,j]acridine CAS N° 224-42-0
8	Dibenz[a,h]anthracene CAS N° 53-70-3
9	7H-Dibenzo[c,g]carbazole CAS N° 194-59-2
10	Dibenzo[a,e]pyrene CAS N° 192-65-4
11	Dibenzo[a,h]pyrene CAS N° 189-64-0
12	Dibenzo[a,i]pyrene CAS N° 189-55-9
13	Dibenzo[a,l]pyrene CAS N° 191-30-0
14	Indeno[1,2,3-cd]pyrene CAS N° 193-39-5
15	5-Methylchrysene CAS N° 3697-24-3

These substances are widely distributed in nature. They are found in:
- Emissions produced by wood and fuel combustion in household heating.
- Gasoline and diesel engine exhaust.
- Waste burning emissions.
- Coke tar.
- Coal tar.

- Industries smoke.
- Wood coal combustion.
- Tobacco smoke.
- Mineral oils.
- Creosote.
- Pyrolysis products
- etc.

Ways of exposure to these substances, due to their wide distribution nature, are quite diverse.

We can mention:

- Inhaling of contaminated air. They have been detected both in dust and soot.
- Contaminated water consumption.
- Consumption of contaminated foodstuffs. In various concentrations these compounds were detected in: smoked foodstuffs, meat roasted with wood coal, vegetables, vegetable oils, margarines, toasted coffee, grated coffee, sausages, cereal and oil grains, flours, bread, meat, seafood, fruits, elaborated foodstuffs, drinks.
- Dermal exposure through contact with wood products treated with creosote, street asphalt, coal tar, dermatological preparations containing coal tar. In normal conditions, the risk of dermal exposure is low, but small quantities could enter the body through contact with oily products contaminated with these substances.

Nitroarenes

Nitroarenes are a family related to polycyclic aromatic hydrocarbons which also includes several substances. Below we summarize two documents published by IARC (IARC, 1989) and by the U.S. Department of Health and Human Services (US DHHS-PHS-NTP, 2002).

Such substances were detected in the following media:

- Diesel motors emissions.
- Toners for use in photocopy machines.
- Kerosene household heaters.
- Household cooking or heating burners, fed with natural or liquefied petroleum gas.

The main ways of exposure is inhaling.

In vehicle emissions, more than forty nitroarenes have been identified. IARC presented a study on fifteen substances (IARC, 1989). In Table 16, the 6 substances were selected by IARC as possibly carcinogenic in humans, five out of which are also included in the 10th Annual Report on Carcinogens (US DHHS-PHS-NTP, 2002) as substances which can be reasonably anticipated as carcinogens to humans.

For the remaining substances, the evidence in experimental animals is either inadequate or insufficient to be classified regarding its carcinogenicity to humans – that is why IARC includes them in Group 3. However, let us not forget that this classification does not imply the lack of carcinogenic risk. Only the substances included in Group 4 of IARC classification are considered as *possibly not carcinogenic to humans*, meaning that the evidence in humans as well as in experimental animals suggests the lack of carcinogenicity in both.

Table 16:   List of the 6 most common nitroarenes

	Name	IARC	10th A.R.C.
1	1.6-Dimethylaminoazobenzene CAS N° 42397-64-8	Ps.C.H.	R.H.C
2	1,8-Dinitroperene CAS N° 42397-65-9	Ps.C.H.	R.H.C
3	1-Nitropyrene CAS N° 5522-43-0	Ps.C.H.	R.H.C
4	2-Nitrofluorene CAS N° 607-57-8	Ps.C.H.	
5	4-Nitropyrene CAS N° 57835-92-4	Ps.C.H.	R.H.C
6	6-Nitrochrysene CAS N° 7496-02-8	Ps.C.H.	R.H.C

Polychlorinated Dibenzodioxins

These contaminants constitute a family of substances called congeners, which, according to the number of chlorine atoms and to their position within the molecule, can constitute 75 different substances. The most commonly known is the 2,3,7,8-Tetrachlorodibenzo-para-dioxin, which also poses a toxicological risk including carcinogenicity.

IARC presented a thorough study on these substances (IARC, 1997).

There are several ways these substances are formed, such as:

a) Chemical reactions

They are found in:

1. Herbicides derived from chlorophenoxyacetic acid.
   It is worth mentioning the 2,4,5-T herbicide, also known as Agent Orange.
2. Hexachlorophene bactericide synthesis. It was used in cosmetics but its use was stopped in the European Union.
3. Chlorophenols synthesis.
4. Herbicides synthesis derived from chlorodiphenyl ether.
5. Hexachlorobenzene synthesis.
6. In the paper industry (paper pulp bleaching process).
7. In the synthesis of inks and pigments.

b) Due to thermal reactions

Formation of dioxins were found in:

1. Incineration of municipal waste.
2. Incineration of sewage sludge.
3. Incineration of hospital waste.
4. Incineration of polyvinyl chloride (PVC).
5. Combustion of Wood.
6. Automobile emissions.

c) Due to photochemical reactions

d) Due to biochemical reactions

Chlorinated phenols transformation

Ways of exposure:
Just like polycyclic aromatic hydrocarbons these substances are widely distributed in nature. Ways of exposure could be:

a) Workplace exposure

1. In the production of 2, 4, 5-T herbicides and Chlorophenols.
2. During the manipulation and application of the 2, 4,5-T herbicide.

3. In the incineration of waste.
4. Exposure in paper and pulp mills.
5. In the steel industry.

b) Risks in population due to industrial accidents, such as the Seveso case in Italy.

c) Environmental exposure to the population in general:
   1. By inhaling. Monitoring in various countries has detected these contaminants in the air.
   2. By consumption of contaminated waters. These compounds were found in drinking water samples.
   3. By contact with contaminated soil.
   4. By consumption of contaminated foodstuffs. Monitoring in foodstuffs detected these products in: bread, cereals, nuts, carcass meat, meat by-products, poultry meat, fish, oils, fat, eggs, milk, milk by-products. In vegetables: horticulture products, fruits, children foodstuffs, margarines, pork fat.

These substances were detected in human tissue. They are fat-soluble and it is interesting to point out their detection in breast milk.

Apart from their carcinogenic effect, these substances also have other adverse effects in health which are worth mentioning. Long exposure could certainly be responsible for other damages to health, which are not necessarily carcinogenic but could also be included among the technopathogenies caused by the substance (either directly or indirectly).

This includes:

- Effects on the skin: Chloracne and others.
- Effects on the liver: Alterations were detected in: 1) Levels of different enzymes, among them Aspartate aminotransferase and Alanine aminotransferase; D-Glucaric acid; 2) Porphyrin metabolism; 3) Levels of lipids; 4) Total Cholesterol and Triglycerides.
- Gastrointestinal effects: Ulcers (chronic).
- Effects on thyroid function. In Holland effects were detected on this gland in infants and it was related to dioxins on breast milk. Elevated levels of Polychlorinated dibenzo-*para*-dioxin in breast milk may alter thyroid function.
- Diabetes.

- Immunological effects.
- Neurologic effects: Neuropathies were detected in people exposed in the Seveso incident. No effects were found associated with dioxins exposure in other people and children.
- Circulatory system effects: There are studies indicating mortality in people exposed to dioxins due to circulatory effects.
- Pulmonary effects: Certain studies (though limited) have shown a relationship between people exposed to dioxins in their workplace and an alteration of the normal breathing functions.
- Renal effects: Even though there is scarce data, a relationship between dioxins and a bladder malfunction has been suggested.

N-nitroso compounds

The N-Nitroso compounds are another major group of substances which are of interest to Technopathogenology due to their potential risk on humans, since various techniques can be involved in the generation of associated technopathogenies.

In 1978, IARC presented a valuable document in which diverse substances of this group were considered (IARC, 1978b). We will base on such document to describe the risk such substances entail.

Even if we mention this group of substances among the contaminants, some of them, and as we will see in each case in particular, were synthesized for industrial applications.

These compounds are widely present in nature.

Their toxic action has been known for many years since the hepatotoxic effect of the N-Nitrosodimethylamine in humans was discovered in 1937. The carcinogenic effect of this substance was first mentioned in 1956.

The detection of severe damage in sheep fed with fish feed that had been treated with sodium nitrite as preservative and the identification of N-Nitrosodimethylamine as the responsible toxic agent, motivated investigating on the levels of such compounds which could be present in foodstuffs for human consumption.

They are very specific compounds concerning the induction of tumours in several species and in different areas within the same species. It thus constitutes a tool to research on the possible mechanisms in which cancer (neoplasias) can be inducted.

Formation and ways of exposure

People can be exposed to these substances in several ways:

- Formation in the environment and subsequent absorption through the air, water and/or food.
- Formation in elaborated foodstuffs and cosmetics.
- Direct formation within the organism through separate ingestion of precursors (amines and nitrites, for example), through foodstuffs, air or water.
- Consumption or industrial products.
- Nitroso compounds are used in industry as accelerators of chemical reactions and antioxidants. The industrial usage of these substances does not only mean workplace contamination for workers but also air contamination, thus posing an exposure risk in people in general through inhalation. Regarding the industry, it was found that the disposal of waste containing amines favour the formation of nitrosamines on the soil, waste and waters.
- Consumption of tobacco.
- Naturally occurring compounds.
- In refrigeration fluids used in the steel industry for the cooling of cutting tools.

Unlike other contaminants we have seen, it is interesting to note that this family of compounds has the potential property of self-generating within the same organism. This increases its potential risk. It has been known for many years (since 1865) that under certain acidity conditions, sodium nitrate can react with the dimethylamine and form the N-nitroso-dimethylamine. It has been suggested that this reaction of nitrites with amines can occur under the acidity conditions found in the stomach of mammals and originate N-nitrosamines – a phenomenon proved in 1968.

Nitrites and nitrates are used as foodstuffs additives – mainly fish and meat – to prevent contamination with the botulinum toxin.

Nitrite can also be used as a color enhancer due to its reaction with haemoglobin (Belitz & Grosch, 1992) (Kapfelsperger & Pollmer, 1982) and as a taste enhancer in the processes of curation and smoking of meats.

Nitrites and nitrates are ingested by humans in water and food contaminated with such substances. Nitrites are also formed in the mouth cavity due to bacterial reduction of nitrates (in this case nitrites appear in saliva). Even though nitrates are not necessarily technopathogenic, they are so indirectly because they can potentially help nitrites formation.

It was discovered that when food rich in nitrates is consumed – such as certain roots or vegetables – the levels of nitrates and nitrites are proportionally increased in saliva.

The reduction of nitrates to nitrites can also continue in the stomach of persons with low-acidity. This characteristic was found to be connected to the etiology of gastric cancer.

Among the compounds that can react to nitrites, the following are found: secondary and tertiary amines, quaternary ammonium compounds, urea, carbamates and guanidines, some of which are of wide distribution in nature. Some medicines containing amino or amides groups also react to nitrites. For example, the Amidopyrine drug, which can react to nitrosating agents and form the N-nitrosodimethylamine. This carcinogenic nitroso compound has been detected as contaminant in medicines having Amidopyrine as active principle. As we can see, this is a case in which a substance does not pose a technopathogenic risk in itself but, due to the chemical reaction generated in the organism, it becomes another substance leading to such risk.

The evidence regarding the feasibility of formation of such compounds in the stomach is given by: a) Detection of Nitroso compounds in gastric juice in vitro and in animal and human stomachs in vivo; b) Observation of acute toxicity as well as carcinogenicity in experiences in which Amines, Amides and Nitrites were simultaneously applied.

Regarding the formation of such substances, it was found it is inhibited by the presence of Ascorbic Acid and α-Tocopherol. This is of high relevance since it is a property that contributes to confirm our proposal on the new concepts or quality criteria (Eguiazu & Motta, 1991, 1992, 1996) which we will refer to in Chapter IV.

There is an interesting comment by IARC in one of its reports that supports our hypothesis that it is better to try to prevent a Technopathogeny rather than try to repair it. In connection to Nitroso compounds, this indicates that even though the carcinogenic potential has been proved on humans, by the time the document was published – and maybe even today – there was not enough epidemiologic evidence. It would be very difficult – or even impossible – for IARC to demonstrate in the population in general a cause-effect relationship between the exposure to low levels of N-Nitrosamines and the incidence of certain types of neoplasias in humans. This great difficulty supports the idea of prophylaxis and the need of a Technopathogenology.

Below there is a list of some nitroso compounds for which there is evidence indicating carcinogenic risk in humans. Following the same criteria as table 8, we also include the Chemical Abstracts Service number.

Table 17: List of some nitroso compounds presenting carcinogenic risk and their presence in the human environment.

Compound	Use and/or Occurrence	Eval.
N-Nitrosodi-*n*-butylamine CAS N° 924-16-3	Use: It has been used in the synthesis of di-*n*-butylhydrazine. Occurrence: 1) Tobacco smoke. 2) Water. 3) Food and feed: Cheese, luncheon meat, cooked and smoked ham, salami-like sausages, bacon-like products, beef meat, fried minced meat. Tinned and powdered soaps, tinned meals. 4) Vapor-phase corrosion inhibitors.	Ps.C.H.
N-Nitrosodiethanol-amine CAS N° 1116-54-7	Occurrence: 1) Tabacco. 2) Cutting fluids: used to reduce the temperature of the metal-tool interface during metal cutting or grinding. 3) Pesticides: In Atrazine formulations. 4) Cosmetics: Facial cosmetics formulations, hand and body lotions, and in hair shampoos.	Ps.C.H.
N-Nitrosodiethylamine CAS N° 55-18-5	Occurrence: 1) Air. 2) Tobacco smoke. 3) Water: Deionized water, waste-water. 4) Food: Cheese, Vegetable and Vegetable oils, Cereal products, Fish, Meat products. 5) Feed: Fishmeal. 6) Alcoholic beverages: Apple brandy, ciders, cognac, armagnac, rum, whiskey. 7) *In vivo*: In human blood both before and after the ingestion of a meal.	Pr.C.H.
N-Nitrosodimethyl-amine CAS N° 62-75-9	Use: In the production of 1,1-Dimethylhydrazine. Occurrence: 1) Air. 2) Tobacco smoke. 3) Water: It can result in the chlorination of drink-ing-water. 4) Soil.	Pr.C.H.

Compound	Use and/or Occurrence	Eval.
	5) Foods: Cheese, vegetable and vegetable oils, tinned fruits, meat and fish, spices. 6) Feed: Fishmeal. 7) Alcoholic beverages. 8) Pesticides: in formulations of 2,3,6-Trichlorobenzoic acid. In various herbicides. 9) Drugs: Formulations of Amidopyrine. 10) *In vivo*: It was formed in laboratory mice. It has been reported in human fluids: vaginal fluids, urine, gastric juice, human blood.	
N-Nitrosodi-*n*-propyl-amine CAS N° 621-64-7	Occurrence: 1) Waste water. 2) Food: Cheese. 3) Alcoholic beverages: Apple brandy, cognac, rum, whiskey. 4) Pesticides: In formulations of Trifluralin.	Ps.C.H.
3-Methylnitrosamine-propionitrile CAS N° 60153-49-3	Occurrence: in the oral cavity of betel-quid chewers.	Ps.C.H.
4-(Methylnotrosami-no)-1-(3-pyridyl)-1-butanone CAS N° 64091-91-4	Occurrence: Tobacco and tobacco smoke.	Ps.C.H.
N-Nitroso-*N*-ethylurea CAS N° 759-73-9	Use: In the synthesis of Diazoethane. Its mutagenic effect has been studied for promoting the growth of various plants.	Pr.H.C.
N-Nitrosomethylethyl-amine CAS N° 10595-95-6	Occurrence: 1) Tobacco smoke. 2) Foods: Smoked horsemeat, luncheon meats, bacon, chicken, complete meats containing mushrooms, cured meats.	Ps.C.H.
N-Nitroso-*N*-methyl-urea CAS N° 684-93-5	Use: 1) Its has been commonly used for the laboratory synthesis of Diazomethane, but it has been largely replaced by other reagents. 2) Its has been studied for use as a cancer chemotherapy agent. 3) Its has also been studied for its mutagenic effects on various plants.	Pr.H.C.
N-Nitrosomethylvinyl-amine CAS N°: 4549-40-0	Occurrence: In apple brandy	Ps.C.H.

Compound	Use and/or Occurrence	Eval.
N-Nitrosomorpholine CAS N° 59-89-2	Use: 1) As a solvent of polyacrylonitrile. 2) As a intermediate in the synthesis of N-Amino-morpholine. 3) It has been found to be effective against micro-bial infections. Occurrence: In solvents: Dichloromethane and Chloroform.	Ps.C.H.
N´-Nitrosonornicotine CAS N° 53759-22-1	Occurrence: 1) Cigarette smoke. 2) Tobacco	Ps.C.H.
N-Nitrosopiperidine CAS N° 100-75-4	Occurrence: 1) Tobacco smoke. 2) Water. 3) Foods: Cheese, fish, meat, spices. 4) Feeds: In samples of rabbit diet, in experimental animal feed.	Ps.C.H.
N-Nitrosopyrrolidine CAS N° 930-55-2	Occurrence: 1) Air. 2) Tobacco. 3) Waste-water. 4) Foods: Meats and fish products, spices. 5) Feeds: Animal feed. 6) In vivo: in blood of persons who ingested cooked bacon.	Ps.C.H.
N-Nitrososarcosine CAS N° 13256-22-9	Occurrence: Foods: Smoked meat, boiled ham, bologna, meat-loaf.	Ps.C.H.
Streptozotocin CAS N° 18883-66-4	Use: It has been investigated as a potential antibac-terial agent, but never used as such commercially. It has been investigated for use in diabetes. It has been used clinically in the treatment of tu-mors of the pancreatic B-Cells. It is active in the treatment of malignant carcinoid tumors.	Ps.C.H.

Bibliography Table 17:

N-Nitrosodi-n-butylamine, N-Nitrosodiethanolamine, N-Nitrosodiethyl-amine, N-Nitrosodimethylamine, N-Nitrosodi-n-propylamine, N-Nitroso-N-ethylurea, N-Nitrosodimethylamine, N-Nitroso-N-ethylurea, N-Nitrosomethylvinylamine, N-Nitrosomorpholine, N-Nitrosonornicotine,

N-Nitrosopiperidine, N-Nitrosopyrrolidine, N-Nitrososarcosine, Strepto-zotocin: (IARC, 1978b; 1987b), *3-Methylnitrosaminepropionitrile, 4-(Methylnotrosamino)-1-(3-pyridyl)-1-butanone:* (IARC, 1985c; 1987b).

To sum up

We have described substances and Techniques related, with real or potential technopathogenic risk. Other Techniques could be enclosed, for example the Techniques applied in drinking water. Although the destruction of microbiological pathogens is very important, the substances used as disinfectants: chloramines, chlorine, chlorine dioxide, chlorite, chlorate, and iodine, as well as the disinfectants by-products: bromate, chlorophenols (2-chlorophenol, 2,4-dichlorophenol, and 2,4,6-trichlorphenol), formaldehyde, MX, trihalomethanes (bromoform, bromodichloromethane, dibrochloromethane and chloroform), and other chlorination by-products: monochloroacetic acid, dichloroacetic acid, and tricloroacetic acid, are substances with potentially harmful long-term effects on humans. Although the evidence is considered inadequate, epidemiological studies have reported "a positive association between the ingestion of chlorinated drinking water and mortality rates from cancer, particularly of the bladder" (WHO, 1996).

We have seen how an uncountable amount of substances, either natural or artificial and of usage or contaminants, can cause technopathogenies by individual action. However, there is another theory in connection to the substances and their joint action:

Theory V: Technopathogeny as a global and additive phenomenon

The short description of technopathogenic risk caused by contaminants, apart from the substances already considered, allows us to support the environment hypothesis of cancer. As we have said before, this hypothesis is internationally accepted as the etiological origin of such diseases. Let us bear in mind that 60 to 90% of neoplasias have as etiological causes factors which are present in the human environment – among them, technopathogens.

The non-evident negative aspects of Technique constitute the critical point to define the study of Technopathogenology.

Once we were open to this approach, we found a myriad of substances causing technopathogenies. We thus incorporated in our study – which had begun with mycotoxins and pesticides – nitrosamines, dioxins, nitroarenes, and combustion products (benzopyrenes). We thus saw the need of an efficient prophylaxis methodology. When we thought of the possibility of all these substances acting at the same time, the elements in common started coming up to light. Some of them had and anthropogenic origin – that is, they were created by humans – and others were not produced by humans – such as mycotoxins and other contaminants. However, as we have commented in the previous chapter, the risk or damaging circumstances were caused by action or omission of the technical human being.

The hypotheses spawned by the study of chemical substances that lead to consider Technopathogeny as an integral problem were the following:

Hypothesis: Chemical Technopathogenies: Is Analytical Chemistry enough for prevention?

We have already analyzed this possibility for the specific case of mycotoxins. We have also observed the limitations with pesticides. We could make this analysis extensive to all the substances.

Analytical Chemistry is a valuable tool to identify them, detect their presence in the environment as well as to prevent exposure on humans. But we have seen the enormous effort involved in using Analytical Chemistry to prevent mycotoxins to prevent only one group of them – aflatoxins. This effort was applied to the development of a new technique, the Self Activated Thin Layer Chamber-Plate, a simple and inexpensive method, which can be applied practically everywhere where there are grains potentially contaminated with aflatoxins. This solved one problem in particular. However, the effort was far too great for a single cause of technopathogeny. Paradoxically, the bigger effort consisted in trying to find simple and accessible means that could be applied in the rural environment to detect minimum quantities. Trying to detect 2 to 5 micrograms per kilo requires a much greater effort than using normal devices.

If only one substance required such a great effort, it would be practically impossible to develop simple analytical techniques for the myriad of natural, artificial usage or contaminant substances which can potentially cause technopathogenies.

In addition, analytical chemistry has certain limitations, as we have said, regarding the capacity of detection of minimum quantities and, even though a no-risk limit could be established for the carcinogenic effect, humans could be not only exposed to one substance but to a myriad of them.

Therefore, the other two hypotheses that contributed to verify this fifth theory were the following:

Hypothesis: Does the fact that further determination is not possible imply that it has no effect?

Hypothesis: What would happen if all the hazardous substances acted in conjunction?

In order to try to find an answer to these questions, we analyzed Prof. Preussman's (Heidelberg) studies on the combined effects of carcinogenic substances. Professor Preussman (Preussman, 1972) proposes a *zero tolerance* for carcinogenic substances. However, we could not find an answer to this question: Which effects do low concentrations of various toxic substances have when acting in conjunction on the human organism, even when being so low individually that each substance cannot be further detected?

What we have stated in the first hypothesis suggests using Analytical Chemistry to identify the potentially risky substance. As we have said before regarding Analytical Chemistry, we see that not only the development of sophisticated techniques is very complex and expensive. We are referring to complex laboratory techniques, as well as to easy to apply techniques in environments where potentially technopathogenic chemical agents can be found but there is no complex laboratory in the area to analyze the samples. Apart from the complexity and the cost of development of these techniques, we also have to consider that no matter how precise the technique is, there will always be a limit of detection. When we added small quantities of aflatoxins that were not detected, we wonder if that could also happen with the rest of the contaminants. That is to say, if small quantities of contaminants in samples classified as free of contaminants are somehow not perceived.

If it is impossible to identify a substance when it is below the levels of detection, it will be even more difficult to identify a large quantity of

substances. Therefore, as we have said in connection to aflatoxins, *it is better to avoid the development of mold rather than detecting aflatoxins*, we could generalize this principle for all the substances saying that:
It is better to prevent the technological error rather than detecting the technopathogen generated by such error.

Thus leading to another hypothesis:

Hypothesis: Is it necessary to eliminate hazardous substances as a form of prevention?

We have proved that this is essential, since each of them could be present in such a diluted way that even though it could not be detected it could constitute a hazard on human health since each substance does not act independently. At a later stage, when we refer to the characteristics of neoplastic diseases and their causal agents, we will further analyze this issue.

So far we have referred to chemical substances and the technopathogenic risk they entail. But not only chemical substances are used or produced by Technique. This is how a new hypothesis came up:

Hypothesis: Are chemical substances the only technopathogenic hazards?

The analysis performed on Techniques using other knowledges (physical, biological) which will be described below, easily permitted falsifying this hypothesis. We have seen that other techniques contribute to what was stated in the fifth theory about the overall and additive phenomenon of technopathogeny.

Technopathogenies and physical factors

There are several technopathogens of a physical nature, such as: radio frequencies, microwaves, electric fields and magnetic fields, etc. normally known as *electro-smog* (International Conference on Cell Tower Siting, 2000). We could also include ionizing radiations, including those generated by nuclear contamination.

We will briefly refer to the risks on health associated with electromagnetic fields and ionizing radiation associated to the exposure to nuclear energy.

Electromagnetic fields

In some laboratory studies it was observed that electromagnetic fields are connected to the following damages on health (NIEHS-DOE, 1995):

- Changes in the functioning of cells and tissues.
- Decrease in the melatonin hormone.
- Alteration of immune system.
- Changes in biorhythm.
- Changes in human brain activity and heart rate.
- Accelerated tumor growth.

Some studies in humans have observed:

- Risk of miscarriage.
- Possible link between occupational EMF exposure and increased incidence of Alzheimer's disease.
- Association between EMF and breast cancer.
- Statistically significant increased risk of several types of cancer in occupational groups. For example: leukemia.

All these effects can be framed within technopathogenic effects.

In connection to cancer, even though lab studies have demonstrated that it is unlikely that electromagnetic fields can initiate the development of tumors, they suggest they can indeed promote the development of certain types of cancer (NIOSH-NIEHS-DOE, 1996). Shortly we will refer to this characteristic of neoplastic diseases, which are highly relevant to our study.

As for the incidence of cancer, breast tumors are mentioned in men and women (NIEHS-DOE, 1995). Also a major incidence of leukemia in children living near transmission towers. A study carried out in Sweden investigating leukemia in children found a significant statistical increase in children living in places where there was an increase in the electromagnetic field (NIEHS-DOE, 1995).

A two-year study on experimental rats and mice did not show carcinogenic evidence in female rats and in mice of both sexes. The evidence in male rats is contradictory since what was found was an increase in the incidence of neoplasms in thyroid glands. This study showed no increase in the incidence of tumors in the areas where epidemiological studies in humans had suggested a connection between exposure to magnetic fields and tumor development (brain, mammary glands and leukemia) (US DHHS-PHS-NIH, 1992b). Another study was carried out in female rats in order to investigate the connection between electromagnetic fields and the development of breast cancer. The rats were previously treated with an initiating substance. However, such effect was not found (US DHHS-PHS-NIH, 1992c).

Even if there was not enough evidence found to establish the causal relationship between exposure to electromagnetic fields and a higher incidence of cancer, neither was evidence found to ensure the lack of risk. Therefore, and as we will see in Chapter IV, doubt makes it reasonably to adopt preventive measures so as to avoid excessive exposure.

Ionizing radiation and nuclear energy

In connections to the risks associated with nuclear energy, several works have been carried out.

Apart from the program developed by the WHO: International Project on Health Effects of the Chernobyl Accident (IPHECA), some authors have carried out studies among which we could mention:

In an article published in 2006, that is, 20 years after the incident, a high incidence of different types of cancer is mentioned. The article refers to a study carried out in Oblast Gomel, Belarus, in people who had been exposed to the radioactive cloud (Langfelder & Frentzel, 2006). Even though most cases were of thyroid cancer (see table below), there were also cases of cancer in the stomach, the lungs, the skin and prostate (in men). In women: breast, uterus, stomach and skin cancer.

In Berlin, Germany, a significant increase of the trisomy 21 (Down Syndrome) was detected.

Table 18: Thyroid cancer in Oblast Gomel (Belarus) after the Chernovyl incident
(Source: Langfelder, E., Frentzel, Chr. (2006)

Age	1973/85 Period	1986/88 Period	Increase
0-18	7	407	58 Times
19-34	40	211	5.3 Times
35-49	54	326	6 Times
50-64	63	314	5 Times
Over 64	56	146	2.6 Times

As we can see in table 18, the biggest incidence is manifested in children and adolescents – 58 times more than the same age group prior to the incident.

Later, we will analyze and develop a hypothesis about how the Science and Technology administration system fails to recognize the actual importance this risk entails. This attitude is clearly described in Langfelder and Frentzel's article (Langfelder & Frentzel, 2006):

> Even though the International Agency of Atomic Energy considers it a case closed, this cannot be minimized in any way. Neither are known the effects produced by the radioactive cloud in Western Europe countries. The problem with the concealing or hiding tactic is that should anything similar occur in Germany or Western Europe, the authorities would not be prepared to control the situation. In Germany, for example, if a situation of this kind occurred, about 6 million people would have to be evacuated. Neither are born in mind other scenarios, such as human error, or what could be worse, a terrorist attack.

In addition, another author includes other countries (Ukraine, Germany, Bulgaria, Belarus, Turkey, Croatia) and describes an increase of malformations in babies (Schmitz-Feuerhake, 2006).

This article mentions that official reports only acknowledge 50 deaths as direct victims of the Chernobyl incident (which includes the *liquidators* or *clean-up workers*: people in charge of protection and cleaning the area after the incident). According to this author, official reports have tried to underestimate the effects of the incident, for example, by minimizing the actual relationship between the increase of thyroid cancer in children and youngsters and the Chernobyl incident.

The author states that this data contradicts dramatically what the scientific literature is constantly publishing. An example is the malformation in children due to prenatal exposure. In countries such as Belarus, Ukraine and Turkey, as in the other countries cited above, an increase of malformations in new born babies was observed (see table 19), as well as an increase of abortions and perinatal mortality. This grave problem is illustrated in table 20. An increase in the Down Syndrome as well as other diseases in children was also observed. Thus the author concludes that the teratogenic effects spectrum through incorporated radiation is considerably higher to what the international guilds of atomic energy had evaluated considering the results of the investigations carried out after the nuclear explosions in Hiroshima and Nagasaki. These investigations were carried out much later after the explosion and it is believed that much of the data taken was not reliable. This is why extrapolating the results found in the Japanese cities is scientifically unreliable. The author also indicates that:

> The simple physical measurements of the punctual and remnant radiation doses, have no relation whatsoever with the real genetic or mutagenic effect of low radiation doses. The biological dosimetry demonstrated that the evaluation of doses through physical parameters is rather coarse and way below the real biological effect of radiation.

Table 19: Increase in malformations observed in new born babies after exposure in womb after Chernobyl incident. (Source: Schmitz-Feuerhake, I. 2006)

Region	Type of Effect
Belarus	
Central Register	Anencephaly, spina bifida, cleft lip and palate, polydactyly, limb shortening, oesophagus and intestine obstruction, various anomalies.
Gomel – Highly contaminated region	Congenital malformations
Gomel – Chechersky District	Congenital malformations
Mogilev Region	Congenital malformations
Brest Region	Congenital malformations
Ukraine	
Kiev – Polessky District	Congenital malformations
Turkey	
Turkey	Anencephaly spina bifida
Bulgaria	
Pleven Region	Heart malformation Multiple anomalies
Germany	
Central Registry of malformations in Western Germany	Cleft palate and lip
Bavaria	Cleft palate and lip Congenital malformations
Western Berlin Annual Report on Health, 1987	Malformations found in still born babies
Jena – Registry of Malformations	Isolated malformations

Table 20: Increase in still births, early infancy deaths, miscarriages and low weight at birth observed after the Chernobyl incident. (Source: Schmitz-Feuerhake, I. 2006)

Region	Type of Effect (*) Postpartum mortality includes still births and mortality of babies the first seven days after delivery
Belarus	
Various chosen regions	Postpartum deaths (*)
Chechersky District (Gomel)	Postpartum death
Gomel	Postpartum death
Ukraine	
Polessky District (Kiev)	Postpartum death – birth rate decrease – premature births
Lugyny Region	Postpartum death
Ukraine (cont.)	
Zhitomir Area – Kiev Region – Kiev City	Postpartum death Birth rate decrease
Germany	
Total (West and East Germany)	Postpartum death
South Germany	Death during early infancy
Bavaria	Postpartum death – Still births Birth rate decrease
Rest of Europe	
Greece – Hungary – Poland – Sweden	Still births
Poland	Death during early infancy
Norway	Miscarriage
Hungary	Low weight at birth
Finland	Premature births – Early infancy children with malformations – Decrease in birth rates – Still births

The article also describes an increase in the incidence of the Down Syndrome (see table 21) and health damages on children who had been exposed during the gestational period (see table 22).

Table 21: Down Syndrome increase observation after Chernobyl incident. (Source: Schmitz-Feuerhake, I. 2006)

Region	Result
Belarus – Central Region	1987/94 increase: near 17%. Significant increase after ninth month.
Western Europe	Increase started the first year after the accident. Reaches 22% in the second or third year.
Sweden	Slight increase in highly contaminated regions (30%).
Scotland – Lothian Region (740.000 inhabitants)	Significant increase in 1987 (twice as much significant).
South Germany	Supraregional evaluation of amniotic fluid.
East Berlin	Significant increase in ninth month.

Table 22: Childhood diseases observed after prenatal exposure to Chernobyl incident (malformations, Down Syndrome and cancer are not included) (Source: Schmitz-Feuerhake, I. 2006).

Region	Type of Effect (Malformations, Down Syndrome and cancer are not included)
Belarus	
Selected regions	Psychological development affected – intelligence affected Speech disorders
Chechersky (Gomel District)	Breathing, blood and circulatory systems organs diseases
Stolin Region (Brest Region)	Diseases in: breathing organs, blood and circulatory system, digestive system, digestive functions alterations.
Belarus – Ukraine – Russia	Psychological disorders, mental retardation, and other mental disorders.
Ukraine	
Polessky District (Kiev)	Breathing, blood and circulatory systems organs diseases
Rovno province	Childhood diseases
Immigrants from the irradiated regions arriving to Israel	Asthma

Apart from the adverse effects already mentioned, genotoxicity studies carried out in Austria, Germany and Norway have detected that chromosomal aberrations – among them dicentric chromosomes – had increased up to fourfold in Austria, two point sixfold in Germany and tenfold in Norway (Schmitz-Feuerhake, 2006).

We must return to what we have already mentioned in relation to accurate analysis as a solution to prevent a Technopathogeny. In this case, and from such approach, prevention could be achieved by framing this phenomenon within Analytical Chemistry. However, there will always be a limit that even the most accurate analysis technique will not be able to detect. If it is impossible to identify a substance, it will be even more difficult to identify a large amount of substances. This is why we say that: *It is better to prevent a Technopathogeny than detecting its potential causal factor.* Considering what we have said in connection with nuclear radiation, we can see that this concept can also be applied to techniques developed for dosimetric measurements of nuclear radiation exposure.

As for the nuclear energy risks, it is worth reading the opinion of the President of the Federal Office for Radiation Protection (Germany) (König, 2006):

> Chernobyl became a symbol of the loss of trust in politicians and officials responsible as well as on economy, but it was also a symbol of loss of credibility in Science. The explanations that scientists gave lacked enough grounding and showed that such explanations were influenced by political and economic interests.

The author concludes: "The risk is not hypothetical. It is real. This is the teaching Chernobyl has left."

Paraphrasing this author, we could say that: *Technopathogeny is not a theoretical lucubration lacking connection with the real world. It is not a hypothetical phenomenon but a real one, and as concrete as Technology itself.*

Based on the articles above quoted and the concepts explained by the author, especially the last one, referring to the credibility of science and to the fact that the risks posed by technique are not hypothetical but real, we can see that our proposal on the need to prevent these non-evident risks in the long term – which we call technopathogenic – is not wrong at all. The fact that what has been done until now is not enough – probably because the problem was not given proper significance thus lacking a specific science – supports this statement. Trivializing and minimizing the problem is like hiding dust under the rug. It may not be seen at the time, but sooner or later its presence will loom out. The German law aiming at the gradual substitution of atomic energy further supports our theory. According to this law, by 2023 all the nuclear plants must be disconnected and the energy they supply substituted by other sources (Stumpf, 2006). This shows how fragile the scientific community opinion is. Two or three decades ago no scientist in Germany would doubt defending the use of nuclear energy. But the energy they defended carried the germ of technopathogeny. When the evidence shown by the facts was undeniable, the scientific community started changing their mind little by little. Nowadays, after Chernobyl, only a few scientists would defend the use of nuclear energy based on that old criterion. Most of them now openly recognize its risks. As we will see later, experience recognizes the need to get rid of old programs or old paradigms.

On the other hand, even though some argue that the accident was caused by a human error since the plant was safe, technique can nevertheless not be separated from the human factor. A highly risky technique which depends on a human error and may, as a consequence of such error, bring about death and harm to an enormous amount of people – and also harm future generations, as we have seen in the comparison with the coal boiler (Eguiazu, 1991) – should have never been created.

Two or three decades ago, the minimization and trivialization of risks estimated by official institutions was usually not contradicted by the scientific community. This is now undergoing a change of paradigm that has many followers within the community.

Technopathogenies in genetic engineering

In order to carry out a thorough analysis of technopathogenic risks, we must also consider unexpected collateral effects of genetic engineering and the genetically modified organisms (GMOs) produced by it. The industry claims that this technique provides different types of benefit, for example, that it enhances turnout and quality (this will be dealt with in more detail in Chapter IV). We do not deny the benefits, the good will, and the efforts put forth on this search. However, this can also cause technopathogenies (Eguiazu & Motta, 2001c).

The genetically modified organisms (GMOs) are currently at the core of a very intense debate, both in our country (Clarín, 2000) and abroad (Parr, 2000). Even though this technique is expected to bring about high economic and ecological benefits, there are many objections to it (Institute of Science in Society, 2000) (Shiva Vandana, 1995). The most enthusiastic about this technique are the official organisms in charge of its approval as well as the companies involved (San Martín, 1987). Almost an 80% of Argentine soy and by-products are exported to the European market, which represents annually about 3000 million dollars (Anonimous, 1996). But the European market is increasingly reluctant to the consumption of GMOs (Mitchell, 1999).

We will now analyze the technopathogenic aspects of GMOs and the risk they entail (Bompiani, 2000).

What are Genetically Modified Organisms (GMOs)?

GMOs are organisms which have suffered a modification in their genome beyond that of classical genetic selection (Hansen, 1999). Genetic engineering is applied to protist, plants and higher animals (Jones, 1999). It began with the modification of bacteria, one of the first being Escherichia coli to which genes regulating the production of insulin was incorporated (San Martín, 1987). In vegetables, most of the work has been carried out in those of economic value, such as soy, corn or cotton.

The following modifications have been carried out:

a) In soy: the resistance to glyphosate, a herbicide (it makes soy more resistant to the increasing doses that must be used due to the adaptation of weeds).

b) In corn and cotton: the resistance to insects through the incorporation of the gene Bacillus thuringiensis, which regulates the production of the specific toxin.

This is not only used in crops. Just like there are advanced techniques of in vitro plant cultivation, animal organisms can be (and have been) obtained from a single cell, whether modified or not.

There are attempts to modify the cow milk composition by modifying the original genome incorporating genes that enhance the presence of substances which are of particular interest or that can act as vaccines.

As we can see, so far there is apparently nothing to worry about genetic engineering when it comes to improve production or to obtain new cultivars, for example. Now let's take a look at the differences between this new technique and the classical methods of animal and plant selection and improvement.

The classical form of selection

These techniques begin with what is known as mass selection. Given a plant population that requires improvement, the seeds of those samples that show phenotypic characteristics that have desirable properties are saved for the following harvest. This process has been carried out since antiquity and it requires no more than basic knowledge. The other technique used is called inbreeding (a plant population is first bred within itself). As the number of homozygote gene pairs increases, a pure line will result from selecting the individuals of interest. The gene sifting allows for the reproduction of those individuals which are of interest and not the others.

Afterwards, these pure lines can interbreed and the hybrid can be obtained (out of which superior characteristics are expected – as better yield, for example). This technique was regularly used until the 70s and through which the high yielding hybrids of today's agriculture were obtained.

However, such technique is considered responsible for producing the so-called genetic erosion through which the genome of a plant which was rich and varied in genes got much of its variability eliminated and with it, the capacity of adaptation to biological avatars. Some genes which were apparently useless to obtain the desired characteristics could have been very useful and get activated in unexpected situations thus saving a crop. Aiming at a better yield or other desirable agricultural characteristics, valuable resistance properties were ignored. As we have seen, this allowed us to formulate a hypothesis – subject to falsifiability – about the fact that the frequent and almost inevitable apparition of aflatoxins in Argentine corn was caused by this modification that did not bare in mind the storage factor as a characteristic to be taken into account by the selector. This means that this was a technopathogenological aspect of classical selection (Eguiazu, 1999a) (Eguiazu & Motta, 2001c).

However, this genetic erosion did not modify the genomes dramatically since the selection was carried out among individuals of the same species. It is very difficult to obtain dramatic alterations through this method since the sequence and position of the genes is not greatly modified.

With the classical techniques of selection of species, only in a few exceptional cases they can be hybridized but still breed barren individuals.

Two known examples are Triticale (breed of wheat and rye) and the mule (breed of horse and she-donkey or mare and donkey). We can ask ourselves then why nature has such strict barriers among species, barriers which were consolidated after thousands of years of evolution. Also, how come even if these species can cross and breed are their descendants barren? Even if they are different species they have similar characteristics, that is, they do not differ as much as a plant species and a bacteria. What is really revolutionary is the incorporation of genetic material in species which completely differ among themselves.

We can then state that even when nobody denies the right of researchers to cross these barriers in order to advance in knowledge, possible unexpected consequences should not be ignored. These technologists cannot ensure that going against nature will not bring about non-evident and not-acceptable collateral effects which can pose a risk on human health.

Genetic engineering modifications

Genetic engineering techniques are characterized by a real gene surgery in which genes are cut and replaced in one species genome, regardless of the fact they come from other species or even from human beings. These techniques allow for an amazing control of the characteristics that the bioengineer wants to implement. Through in vitro cultivation of plant callus, there is acceleration in the growth of generations of organisms, and of seedlings generated from a single cell taken from the plant callus through the adequate hormonal stimulus, even though this is not exclusive of genetic engineering – it can also be carried out in common plants (Brown, 2000).

What is being said in favor of extended usage of GMOs?

Arguments in favor of this technology

We will now see six arguments generally used to support this technology.

1) Freedom of research and free choice of the object of study

If there is a possibility of crossing the barriers of species and obtaining useful organisms, or by shear curiosity and advancement of knowledge, why should we not do it? Hasn't everything knowable the right to be known, and what's more, to be applied? Any attitude against this is a-scientific and obscurantist. Ecological organizations play with the general public's emotions generating collective hysteria turning the public against this without scientific proof.

2) Economic

The use of GMOs allows for saving in the use of pesticides and provides extra yields in crops. The labeling (identification) of a batch as transgenic is useless and expensive since it implies separating the crops in the field. It is irrelevant for consumers to know whether they are consuming transgenic food or not. It would be unnecessary to explain this to consumers. It is just another technique – such as hoe or disc plough. Advocates say it is expensive to separate the crop (for example, transgenic soy from non-transgenic soy) and force producers to do so.

3) Ethical

GMOs will allow us to increase food production to feed the hungry in the world.

We can also incorporate characteristics that enable mass consumption in poor areas, include elements which are currently lacking, such as genes that increase the content of iron in rice, or a vaccine in bananas which are massively consumed in poor areas.

Just like there are advanced techniques of in vitro plant cultivation, cloned animal organisms can be obtained from a single cell, whether modified or not. We can use this technique to clone humans in order to use their organs. The human clone is only a tissue that can be killed or used at will as an organ whose carrier has died.

4) Environmental

The use of GMOs will allow for a reduction of pesticides – especially by the use of plants that possess the gene that regulates the pesticide toxin, for example, the one generated by *Bacillus thuringiensis*, reducing the impact on the environment. The best and most specific control of insects will provide a better quality to grains and environment by not destroying beneficial insects.

5) Protection of health

This reduction in pesticides would considerably reduce the risk on applicators and consumers. A better control of insects would also avoid the entrance of Aspergillus flavus infection in corn (which produces aflatoxins and causes cancer). The GMOs technology is completely safe since it controls the gene and the characteristics it incorporates. Vaccines in plants and milk can also be incorporated thus benefiting health. We should not worry about transgenic foodstuffs, since they are substantially equivalent to the original plant or organism and so far no damaging effects in humans have been proved.

6) Institutional

In developing countries it could be said that we should trust organisms of control that work with responsibility and in collaboration with the most important transgenic centers in our country which work closely with their international counterparts. In addition, the extremely strict Science and Technique system and ethical scientists are saying that the GMOs are innocuous, that we must trust both them and the relevant institutions supporting them.

Who defends these reasons?

These reasons are usually given by the advocates of this technology – mostly working in the companies producing these seeds and their related supplies. They are also given by official organisms of control and by the research centers developing GMOs (Eguiazu & Motta, 2001c).

Arguments against the extended usage of GMOs

A concept that arises here (and maybe in every technique) is the doubt as to whether the controls on these technologies are honest and efficient enough to avoid getting out of control (Thurau, 1989).

Although the GMOs are considered a possible solution for the shortfall of cereals for feeding the human population predicted for a near future, "there is considerable disagreement about the advisability of using such crops, particularly in Europe" (Purchase, 2004).

Which are the reasons used against a complete freedom to use this technology?

1) Health risks

About this aspect, an author (Purchase, 2004) mentions that:

> Obviously the safety of the food derived from the GM crops is a primary consideration. Safety assessment relies on establishing that the food is substantially equivalent to its non-GM counterpart and specific testing for allergenicity of proteins and toxicity of metabolites and the whole food.

There are human health reasons to forbid its usage, unless there is a prior strict technopathogenological control (Ewen & Pusztai, 1999b) (Feldbaum, 1999) (Lachmann, 1999).

It has been proved that GMOs can be allergenic in some cases. It is also feared that the incorporation of a strange gene can produce unexpected interactions with metabolic regulations that can lead to the production of harmful substances. This is the case of toxins that appear in crops which would otherwise not produce them. Arpad Pusztai's work (Anonimous, 2000b) (Berger, 1999) (Brown, 1999) (Rhodes) produces the falsification of the GMOs innocuousness hypothesis.

This researcher discovered that certain transgenic potatoes, to which a gene of another species had been incorporated (Galanthus nivalis), which acted as a pesticide through a specific lectin, had unacceptable collateral effects on lab rats. These collateral effects were, for example, major alterations in intestine villi. Had these potatoes been used for human consumption, negative effects in humans would have been expected (Ewen & Pusztai, 1999a).

In general, it is said that modifications produced in the organism when alien genetic material is incorporated are so small in relation to the amount of original genes that it determines that the genome prevails practically untouched and we could speak of a substantial equivalence. This would mean that the transgenic modification will not alter the substantial elements of the species. In other words, the transgenic element would be substantially equal to the same species unmodified. This would be correct if the modifications were of such nature that they would not imply an unexpected risk on the consumer. But we cannot speak of a substantial equivalence. If the modifications produced unexpectedly by the incorporated gene are harmful, they will not be substantially equivalent to the original non-harmful species. The adverse consequences of this unexpected non-equivalence (technopathogenies) are not excluded enough beforehand (Sanders, 1999) (Watson, 1999).

As part of the genetic modification technique, antibiotic resistance genes are incorporated – of interest only as indicators in an intermediate stage, in order to ensure that the gene of economic interest has been incorporated. This means an unnecessary load of antibiotic in the human trophic chain. It is not clear whether they could generate bacteria strains which are excessively resistant to antibiotics as in the cases of consumption of antibiotics for therapeutic reasons. It is thought that the synthetic genome obtained can be transferred completely or partially to other organisms (Gebhardm & Smalla, 1998) increasing the uncertainty on potential risks (Bateson, 1999) (Beringer, 1999) (Crawford, 1999) (Fisken, 1999) (Horton, 1999a, 1999b) (Klug, 1999) (Mercer, 1999) (Mitchell & Bradbury, 1999) (Pirisi, 1998) (Sanders, 1999).

Other reasons

These are some of the reasons supporting a criterion of precaution in the development of Genetically Modified organisms (GMOs) (Asscher, 1999) (Greenpeace, 1998):

2) Freedom of research and free choice of the object of study

Even if it is important that the advancement of knowledge and its application move forward without restrictions, not everything knowable has the right to be known, and not everything that is doable must be done.

All this is supported by recent examples related to the atomic bomb. The atomic bomb was the consequence of the naive belief of scientists that knowledge would correct itself and everything would be for the better. Another supporting argument states that upon the advancement of knowledge in risky areas or even harmful ones (armament) it would be better for scientists to self direct their object of study, thus avoiding to insist in questions that may lead to highly risky results on humans. Not every advancement in knowledge, just for the sake of advancement, is positive.

3) Economic

The arguments against refer essentially to the fact that the development of GMOs is a great business for multinational corporations which develop and commercialize them. They expect a return of the money invested in their research and development. This benefit will not reach agricultural producers nor consumers, who will not pay less for flour elaborated with Bt-corn or soy by products elaborated with transgenic soy resistant to glyphosate. It is also said that the fact that importing countries consumers may turn against the consumption of GMOs – Europe, specifically, where most part of soy production is consumed – risks the producing country's economy if importers cede to the consumer's pressure. To support the frailty or indeterminacy of the economic justification as an example we can resort to the well known case of bacteria modified with insulin producing genes. It was found that the final product did not turn out to be as profitable as expected (San Martín, 1997).

4) Ethical

It has not been sufficiently proved that the consumer obtains additional benefits (Anonymous, 2000a) (Hansson, 1999). We cannot say that the hungry of the world are eating more or better thanks to transgenic food, since it is not inexpensive and the problem of hunger will probably remain as it is today: it is a problem of distribution rather than quantity. The hungry have no currency to pay for food and they will most likely remain hungry. The ones who own foodstuffs prefer to use it to feed developed world animals rather than sell it for very little money or for a symbolic price to the hungry of the rest of the world. Neither was the consumer asked for prior consent as it is done in the first human trials of any medicine or risky technology. Consumers must know they consume foodstuffs elaborated with transgenic raw material and the supporters of this position agree that this must be clearly specified in the label. Consumption is random. The Hans Jonas principle of responsibility (Jonas, 1984) so far cannot be applied, since it cannot be scientifically proved that there will not be collateral effects after its usage (Druker & Roth, 1999) (Holden, 1999).

Another point is connected to the usage of human genetic material to be incorporated in cells of superior animals or to produce a hormone of an interest in particular, since it is not clear yet whether it would be the same as using human parts in animal transplants. This is critical when there is talk of the possibility of cloning a human being to use the parts of the embryo. Religious ethics, especially Catholicism, believe that (Nuñez de Castro, 2000):

> An embryo is a complete human being and it must therefore be fully respected, whether it was conceived by natural means, in vitro or by cloning.

5) Environmental

It is feared that these techniques generate superplants hard to beat. It has been demonstrated that some wild crops hybridize with GMOs bringing about unpredictable consequences (Anonymous, 1999) (Mayer & Meister, 2000) (Mikkelsen, 1996). The toxin present in Bt-gene corn for insect control can be harmful to useful insects (Elmore, 2000) (Greenpeace, 2000) (Losey, 1999).

In some cases, there is a suppressive effect in the incorporated gene that requires the need to apply pesticides (this is what happened with cotton plantations in the USA). This makes it necessary to apply pesticides in spite of the Bt-gene.

The apparent advantage of the GMOs would not last indefinitely. The insect would get adapted to the incorporated gene which would require the need to go back to normal pesticides.

Also, there is evidence indicating that RR-Soy (which is resistant to glyphosate active principle) might threaten agricultural production (Greenpeace, 1996) since the crop gradually gets more resistant to increasingly higher doses of the pesticide. This resistance has a limit (Preciado Patiño).

6) Institutional

Official institutions that allow for the usage of these organisms are not always reliable.

An author (Purchase, 2004) says that:

> The public's perception of the risk of new technology is critical to its acceptance. In turn their perception of risk depends on the credibility of the source of the information and trust in the regulatory process. In many countries the public appears to have lost its trust in the scientists and government dealing with genetically modified food, making the acceptability of genetically modified crops uncertain.

184

Another example of this loss of trust is the high tolerance to pesticides of risk. In Argentina the use of some pesticides was allowed in spite of being considered carcinogenic in developed countries. There must have been an official institution that authorized or allowed the import of such pesticides.

The fact that official institutions have released transgenic crops is connected to yielding to the pressure of interested corporations and research institutes. You cannot be both judge and party and national agencies have decided under the pressure of interests. Something similar happened in the USA with the Food and Drug Administration (FDA) (Druker & Roth, 1999) when authorizing the use of transgenic soy.[2]

The ethics of the Science and Technique system and their principal actors is not always what one would expect. This questionable ethics could smudge the transparency and publication of the collateral aspects or indetermination of some technology if it does not favor the major economic investment claiming for urgent return. Neither the principle of substantial equivalence would make institutional sense. The fact that most of the discoveries are patented by the companies that develop them is contradictory with the idea that the transgenic is substantially equivalent to the original crop. If it is equivalent, why should they patent it? It would seem that the *manufacturers* of these transgenic products would reason this way: *Our product is substantially equivalent regarding its possible risks but it is at the same time substantially non-equivalent regarding the positive effects we have incorporated in it.* This is the only way we could understand the concept of substantial equivalence. Now, from the logical point of view we can see that this concept does not make much sense.

The disadvantage entailed by this kind of technology is also discussed by other authors.

An author (Buntzel, 2006) mentions that on the one hand, the benefits would not reach producers – especially small ones – and, on the other, the valuable craft of cultivation – transmitted from generation to generation – will be inevitably lost. The excessive simplification of something that is so complex and diversified will not favor the sustainability of agriculture in the long term.

---

2   FDA documents prove that the institution ignored the scientist's warnings concerning the safety of consumption of transgenic organisms.

As its name indicates it, agriculture is the culture of biological organisms, which are amazingly different and variable. Sometimes, the in-depth knowledge of a living organism out of which humans obtain benefits has led to the slow accumulation of intergenerational knowledge. This knowledge can get lost in one generation if it is ignored, in this case, when this knowledge is replaced by the simplicity of the machine and a chemical product.

Other researchers specialized in social or political sciences can surely carry out more profound analysis regarding the *technological dependence* on big corporations. We have even heard about conventional selection that the best plant breeder is the one who *discards a lot and retains only a little*. Discarding a lot implies losing genetic variability. This is known as *genetic erosion*. If such variability is needed in the future, the solution will be found in big corporations or in the varieties they produce. This is referred to conventional selection, but also applies to GMOs.

Which is our position as technopathogenologists?

In the reading included in Chapter IV in connection to Technopathoge-nology and its contribution to a strict regulation of international commerce of risky substances (in this case, pesticides), we will mention that in a meeting where we dealt with such topic we manifested the following principle: if in doubt, choose what benefits humans (Eguiazu, 1996). We were referring to whether risky pesticides which were banned (or suspected of being risky) in developed countries should be used in developing countries. We could apply the same principle to GMOs. In such meeting we had to oppose to the official position which stated that risky pesticides were to be used until developing countries had their own and exhaustive toxicological studies (Eguiazu, 1988). The government position included the concepts of sovereignty and automatic exclusion: we could not adopt the position of the developed country automatically because on the one hand, we did not know whether the prohibition was objectively funded and, on the other, the automatic adoption of another country's criteria would attempt against national sovereignty.

This suspiciously favored the usage of the risky substance. In the case of GMOs, the substantial equivalence principle is equivalent to the principle of let's use the product until negative effects appear which was used in the case of pesticides (or even the less serious argument of sove-reignty).

Our principle will be *In dubio pro homine*. If in doubt let us favor the common folk, poor and ignorant, who will perish as a hamster by the flaws or doubts of the system and by the arrogance of scientists who dogmatize the infallibility of their method and the innocuousness of their technology. This is the precaution Principle.

Any other principle would not be ethically sustainable. This means an undetermined moratorium on use of the substance until there is enough scientific proof of its innocuousness – not just reasoning about a probable innocuousness and even less blind faith in the infallibility of scientific method. Proof must be experimental and presented in such a way that it can be falsified. Consumers must be able to have access to such proof in a transparent and immediate way. The absence of factors that can cause technopathogenies must be thoroughly proved since, in Prof. Beck's words, "The non-verification of an existent does not mean the verification of a non-existent."

To sum up: there must be evidence of a thorough technopathogeno-logical research prior to sending the GMOs to cultivation. If there is no such evidence, our position is to adopt the precaution criterion already indicated (Christie, 1999).

Technopathogeny in other fields of Technique

We have already analyzed the technopathogenic risks associated with chemical, physical and biological factors.

Even though we have not explored this area yet, the study of tech-nopathogenic risks would not be complete if we didn't mention that just like humans, as Prof. Beck analyzes (Beck, 1970):

> Humans are dominated by the ideology of doing everything through technique: in the field of physics through physical technique and chemical technique, in the bio-logical field through biotechnology

So, we must also include other two techniques from the field of culture considered by Prof. Beck: Psychotechnology and Sociotechnology.

The first is defined as the branch of practical psychology which, bear-ing in mind the results obtained through psychognosty – that is, by know-ing through scientific and accurate means the psychological behavior of a person through the study of its diverse scientific and professional aptitudes – aims at treating and orienting individuals adjusting to their psychic aptitudes (Diccionario Enciclopédico Ilustrado de la Lengua Española, 1962). We can then think of which errors in this technique can generate psychological factors that can harm the individual or a social group. We could consider it as a form of Iatrogenesis of Psychotechnology.

Also, Sociotechnology is defined as the "transformation of the ways of society through rational methods, for example, the destruction of society structures to construct new structures" (Beck, 1979a). We can then think of defects or imperfections in the procedures or techniques applied for the transformation of society or for the construction of new structures of society that lead to unexpected harm within the society itself.

V.   Technopathogeny: Preliminary analysis of the situation

Summarizing what we have seen in this chapter so far we can see that all these topics – from mycotoxins to Genetic Engineering – share three fundamental characteristics:

a) They have been originated in or caused by Technology.
b) They have a consequence or effect in common: harming the human health.
c) In spite of the previsions of Science and Technique that assured its non-existence, they were manifested when the technique was applied.

Let us add (and it is interesting to highlight it since it is a valuable contribution to Technopathogeny) what we have already mentioned regarding cancer and neoplasias: that there are 200 diseases grouped under cancer, and that it is a multifactor disease regarding its cause and multistage regarding its development process. Nevertheless, even though cancer maybe one of the most significant hazards to health, it is not the only type of Technopathogeny. This characteristic of neoplastic diseases let us see that the diversity of factors generated by technique that can damage health will not act by themselves, neither will they be associated with a specific damage on health. As we have said before, these charac-

188

teristics of neoplastic diseases and of factors causing them imply that even if the carcinogenic property is discovered, it is very difficult to prevent their risk. Even if there is legislation forbidding its usage – if a carcinogenic substance is used in a technique – or making a compulsory analysis and control if it is a contaminant – if the person was already exposed during a certain amount of time, he or she might end up getting the disease. This example further supports the notion that a correct or anticipated prophylaxis in technology would be the logical road towards successful prevention.

In addition, the cellular events involved in the manifestation of neoplastic diseases was what allowed us to support the idea of using the concept of Biopathological instead of the previously considered Ecotoxicological. As we have explained, the latter is closely linked to Ecology. The concept Biopathological comes from the term *pathobiological* which we have already used. This term is used in a study on tobacco smoke aldehydes to define the harmful effects generated by these substances. Some examples are:

- The reduction of clonal growth in epithelial cells
- Damage of DNA
- Mutation
- Inhibition in the repair of damaged DNA

Such effects are related to the initiation and promotion of the carcinogenesis process caused by aldehydes (Grafström *et al.*, 1987). That is to say, effects manifested in the long-term. This is why we can make the concept of Technopathogeny extensive not just to substances but also to any other factor present in the environment capable of generating or inducing cellular effects as the above mentioned as well as other similar effects which could cause a technopathogeny. We could also consider such factors as determinants of the biopathological quality in the human environment.

Even though we will later propose a hypothesis involving Ecology, we could say that Ecotoxicology is the science that studies the effect of xenobiotics in the ecosystem. By extension it was used many times as the science to study the behavior, for example, of pesticides in the environment and the residues left on the water, soil, air, organisms and food. However, Ecology as a science focuses more on the xenobiotic effect of organisms. It says nothing of its importance in terms of its concrete effect in humans, as well as on the condition of such effect. This is why the term Biopathological is much more accurate than the term Ecotoxicological. In Chapter IV we will further discuss the issue of the quality of human environment. Even if the knowledge of a substance and its effect on organisms or the ecosystem is important, the main interest of Technopathogenology is centered on the capacity of the substance to reach exposed surfaces of humans and have a <u>non-evident</u> concrete negative effect. Of course in order for the xenobiotic to reach the exposed surfaces in some cases it needs the ecosystem trophic chains but the impact on it would be secondary to our aim and its study is the object of Ecotoxicology. Ecotoxicological information can be valuable twofold: It can provide information on the biological transport of xenobiotics and it gives the possibility of resorting to organisms of the ecosystem that manifest the effect of the substance as biological indicators. Apart from the information provided by this science, we are interested in the information generated by human toxicology and, of course, the circumstance in which the substance is used and its possible relationship with the product to be consumed.

What we have described so far allows us to propose a sixth theory:

Theory VI: Prevention is the only reasonable way
for the technopathogeny phenomenon

Because of what we have already described, we should not speak only of factors present in the human environment being the human environment a vector, but of negative effects coming from chemical, physical or biological factors whose individual adverse effects may not be detectable. But, as we have said before, what happens when such adverse actions are combined? Why does a fronton wall have to be that strong if it only has to bear a small, light ball hitting it?

We thus saw the need of an efficient prophylaxis methodology. When referring to the technopathogenic risk specifically in relation to substances we started weighing the possibility of focusing our research on prophylaxis. But when we actually grasped the global problem of technopathogeny, we realized the only reasonable way to find a solution we could come up with was prevention – a rather unique form of prevention.

We very clearly saw that among all these measures of prophylaxis the individual pathogenic risk factors could not be determined – which would allow to determine which had to be stopped from reaching humans. This would take too long and it would be too late to save lives. There are certain toxicology tests such as the Ames test and other more modern tests that can, for example, provide for an early detection of potential harmful substances. As a result of our INCABIE program a book with indications and prophylaxis of mutagens in the environment focusing on the usage of the above mentioned test was published.

The fact that there are so many substances of use, as well as contaminants, that can have a technopathogenic risk, a complete analysis of a foodstuff in particular, for example, to identify all the risky substances present in it would always be imperfect and enormously complicated. This is why we think it is more realistic to take a sample of a foodstuff and supply it to a living organism. Even though the risky substance or substances are below the limit of detection, it is reasonable to think that they would manifest their effect acting either independently or in combination. Moreover, if the foodstuff proves positive in the bacteria trial, we might not be able to identify the substances responsible for it, but at least we could determine that such foodstuff has a mutagenic factor. It could also be used as a primary test to later determine the mutagenic factor of a substance.

Taking Chemical Technology as an example, the concrete fact is that humans produce substances hastily with a useful aim, but when it is proved that such substances are harmful, the honest practise would be to retrieve such substances from the market. However, there are unethical practices which, instead of terminating the manufacture of a harmful substance, send it to countries where there is still no legislation that controls or prohibits such substance.

This is a very inefficient method and it leaves behind plenty of suffering. This is similar to planting a fast growing tree and then trying to get rid of it by plucking one leave per day. It is a very primitive method.

This led to the following question: What should total protection be like?

Total protection means, among other things, a change of paradigm – for example, by adjusting the concept of quality to protect consumers rather than business. In connection to this, we have proposed a few new quality criteria which, although connected to food, could be extended to the whole human environment (Eguiazu & Motta, 1991, 1996) – which we will deal with more thoroughly in Chapter IV.

On the scientific level, total protection means a change of scope, a search for scientific and technical methods that allow for an effective prophylaxis.

Some philosophers saw the need to produce changes in science. For example: According to Kuhn, this need of changing the scope or, as he calls it, *paradigm*, (Kuhn, 1995):

> It is an irrational process produced not by a rational well-supported discourse, but by the historical clash of generations, that is, among defenders of the old paradigm against defenders of the new one.

Lakatos (Lakatos, 1982), on the other hand, goes back to Popperian falsifiability and proposes a revised version:

> A theory will be eliminated only when it can be replaced by a new theory that not only explains the previous theory's achievements but also presents the capacity of predicting surprising new facts.

Feyerabend (Feyerabend, 1986), Popper's disciple, considers that:

> Science is closer to myth than science philosophers want to admit. Therefore, science must not become a State aggressive philosophy and become an instrument of an almighty State.

These are the arguments we use to support our proposal, which we consider more self-explanatory and thorough. The old program, which ignored the technopathogeny phenomenon, is thus substituted by the new program incorporating this phenomenon. Had we achieved this aim, it was due to:

- Not because the rational nature of our proposal, but because of the strong defense of our paradigm against a system or generation that tried to stop it from happening.
- Having proposed and supported new theories that allow tackling the technological problems with the efficiency needed, eliminating fallacious theories that tried to justify it.
- Our contributions to other existing proposals and other disciplines or multidisciplines which also try to remedy it or mitigate the phenomenon.

192

- Having survived an almighty Science and Technique system which, as instrument to exercise its power, turned into ideology scientific criteria only supported by authoritarianism – a system which reserves the right to decide what, how, when, where and with whom a scientific activity can be carried out.

Going back to the tree example, we can say that we started with leaves, but without plucking them. We climb down through them and we pass on to branches, and then on to thicker branches and then to the main trunk. So, as we distance ourselves from the leaves we get to the trunk. And this is how we get to the critical point of our research since climbing down the trunk we find the tree roots, in other words, the central point where the problem can be tackled. Prevention must be sought for in the roots of the technological germinal matrix.

We can then go back once again to the tree example, to analyze the need of an effective prophylaxis. Let us consider a fruit tree. If after planting it, waiting for it to grow and bear fruit we discover that the fruit quality is not good and we then realize that the soil where we planted it was not adequate, there is nothing we can do once the fruit is mature; we cannot improve its quality. What we can do is to take measures for the following harvest (fertilize the soil, etc.). This is how science and technique sometimes works.

We can compare bad quality fruit with substances which are found to be carcinogenic, mutagenic or teratogenic after their application. These unexpected effects are consequences of a series of previous mistakes that go back to their roots, that is to say, the way in which science is made.

The architect example

In one of our papers we used the architect example. An architect can detect an error or omission in a plan (designed by him or her or by somebody else) and correct it. By observing and detecting the defects (errors in calculation, for example), the architect can prevent the construction so that such mistakes are not translated into flaws that may cause the structure to collapse (Motta, 1994). In our field of study, we have perceived the need of a science that detects the errors in the symbolic *plan* of a technique in concrete that can cause a technopathogeny.

In our work, we have observed that every time we managed to clarify a part of the phenomenon, we automatically found a lateral question which allowed us to further investigate. It would have been a lot easier if we hadn't found that lateral question and had continued trying to find only the answer to the original question. For example, in the case of mycotoxins, instead of trying to further investigate the secondary question – irrelevant to Technopathogenology – which arose later (on molds). That is to say, if we just kept the thread we have pulled from Goblot's skein without further pulling, we would have reduced the original phenomenon and kept on producing articles only on that aspect of the phenomenon. But the questions that arose digressed from the relative comfort of the established discipline. And we chose to keep digging in the skein. We chose to repeat this procedure many times until we finally were able (after our first attempt on framing the phenomenon in the various disciplines, as we will further discuss later) to verify the aporia that there was no existing discipline to study the phenomenon so we had to create it. We then arrived, as the term defines it, to the logical difficulty of trying to frame the problem in a science that still did not exist.

This way, and using our experience with mycotoxins – the use of an analytical technique to detect a natural toxic substance that has a negative effect (hepatocarcinogenic) – we arrived to an unexpected conclusion. This conclusion was that in spite of dealing with a natural substance, such substance was produced or favored by the action of human technique. This way, the problem fell out of the scope of natural sciences to become an undesirable consequence of an ill-conceived technique. Technique, by action and omission, was much more relevant to the genesis of the toxin and the actual harm produced by it than its observation in the natural sciences fields. Therefore, it was included within the family of various techniques that produced negative side effects on humans in the long term thus stressing the need of a complete prevention of this phenomenon.

VI.   Searching for a solution

The need of a science that allows detecting and avoiding the Technopathogenic phenomenon is undeniable (Motta, 1994).

We have already mentioned that the Greeks considered that through what is true all other goods can be reached. We could add to this that (Goblot, 1943):

> Because of this, the Greeks try to find a Cannon and a τεχνη (Techne: Art or Technique) in everything. As we have said before, "The ambition of the Greeks consists in executing all their tasks according to clear, certain and well funded rules."

But the problem is enormously complex. The question that comes out of all this is: which are the Cannon and Technique with which to handle the technological process in such a way as to avoid altering the proportion and correspondence (harmony) among the elements of the human environment and humans themselves in such a way that they are not harmful to their own lives? Which are the Cannon and Techniques that allow to rule science in such a way that the knowledge used to develop new techniques is authentic and strictly true?

Going back to the architect analogy, there is a law which the architect cannot neglect: The Law of Gravity. This determines the adequate structure and elements needed in a construction in order to avoid accidents.

As we can see, the situation is simple for the construction technique, but this is not so for many other techniques. As we will see at a later stage, Prof. Beck states that there are certain laws which may not be as tangible as the law of gravity but which must be respected. Whether known or not, if such laws are not respected, there would be unexpected collapses. Beck thus proposes caution in technological progress.

A substance which, as cultural object was synthesized or created by humans to satisfy a need in particular, causes a negative side effect on health after being used, is certainly a badly known object. So, which Cannon and which Technique make objects built and adapted by humans known?

Even though the problem is complex and well conceived techniques which are completely innocuous to humans are difficult to obtain, the Technopathogeny phenomenon is undeniable and it has serious consequences. This is why the sooner the problem is tackled and dealt with, the better the detection and prophylaxis of technopathogenic factors will be. This is why the problem must be tackled in the early stages of the technological development.

Having supported the need of prevention to avoid a technopathogeny, a new theory arose:

Theory VII: A new discipline – Technopathogenology – is needed to get the efficient protection against technopathogeny.

This is the hypothesis that led to it:

Hypothesis: Why is a new science required for the study and prevention of Technopathogeny? Couldn't this be framed within one of the existing disciplines?

As we have seen, it is not enough to frame the problem within the existing disciplines in order to prevent the problem of mycotoxins. We could say the same thing about pesticides. But, why is it that a new science is required to deal with the problem of technopathogeny?

In order to postulate this theory, we had to deal with a new problem and answer to the question presented in this first hypothesis and, just like we did with a problem in particular (mycotoxins), analyze whether technopathogeny could be framed within the existent disciplinary framework.

VII. Technopathogeny. Searching for a disciplinary framework

Now, going back to the question that triggered our investigations, *cause and effects of contamination by mycotoxins in humans,* we realized it derived from various fields of expertise which led us to different paths and would make us experts in another field of study. The questions that come up are the following:

Which type of discipline do we need to study this phenomenon?

Or rather, going back to the labyrinth analogy we used when trying to find a framework to study mycotoxins: Which is the way out of the labyrinth?

Neither question can be answered yet.

The void is self evident when verifying that the question on aflatoxins resisted to be framed within other existing disciplines. In addition to this, indirectly, our research allowed other disciplines such as physiology, mycology, plasma chemistry, etc., to also carry out punctual projects on aflatoxins as a side research. This confirmed the idea that we were unveiling a phenomenon of a much higher relevance than a simple grain fungal contaminant.

What we managed to unveil was so important that it enriched other disciplines. However, the discipline the subject of study required was still to be developed.

The enormous disciplinary orphanage comes then to light, since the main causal question remains unanswered.

At this point, and going back to Lakatos' concept on research programs, we can ask ourselves: Wasn't our perspective on aflatoxins the beginning of a program which fit Lakatos' concept of research programs? But wasn't this program which was considered a program on aflatoxins or on the family of similar substances called mycotoxins, just a program within the Health and Human Environment, or Technology-Human Environment and Health frameworks? This is why our initial research was so successful among other disciplines – while, at the same time, it left us unsatisfied since our initial question could not be answered.

This also explained why the reports on our work were so poor – we were failing to frame the question within an existing discipline. Wasn't then the problem the initial thread in Goblot's skein (Goblot, 1943) or the tip of an entangled yarn ball in Morin's concept? (Morín, 1995).

After this trial and error process to frame our object of study, the only thing we had was a feeling of orphanage, and not just an intuition or gut feeling, but a certainty grounded on the collection of negative reports our work had received. We received such reports when we asked for evaluations, either for scientific reports or to ask for subsidies or tools we needed for our program.

We called them tangential or not core reports because we had sent the proposal to experts on other disciplines, who gave their opinion from their point of view but without reflecting on what our actual object of study was, that is to say, on which object they actually had to focus.

The feeling of orphanage could be compared to a writer whose manuscripts were evaluated by a calligraphist, who could say, for example, the r is mistaken for an n, or by a copy editor, who could say it has spelling mistakes, or the grammar is bad, when only a writer could really evaluate whether the work was of some literary value. This example illustrates the problem of the above mentioned evaluation flaws.

The collection of these reports *about what it was not or was not done and should have been done* with the logical negative consequences (and which was patiently kept for thirty years) allowed us to recognize the need of a correct evaluation to our question and finally support the need of creating a specific discipline. It was amazing how the scientific system was automatically using the mechanism of *returning to the old program* or *to the old paradigm*. This procedure is often applied deliberately – as we will see in Chapter IV – to control the researcher and the advancement of knowledge.

There must be then a profound change of paradigm, since it was always taught in classical science that the accumulation of knowledge generated by basic science would eventually lead to new technologies which would be useful to humans. In this old paradigm the finality nature of technique was not borne in mind. It was considered a consequence of the growth of science, in a mechanical and blind manner, similar to the division of cells. The possibility of a gestational flaw in the technique was not taken into account. Although this might seem an exaggerated statement, this was a consequence of methodologically ignoring that it was developed by human mind.

The new paradigm that positions Technique within the cultural sciences rather than in natural sciences recognizes the essentially human and practical nature of Technique (Eguiazu & Motta, 2000) and as any idea that is later materialised, the innate frailty and fallibility of any creation or human development must be recognized.

Sketching the discipline

Having mycotoxins as a starting point, being them a real or relevant problem to humans – which is why we were interested in researching on

198

it – and analyzing other techniques with the same relevance, we realized that in every case there is a technique that poses a risk on humans either by action or by omission. In the case of mycotoxins, by action (by genetically weakening or eroding the grains) and by omission (by not bearing in mind the adequate storage conditions this weakened element requires). Aflatoxins had the fascination Morin attributes to a complex and ill reducible reality. It was part of a vital technology to humans – agriculture – which, in spite of the most modern aspects that present it as apparently self-sufficient and invincible, it is not more than a millenarian culture humans have been developing since their very origin. This technology does not differ much from the old bow and arrow technique and, just like it was substituted by new killing technologies, agriculture must also be substituted by others which have advantages of current technologies. This way, in a Heraclitan flow in which *the new substitutes the old* there is a being – in Parmenides conception – a being that is actor and spectator in this technologic flow who suffers from its consequences: the human being.

But the *question on Technique* always remained unanswered. In spite of being technicians we realized we were on slippery ground when we asked ourselves about technique. Our postdoctoral work (1990-1993) with an expert on technology and culture, Prof. Dr. Heinrich Beck (University of Bamberg, Germany), based on his work Kulturphilosophie der Technik (Beck, 1979a) – which we considered the most relevant to support our work – allowed us to sketch the science we called Technopathogenology.

According to Dr. Beck,

Any technique – be it a simple Neolithic tool or a sophisticated computer – is a human craft and the human, its author, is fallible and can be a subject of passions, which can be noble and honorable or ignoble and disgraceful.

This influences both the creation of the object and its usage and approval.

We wonder then, can this fallible human pass its fallibility onto the object? Prof. Beck's concepts allowed us to place Technopathogenology within Technology, excluding the disciplines where we could have framed it (Ecology, Medicine, Anthropology, Environmental Toxicology or Ecotoxicology) since framing a *technical science which can entail negative collateralities* within the Technology framework is more suitable and enables the direct approach. Following this criterion, the question on aflatoxins could be rephrased as follows: *How much of the effect caused by aflatoxins is a consequence of an ill conceived and badly applied technique?*

This question could already be approached from the right perspective avoiding focusing on a simple answer to the question, leaving the impression that it was somehow solved but not thoroughly dealt with. In this case, the question can very easily digress to, for example, an experimental questioning on carcinogenesis, but what is relevant here in the technopathogenological sense is: according to the technology including it, does it actually entail a risk for humans or not?

Therefore, and in reference to the collateral effects of pesticides, the following question can be posed:

Apart from the experimental harmfulness of a pesticide, according to the technology used, does it entail a risk to humans?

For both phenomena the following can be asked:

How much of the aflatoxins and pesticides negative collateral effect is caused by errors of conception? The same question could be asked about medicines, chemical substances, etc. What about contaminants in general? What about the substances that neutralize the negative effect of contaminants, such as certain antioxidants? There were still other questions in connection with the intellectual and material work invested in the generation of knowledge. Such questions were: How much of this investment must be placed not in natural sciences tools but in the investigation of ethical and legal causes in order to detect and prevent the problem efficiently? How much of this intellectual work is focused on investigating whether the problem of contamination caused by technique is a global effect of multiple of small or big errors of conception or application of technique in humans?

This risky and incisive approach seems to be the most suitable to obtain relevant results with very little economic investment. Technopathogenology could therefore provide a solution for the problem: *Humans create techniques that, apart from the positive aspects, have unexpected collateral effects that turn against them.*

Therefore, and because this phenomenon is originated within technique, the study must be approached by Technopathogenology, a new discipline for a transdisciplinary phenomenon which is essentially human (Eguiazu & Motta, 2000) and whose utmost and most noble aim is that within the proper conception of technique – within the knowledge used for its development – the potential voids that might cause technopathogenies can be discovered (Eguiazu, 1999b).

This is like the architect example, who can detect a flaw or an error before the structure is built and avoid this error – which might cause the building to collapse – from passing onto the construction.

That is, a prospective discipline that aims at detecting the phenomenon before it is actually manifested.

We can then define Technopathogenology as the science that studies, among other technopatogenic phenomena, the process of Technopathogenesis: a set of stages or processes in succession that lead to the manifestation of a technopathogeny and, because it is of such a complex nature, cannot be fragmented because it integrates elements from Natural as well as Abstract Sciences (Ethics, fundamentally).

The concept of technopathogenological research is, in its broadest sense, the unconditional search for knowledge *without limits*. We say without limits to avoid impediments to reach the causes of the phenomenon (Eguiazu & Motta, 2000).

We have seen that certain problems in particular, those related to mycotoxins and pesticides, cannot be prevented efficiently by existing sciences. This is why we are speaking of the need of a new science for them. We must now support the idea that the general problem of technopathogeny is that it cannot be efficiently prevented within an existing discipline framework, or within a multidisciplinary framework.

The following hypothesis will attempt to answer such question: Why is a new science required for the study and prevention of Technopathogeny?

We will see then the attempts of framing it within different frameworks.

Hypothesis: Can prevention be achieved within the Philosophy framework?

We observed that the essence of the apparition of aflatoxins in grains was its unpredictability, that is to say, the substance that appeared in a mass-consumption product and caused (or was one of the causes of) a serious illness in humans had not been predicted. Analyzing another series of similar phenomena we can observe that what the apparition of carcinogenic pesticides had in common with the apparition of aflatoxins and mycotoxins in general was the unpredictability, that is to say, in spite of the previous scientific studies, the pesticide turned out to be unexpectedly carcinogenic. Thus the question: Wasn't this late and unexpected apparition something immanent to these phenomena or concrete technological products? Wasn't there a lot more in common between separate phenomena such as the apparent spontaneous or *natural* apparition of aflatoxins, the presence of a carcinogenic pesticide in foodstuff, the formation of a nitrosamine in foodstuff and the presence of dioxins in the air than the apparent differences between them? Which is the idea that unifies all these phenomena? Is it that in spite of the scientific system and the precautions taken, the problems could not be foreseen? In relation to this question, we will later see the analogy of the fisherman's net.

Also inspired by Prof. Beck's work, we passed on to try to frame the discipline with a radically different methodology: within Philosophy. But here the final objection was: *very well, we have located and defined the problem. We have defined it as immanent to technique, but the problem itself is not abstract; it doesn't lie in the formal world but it is concrete, empirical.* Here Philosophy provided us with a term: teleology. That is, it made us see the teleological or final end of Technique. And here we find the answer to the initial enigma: why the phenomenon cannot be studied within an Ecology framework, among other sciences. Technique, in all its manifestations, and its modern sister Technology – we are saying modern because in the Antiquity knowledge was obtained by empiricism – have something in common: they are both obtained by human effort and understanding to obtain a concrete and useful aim.

Technique equals knowledge, whether it is empirical or rudimentary, either to manufacture a primitive distaff or to develop the space shuttle. Both the simple distaff and the sophisticated shuttle have something in common: they were both produced by the human mind. Techne, as it was defined before, means *art*, that is, the ability to do something and, indirectly, it is the synonym of something developed by the mind, a mind that has ideas, that takes what it knows and applies it over and over again, corrects its mistakes and keeps on trying and changing the original idea every time the concrete object contradicts it. During this constant movement is that Technique (first) and Technology (later) are created.

Even though for our problem in particular it is Beck's work that better adjusts to the phenomenon of technopahogenology, several thinkers have been working on the problem of Technique for many years. Authors such as Huhning, Kapp, Engelmeyer, Ortega y Gasset, Heidegger

Mitcham (Mitcham, 1989) have dealt with it from a philosophical perspective, even though some of them came from the field of Technology. Heidegger's and Ortega y Gasset's works on Technique are well known.

There are others, like Prof. Mitcham, whom we have already mentioned, who have worked on technique trying to separate its more essential aspects from the interaction between science, technology and society.

Several authors have worked on science' fallibility. Karl Popper expresses its tentative, temporary character (Popper, 1973). Feyerabend calls for the avoidance of any dogmatic acceptance, of any absolutisation of its results (Feyerabend, 1986).

Inspired by Prof. Beck's work Kulturphilosophie der Technik, we, as technologists, became interested in the analysis of Technique as a cultural phenomenon. Considering the fallibility of science, we study Technique as a cultural object. Technique, independently of its degree of complexity, becomes a humble, fallible object.

This aspect is of crucial importance, since it is through it that Technique can anytime manifest negative collateralities; furthermore, they can be unexpected, or even considered impossible, but regardless of this certainty, they still appear.

We basically want to contribute to the problem of technique immanent colleraterality by trying to provide methical solutions for technologicists.

This phenomenon (and similar phenomena), can't be framed within Philosophy, given its empirical character.

Hypothesis: Can prevention be achieved within the Ethics framework?

Because of what we stated in the fourth thesis, it would seem that the technopathogenic problem was purely an ethic one.

In connection to Technopathogeny, we have discussed ethical misdemeanors in the Science and Technique system, as well as attitudes regarding truth that are both ethical and unethical. We even discussed the need of an ethical objector to denounce the actions of companies or organisms that can be harmful to humans.

Going a bit further on this issue, we could arrive at the conclusion that this Technopathogenic phenomenon should be framed within the Ethics framework in order to achieve prevention. We could arrive to such conclusion after realizing how easy it is to find faults regarding scientists' ethics. Thus, practically without doubt, we could say that we have come to the sad realization that Science, far from liberating humans, is attacking their dignity and threatening their existence (Gomez Perez, 1986). It would seem that in some cases, the temptation of knowledge is so strong that it can even lead to losing one's mind (Gomez Herrera, 1984).

There are enough examples of this state of mind (Herranz, 1982):

a) Experiments in concentration camps.
b) New highly risky contraception methods trials in third world countries.
c) Experiments with human embryos that ultimately cause their death.

Experiments in developed countries such as:

a) Experiments with poor black people, leaving without treatment a witness group to study the development of a disease.
b) Injection of cancerous cells in geriatric patients.
c) Inoculation of hepatitis virus in mentally retarded children to obtain comparative results.

All this can be explained by a progressive insensitivity of scientists to ethical norms which makes scientists gradually move away from the right decisions. There is also a strong idea in the scientific world that there are lives that are not worth living or that there are beings whose lives do not matter anymore, or that the deaths of a few can save millions. This ideology was systematically applied in experiments carried out by totalitarian regimes on those who were considered *sub-humans*, such as crippled or mentally retarded people.

It is interesting to note the parallelism between these experiments carried out by a racist regime promoting eugenics with other experiments carried out in developed countries many decades later. In both cases, experiments were applied on formally declared *sub-humans*: colored people, old people, defective or mentally retarded children.

What we are dealing with here is not a question of democracy or totalitarianism but the ideology sustained by scientists and the scientific world. Let us not forget that racism applied by totalitarian regimes had already been put into practice back in the 19th century through the humiliating classification of immigrants according to their ethnic origin in a democratic country.

Scientists repeat the same experiments whatever political system they belong to. This is caused by the methodology reductionism of scientists which can blur their vision of the world and take them to subscribe to a *scientific creed*. They turn science into a revealed religion.

The vision of the world becomes blurred. The sense of reality is lost – scientists cannot see that what they have in front is a human being, not an object of study.

The dramatic reduction of a phenomenon, without considering other factors, leads to amazingly successful results. The results become clearer and more differentiated when *parasite factors* or interferences are eliminated – one of them being, perhaps the most important one, the ethic or moral factor.

Some scientists who have lost their ethical conscience turn experimental science into a supreme value, a magic formula, which leads them to develop great arrogance.

This arrogance leads to construct, in some cases, a society based on a *scientific religion*.

When we later analyze the Innocuousness Hypothesis of the technological object, we will quote some philosophical conceptions.

We will see that Galileo considered that humans should reign over nature by subjecting it to their will. Or, as Descartes says, that the possession of the method would be the way for humans to become masters and possessors of nature (Descartes, ed. 1945). We could say that scientificism is the idea that pervades our times. This ideology reaches its riskiest point when science believes it has the sole right to give its opinion on ethical matters. Applying a scientificist ethics, science would also rule in ethical values concerning human beings.

This Comtian pretence, as a principle, cracks day by day with the verification, for example, of the technopathogeny phenomenon – which constitutes the hardest blow against the arrogance of scientists and modern technologists.

If we consider that such anti-ethical attitudes, along with what we could call *scientist's pride*, lie within technology, we could say that Technopathogeny is simply an obvious consequence – a phenomenon which scientists with such attitudes care little or nothing about.

It would seem reasonable to think that Technopathogeny is an immanently ethical phenomenon and that Ethics could be the science that studies it.

There have been huge efforts devoted to fighting against ethical misdemeanours that affect human health (Westerholm, 2004).

As we will see in Chapter III, ethics is important during the genesis, development and application processes.

It is especially important concerning the possibility of, for example, publishing fake or imperfect results, due to the scientist's negligence or in the development of technologies that are sent to the market before there is enough proof of their innocuousness. But during the generation of knowledge stages, the ethical faults could only accentuate a phenomenon which is immanent to the system and cannot be stopped, no matter how many precautions are borne in mind and how ethical and professional the scientists are. Such scientists would be lacking the concepts or tools that must be considered in the early stages, all of which will be described in Chapter III when we speak of the methodology of Technopathogenology.

The ethical faults also play a very important role in two well defined stages that come late in the scientific-technological process.

The first one comes at the end of the development stage of a technological product, when it is decided that it must be tested in humans. Many times, the tests are carried out without a full, well informed consent of the subjects involved. This can happen with medicines like contraceptives, which, while included as part of social programs, they are in fact being massively tested on poorly educated populations. If no negative collateral effects are observed, the product is then used in the developed world.

The second stage in which the ethical misses have a very important role is when the cause of a technopathogeny in particular is unveiled due to the regular use of a technique or scientific research.

In this stage, the following technologies are to be distinguished:

a) Technologies in which the cause of a Technopathogeny has been unveiled by humans after being, unknowingly, the last experimental animal.

b) Technologies in which, although there is still no epidemiologic evidence in humans, scientific research keeps finding more evidence of its carcinogenic, mutagenic or teratogenic effect, increasingly falling in the high risk technologies category as, for example, the technologies applied to the production of food (Belitz & Grouchy, 1992).

The first case is not very common. When a technology is unveiled by epidemiology, the cause of the technopathogeny is revealed after such long time that the product can be easily recalled from the market because the market dynamics has made it lose its profitability. The ethical fault would appear if a product is voluntarily recalled form the market and, knowing it is a banned product, it is exported to another country where either ignorance or a tolerant establishment allow for its indiscriminate use. This is what happens with some medicines and pesticides (Eguiazu, 1988) (Langbein *et al.*, 1989). On this last case, in Chapter IV we include a complete reading on the subject.

The second case is the most common. It involves products which are used but which have no evidence of having either sufficient or limited evidence of their carcinogenic effect. The experimental continuous toxicological work performed on the product while in use increases little by little the evidence of its risk. The most common ethical faults here are minimizing the scientific evidence and applying political pressure on buying states to delay restrictive legislation. If there is a restrictive legislation on one part of the world, the product will be sent to a region where such legislation does not exist. Bribing is very common among officials in underdeveloped countries to allow the import of substances which are forbidden in other countries. The argument for allowing the import of such products is that as long as there is no epidemiological evidence about the harmfulness of such products, they can continue to be used. Let us remember the example of the pesticide when we referred to Doubt as an attitude regarding the truth and its incidence in Technopathogeny.

It is obvious that the element that is missing from the entire reasoning is that the involuntary experimental animals used are concrete human beings. These concrete human beings, which have been subjected like hamsters to a technopathogenic effect, can never be paid back for what they have suffered – even if the producer or the one who allowed the substance recalls it from the market. The technopathogenic effect lasting for months or even years, which affected many people, cannot be taken back from people already affected by simply recalling the product from the market because of the already mentioned characteristics of neoplastic diseases.

Now we can ask ourselves, is this really an ethical problem? In order to prove it is not, we can consider the following statements:

- Above all, the problem of Technopathogeny was grounded and created by Technology. It was supported by Technological/Technical facts.

- The problem is not knowing the collateral effects of the primeval object. Ethics is relevant when the existence of lack of knowledge is known, but as long as the substantial failures of the technological object are not known, the problem is reduced to a failed gestation.

- Even though Ethics, like other disciplines, does have an influence, after thoroughly analyzing the phenomenon we arrived to the aporia that the phenomenon we are dealing with is not an ethical phenomenon but a phenomenon in itself – it is neither chemical nor biological or philosophical – it is a technological phenomenon we have defined as Technopathogeny.

- The enumeration of good neutral reasons is the core of Technopathogenology. Quoting Professor Jacobsson, in many of these cases the term ethics is so much used that it ends up being trivialized or *kidnapped* from its original sense (Jacobsson, 2004).

- We believe that reducing the problem of Technopathogenology to Ethics would be like trivializing the term, as the term Ecology would also be trivialized if we reduced the problem to such discipline.

- As we will observe in Chapter III, Cultural Anthropology is one of the basic sciences that allow us to humanize Technique as the work of humans, but we can also see that the eagerness to generate knowledge and construct work is a human attitude as well.

- It is interesting here to go back here to Prof. Heinrich Beck's concept (Beck, 2000):"The non-verification of an existent does not mean the verification of a non-existent."

The fact that the existence of something cannot be proved does not mean that such thing does not exist. This can be applied to many substances which are risky to health. As we have said before, analytical chemistry is a valuable tool to detect small residual quantities of substances, for example, in food. This way, acute or chronic risk by exposure can be predicted. But it is also true that analytical techniques have a limit of detection and, paraphrasing Prof. Beck, the fact that analytical technique does not prove the presence of residues in foodstuffs does not mean that there are no substances there. These quantities may be small enough so as to be irrelevant from the acute toxicology perspective, or they may be short-lasting to cause an acute intoxication, but this does not apply and here what is important is the analytical limitation to substances of carcinogenic risk. It is worth remembering here Professor Preussman's proposal (Preussman, 1972): zero tolerance for carcinogenic substances.

- Following Prof. Beck's concept we can say that modern technique generates environmental factors which are risky to health (or technopathogens), and even though they do exist, modern technique cannot detect them. This supports our conclusion that it is during the generation process and, above all, during the application of knowledge that the scientist and the technician must be especially careful.

- Another interesting concept is the one of "writing the score of nature," a concept by J. von Uexkull referring to Biology (von Uexkull, 1983). Through this analogy, we could say that studying a technopathogenic phenomenon by breaking it up in the existing disciplines would be like interpreting a symphony where each instrument acted separately and independently. Only with a guiding mechanism can the director of an orchestra achieve a harmonic interpretation. In this case, Technopathogenology would be the *director* of the study. The knowledge obtained from other disciplines together with its own generated knowledge, allow it to tackle the problem adequately and harmoniously.

- The last reflection on the subject is that ethics cannot solve the basic problem on its own. This basic problem proves the low quality of the technological product as well as the poverty of the method used to generate knowledge. As we could say when referring to Philosophy or any of the other disciplines we will refer to later, in order to achieve prevention of the technopathogenic risk, the technologist's or technician's intellectual background should be more related to a technopathogenologist than to a specialist in Ethics.

Hypothesis: Can prevention be achieved within the Science,
Technology and Society framework?

In 1994 we discussed the problem with experts in Science, Technology and Society at Penn State University (Pennsylvania, USA).

We then tried to frame the problem of Technique in terms of its collateral effects, but we did not manage to find an approach that was precise enough. The fact that this movement was oriented towards Social Sciences gave more room for the impact on society of technological developments than for this simple question: Why are there unexpected collateral effects in Technique?

This question, which was more connected to the Eureka! of the inventor, could not be easily framed within Social Sciences, which, in spite of this, can help measuring the social, historic and political consequences of Technique. Likewise, Technopathogenology can also contribute to Social Sciences in relation to the implications that Technopathogeny has in Society. In Chapter IV we include readings dealing specifically with how Technopathogenology can contribute to society: consumer protection, teacher's instruction, among others.

Hypothesis: Can prevention be achieved
within the Health Sciences framework?

If the technopathogenic phenomenon speaks of adverse effects on health, we could say that its study can be approached from Medicine or from some of its branches: Workplace Health, Epidemiology (especially Environmental Epidemiology, very close, but still not convincing), Toxicology and Bioethics. Let us analyze these last three possibilities.

Epidemiology

This science, especially Environmental Epidemiology, since searching not for a pathogen as a cause of disease but for a series of chemical and physical causes, could explain the first planes of technopathogenologic investigation but not the most profound ones. The human character of the cause that lies deep in the creation process of a technique – with its ethical and cognitive implications – cannot be grasped.

Both Environmental Epidemiology and Occupational Epidemiology are two valuable tools to detect factors originated within technology that can be responsible for damages on health in the long term. In the examples given about synthesized or contaminant substances, when seeing its classification of carcinogenic risk, some levels would include the existence of evidence in humans. To verify this, an epidemiological analysis is required in order to provide a more reliable cause/effect relationship result. Once the risk is detected, measures to prevent future damages can be adopted. Both areas of Epidemiology contribute to detect and prevent factors which originate in Technology – either potential or real – that cause technopathogenies. We proposed our program, which combined Epidemiology and Technopathogenology, to be considered in the Environmental and Occupational Epidemiology program of the World Health Organization. In 1989, our program was included in the Environmental Epidemiology Network (WHO, 1989).

Notwithstanding the contribution of Epidemiology to the prevention of technologic risk, we consider it has a few limitations:

1. The damage has to have already manifested itself.
2. Many times it is difficult to establish a relationship with the causal agent.
3. It needs a determined number of affected people for the results to be significant.
4. The carcinogenic agent may not be concentrated enough so as to generate a statistically significant response (Neutra *et al.*, 1992).

Because of the first limitation, within the general context of Technopathogeny, Epidemiology will lose relevance. This is really so because, as the document prepared by the Office of the Technology Assessment (USA) (Congress of the United States – Office of the Technology Assessment, 1981). in 1981 mentions:

> Epidemiology has established a connection between the amount of substances and the incidence of cancer in humans. However, Epidemiology is limited as a technique to identify carcinogens because neoplasms are generally manifested after years or decades of exposure. If a carcinogenic agent was identified 20 years after commencing or generalizing its usage, many people will develop cancer even if the usage of this substance is immediately banned.

To support the second limiting factor, we could go back to IARC's comment on Nitrosamines: it would be very difficult – or even impossible – to demonstrate in the population in general a cause-effect relationship between the exposure to low levels of N-Nitrosamines and the incidence of certain types of neoplasms in humans.

For the third limitation, we could mention the already proved influence of the *host factors* as genetic causes that may be particular to a person and the incidence of cancer. We could think that, given a population in particular, *weak* persons would get sick and, because they are not many, the number would be irrelevant to Epidemiology. Even then, Technopathogeny cannot be underestimated.

Maybe the most suitable framing would be within the so-called *Health Sciences*, since the question refers to a program on health and technology.

Framing a science that deals with the negative side effects on health within the Health Sciences would be relatively better than framing it within the sciences we tried during the previous pilgrimage. However, there are some objections here: the so-called Health Sciences are more focused in curing than in preventing and, even if they do prevent, they do not know Technique as such, they have a – sometimes limited – knowledge of techniques within their field of expertise

Therefore, all these sciences cannot fully provide for the right framework since they lack Technique as an object of study.

Toxicology

According to its definition, Toxicology is the branch of medicine that studies poisonous substances (which, introduced in an animal organism can cause death or serious injuries), their effects and antidotes. If we bear in mind this definition it would seem that the field of action of toxicology would be reduced to poisoning due to food intake, fungi or botulism, to the study of serpent poisons or to acute intoxication by chemical substances.

The evolution of technology and the subsequent risks on health it entails has led to a significant progress in this field of medicine.

Nowadays there is more interest in studies referring to the long lasting effects of poisonous substances to the organism in general, as well as the effects in organs or specific systems. This is how different branches of this discipline have developed: Carcinogenesis, Genetic Toxicology, Immunotoxicology, Reproductive Toxicology, Neurotoxicology, etc.

In addition, the methodologies for the detection of toxicological effects have also improved. The development of new models is currently so vast that each of them requires a specific specialization.

As we have also seen, the development of cancer is a process in which different stages are involved. Even though some agents have an Epigenetic effect, because their action in causing cancer does not involve interaction with the DNA, in general, the studies carried out in human tumors have shown that different types of genetic changes occur in tumor cells.

As we have already mentioned (US DHHS-PHS, 1984):

> Sufficient evidence exists that the process of carcinogenesis, and in particular initiation results from mutational changes occurring in somatic cells. Mutation is used in the broad sense as a change in DNA or chromosome structure that is heritable at the somatic level. It may include specific changes in DNA sequence, i.e., point mutations (based substitution, frame shift), deletions, insertions, gene rearrangement and gene amplification as well as gross chromosomal changes, i.e. translocations, aneuploidy, etc.

The initiation stage is an early event in the development of neoplasms which can involve a mutational change within the genetic material of the cell (Congress of the United States – Office of the Technology Assessment, 1981).

The agents interacting with the DNA causing mutations, damage in the DNA (Kohn), chromosome aberration or sister chromatids exchange – DNA band rupture (Scott, 1991), are called Genotoxic substances.

It is mentioned that the participation of such changes in the early or late manifestation of cancer is unknown. Its influence on the different stages of cancer is also unknown. However, it is accepted that the consistency with which these changes are manifested in different types of tumors and their specificity at a molecular and chromosomal level, provides a reasonable basis that justifies the development of trials that study the genetic exchanges in somatic cells (one of the many substrates used for these studies) as table 24 shows.

The following table shows some cases which relate events on the genetic level to the development of certain types of neoplasms.

Table 23: Type of genetic event and its relationship with the relevant neoplasm.

Type of genetic change	Example
Gene mutation	Human bladder tumor
Chromosomal translocation	Burkitt's lymphoma
Chromosomal deflection	Retinoblastoma
Aneuploidy	Chronic lymphocytic leukemia
Gene amplification	Neuroblastoma

So far we have underlined the relevance of the genetic changes caused by exposure to genotoxic agents in connection with the development of neoplasms, since they constitute a typical example of technopathogenies. However, it is worth noting – also because of its technopathogenic relevance – that many diseases, if not most of them, are originated in our genes. They do not only determine, among other characteristics, how foodstuffs are efficiently processed, but also, how hazardous substances are detoxified and how the organism responds to infections. When genes are acting adequately, the organism is developed and works normally. But the alteration of a gene or even a fraction of a gene can cause malformations, diseases or even death. It is believed that about 4,000 diseases have their origin in mutated genes coming either from the father or the mother (NIH-NCI, 1995).

In the following chart, we present a classification of the systems of study applied to Biomedicine, a discipline which also studies the development of new medicines, diseases, addictions, etc. (US DHHS-PHS, 1995). Even though in this classification bacteria and yeast are grouped within the in vivo studies, they are generally considered as in vitro studies because they are cultivated within a laboratory.

The systems can:
I: use living organisms
II: not use living organisms

I. Systems using living organisms

A) In vivo Studies: Systems that use the totality or integrity of a species be it unicellular or multicellular.
This includes:
- Clinical studies: Epidemiologic studies in humans.

- Studies in superior vertebrate animals: Usage in non-human primates.
- Studies in other vertebrate animals (warm blooded or cold blooded). This includes: dogs (Means *et al.*, 1988), guinea pigs (Fedan, 2001), rats, mice, hamsters, ferrets (Wishnok *et al.*, 1987), rabbits (George *et al.*, 2002); birds: ducks (Vesonder & Wu, 1998), hens (Carrington *et al*, 1988), fish (Pritchard & Bend, 1991), frogs (Burkhart *et al.*, 2000), snakes (Schmäll & Scherf, 1984), etc. We include the bibliographic reference for the least common used.
- Studies in invertebrate animals:
  1. Insects, for example, the Drosophila melanogaster.
  2. Aquatic organisms.
- Studies in microorganisms:
  1. Bacteria: for example the Salmonella o Escherichia group.
  2. Yeast: for example the Sacharomyces group.
- Studies in superior plants: About ten species are mentioned, among them: beans, onion, barley, corn and soy. The observations can be carried out either in the root or in the pollen tube (IPCS, 1985b).

B) In vitro Studies: Use of organs or culturing of human or animal cells cultured in artificial environments. Some of them are listed in the table below.

Apart from the organisms mentioned in this classification, the following table lists other substrates mentioned in the literature as being used. These other systems can be used in these studies, where relevant, either in vivo or in vitro. As it was indicated for studies in animals, there is a bibliographical reference for further reading:

Table 24:   Some substrates used in in vivo and in vitro cell and multi cell studies.

Substrate		Reference
Chick Embryo	*in ovo*	(Swartz 1985)
Chicken Hepatocyte	*in vitro*	(Ferioli, et al, 1986)
Chinese Hamster Lung Cells	*in vitro*	(Sofuni, et al, 1990)
Chinese Hamster Ovary Cells	*in vitro*	(IPCS, 1985a) (Sofuni et al, 1990)
Cultured Cardiac Myocytes	*in vitro*	(Tirmenstein, et al, 1997)
Drosophila Somatic Cells	*in vitro*	(IPCS, 1985a)
Epididymal Sperm of Rats	*in vitro*	(Lowe, et al, 1998)
Germ Cells of Male Mice	*in vitro*	(Lowe, et al, 1995)
Human Bronchial Cells	*in vitro*	(Grafström et al, 1987)

Substrate		Reference
Human Fibroblast	*in vitro*	(Huang, et al, 2003)
Human Keratinocytes	*in vitro*	(Germmolec et al, 1996)
Human Lung Cancer Cell Lines	*in vitro*	(Schuller, et al, 1987)
Human Peripheral Lymphocitoes	*in vitro*	(Channarayappa & Ong, 1992)
Human Testicular Cells	*in vitro*	(Chapin & Phelps, 1990)
Human Uroepitelian Cell Lines	*in vitro*	(Swaminathan, et al, 1996)
Hypothalamus	*in vivo*	(Schallet, 2004)
Late-Step Spermatids of Mice	*in vitro*	(Wyrobek, et al, 1995)
Mammalian Cells	*in vivo – in vitro*	(Witt, et al, 1992)
Mouse Bone Marrow	*in vivo*	(Philips, et al, 1991)
Mouse Embryos	*in vitro*	(Hansen & Grafton, 1994)
Mouse Hepatocytes	*in vitro*	(Mirsalis et al, 1989)
Mouse Liver	*in vivo*	(Swartz & Schutzman, 1986)
Mouse Ovaries	*in vivo*	(Swartz & Mall, 1989)
Mouse Uterine Tissue	*in vitro*	(Liu, et al, 1995)
Rat Alveolar Cells	*in vivo*	(Ghanem, et al, 2004)
Rat Bone Marrow	*in vivo*	(Shi et al, 1992)
Rat Embryos	*in vitro*	(Hansen & Grafton, 1994)
Rat Hepatocytes	*in vitro*	(Mirsalis, et al, 1989)
Rat Liver Enzymes	*in vitro*	(Rabovsky, 1986)
Rat Lung	*in vitro*	(Michiels, et al, 1989)
Rat Lung Cells	*in vivo – in vitro*	(Whong, et al, 1992)
Rat Lung Enzymes	*in vitro*	(Rabovsky, 1986)
Rat Primary Lung Cells	*in vitro*	(Waong, et al, 1990)
Rat Spleen Cells	*in vitro*	(DeBord, et al, 1995)
Rat Tracheal Epithelial Cells	*in vivo – in vitro*	(Zhu, et al, 1991)
Somatic Cell	*in vitro*	(Albertini & Hayes, 1997)
Syrian Hamster Embryo Cells	*in vitro*	(Tu, et al, 1992)
Syrian Hamster Kidney Cells	*in vitro*	(Seemayer, 1984)

Below we describe some of the effects observed in the different systems:

Table 25: Some of the end points observed in the different studies.

Effect	Description	Reference
Aneuploidy	Addition or loss of one or more chromosomes from the haploid (i.e., meiosis) or diploid (i.e., mitosis) number. I.e., 2n+1, 2n-2, etc.	(IPCS, 1985b)
Apoptosis	One role of the programmed cell death (Apoptosis) is the removal of cells with DNA damage from the population. Classically, apoptosis is recognized as an effective mechanism by which cell numbers are regulated during development and differentiation.	(Morris, et al, 1995)

Effect	Description	Reference
Carcinogenesis	The process by which normal tissue becomes cancerous.	(U.S. DHHS-PHS-NTP, 1985)
Carcinogenicity	The power, ability, or tendency to produce cancerous tissue from normal tissue.	(U.S. DHHS-PHS-NTP, 1985)
Citotoxicity	This process enclose endpoints related to the cell death such as loss of colony-forming ability or cell lysis, whereas other are not necessarily associated with lethality, e.g. growth inhibition, cell-cycle delay, reduction in mitotic index and metabolic changes.	(Scott, et al, 1991)
Clastogenicity	Physical or chemical chromosome breakage	(IPCS, 1985b)
Cytogenicity	The Cytogenetic assays evaluate the sister chromatid exchange and the chromosomal aberrations.	(Margolin, et al, 1986)
Deflection	Chromatid or isochromatid aberration in which part of a chromosome is missing as a result of a break; the deletion my be from the end of the chromatid, i.e. terminal, or from the middle of the chromatid, i.e. interstitial.	(IPCS, 1985b)
Dicentric	A chromosome with two centromeres. A chromosome aberration.	(IPCS, 1985b)
Genotoxicity	This process encloses endpoints such as: Gene mutation, chromosome aberrations, sister-chromatid exchange, DNA-strand breaks	(Scott, et al, 1991)
Micronucleus	Small fragment of chromosome material visible during interphase outside and separate from the main nucleus; may occur as result of a chromosome fragment or a whole chromosome that detached from the spindle during mitosis.	(IPCS, 1985b)
Mutagenicity	The capacity to induce mutations or permanent change in genetic material (the material controlling transmission of hereditary characteristics)	(U.S. DHHS-PHS-NTP, 1985)
Sister Chromatid Exchange	An apparently symmetrical exchange of material between sister chromatid.	(IPCS, 1985b)
Teratogenicity	The capacity to induce Teratogenesis: malformations, monstrosities, or serious deviations from the normal type in organisms.	(U.S. DHHS-PHS-NTP, 1985)
Translocation	Isochromatid rearrangement resulting from an exchange of material between two chromosomes	(IPCS, 1985b)
Unscheduled DNA Synthesis	The synthesis of DNA during the excision repairs of DNA damage and as such is distinct from the semiconservative replication that is confined to de "S" phase of the eukaryotic cell cycle.	(IPCS, 1985b)

Different endpoints can be observed in different substrates. For example, some micronuclei can be the object of study in mouse bone marrow (McFee *et al.*, 1994), human peripheral lymphocytes (Channarayappa & Ong, 1992), mammal cells (Gu *et al.*, 1992), rats lung primary cells (Whong *et al.*, 1990), male rat germinal cells (Lowe *et al.*, 1995), etc.

II: Systems not using living organisms.
- Development of mathematical models
- Computerized simulation models (Studies In Silico)
- Image Technology: For example, the usage of nuclear magnetic resonances.

According to the duration, they can be (Witt *et al.*, 2000):
- Short-term tests: Less than 30 days.
- Prechronic or subchronic trials: A few weeks up to 6 months.
- Chronic or long-term tests: 1 or 2 years.

We know that the chronic tests in rodents are more reliable in the extrapolation of the results to humans. However, given the number of substances, time and cost these trials imply, a fundamental aim of Toxicology is to develop simple methods, as the ones described in table 24, which are short-termed and inexpensive. There is a large number of scientists devoted to this task, which would make the tests reliable. This would provide quick, inexpensive tests whose results can be extrapolated to humans, allowing for accurately determining the potential risk factors.

With all this in mind, a meeting was held in 1981 by the International Program for the Evaluation of Short-term Tests for Carcinogenicity in order to evaluate the most adequate in vitro tests for this purpose. More than 90 tests were presented. This meeting confirmed that the Salmonella thyphimurium test is the most adequate primary test to detect potential carcinogens and mutagens. Nevertheless, it was also discovered that this test does not detect – or finds it difficult to detect – some substances with carcinogenic effect in rodents. Therefore, it was proposed that the Chromosomal Aberrations test, along with the Salmonella test, could provide enough primary proof for the detection of possible carcinogenic substances (IPCS, 1985a).

Later, in 1983, a new meeting was held to validate the in vivo short-term tests in order to identify potential carcinogens. More than 60 tests were analyzed. The results cast light on the important role of in vivo short-term tests in the evaluation of potential carcinogenic risks. Once the in vitro genotoxicity is proved through the use of the above mentioned tests, the other tests can be applied. If the agent is still active in the in vivo tests, there are greater possibilities that such agent presents a carcinogenic or mutagenic risk in mammals, including humans.

It was decided that the mouse bone marrow micronuclei test was the most adequate assay for primary *in vivo* testing for this aim, and the rat liver assay for unscheduled DNA synthesis suggested that it could be complementary to the micronuclei test (IPCS, 1990).

The World Health Organization presented a thorough study on short-term tests to detect mutagenic substances as carcinogenic (IPCS, 1985b).

Even though short-term tests have many advantages, they are so far still unable to establish accurately the potential risk in humans. This is why this criterion considers adopting a large amount of short-term in vivo as well as in vitro tests. The four tests above mentioned are proposed as representative tests. If the four tests results turn out to be positive for a factor in particular, then it could be estimated that such factor is potentially risky on humans.

In relation to Genetic Toxicology and Mutagenesis, the National Toxicology Program (USA) uses the mutagenesis in *Salmonella typhimurium* and the induction of micronuclei in bone marrow cells or peripheral blood erythrocytes, of mice (*in vivo*) (US DHHS-PHS, 2002).

With the database on toxicological effects, mutagenesis and carcinogenesis, a relationship has been established among various functional groups and parts of a molecule and their toxicological effect. This led to another attempt to predict potentially risky effects on humans called Structure/Activity Relationship.

The advances in Biotechnology and Molecular Biology in relation with developing an accurate predicting methodology, allows for the constant development of new methodologies. In biotechnology, the development of transgenic rodents and transgenic aquatic organisms (US DHHS-PHS, 1995), for example, led to the development in Molecular Biology of a relatively new field in toxicology: Toxicogenomics. This is a sub-discipline of Genomics, which applies its knowledge to identify and evaluate the effects of the xenobiotics on the general spectrum of genome (Amin *et al.*, 2002). It is the scientific field in which researchers study how the genome responds to environmental stressors or toxic substances. It includes the studies of Genetics, Transcriptomics, Proteomics, Metabolomics, Bio Computer Sciences and Conventional Toxicology (Walter *et al.*, 2003).

Another effort of Medicine in the field of Epidemiology or Toxicology is the search for Biomarkers in humans to identify potential damages due to being actually or potentially exposed to certain techniques. According to its definition, (IPCS, 1993):

> The term *Biomarker* is used in a broad sense to include almost any measurement reflecting an interaction between a biological system and an environmental agent, which may be chemical, physical or biological.

Such biomarkers can be (IPCS, 1993):

- Biomarker of exposure: a substance which a person may be exposed to and/or the substance resulting from its metabolism.
- Biomarker of effect: Measure of biochemical, physiological and behavioral alterations, or other alterations within the organism that can be associated with a possible damage on health. They can be identified in the blood, kidneys, lungs, reproductive organs, etc.
- Biomarker of susceptibility: Indicators of an inherent or acquired capacity of the organism to respond to the incidence of a specific xenobiotic substance.

With this brief description, we can see that it is undeniable that Toxicology is concerned about technologic risks and their prevention.

In connection to Toxicology, it is very interesting to mention that there are scientists who try to diminish the incidence of environmental contaminants to the risk of cancer and that animal studies are irrelevant to predict risks of cancer. For example, Tomatis *et al* comment that according to some authors (Tomatis *et al.*, 2001)

> The exposures to industrial and synthetic chemicals represent negligible cancer risks and that animal studies have little or no scientific value for assessing human risks.

We share the criteria of Dr. Tomatis *et al*, when they say that:

> Our conclusion agrees with the International Agency for Research on Cancer, the National Toxicology Program, and other respected scientific organizations: in the absence of human data, animal studies are the most definitive for assessing human

cancer risk. Animal data should not be ignored, and precautions should be taken to lessen human exposures. Dismissing animal carcinogenesis findings would lead to human cancer cases as the only means of demonstrating carcinogenicity of environmental agents. This is unacceptable public health policy.

We agree with the last sentence.

Nevertheless, even though this discipline is a valuable tool to prevent Technopathogeny, it has not yet focused on the actual roots of the phenomenon. Let us remember the tree analogy we used when we saw that the only possible way for the technopathogeny phenomenon was to analyze it as a complex phenomenon, without reducing it to a mere toxicological problem for whose prevention other considerations are required, apart from the toxicological ones, as we will see in Chapter III. Following this example, toxicology would only pluck out the defective fruits of the tree as they appear. It would say nothing of how to develop a tree that does not bear defective fruit.

Bioethics

Bioethics is another discipline related to health sciences which, considering its name, would lead to think that it is suitable to study Technopathogeny. If Technopathogeny involves harm to health, that is, to life, and if in the apparition of factors generated by Technique causing such damage there are ethical causes, we could include Technopatogeny into the field of study of Bioethics.

However, and bearing in mind some aspects of this discipline, we think that there are some arguments to consider that this science is, once again, not adequate to study this phenomenon.

Let us consider some quotations and concepts defining Bioethics (Chadwick & Levitt, 1997):

> Bioethics is defined as the study of the ethical, social, legal, philosophical and other related issues, arising in health care in the biological sciences. It is thus a multidisciplinary field of study.

It is also considered as an interdisciplinary field of study (Bracalentti & Mordini, 1997).

As an Interdiscipline (Bracalentti & Mordini, 1997):

Bioethics is a field of studies that involves professionals from different disciplines, among them, Philosophy, Medicine, Law, Psychology, Theology and Sociology. Ethical analysis were developed as a valuable tool for the evaluation and administration of new technologies. Biomedical ethics has been long considered of interest to national parliaments.

In another article (Pompidou, 1997) it is mentioned that:

The development of new biomedical technologies addresses both the very first stages of conception and also the terminal stages of life.

"New knowledge thus leads to new abilities and creates new risks."

The characteristics of multifactorial diseases, and in particular of the genes predisposing to diseases, are leading us away from classical preventive medicine towards a so called 'predictive' medicine which threatens the uncertain nature of the pathological risk.

"The danger of eugenic practices or the temptation of medicine guided by personal convenience justify research on medical ethics" (Pompidou, 1997).

Research in biomedical ethics should be not only addressed to evident risk, "but it must also try to anticipate potential risks, in particular the so-called 'indirect' risks whose consequences are not immediately obvious." It is mentioned that this type of risk is more complex and two principles are mentioned in connection to this: *Caution*, which implies looking for a demonstration or proof of the absence of risk in technology and the principle of *Learning from experience*. The latter is often disregarded due to the contradictory attitudes of the experts. On the one hand, we find the enthusiasts, who want to advance too fast and, on the other, the critics, who place obstacles (Pompidou, 1997).

The development of ethics in biomedical research establishes the question of the relationship between science, ethics and society. Biomedical Ethics is connected to the evolution of society and must involve drawing other disciplines nearer, an interdisciplinary approach. This entails the confrontation among scientists, politicians and the public opinion. A strategic approach in biomedical research is essential (Pompidou, 1997).

Another author says (Bardoux, 1997):

The research on biomedical ethics addresses general standards for the respect of human dignity and the protection of the individuals in the context of biomedical research and its clinical applications.

In this short description we can see that Bioethics is only focused on Medicine, biomedical research and/or Technologies applied to health and on preventing risks caused by such technologies.

The decisions based on an apparent scientific knowledge, which might lead to abort fertilized ovules with apparent future malformations reveal the incapacity to understand the substantial indetermination of the scientific knowledge.

Mount Taygetus, where malformed babies in Antiquity were eliminated because they would be unsuitable for war, has become *Genetic Taygetus,* where the chromosomal map can decide who lives and who does not.

Just as in the Antiquity any malformed baby unsuitable for war could have been a potential Socrates or Aesop, the current myopia of the chromosomal map could disregard human potential in the eliminated ovule (Eguiazu, 1991).

Once again, even though Bioethics provides invaluable knowledge in the field of medical technology and in the handling of human life from its conception until its death, and even though it can take into account immanent and hidden risks – as the ones we defined as causing Techno-pathogenies – in the case of this discipline, the risks borne in mind are only those related to technology and medical decisions.

Moreover, if we circumscribe the risks to purely ethical reasons and if each Technique approached its prevention independently, we would have to think of a Chemical Ethics, Physical Ethics, Electro-Ethics, Cyber-Ethics, etc. We could even reduce everything to Technique and speak of *Technoethics*, but it would still be a narrow concept which, as we have said when we referred to ethics, even though in the generation and manifestation of the phenomenon there is a strong ethical component, not all the causes of Technopathogenies are ethical.

Hypothesis: Can prevention be achieved within the Ecology framework?

When we consulted an ecologist on the problem with mycotoxins, he expressed that he considered technological risks – whether acute or chronic – were caused by contamination and the problem was the lack of police control of emissions. That is to say, even if he considered Technopathogeny as a phenomenon, for him it would only be a police problem.

We can see that in the Ecologist's eyes, the problem with contaminants is not an Ecological problem, but a control problem. We could think then that just like a natural contaminant risk could be prevented through control, the same could be applied to the problem of Technopathogeny.

Even though he is using an argument we do not agree with, the ecologist considers Technopathogeny is a problem that cannot be approached from the ecological perspective.

Other ecologists, on the other hand, include the study of contamination in a branch called Human Ecology. This is what inspired us, at the very beginning, to think that this new phenomenon – which we still had not fully glimpsed yet – could be approached by a discipline which was a branch of Ecology and which we defined as Anthropo-Ecology. At first we considered that Anthropo-Ecology could be the scientific discipline that postulated the fundamentals of human habitat (SAGUF, 1983) thus establishing a relationship between Technical Humans and their habitat and the prophylaxis of its deterioration (Eguiazu, 1985). Our proposal seemed to us even more consolidated through the recognition of our program by the Swiss Academic Society for Environmental Research and Ecology (SAGUF). However, the concept of Anthropo-Ecology, just as what happened with Ecotoxicology, was later considered inadequate.

The first objection to use a classical science such as Ecology to study Technopathogeny is that this science is not focused on humans but on the Ecosystem. Humans are taken as just another *organism* interacting with the others. Ecology is just another science that can describe the mechanism of interaction among the organisms and their environment. It could study the negative effects of Technique in the ecosystem and the causalities or alterations that can affect or not humans. Ecology studies all the links of the environmental chain without focusing on the first – Technique – and on the last – humans.

Given its origin in Haeckelian biology, Ecology cannot grasp the concept of Technique since, as a biological science it reduces and excludes as object of study a cultural manifestation such as Technique. Ecology can, however, study the consequences of the application of a technique in particular on the ecosystem, but it does not try to arrange its effects in order of importance since, as we have said before, humans are taken as just another part of the system. Ecology can neither say anything in connection to prospective effects on humans' exposed surfaces. It only studies the environment – it has no means to study harmful effects on humans.

Ecology could be an auxiliary science in the problem of Technopathogeny. When studying and measuring the effects of contaminants on flora and fauna (sea, lake, etc.), Ecotoxicology provides valuable indicators or markers for the prediction of potentiality of risk of such contaminants in humans. However, in spite of its undeniable importance to detect and prevent damages in the ecosystem, it is not an indispensable discipline to frame the technopathogenic problem.

This can be particularly seen in two examples of Technopathogeny: Thalidomide and the Minamata disease.

Thaliomide is an active principle of a medicine which was prescribed to pregnant women to relieve morning sickness symptoms during pregnancy. This substance was passed onto the fetus through the placenta causing severe teratogenic effects. Where is the Ecosystem? Where is Ecology? This is a typical case of technopathogeny but there is no room for Ecology here.

The Minamata disease was caused by mercury poisoning in children and adults, carried by marine trophic chain (working as biological transport) and ingested by humans through foodstuffs. This is a case of technopathogeny where Ecology (Ecotoxicology) is also involved, because Ecology is required to study the complex trophic chains: *Phytoplankton – zooplankton – small fish and marine animals – big fish ingested by humans,* through which the contaminant concentrated in the tissues of fish to such a high level that they intoxicated humans.

As for Ecotoxicology, it is worth mentioning the remark of a specialist in this discipline who, when asked about the Chernobyl incident, declared: *I am not a specialist in Chernobyl.* Apart from the limitations manifested for Ecotoxicology, we can also conclude that according to this specialist, we would require as many specialists as technological problems there are.

It is clear then that, in connection to Technopathogeny, Ecology is an auxiliary science. It is a widespread error to frame this problem as an environmental problem. From this perspective, there is no answer to the question on the relationship between Technique and Humans – the first and last elements of a relatively long chain of causalities which are themselves indeed object of study of Ecology.

It would seem that this science is still, in essence, mechanicist and that the mechanical model now is applied to the ecosystem. Using it as a leading science to study the problem of Humans and Technique would not provide convincing answers thus leading to the ecologism dead-end, in which the ecosystem, without humans, becomes object of political affirmation. In spite of the many efforts to frame Technopathogeny within this science, our discipline cannot be studied from this perspective. This is why it is now preferred to speak of Environmental Sciences when referring to the Human Environment and Humans – which we will refer to later – and to speak of Ecology when referring to the science of the ecosystem.

However, there have been efforts to establish a Human Ecology from the Social Sciences perspective – but still without considering the problem of Technopathogeny as such (Jungen, 1985) (Tengstrom, 1985).

We have seen that the initial phenomenon, aflatoxins, could not be framed within Ecology because there was a technological factor that had generated it, a mechanicist and not finalist factor that Ecology cannot account for. Likewise, the general phenomenon, Technopathogeny, could not be accounted for either. As part of Biology, Ecology cannot incorporate the phenomenon of Technique.

The Haeckelian mechanicism lacks room for the human spirit – which is fundamental in Technique. Technique therefore escapes a possible framing within natural sciences and becomes an object of study of the science of humans' objects. Science is made out of humans' teleos, out of the constant search for the finality in the thing when *fighting for being*, the fight for transcending and *being there* (Heidegger). Biology and its sciences explain living matter but not teleos, the finality, which is essentially human. Teleos implies election and will, which a bacteria or a tree cannot possibly have.

Our argument on the impossibility of Ecology approaching the study of Technopathogeny can be summarized in the following chart:

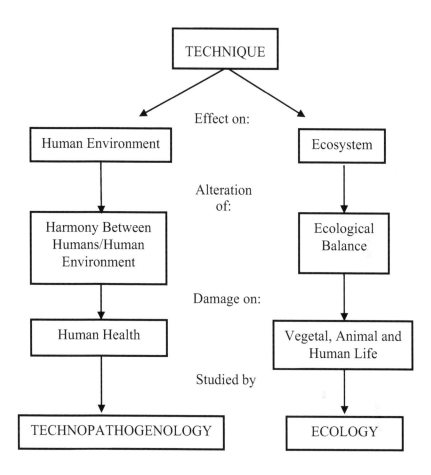

Chart 1:   Effects caused by Technique and its consideration according to Technopathogenology and Ecology criteria (Motta, 1994).

Apart from what we have already discussed in connection to the differences between the concepts of Human Environment and Environment, Ecology incorporates the concept of Ecological Balance, in which Technopathogenic effects could be erroneously included. Nevertheless, the effects
of Technique on animals, vegetables as well as on humans are studied under the concept of Ecological Balance. For example: oil spills and their effects on sea flora and fauna; acid rain and its effects on forests.

By considering the concept of Human/Human Environment harmony, Technopathogenology studies the alteration Technique produces on

the proportion and correspondence between the Human Environment/Human elements that make life possible.

As for the negative effects of Technique, humans are the most affected. In the chain of negative effects, humans deserve priority.

As we have mentioned before, the negative effects that Technique can cause on humans are too wide, complex and relevant to be diluted in a group of negative effects on animals and plants.

From the ecological point of view, humans are just one part of the Ecosystem. Since this science only deals with factors belonging to the environment, given its conceptually limited nature, it cannot incorporate elements which are included within the concept of Human Environment. Among the aspects which are not analyzed by Ecology and which are highly relevant, we can mention: medicines, foodstuffs additives, veterinary medicines, medical treatments, workplace exposure, etc.

Of course we must not forget that the preservation of biological diversity is also important since in the chain of causalities their alteration can end up having a negative effect in humans (Motta, 1994).

To sum up, given that Ecology studies the interaction of organisms among themselves and with the environment, it cannot provide an answer to:

a) Humans within the organisms/environment interaction framework.

b) Technique as a causing factor.

c) The negative effects on human health, especially long term and non-evident effects (Eguiazu, 1991). This science cannot provide answers to the phenomenon of these unexpected effects whether they were caused by action (presence of a contaminant, for example), or omission (which is much harder, for example, due to lack of a vitamin in certain foodstuffs, for example).

Hypothesis: Can prevention be achieved
within the Environmental Sciences framework?

Having analyzed and not found the adequate framework within Ecology, it was considered whether the study and prevention of Technopathogeny could be included within a framework which is more specific than Ecology: Environmental Sciences.

At first, and accepting temporarily the criteria, though erroneous, that Technopathogeny is an environmental problem, it was analyzed what would happen with projects that included an environmental approach. For example, analyzing problems such as environmental contamination, acid rain or global warming.

Our experience has shown us that conforming a specific committee to approach these questions is very much resisted by the evaluators of other classic disciplines – maybe because they fear that the value guidelines applied to their own disciplines would lose universal entity and, why not, power within the system as well.

Since the same criteria applied in, for example, basic chemistry, molecular biology, aerosols physics or plasma physics, cannot be applied to environmental sciences, it is thought that the environmental question lacks scientific rigor. Such rigor is necessary to preserve the quality of the scientific product required in these disciplines which are already consolidated.

Another argument to disqualify environmental proposals is that they lack clear hypotheses – such as what are indeed found in basic and consolidated sciences.

It is also usually said that there is no methodology, or that it is obscure or undetermined. In some cases, complex research projects (like environmental projects) are criticized as cryptic.

It is usually said that when a researcher coming from the so-called hard sciences asks for an interdisciplinary evaluation that includes the so called soft sciences when dealing with an environmental question, he or she is only trying to evade the evaluative rigor of hard sciences.

This kind of distrust leads to disqualify methodologies which are generally simplified because they are considered elemental and lacking scientific rigor.

However, there is a particular rigor and entity in the effort required to bring to light the environmental problem. They are both necessary for the recognition of what is essential in a given environmental problem, i.e., its critical core. There is such effort and dedication involved that in general a problem that has been hidden for a long time manages to be elucidated. This problem, brought to light, can be of such scientific density that later, systematically, the classical consolidated disciplines appropriate the whole or part of it and continue researching it, each of them with their own methodology.

Once the problem is elucidated, once what deserves to be investigated is made clear, each of the specialists can apply the whole methodological artillery of their own consolidated discipline. They can then obtain results that are much more harmonious than the ones barely sketched by the environmental researchers, no matter if they were the ones who raised the question that started the whole thing, even if the entity of such question was systematically denied by the system.

That same system, however, now through consolidated disciplines, extensively uses the new line of knowledge the environmental researcher has opened.

We can therefore see that even if we considered Technopathogeny to be an Environmental problem, there would still be evaluation difficulties. It would also seem that other phenomena typical of these sciences must face evaluation difficulties already described for the Technopathogeny phenomenon (when we referred to the search of a disciplinary framework for the phenomenon and the poor evaluations our work received if we did not frame the question within an existing discipline).

Seeing the difficulties entailed in tackling environmental problems, we finally arrived at the question whether there is a consolidated discipline for those who attempt to do it.

Ecology and Environmental problems

We have considered inadequate to include the Technopathogenic problem within Ecology. However, generally speaking, it could be said that Ecology, as a science, can provide solutions to the so-called environmental problem. Even if this is so, we consider that although part of the environmental problem can be solved through Ecology – going back to the analogy of the puncher and the plane – part of the problem can remain in the plane without being even considered.

However, the ecologist's puncher would be much more adequate to elucidate the problem than the physiologist's. Nevertheless, Ecology cannot grasp the role of culture as well as the human creative output in general. What this means is that given that Ecology cannot grasp the role of culture, it can neither grasp the role of technique and its most modern expression – Technology – in the environmental problem.

Therefore, there is a need for another discipline other than Ecology that includes the role of technology in the environmental issue.

230

Environmental questions and their disciplinary framework

We can see that the environmental problem can be studied both through a multi and a transdisciplinary approach. If so, it can happen that, since there are researchers that for a long time do research related to part of the environmental problem using a rigorous methodology, they can extract and categorize the common elements in the phenomenon and, after taking apart such common elements, they can arrive to a transdiscipline. This implies proposing a new environmental science. Maybe, in a more modest manner, one of the so many environmental sciences that contribute to solve part of the problem can be chosen to tackle the whole problem.

Some authors do not accept this possibility since they consider this would mean going back to an individual discipline. What they want to avoid is repeating the same story for future new situations or problems which, being impossible to frame within the existing disciplines, may be partly left unresolved. In Chapter III, when we analyze the attempt of approaching the study of Technopathogeny from a multidisciplinary perspective, we will observe something completely unexpected. The result, following these authors' criteria, is completely the opposite. In order to study the environmental problem, all the intellectual circles should be imbued in the so-called environmental paradigm, in order to achieve an apparent conversion to new schemes of thought. This last idea is perhaps the one that generates the most distrust from hard sciences evaluators since the vagueness of the proposal would disgust the scientific method.

Maybe the most suitable way to make the environmental problem to be accepted within the hard sciences, would be promoting the development of specific sciences. Therefore, instead of speaking of a diffuse environmental science, we would refer to several environmental sciences, each of them *clara et distincta* from the others.

We could then speak of, for example, Environmental Chemistry, which a classical chemist would not find it difficult to accept, or even of Environment-Analytical Chemistry which would be easily accepted by a chemical analyst.

An example taken from other disciplines is Environmental Law, which, as it has been demonstrated, can be accepted by the Law specialist.

Each of these disciplines would have an accurate object of study and contain a collection of specific methodologies.

Even though the environmental problem can bring about a change in the approach of classical problems, it can also consolidate scientific disciplines that contribute methodically to the advancement of knowledge while contributing to the mechanisms of recognition of the genesis and prophylaxis of the problem.

In order for this to happen it is crucial that the representatives of old and consolidated disciplines accept the inclusion of new peers in the examination boards.

Being a biological science, Ecology cannot tackle the solution of the environmental problems by itself – nor can it do it for technopatogenic problems. If it did, it would leave a great void in everything that is related to culture. Culture is closer to Anthropology than to Ecology, and Technique is part of Culture. We then have to ask ourselves where to place Technique within the environmental problem and which is the specific science that has as object of study Technique as a relevant factor to the understanding of environmental problem.

This does not invalidate the valuable efforts to develop a Human Ecology as a specific science to explain many of the problems that arise from the relationship of certain communities with their environment, as we have mentioned above when we discussed the attempt to frame Technopathogeny within Ecology.

Technopathogeny and environmental problems

Analysing technopathogeny and the environmental problems together, as well as the need of specific disciplines for their study, it would seem that according to some scientists' and epistemologists' criteria, methodology is the most important element for a science to be considered as such. This was our case: among the opinions, comments and critiques our proposal of Technopathogenology received and which we are enclosing in the annex, one of criticized aspects was methodology.

When dealing with a science in formation, maybe it would be more adequate to focus on the correct object of study rather than an accurate and complex methodology, which can indeed be found in classical disciplines.

In the case of a discipline in formation, an exact methodological characterization that reduces it to a related discipline can denaturalize it completely. This would mean pressuring an original project to frame it within an existing discipline and it would require its reformulation and mimetization into a similar project that can be framed within one of such disciplines. This framing pressure is quite common when asking for formal support or working tools in State structured scientific institutions. Many times, and moved by the interest in developing their project, environmental researchers reduce their question to a related discipline. The reduction is usually done wrongly and hastily or for convenience reasons. Both decisions lead to wrong roads. We can finally see that if a problem is not approached through an existing discipline, that is, if the framing is not authentic, it can paradoxically threaten the advancement of the knowledge it is trying to obtain. The system has such an enormous inertia that it could be defined as conservative or fearful of any new idea. It prefers insipid research projects (so well described step by step that the results can be guessed beforehand) rather than real adventures of knowledge.

Extremely precise descriptions can provide a wide amount of safety for an evaluation. However, they do not always guarantee an advancement of knowledge; on the contrary, they offer more of what is already known with expected conclusions.

Maybe the most exciting factor of the problems is that they are what they are and their solution has a good margin of personal inventiveness.

This leads not only to the consolidation of the existing knowledge, but also to ascribing to the audacious conjecture of its existence as a problem and independent object of study.

We ignore the complete magnitude that environmental problems associated to Technique can have. But we do know the magnitude of its adverse effects that manifest themselves in the long term on human health.

Until this level of our analysis and for the last of the effects produced by Technique, we consider the need of a new transdiscipline: Technopathogenology, a science that, ontologically, lies within Technique, its field of application falling within preventive health. Technopathogenology relates only tangentially to the so-called environmental sciences in the sense that many technopathogenies require the environment to reach humans' exposed surfaces. Considering the concept of environment from the ecological perspective, the technopathogenies generated by foodstuffs and medicines would be excluded from this since they enter the human body without *previously passing through the environment*. On the contrary, technopathogenies generated in the air and water do need to pass through the environment first.

Not finding a positive answer for this hypothesis, if prevention cannot be obtained within this science or group of sciences' framework, we can then formulate the following hypothesis:

Hypothesis: Can the Technopathogeny problem be considered an environmental problem?

This question is valid considering that certain problems such as environmental contamination, acid rain or global warming are originated within Technique.

However, and because of what we have already mentioned, the Technopathogeny phenomenon includes factors that would very unlikely be included within Environmental Sciences such as medicines, foodstuff additives, etc.

Environmental Sciences consider the environment from an ecological conception whilst, as we have mentioned before, Technopathogenology resorts to the much wider concept of human environment.

Environmental Sciences can consider, apart from the adverse effects towards the environment, the damages on health caused by certain phenomena, but Technopathogenology is more specific regarding the damages on health, which must be non-evident, must manifest themselves after several years or generations, etc. We can compare this to what we have already mentioned in connection to Ecology.

Similarly to what happens with the problem of Iatrogenesis in Medicine, certain problems that might interest Environmental Sciences could also be included within the Technopathogenology framework.

This way, a discipline that includes the study of the immanent and hidden errors or defects within Technique that can lead to negative consequences to human health can contribute, as in fact it does with other fields of study, to environmental sciences.

If technique as a phenomenon has such an entity, the following question would be valid:

Hypothesis: Wouldn't this object of study fit more within Anthropology?

We then carry on trying to imagine not only in which science or group of sciences to frame our object of study but also trying to find a discipline or science that casts some light on the method of our science.

234

Even though Anthropology provides a thorough answer to the human creative act – from the most elemental to the most complex – and in some way humanizes technology, it lacks elements to recognize technology as a science, since it entails a different background and methodology.

Cultural Anthropology, as we will see in Chapter III, is the science that allows us to change substantially the framing of Technique as a self-sufficient and powerful entity and consider Technique as the consequence of a fallible and tentative human act. However, it is not enough to provide a framework for a science that studies the unexpected collateral effects of Technique.

Hypothesis: Wouldn't this object of study fit more within the Social Sciences framework?

We once sent an article to a journal dealing with Social Sciences, but it was disregarded by the evaluators since they considered our field of study did not fit within their framework.

The evaluation of our work stated that it did not belong to Social Sciences.

Nevertheless, we considered that such evaluation was biased, narrow and emotional and ideologically hostile. Similar articles were sent to and published by the German journal Umwelt-Medizin-Gesellschaft (Environment, Medicine and Society), which also includes social aspects, as shown later.

Notwithstanding, we came to understand the criteria of the first journal since the object of study of Social Sciences is human society, that is, gregarious humans and their consequences. How is this connected to Technopathogeny? An isolated human, such a Robinson Crusoe, could develop a technology which could carry the technopathogeny germ even when it would have no connection to society since the isolated human is still not associated with other humans and has not created institutions yet. That is to say, Technopathogeny is a phenomenon connected to the human creative act. An isolated human can generate Technopathogenies, however simple the technology is. This means that Technopathogeny cannot be framed within the Social Sciences framework.

This was corroborated by interesting discussions with the sociologists Ulrich Beck in Bamberg in 1993 and with Ivan Illich in Penn State, Pennsylvania, in 1994. They both coincided that the phenomenon could not be framed within the Social Sciences framework. Also, Prof. Hans Gadamer in Bamberg in 1990 had already indicated that Technopathogenology had to be framed within a different field. Professor Heinrich Beck, through his concept of technology and culture, also helped enormously – as we have already seen – to understand how distant the concept of Technopathogenology was from Social Sciences.

On this framing alternative, another element that supports the idea that our field does not belong to Social Sciences is the German journal that published our thesis on the creation of this new science (Eguiazu & Motta, 2005b, 2005c). This journal includes articles on the Environment, Medicine and Society. It is interesting to note that even though the journal was interested in publishing our work, it included it under the *Global Survival* section. This means that the evaluators who did comprehend the aim of our science considered it did not belong within the Society section, nor within Medicine or Environment, but saw it as preventive methods to make human survival easier.

Hypothesis: Wouldn't it be possible to study it as well as efficiently prevent it using the disciplines, multidisciplines and processes that deal with Risk Analysis?

There are other new and interesting proposals, be it disciplines, multidisciplines, processes or criteria developed with the intention of approaching this problem in a more specific way.

As examples we could mention Prof. Jacobsson's proposals (described in the section dealing with Prof. Jacobsson's critiques and recommendations included in the Annex):

Technology Assessment
Environmental Impact Assessment
Cycle of Life Assessment

and Prof. Rammert's proposal: (Rammert, 1991)
Genesis of Technique (Technikgenese).

Many other specific proposals on risk are mentioned in a Lexikon (Anonymous, b):

Risk Control
Risk Calculation

Risk Recognition
Risk Management
Alternative transfer of risk
Decision under risk
Decision under unsafety
Exposure
Tolerance to errors
Planning of Risk Areas
Risks
Catastrophe prevention
Risk relative reduction
Risk Analysis
Aversion against Risk
Risk management standards
Risk Manager
Risk neutrality
Preference of Risk
Prize to Risk
Typology of Risk
Safety rate
Alarm systems
Management of person responsible for Quality

Below we will analyze some of these proposals. In the Annex we will discuss Prof. Jacobsson and Prof. Rammert's proposals.

Hypothesis: Wouldn't it be possible to study the risk as well as efficiently prevent it using Risk Assessment and Risk Management?

Humans became aware of the risks entailed by Technique and started envisaging the need for Risk Assessment and Risk Management, and based on that, establish Risk Management measures.

Both are considered as a process (Ris & Preuss, 1988) or as a multi-discipline (IPCS, 1999a).

According to their definition, Risk Assessment and Risk Management are new terms that can be used to describe how decisions are taken in the environment field and in the public health protection related to it. (Ris & Preuss, 1988)

The World Health Organization, through its International Program on Chemical Safety (IPCS) has presented a detailed study of these new processes (IPCS, 1999a).

Chart 2 clearly summarizes the characteristics of such processes.

Risk Assessment

Using the work presented by the WHO (IPCS, 1999a) as reference, we can see that:

Risk Assessment is defined as a scientific evaluation, ideally quantitative, of potential effects with certain concentrations of exposure.

The model of the National Academy of Science is mentioned as a useful tool for Risk Assessment.

This model includes four stages:

1. Hazard Identification
2. Dose-Response Assessment
3. Exposure Assessment
4. Risk categorization

1) Hazard identification

During this stage, the importance of the tests related to the adverse effects on humans is evaluated based on the toxicity data and the mechanisms of action of the agent in question. Let us remember the levels of classification adopted by IARC. This data provides the necessary information to estimate whether the agent can represent a risk for human health and in which circumstance can the risk manifest itself.

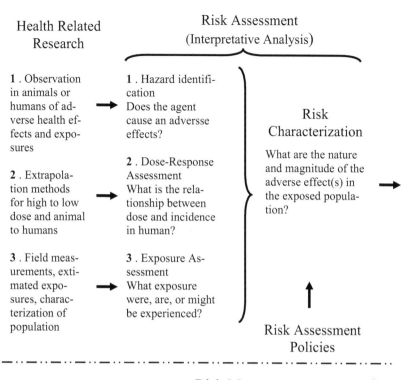

Health Related Research

Risk Assessment
(Interpretative Analysis)

1. Observation in animals or humans of adverse health effects and exposures

2. Extrapolation methods for high to low dose and animal to humans

3. Field measurements, extimated exposures, characterization of population

1. Hazard identification
Does the agent cause an adversse effects?

2. Dose-Response Assessment
What is the relationship between dose and incidence in human?

3. Exposure Assessment
What exposure were, are, or might be experienced?

Risk Characterization

What are the nature and magnitude of the adverse effect(s) in the exposed population?

Risk Assessment Policies

Risk Management

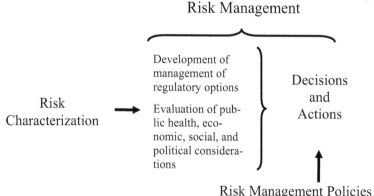

Risk Characterization

Development of management of regulatory options

Evaluation of public health, economic, social, and political considerations

Decisions and Actions

Risk Management Policies

Chart 2: Elements involved in Risk Analysis and Risk Management (Source: Ris & Preuss, 1988)

239

The data used for the Hazard Identification is taken from:

- Humans: volunteers; epidemiology.
- Animals: It includes short-term tests, sub-chronic, chronic, development and reproductive toxicology, immunotoxicology and carcinogenesis.
- In-vitro studies: They include the use of mammals' cells, bacteria, cultures.
- Structure/Activity relationship: A substance with a functional group in its molecule associated with a determined toxicological effect can predict whether another substance with the same functional group can have the same toxicological effect.

2) Dose-Response assessment

This stage tries to establish the relationship between the dose of an administered product and the adverse effect on health.

A threshold or concentration level of a substance is established. If the concentration level is below such threshold, it will be considered innocuous. However, as Prof. Preussman proposes, there is no threshold level for other effects, such as mutagenesis or genotoxic carcinogenesis (which includes chromosomal damage).

This is why it is said that there is not a *no effect threshold* for carcinogenic substances.

For those substances that have a threshold, it is estimated that there is a level of exposure under which no adverse effects can be observed (No Observable Adverse Effect Level, or NOAEL). Reference doses are usually established.

There is no agreement as to which methodology should be applied to assess the risk of substances without threshold.

3) Exposure assessment

This stage aims at determining the nature, magnitude, duration and frequency of the exposure experimented or expected for the substance in different conditions (IPCS, 1999b). This is a complex stage that establishes mathematical equations, statistic models, sampling methodologies, etc. (IPCS, 1999b). In order to evaluate the exposure, the following elements are measured: levels of concentration in the environment, personal exposure as well as the already mentioned biomarkers, including substances or metabolites detected in the organism produced by exposure to a substance.

Within the environment, emissions, routes and speeds of a substance, its transformation or degradation are measured in order to estimate the concentrations to which human populations can be exposed.

The results obtained allow estimating the intensity, speed, duration or frequency of the exposure. However, the toxicological result of an exposure will depend on the internal dose and not on the level of external exposure.

4) Risk categorization

In this last stage of Risk Assessment the information obtained from scientific tests and supporting data is processed in a comprehensible language for the management specialists to adopt the adequate measures.

This stage includes the evaluation and integration of scientific tests used to estimate the nature, importance and magnitude of risk for humans or the environment (including uncertainties that are naturally expected from exposure to a concrete agent in specific circumstances).

Risk Management

This is the last stage in risk prevention. Here certain measures must be adopted, for example, to decide whether an agent with an associated risk in particular must be eliminated or reduced. During this stage, the adoption of certain measures is indicated: regulatory, non-regulatory, economic, consultative and/or technologic.

Some aspects to consider in the decision making process include: Legislative, politic, economic, technical viability, risk population, size of population, duration and magnitude of risk, comparison of risks, repercussions for trade, resources, quality of scientific information. According to such elements, decisions can vary greatly.

This is described as a complex multidisciplinary process, rarely codified or unified and sometimes lacking structure.

In connection to this process, according to a United Nations Report on the Environment (PNUMA, 1985b).:

> We all know that there are no innocuous chemical products, but innocuous ways to manufacture, handle and utilize them ... Innocuousness or chemical safety does not mean complete absence of risk, but management of such risk.

241

At the public acceptance level, the management measures adopted regarding perception and communication of risk are also important.

When referring to the adoption of legislation during this stage, we can reiterate what we stated regarding the importance of Jurisprudence in the prevention of the problem of mycotoxins. When we discussed this we concluded that legislation can contribute to control but not to effective prophylaxis (Eguiazu, 1993).

We could say the same of Technopathogeny in general, and think that a strict juridical structure could force those who apply the technologies to control contaminants, thus effectively stopping such contaminants from reaching consumers. We have postulated the possibility of developing a Law of Technopathogeny (Motta & Eguiazu, 1989). However, we arrive to the same conclusion: legislation can contribute to controlling the problem, but efficient prophylaxis will not be obtained. The law could not avoid the defective Technique to be developed.

Based on our description we can observe that the Risk Assessment and Risk Management processes are a valuable contribution to the prevention of technologic risks. Evidently, although Risk Management can detect technologies that are risky to humans, since this stage requires the later Risk Management, we can see a difficulty or problem in this point. It will barely be efficient enough so as to achieve an adequate prevention. Maybe this is due to the fact that when evaluating if a technique that has already been developed *should* be banned, the money that has already been invested in its development will put pressure to avoid making any ban effective.

Just like other disciplines, these processes can also use Technopathogenology as a tool.

The complexity of these processes, especially during the risk evaluation stage, also reveals the complexity of the problem it is seeking to prevent. These are some of the differences between Technopathogenology and Risk Management to consider:

- We can see that these processes, whether agents, physical, chemical or biological, aim at the existing problems.
- They analyze a concrete problem, estimate its risk and, if they discover it, they act to prevent it. They do not continue, as Technopathogenology does, investigating the causes that motivated the manifestation or genesis of the problem.

- Risk Assessment and Risk Management evaluate the potential risks of technological factors on the human environment and on humans. They are not concerned with the development of techniques which are free of risks.
- The position of these two processes in connection to certain technological risks (like contaminants as aflatoxins, or foodstuffs elaborated with transgenic products, among others) is not clear.
- Includes the environment apart from humans.
- Once the agent is known (for example, with the evaluations carried out by IARC), to evaluate the risk on humans, they need to detect its presence in the environment: water, air, food, soil, etc. In order to do so, they need to resort to analytical techniques, with the difficulties and limits of detection inherent to them.
- Based on toxicological studies and once the risk is identified, they develop more studies and adopt measures in order to avoid such risk. They focus on what we could call *Risks by Action*, or rather, *Evident Risks by Action*. These processes do not bear in mind aspects Technopathogenology does consider: *Non-Evident Risks by Action*, neither the risks entailed by the absence of factors (which we will refer to when we deal with new quality criteria, including Biological Quality) which we could call *Risks by Omission*.
- These reasons make these processes – just like Epidemiology – lag behind technologic risks. They are just trying to mitigate them.

Hypothesis: Wouldn't it be possible to study it as well as efficiently prevent it from the Technology Assessment perspective?

A proposal that was also borne in mind due to its similarity with Technopathogenology is Technology Assessment.

Apart from what was indicated by Prof. Jacobsson that this proposal "tries to study the balance between the positive and negative effects of the introduction of new technology," in general what it evaluates is the impact of factories or technological buildings in certain geographical areas. For example, we could mention the problem of the establishment of big pulp mills in the Uruguay River, the border between Argentina and Uruguay. A Technology Assessment can evaluate the cost-benefit ratio between the positive and negative aspects of locating the factory in such area. But it says nothing about the gestational process of the technology used, since it is seen as a completed technology. Another example is thermonuclear power stations. In this case, Technology Assessment evaluates the impact power stations could have in specific geographical or populated areas.

Technopathogenology would evaluate the creative process and the risks on human health. Technology Assessment evaluates the finished reactor; it does not question its existence or its need. Technopathogenology would have detected unacceptable risks on human health, proposing the need to stop the project. Another example is Chernobyl. A technopathogenologic assessment would have avoided the incident since the reactor would have never been built. When a nuclear reactor is built it is done knowing beforehand the enormous risk the manipulation of nuclear energy entails. Even though Science and Technique develop all the safety methods for the probability of a catastrophe to be extremely low, there is still a possibility of a catastrophe due not to technical causes but to human errors. The human element cannot be disregarded since Technique needs a human being to apply it. This dependence on humans and the risk of human errors provide enough grounds to reject the technique and search for another, less sensible to human error. It is common sense that certain sources of energy, such as eolic turbines, are more tolerant to human errors since they do not entail catastrophic effects.

We can clearly see the difference between Technology Assessment and Technopathogenology in the US Senate definition (1972) of Technology Assessment quoted in Christian Fuchs' Internet article on Technikfolgenabschätzung (Technology Assessment) (Fuch, 1972):

> Technology Assessment is a term, used to identify a process for generating accurate, comprehensive and objective information about technology to facilitate its effective social management by political decision-makers. Specifically, technology assessment is the thorough and balanced analysis of all significant primary, secondary, indirect and delayed consequences or impacts, present and foreseen of a technological innovation on society, the environment or the economy.

Let us analyze some of the most relevant aspects of the definition:

The observed object: Technology: Observed aspects: All the consequences or impacts of its usage.

a) *..a process for generating accurate, comprehensive and objective information about technology...*

We can see here that the concept of science is disregarded. There is reference to the idea of *process*, a term also used for the definition of Risk Assessment and Risk Management.

However, Technopathogenology is a science.

Just like Risk Assessment and Risk Management, Technology Assessment would be a broad multidisciplinary study, broader still than the former since it would include other aspects apart from analysing risks. We consider that Technology Assessment can include Technopathogenology.

b) *..all* significant *primary, secondary, indirect and delayed consequences or impacts...*

By *all the consequences* we can see that the goals cover an extremely wide field: Society, Environment, Economy, etc.

Among them, Technopathogenology is interested in the aspects related to adverse effects on human health, and within those, the non-evident effects. The aspects from technology studied by Technopathogenology are clearly more restricted.

c) *..significant (...) consequences or impacts*

The definition does not specify what is meant by *significant*. Significant is something that is important because of what it represents or the value it provides. Technology can have impacts that are not considered significant to Technology Assessment. Evidently, the vast field of aspects considered by Technology Assessment can imply that some impacts are left aside or not considered since the first evaluation that must be carried out before the positive and negative aspects of the technological innovation are even considered is about whether such innovation is of value or not. For Technopathogenology, any non-evident effect on health is significant. Human health cannot be assigned a value that is negotiable. Some diseases are more serious than others, but Technopathogenology does not justify accepting an adverse effect of Technology because the illness it causes is not serious. It neither accepts considering damage significant only when a large amount of people are affected.

d) ...consequences or impacts, present as well as expected

The idea of *expected* makes reference to the evident, whether positive or negative.

Technopathogenology studies the adverse effects on human health, and within those, the non-evident effects.

e)...balanced analysis (...) of a technological innovation...

The *technological innovation* analysis requires the technology to be finished. As we will see in Chapter III, even when Technopathogenology investigates and proposes criteria to prevent possible technopathogenies when facing a Technique already developed, it also aims at reaching the process of creation of a new Technique.

In addition, the concept of *innovation* refers to a novelty or something new, a novelty that is introduced in something else. As Prof. Jacobsson explained to us, Technology Assessment analyzes the introduction of a new technology. This means that it would not analyze technologies that are already being used.

Technopathogenology, on the other hand, can evaluate technologies that are being used and investigate factors which can potentially generate technopathogenies in order to propose measures for their prevention.

f) ..of a technological innovation...

Technology is a vast field of study. The concept of Technology is applied to practically every branch of human activity. Not only in production processes. Technology is referred to when new medicines, new medical treatments or new medical diagnosis methods are developed. When it is applied in schools, this is referred to as technology being applied. Technology is present even in artistic manifestations.

We do not know whether the application of technologies such as veterinary drugs or a foodstuff coloring is analyzed by Technology Assessment. Since the field of aspects of technology observed by Technology Assessment is rather vast, some aspects can be left aside. Maybe, because of that too, some Technologies can be left aside also. The development of a new food colorant is a technological innovation. This can have consequences on human health. Now, is this an object of study of Technology Assessment? A new product for building or decorating a household is a technological innovation, but is this studied by Technology Assessment? The field of technological innovations is vast, but Technology Assessment seems to study only big technologies, such as chemical plants, thermonuclear power plants, fossil fuels power plants, paper mills, etc.

Technopathogenology, however, studies any kind of innovation, be it a medicine for humans or animals, an electronic device, a pesticide, a process to obtain oil from oleaginous plants, etc. It can do it because it is limited to studying in each case only the non-evident adverse effects on human health.

We can also add here what we already said when we referred to Risk Assessment and Risk Management. Technology Assessment would focus on what we could call *Risks by Action*, or rather, *Risks by evident Action*. What it does not bear in mind are the aspects considered by Technopathogenology: unexpected risks, risks which, within this framework we could define as *Non-evident risks by Action*. Technology Assessment does not consider either the risks entailed by the absence of factors (which we will refer to when we deal with new quality criteria, among them Biological Quality) such as the diminishing or loss of vitamins – what we call *Risks by Omission*.

A veterinary drug and a food colorant, for instance, are elements involved in techniques to heal an animal or to make a foodstuff acceptable respectively. But it is not clear whether these types of technologies are contemplated by Technology Assessment.

For example, some of the aims or lines of evaluation of this proposal include:

1. Data processing, information and communication technologies utilizing expert systems.
2. Optic laser technologies and microelectronics.
3. Micro system technologies.
4. Communication, media, printing, publication services.
5. Technology and society; ethics, values, attitudes.
6. Technology and economy.
7. Technology and law.
8. Technology and sustainable development.
9. Institutionalization of Technology Assessment.
10. Technology monitoring and technological forecasting.
11. Research and development assessment.
12. Future studies.

The following table summarizes the most significant differences between Technology Assessment and Technopathogenology.

Table 26:   Differences between Technology Assessment and Technopathogenology.

Technology Assessment	Technopathogenology
Is a process. It comes from the interaction of various disciplines.	*It is a science* for Technology to reflect upon itself and its own fallibility.
Because of its aims, the participation of various disciplines is necessary in the observation of the *finished object.* It tries to solve the problem in a *multidisciplinary* way.	The object of study surpasses the existent disciplinary field – it is a *Transdiscipline.*
The *concept of Technique and Technology* follow an *economic utility criteria*	The *concept of Technique is philosophical a*nd it is originated within humans' own cultural activity (Prof. H. Beck).
The *ontological place is centered on technological effects and collateralities.*	The *ontological place is technique itself* as a human cultural object.
It usually analyzes a *technology which is already finished.*	It begins in the *germinal or gestational stages* of Technique, much before it is produced or finished. It can also provide knowledge during the developmental stages of a technique and during its application.
The *object of study* – the effects of technology – is *vast.* It covers Society, the Environment, and Economy.	The *object of study* – the effects of technology – is *specific*: to study the negative effects on human health. The phenomenon is studied in a systematic and preventive way.
The control or diminution of negative aspects of Technology on *human health* is only *one among several* aspects it studies.	The study and prevention of non-evident negative aspects on *human health* is the *only aspect* it studies.
It develops a methodology for a problem which has a general impact.	It concentrates on the development of a methodology to prevent non-evident negative risks on human health.
The uttermost interest is the acceptance or promotion of acceptance by the general public.	There is no interest of influencing the general public through a pro-against risk evaluation. Furthermore, there is no interest of making propaganda for the application of a Technique in particular.
It does not concentrate on the reasons or consequences coming from the fact that Technology uses bodies of knowledge with voids, which are potentially responsible for its defects, which are, in turn, responsible	It concentrates on the question *why is it that the knowledge employed in a technological development can have faults or voids which are later responsible for the defect in Technique?* It studies the

Technology Assessment	Technopathogenology
for damages on human health.	seemingly non-evident technological consequences to try to discover where the gestational flaws lie.
Technology Assessment is a term, used to identify a process *for generating accurate, comprehensive and objective information about technology to facilitate its effective social management by political decision makers.*	It is a neutral science. Political decisions are not taken into account. It is only interested in the creative process in itself, in order to bring to light the weak points of Technique where the gestational error lies in order to try to overcome them or correct them.
It *does not study the creative process of new objects.*	It *studies the creative process of new technological objects* in a prospective manner.
It resorts to different specialists in order to solve a concrete risk problem.	It provides the specialist with intellectual tools to study the phenomenon.
It can present situations or cases that lead to framing difficulties since its aim is too vast.	It has no difficulty in framing the technopathogenic problems. It has its own methodology and its own tools to achieve prevention. It is not part of Technology Assessment, but it could be used by it.
It aims at studying *Risks by Action* or rather, *Evident Risks by Action,* the most important being short-term risks. Non-evident risks by action or long-term gestational risks are not considered.	It aims at studying *Non-Evident Risks by Action.* It is interested in long-term risks.
It does not take into account *Risks by Omission*	It considers *Risks by Omission* as risks that can be caused by the absence of factors that can affect the biological quality of foodstuffs. The application of certain Techniques can imply, for example, diminishing the vitamins of foodstuffs, which is highly relevant to human health.
It takes the idea of *Environment* in its classical conception. A medicine or a foodstuff additive are part of concrete technique, but they can hardly be focused, framed or included within this discipline.	It uses the concept of *Human Environment* (it makes reference to whatever can reach the exposed surfaces of humans: skin, digestive and respiratory system) as opposed to the concept of Ecology. This enables the inclusion of medicines or foodstuffs additives, for example.

Technology Assessment	Technopathogenology
It *mostly includes major technologies*, for example: Chemical industries, steel industry, nuclear reactors, etc.	The concept of Human Environment allows to efficiently focus on the damage on health with technological etiology. *It does not limit itself exclusively to major technologies* – it can investigate, for example, the consequences of the development of a new plant variety.
This proposal can overlap with others which are also considered multidisciplines and which also approach the study of risk: Risk Assessment, Risk Management, Environmental Impact Assessment, Cycle of Life Assessment, Technological genesis, etc.	The other proposals are not included in Technopathogenology because it focuses on a strict and well-defined object of study – which is actually the object of study that other disciplines disregard. *It studies a phenomenon which is not considered by other proposals.*
The ethics of the Science and Technique System is not included as a subject of analysis in the decision making process.	The *Scientists'* and the *Science and Technique system's ethics* become an object of study. Ethics is included because it is considered a co-causer of the Technopathogenic phenomenon.
It aims at helping social administrators and supporting political decision makers.	It is not interested in social administration.
It *decides* whether a Technique can be applied or not since it is connected to political decision makers. It has power of decision.	It *does not decide* whether a technique can be applied or not. It only provides knowledge and evidence to decide on it.

Another interesting difference with Technopathogenology, is that Technology Assessment is accused of *curving technological development*. This is because the assessment of a finished technique can lead to banning its usage or, in the best of cases, restrict or delay its application. In fact, the Technical Object is studied in the last stages of its development and the idea of banning its usage *disappoints* the system and its economic expectations. Technopathogenology can also be called upon to evaluate potential technopathogenic risks in Techniques which are already finished. However, its principal aim is to develop techniques which are free of the errors that can lead to technopathogenies. Through an adequate method, the techniques generated will not entail risks on humans. Any well conceived technique will not be eliminated or restricted. Therefore, Technopathogenology does not curve the progress: technology creators internalize the paradigms and any possible defect can be neutralized on time and at a minimum expense. The critique on Technology Assessment is precisely that its aim is to stop a technological object – an

250

object which has generally been heavily invested on and on which there is a capital return expectation – and whose inertia is almost impossible to stop. The efforts to stop it only generate resentment from those who enthusiastically invested on its development not knowing they were developing such a defective object. Technological objects are chaotically created and their defects are discovered too late. By the time Technology assessment acts, the technopathogeny has already occurred. However, as we have seen, Technopathogenology acts in a completely different manner: a preventive vigilance that neutralizes one by one every single tiny error.

Technopathogenology does not curve development since it analyzes objects which do not exist yet. It *tackles* Technique at a stage which is prior to concretion. There is no disappointment at economic expectations, since the development was stopped before the expectations were created.

Technopathogenology and Technology Assessment – The hydroelectric power plant example

In order to further explain the differences between Technopathogenology and Technology Assessment, we will analyze the example of a hydroelectric power plant.

Technology Assessment

Following the criteria used for its definition, Technology Assessment would consider:

Environmental impact

Because of the dam formed and the microclimatic alterations in the area: Effects on plant and animal species. Need to eradicate some species.

Impact on society

a) Due to the need to relocate population: Problems of uprooting, cultural change, changes in human relationships. Housing problems when relocating in households which do not respond to the needs or preferences of the people, etc.
b) Due to relocating people in new occupations.

c) Due to the affluence of new people in the not relocated populations near the power plant. Alteration of local habits.

d) Polluting and highly risky fuelling methods such as fossil fuels and thermonuclear power plants would be avoided.

e) Risks on human health. The evident or expected risks would be the ones mainly considered – practically limited to the power plant workers (risks which can be reduced to the bare minimum with the adequate hygiene and safety measures). Risks associated with engineering problems: collapsing, leakages, etc.

Impact on economy

Local, regional, and nationwide:

a) Need to provide new jobs to relocated people.

b) Generation of new jobs (directly and indirectly).

c) Impact on general economy due to the advantages of having a new source of energy and avoiding the dependence on fossil fuels, etc.

Technopathogenology

It would evaluate technopathogenic risks for consumers and for occupationally exposed people (the most significant risk group).

The most important aspects would be:

Physical Factors: Electromagnetic fields generated. Risks for consumers that live near high tension lines and for plant workers.

Chemical Factors: Products used in the plant: Lubes, refrigerants, generation of ozone, etc. Principal risk for plant workers.

Biological Factors: Associated with the dam and microclimatic change in the area.

Cultural or Psychological Factors: Evaluation of psychological implications due to changes in lifestyle.

Once the risks are assessed, prevention methods would be proposed.

VIII. Other aspects of the Science and Technique system that contribute to further support the need of this new discipline

So far we have referred to: theories connected to concrete factors of technopathogenic risks, failed attempts to frame technopathogeny within existing disciplines and the need to create a new specific discipline. Below we will present another theory that could be considered as *marker* or indicator of the disciplinary void for this phenomenon:

Theory VIII: The evident difficulties of the evaluation system to frame Technopathogeny indicate the disciplinary void for its study

When we referred to the disciplinary framing of the Technopathogeny phenomenon, we described the normal way of making science within a specific discipline (for example, physiology, physics, chemistry, etc.). Now, what happens when there are no specific phenomena which can be easily incorporated in the classical divisions of science (Biological, Chemical, Physical, Agricultural, Earth, etc.)?

In this case, and according to our experience, we can expect great difficulties due to the nature of the evaluation process.

This led to a new hypothesis:

Hypothesis: Can the difficulties within the evaluation system indicate a void in the disciplinary system that makes it difficult to frame a new phenomenon?

Every evaluative process implies determining one or a group of qualities to consider in a determined object in order to judge it. A research project and the proposal of study of a new phenomenon are objects which can be judged.

The existing disciplines provide a group of values that can be considered by an evaluator to judge the proposal of study of a phenomenon. If this fits within the existing disciplines, the project can be accepted or not, but there will be no inconveniences for its evaluation. However, when a phenomenon is new for the evaluator, certain inconveniences can arise that can lead to rejecting the project – not for being of little value or for having deficient aims, but because the evaluator has no parameters for its analysis. Therefore, the easiest attitude is rejection. In connection with this and as proof that pursuing the new is something that has existed throughout history, we can quote Voltaire: "There is no truth that has not been persecuted from its birth (Voltaire).

We have experienced this difficulty ourselves when we proposed Technopathogeny as object of study. This encouraged us to make a more thorough study of such difficulty which we include as a reading in Chapter IV (Cultural Clash of Technopathogenology in the Scientific System). We speak of culture because it implies the value that humans give to an object.

When studying mycotoxins, we encountered difficulties when we tried an anthropo-ecological approach, especially when trying to frame it within known and consolidated disciplines which were part of the Science and Technique System.

Back then, and after our research, mycotoxins became a known object of study. They were included in several research projects from different perspectives or disciplines, but not following our proposal to study them in connection to their prophylaxis and its influence on human health. All these projects in consolidated sciences received funds, but our proposal did not.

If this is analyzed superficially, it can be read as stealing ideas, but from a different perspective, it is understandable that whoever is in a consolidated (or aged, according to Lakatos) program, falls in the temptation of appropriating an idea that can enrich it. The compensation would be to help whoever came up with the idea to freely develop his or her own program. Selfishness both of people and of the system manifests itself in the following: Join our program or be left out. No thank you for the new idea. The authoritarianism for the new enriched program is monolithic and must not make any exception for fear of showing weakness. Therefore, whoever has a program that fosters new ideas must be in a constant fight against disciplinary reduction and corporative inclusion.

The evaluators did not understand that the detection and prophylaxis of aflatoxins risks could be of interest to receive financial support. It was a program with individual entity.

It is obvious that when the system does not understand the reason or orientation the researcher gives to his or her work, it prefers that the work be approached by consolidated disciplines. We could define such attitude as an *automatic mechanism of reduction.* Or to an excessive conservative attitude which prefers accepting small variations of what is already known rather than something substantially new.

In an attempt to try to see these facts objectively in order to give adequate judgment, we could perhaps say that our question on detection and prophylaxis to protect consumers from the non-evident immanent risks of technique did not fit within the scientific structure of the science and technique system. The evaluators were only interested in the aspects that linked this question with other branches or other existing disciplines. This explains why our project was not approved by evaluators as a scientific question: it could not be measured by any evaluation method. This was a problem since, because of the way we presented the question, it could not be answered by any discipline.

Let us go back to the example of the plant species to be studied by two researchers: one would do it from the point of view of medicine, and the other from the point of view of taxonomy. If the system only accepts the analysis of the latter, the questions that the former asked will be unanswered.

This means that since there is no branch of science or discipline that can focus on the detection and prophylaxis of environmental effects caused by technology and carried through water, air and foodstuffs, the existing disciplines should be the ones leading the advancement of knowledge in the field.

This short reflection on the characteristics of the evaluation system is very interesting since it shows the difficulties that arise when trying to approach research from certain perspectives. Maybe the aim of our proposal was not understood and those who decided on the subsidies – with a conservative criterion – preferred to subsidize the known and not support the unknown.

We have noticed evaluation difficulties in connection to Technopathogeny both in the scientific and academic worlds. Regarding the former, every single project presented to evaluation committees in order to apply for financial aid for research was systematically rejected. The argument used was that there was already a discipline to study the phenomenon. But what the evaluators considered as already existent was only a discipline that could perhaps approach part of the question. We were forced to reduce the question to such extent that its nature was completely altered. The only possible alternative – though unacceptable from the intellectual perspective – was to frame the phenomenon within an existing discipline, overcoming our disgust for having to leave a major part – or the core part – of the phenomenon without being studied.

Our discipline was also rejected in the academic world. Our attempt to try to include it in the curriculum of a technological degree was flatly rejected. Even the possibility of including the aims of our proposal in a consolidated subject was rejected (Eguiazu, 1998).

The attitude of evaluators both in the scientific and academic fields was the same: *I reject the proposal because I do not understand it. It must adjust to what I know so that I can accept it.*

We have mentioned this difficulty in this hypothesis because it proves that the phenomenon is new and that there is no discipline that can approach its study. In a way we are taking responsibility off the system's shoulders, giving it the benefit of the doubt. It is reproachable, however, that the system is impervious to new proposals. If the system's criterion was the progress of knowledge, this should be unacceptable. The basic principle of the university system – the advancement of knowledge passing it on to students without restrictions – is bastardized here.

When we referred to the attempts of framing this phenomenon within an existing discipline, we said that each presented project produced a statement on *about what it was not or was not done and should have been done* and the logical negative consequences. We have also said that the collection of these reports patiently kept for thirty years allowed us to recognize the need of a correct evaluation to our question and finally support the need of creating a specific discipline. We could summarize this difficulty stating that *the system evaluates what was not done because it cannot evaluate or fears the evaluation of what was in fact done.*

We can add as well that there was also a good deal of pride and cowardliness in the evaluators. Pride, because they are ashamed of admitting that they do not know something; and cowardliness, because if the magnitude of the problem and the human and social implications are understood, they fear either being intellectually overcome or severely criticized by the authorities who do not want the research to be carried out.

Hypothesis: Why is there reluctance in the scientific system as a Technical/Productive entity to recognize and accept Technopathogeny as a new phenomenon?

In general, the lack of knowledge of the new and the doubt generated by the new leads to certain kind of reluctance for its acceptance. With time, the positive aspects of the new can be proved and it can then become accepted. Technopathogeny as a phenomenon and Technopathogenology as a new scientific proposal are no exception.

Apart from the cultural differences we mentioned in the previous hypothesis, the difficulties that arose while we developed our project – which would lead to another work we will briefly describe in the first reading of Chapter IV – prove such reluctance. Evaluation difficulties, no acceptance of the projects, etc., motivated the need of an Ethical Objector in Science and Technique (this will also be discussed in Chapter IV).

The reluctance of the system is manifested not only in coercing the researcher to *adjust* his or her ideas to the existing disciplines, but also in the attitude of the corporation telling the researcher that his or her ideas are already being studied by other disciplines. If it does not exist, the system can readily create it resorting to the most ridiculous acronyms. The researchers' wit would be to incorporate in a consolidated program, let's say, physiology, an acronym including this new idea in its science. This can ensure innovation in his or her ageing program. For example, if a researcher has an original and relevant idea, the physiologist will try to incorporate it with the prefix or suffix *physio* to say which field is already studying that area. This would lead to such strange terms as *physiopathology* or *pathophysiology, technophysiopathology, physiotechnopathogenology, environmental physiology*, etc. This way, the researcher of the corporation ensures that he or she will receive new funds for incorporating the new idea to his or her ageing program. What is not said is that if the idea in fact is suitable to have its own program, the researcher will find it difficult to defend it and develop it without funds. The funds will be destined to the old, rejuvenated program with the *aesthetic surgery* performed by the change of name. Putting it bluntly, the robbery of the idea will pass unnoticed. The ageing program that has *borrowed* the new idea will receive the subsidies for its research. If the researcher who had the original idea, being deprived of it and disillusioned, weakens, the original program will fail. The only thing that remains is the illegitimate acronym as the sole *owner* of the new idea to develop. If the researcher does not weaken and strongly defends his or her idea, he or she will become an Ethical Objector – a subject we will discuss in the eight reading of Chapter IV.

In connection to this hypothesis, in Chapter IV we will also discuss the new concepts of quality, the cultural criteria of Science and Technique and the protection of consumers – all of which must be considered for the prevention of Technopathogenies.

One of the cultural criteria of the technical/productive system we have considered is the motto of Chicago World's Fair on Technological Innovation (1933) (San Martín, 1990): "Science Finds, Industry Applies, Man conforms."

This phrase allows us to understand the frame of mind at the time and the euphoria and enthusiasm towards Science, Technology and Industry. Such euphoria and enthusiasm numbed any possibility of criticising the so called myth of progress. It was believed that there was some kind of permanent and eternal progress which any technological innovation would bring about. In this sense, humans should accept any technological innovation without reluctance. In other words, they should conform. This blind faith in progress was so big that they believed it would be possible to modify on the spot any error incurred by Technique or to convince whoever opposed to progress to change his or her mind. Any determination of humans who did not fit within the rules of science, industry and technology was considered a rebellion or anarchism against progress.

In connection to our project, it is easy to understand why there has been such reluctance to accept it.

This reluctance can also be observed with concepts coming from the system itself. Apart from the fallacious concepts to justify the damage incurred by technique, we could mention, for example, that our hypothesis on mycotoxins contradicts the old argument that minimizes the apparition of contaminants of industrial origin saying that aflatoxins and mycotoxins have always existed in nature: since human beings have survived those contaminants, they will also survive other contaminants (Frank, 1980-1983).

This is an opinion supported by many scientists who ignore that even though these are natural contaminants, the way they enter humans and the damage they cause have a technological nature. There is an interesting example on the technology of uranium in connection to this.

This is a natural component, but since it is distributed in nature in specific areas and it is not concentrated, the circumstance of exposure on humans is very unlikely.

If humans are aware of the areas where uranium in its natural state is found in relatively large quantities, they can avoid exposure (as they would avoid living near a solfatara, which continuously emanates sulphurous gases).

In this case, Technique is responsible for uranium to be: enriched, concentrated, turned into the critical mass of a reactor, taken to special circumstances of uncertainty and be placed near populations which are told there is no risk whatsoever since it is meant to be under control. When the defect is manifested as accident, as in Harrisburg or Chernobyl accidents (insidious the former, spectacular the latter), the first reaction of Science and Technique is of stupor and denial. The scientific/political power denies responsibilities. In other words, it lies.

In general, all the radioactive contaminations have a slow long-term negative effect on health which can manifest itself after many years or decades. As we have mentioned before, a decade after the Chernobyl accident the WHO published a report on the accident and its consequences prepared by the International Program on the Health Effects of the Chernobyl Accident (IPHECA).

This program was developed to support the national programs, to watch the health consequences of the accident and indicate activities needed in the future to ensure that after this incident all possible information be obtained. As long term adverse consequences to health, thyroid cancer and leukemia are mentioned. A significant increase of thyroid cancer in children was registered, but when the report was published (10 years after the incident) there was no significant increase in leukemia cases. However, the study includes a brief period of time – it is mentioned that more than 10 years are necessary for hemopathies to manifest at a maximum point. Long term studies are recommended on this subject. On the psychic level, even though it could not be established to what extent radiations could have contributed to such manifestations, there is proof of mental retardation and anomalous behavior in children who were exposed to radiation while in the womb (WHO, 1997). Another criticism was seen in an article published by INES in 2006, which clearly states the lack of sustainability of nuclear energy since its risks are much higher than its benefits (Mian & Glaser, 2006).

When we referred to the risks of Ionizing Radiation by exposure to nuclear energy, we mentioned that other authors expressed the reluctance of the system in recognizing both the damages of the Chernobyl accident and the risks of the exposed.

It is interesting to go back to table 2, which showed that according to scientific evaluations, the possibility of a nuclear plant accident would be the same as an aerolite crushing the earth and killing 100 persons (approximately once every 100,000 years) (Gassen, 1988).

Going back to the solfatara example, we can say that humans living in big cities live near a technique-generated solfatara without knowing so: due to environmental pollution, a slow (unlike the risks presented by nuclear material) and insidious effect of sulphur oxides is produced in the organism.

Here the argument of those who minimize the importance of industrial pollution using nature as an example shows its lack of soundness (Eguiazu & Motta, 2000).

The denial of risks causes that, in general, it takes a while from the moment a technopathogenic harm is detected until it is attributed to the technology that caused it and even more until the technology is detected and recalled.

This means that real damage will necessarily occur: the relatively long time of usage is a fact. Once the damage is proved – sometimes in humans, such as the bovine spongiform encephalopathy – the system starts slowly backing up the technology. This backing up is sometimes not done immediately after the effect is known – there is some kind of inertia or even a deliberate hiding of the detected negative effect. In general, panic or damage to the economy is avoided. If there is a high pressure of voters, the measures are taken faster, thus leading to economic loss, as was seen with the cremation of livestock in England (Eguiazu & Motta, 2001a).

Can the evident be denied?

We have seen the urge of changing the existing criteria, an urge that was not brought about by the quiet acceptance of more solid theoretical arguments but due to the evidence of facts, especially the apparition of a phenomenon: the inherent and hidden collateral effects of a technology.

Neither Technique/Industry/Corporations, even less the Scientific system can continue with this indulging attitude, admiring The Emperor's New Clothes (Andersen) when the emperor is in fact naked, admiring technique/technology while having proof of the deficiencies it can have. There are of course some differences. In the famous story, anyone who acknowledged that the emperor was naked would show he or she was stupid and unsuitable for his or her job. Everyone knew that the emperor was naked but no one dared to say it out loudly. In the case of immanent and hidden risks of Technique responsible for Technopathogenies, we do not know whether any technician or scientist was aware of them but did not dare to talk fearing *sticking his or her head out*. Furthermore, the child in the story who, carried by his innocence, cried *the emperor is naked* received no punishment because of his innocence. On the contrary, the whole village was relieved to finally recognize that the emperor was naked. But in Science and Technique, speaking out that Technique is not that wonderful, crying out *Technique can cause non-evident risks!*, infuriates the *tailors of technique*, because what this means is that their technique is not *as wonderful* as they believed. It all ends as if in the story the child would have been silenced and punished. The tailors' anger exposes the denouncer – an ethical objector – which entails certain risks, as we will see in Chapter IV.

Instead of punishing objectors, scientists or technologists should promote them. Scientists or technologists should recognize that there is an underlying phenomenon in the Technique they are developing – a Technopathogeny – they cannot get rid of and that must be excluded a priori (Eguiazu & Motta, 2000).

It is a proved fact that in spite of the precautions Science and Technique take, several technologies have surprisingly unacceptable collateral effects.

Their apparition surprises and reduces the Science and Technique system, which usually avoids investigating what causes them. A unidirectional reaction is then produced: secondary causes are investigated and there is an attempt to repair the damage caused. But there is no retrospective investigation on the uttermost cause. Humans end up being hamsters. It would seem that the *reparation of theories* mechanism, justified by the concept that science is self corrective, is continuously employed. This mechanism is very much used in Science and Technique in order not to abandon theories which do not necessarily fit with the facts, to support the hypothesis or theory of innocuousness of the concrete technological object. In Chapter III we will thoroughly analyze the *theory of innocuousness*. This innocuousness becomes a *must* (Jonas, 1984) of any technology that passed the safety tests, first through the strict evaluation of its scientific grounds by peers and then through the strict tests on safety which the system applies to concrete techniques.

The facts show that the apparent safety or infallibly of the method is not always so. This was particularly complicated in the discussion of transgenic safety regarding the example of Arpad Pusztai's falsification (Pusztai, 2000), which we will refer to when we discuss transgenic foodstuffs.

Had Pusztai not carried out his experiments or the civil courage to expose them in the media, those potatoes would have surely passed all the safety measures the relevant ministries imposed and consumers would have probably ingested them. Once the symptoms were found, it would have been much cheaper for the establishment that marketed them to find an underlying cause for the disease which differed from the truth (the real cause can lead to lawsuits and it is better to keep it unrevealed). Under these circumstances, the consumer has to conform not only to a low quality product, but to a harmful one. Paradoxically, on the other end of the trophic chain, the producer can consider the possibility of using this product due to its extraordinary resistance to nematodes or insects, for instance, or due to the high turnout. We will go back to this at a later stage.

Another interesting question is:

Hypothesis: Technopathogeny. Is this a phenomenon for epistemologists or for technologists?

Let us accept that Technopathogenology is a necessary discipline to bring prophylaxis to proved facts which imply damages on health after the application of new technologies which were thought to be innocuous. Even then, it could be argued that it is a question of humanitarianism or of extreme human health. Strictly speaking, it would be like wanting to protect someone from getting hit by a hard object that might fall off a building by asking the person to stay permanently at home. If the person does not go out into the street there is no risk at all, but then the subject is completely immobilized and loses the possibility of carrying out the simplest activities. Technopathogenology could then be a beautiful object of study for theory epistemologists, but not a discipline for technologists with practical implications.

According to our thesis this is not so, and, as we will see further on, it even has economic implications. Technopathogeny is a phenomenon that must be known by technologists who, with the bases or elements provided by Technopathogenology, will be able to take measures in order to eliminate or reduce risks.

IX. Conclusion

To conclude this Chapter we could then say that starting with a problem in particular – a natural contaminant – and then moving on to engulf Technique in general, we found that the Technopathogeny phenomenon could not be framed within the existing disciplinary system. In the case of aflatoxins, it was a failed attempt to incorporate the phenomenon to different disciplines. It was also a failed attempt – due to the lack of a discipline within the academic/scientific field – to try to develop a sub-field within the grain-post-harvest-handling field (for example, the quality and conservation of grains) to study these contaminants: the technopathogenic analysis proposed was flatly rejected by the evaluators (Eguiazu, 1998).

Our findings throughout thirty years of investigations were neither perfect nor irrefutable. What we found in this path allowed us to sketch a theory – a theory which, as every theory, is an attempt to approach falsifiable knowledge.

We have seen the logical connection between hypothesis and theories that enabled us to arrive to the conclusion of the impossibility of framing, a connection that arose in an unforced and natural way. We were not obsessed with the idea of creating a new science. The need arose as an *a posteriori* consequence, since the knowledge came from or depended on experience or, in other words, was a reasoning that arose from the effect to the cause or from the properties of the thing to its essence. The idea of a science is babbling and tentative. Our detailed description of attempting and failing to frame this discipline within existing sciences led us to slowly and unwillingly conceive the idea of a new science. We believe we have covered all the possibilities of framing it within the existing sciences. Applying the falsification criteria of a hypothesis or theory, we carried out an analysis trying to demonstrate that our proposal was unnecessary. But it did not prove unnecessary at all, and we had no choice but to accept the need of a new science. In other words, we tried to falsify our own postulate asking ourselves whether our science was actually necessary. We would like to insist that this study is the product of 30 years of work that ends up with this proposal.

We have considered several disciplines to try to frame this phenomenon. We are not saying that the analysis was complete. In some disciplines the analysis could have been more thorough.

We could go back to the labyrinth analogy: in science, the search for an answer of a new problem is like introducing the problem or the question in the labyrinth. Each path corresponds with a discipline and the solution to reaching the core of the problem is in choosing the way that allows to reaching the centre of the labyrinth. In this centre of the *disciplinary labyrinth* is where the adequate discipline would be found. As we have seen, every alternative of framing we studied – Philosophy, Biology, Ecology, etc. – were dead end paths: none of them reached the centre.

Another analogy could be a sick person trying to recover his or her health. The correct way would be to consult a general practitioner first who would, in turn, indicate which specialist to consult. But patients usually consult the specialist first. If they see a problem in their skin, they would consult a dermatologist. But the dermatologist will most probably treat the problem from the point of view of his field and may never arrive to the actual cause of the problem. The symptom that the patient observed on his or her skin can be the manifestation of another problem – hepatic, for example. These analogies can be found in other fields (plants, animals, etc.). Something similar could have happened with Technopathogenology. Even though our intuition led us to the need of a new science, we tried *consulting* different fields first: Philosophy, Biology, etc. All of them could have analyzed the problem of Technopathogeny, but none would have arrived to its root. The final aporia led us to conclude that just like a sensible patient should first consult a general practitioner to be recommended the adequate specialist, technopathogeny should be treated by a specialist too: The technopathogenist. The evaluative system, however, by observing only the problem on the outside, oriented it to the discipline which seemed to lay closer to the problem. In some cases, this lacked adequacy to such an extent that the decision was sometimes taken by some clerk who derived the project to the Commission whose name resembled the title of the project in some way. Once the project entered the evaluation process and was in the hands of a group of experts, there was no going back, which is what happened with mycotoxins. By seeing the project dealt with a fungus, the evaluation system assigned it to Mycology or Biology. But a thorough analysis of the problem allowed us to see that it was essentially a technological problem; furthermore, it deserved a specific science for its study. We could say that at first we saw aflatoxins as an indicator. In chemistry it is common to use indicators to measure, for example, the acidity or alkalinity of water, which, in general, react by changing color. In general, indicators show an underlying phenomenon – in this case, chemical reactions – that determine the acidity or alkalinity of water. Baring this example in mind, we could say that specialists saw aflatoxins as an object of study in itself that could enrich their disciplines. But it is as if they were only interested in the fact that the water color changed and use it to dye fabric. That is, they only saw the *profitability* of the idea, typical of an *aloentic* system, as we will describe in the first reading of the Annex. To them, the problem with aflatoxins was a profitable idea. They rushed to ask for subsidies, which they obtained, while we kept on thinking on the question, which is the underlying phenomenon this indicator is showing? Why does the water change color with the indicator? In the case of aflatoxins: Why do aflatoxins appear in grains? Which is the underlying phenomenon?

Going back to the comparison with the general practitioner, we wonder whether in Science and Technique there should be a general practitioner scientist to guide young researchers with innovative ideas to which specialty to resort to in order to approach their investigations. Many topics might lose sight of their aims due to the wrong approach to the subject – due to a premature derivation of the problem.

In connection to risk in particular, we have seen that there are other new and interesting disciplinary or multidisciplinary proposals developed with the intention of approaching the problem in a more specific way (not considered in this chapter). We believe that a thorough analysis of each of them would lead to another extensive chapter of this book. We hope that the proposals selected to its analysis provide enough grounds to support the limits to achieve an adequate prevention of the problem.

We have supported the fact that after this peregrination throughout disciplines we could not find an adequate place to answer to our question on Technopathogeny. Just like the problem with aflatoxins, trying to frame Technopathogeny within various disciplines was also a failure. In the best of cases, the help obtained from the disciplines is partial. The *atomization* of a complex problem – Technopathogeny, in this case – only dilutes the essence of such problem. It will hardly contribute to find a solution. We therefore had to think of building a new place in the disciplinary town for our question to dwell.

We could compare our search with a hound searching for a trail in an apparently chaotic way. It will sooner or later find its prey even if its master, though mistakenly, leads it through a different path. The hound will even abandon its master to find its object, baring the master's insults for not responding to his call. The hound will search for the object even if its life is in danger, even if gets wet or muddled. Similarly, we could say we search for Technopathogenology no matter how reluctant the scientific system is (which, as we will see in the first reading of Chapter IV, behaves as if it were the *master* of the researcher). This *master* tried in vain to separate us from our trail, from that *motivator* we cannot describe and which made us bare the aggressions to such an extent that we became Ethical Objectors.

We were thus able to confirm the concept, the void of knowledge and the nature of the intellectual progress achieved with Beck in the proposal of Technopathogenology.

To answer our Theory VII, the uttermost aim is to include the risks of technique in a technological program since the aim of Technique cannot be severed from the concept of doing it well that lies within its nature, i.e. the lack of technopathogenies. This new place in the disciplinary town to study the phenomenon of technopathogeny is a science that must be part of Technology: Technopathogenology.

CHAPTER III

Technopathogenology – The science and its method

'To protect present and future Humans'

I. Introduction

When we finished our Introduction, we said that following the principle of Ancient Greeks, the aim of Technopathogenology is to contribute to the establishment of the *canons* which Technology should respect, so that the generated change does not lead to adverse effects of late manifestation in human health. Such change should not *neglect* the environment or fellow living creatures, which are many times not the direct beneficiaries of the work created by the Technical Man.

We chose the epigraph *to protect present and future Humans* for this chapter – in which we will describe our disciplinary proposal – as a principle and commitment that must guide the search for knowledge in our discipline and also should guide any technological change.

In the previous chapters we have dealt with the two first epistemological criteria to support the need for a new science. We have defined both the phenomenon and the theories that showed its disciplinary orphanage. We have also observed that this phenomenon has its own identity or singularity as well as such a large magnitude or dimension that calls for a new science. In this chapter we will analyze the methodology and tools proposed for the study of this new phenomenon.

II.   Technopathogenology: The science

Technopathogenology. The search for similar scientific situations

We have found similarities with the origin of Technopathogenology in the science developed around the study of the soil (Eguiazu & Motta, 2000). We do not know whether the person or persons who supported its creation had to go through the same disciplinary pilgrimage we had. Due to its characteristics and constitution, one could think that soil, as a phenomenon, could be approached by multiple disciplines: Geology, Biology, Physics and Chemistry. However, the soil is not studied by a set of isolated disciplines which are artificially integrated – which would make it a multidisciplinary study. The soil is studied by a specific science: Edaphology.

Another science in which we have found similarities is Criminology. Even though it is not that much an empirical science, it is based on empirical evidence to clarify the phenomenon. In this case, the cause of the empirical evidence found is tracked down until the crime is solved. As we will see later, this example is applied as a contribution to support our methodological proposal for Technopathogenology.

It is perhaps in the method applied by criminology – at least during the diagnose stage – where we find similarities with Technopathogenology. But during the prospective or germinal improvement stage (of technique as an object), Technopathogenology will be more akin to formal sciences.

We have mentioned as example two sciences: Edaphology and Criminology. The question we can ask ourselves is: why do people approaching the study of a new phenomenon experiment the need to build a new disciplinary field?

In order to answer this question we believe it is interesting to bear in mind a concept by Kuhn on "Anomalies." Some may postulate another – maybe more adequate – criterion, but we consider it is interesting to think that the developers of Edaphology and Criminology realized that the phenomenon they were studying presented an anomaly that made it impossible to frame it within the existing disciplines.

Let us analyze then T. Kuhn's concept.

"Persistent anomaly" or the key to innovation

This concept was postulated by Kuhn (Kuhn, 1995) to describe the general process of innovation or discovery. According to the author, any innovation or discovery needs the researcher or discoverer to have a prior feeling that something is wrong, a feeling which returns again and again to his or her field of study and which we could describe as an *ostinato*.

The researcher can try to eliminate it at first, so that it does not dampen what he or she is expecting to see in his or her experiment. But the annoyance comes up over and over again, dampening the expected theory, thus ending up being recognized as a phenomenon in itself. The persistent anomaly is only the manifestation of a phenomenon which is not very much known that appears along with one which is known. Time, the persistence of this anomaly, and the intuition capacity of the innovator to recognize in such anomaly something more than an annoyance, make the innovator change focus towards such anomaly. The discovery is thus produced.

It is interesting to apply Kuhn's concept to the phenomenon of Technopathogeny. We can then ask ourselves: When, according to Kuhn, do we speak of *anomalies*?

Because some of the sciences involved in technological development are framed or self-defined as *exact sciences*, when applying the *methodological rigor* to the development of knowledge created by them – unlike other ways of obtaining knowledge, such as empirical knowledge, which is an anathema for these exact sciences – we could say that the normal science works in paradigms and thus state that: *Technology is the product of the methodical and exact doing of the scientist, which is why it is innocuous.*

Kuhn's anomaly applied to a persistent collaterality shown in Technique is the phenomenon of Technopathogeny. If the statement above quoted was correct, Technopathogeny would not exist.

Now, what does this mean? Which are the intuitive conception and the clash of generations Kuhn is talking about when he says that the change of scope or *paradigm*, as he calls it, (Kuhn, 1995) is:

An irrational process produced not by a rational well-supported discourse, but by the historical clash of generations, that is, among defenders of the old paradigm against defenders of the new one.

The answer is very simple: the initial idea of Technopathogeny was not conceived by logic but by intuition – an idea which was later proved in some techniques (by induction of observed cases and then postulated to technique in general by deduction of many other observed cases). Its recognition by the scientific community will come as a consequence of the generational clash of researchers.

Which were the particular anomalies we detected that gave us the *gut feeling* that there was *something else*? Which were the anomalies that permitted us to say *there is something going on here* or to ask ourselves, *is there something unexplainable going on just with what we have in our hands*? The anomalies in the two first research topics were: in one, the different susceptibility of sunflower grains to biological deterioration and to the apparition of aflatoxins and, in the other, the lack of relationship between acute and chronic risk (carcinogenicity) in the case of pesticides.

Kuhn is right when he criticizes Carnap or Hume's inductivism, but also Popper's deductivism. According to Kuhn, the anomalies within a paradigm can only be resolved because more and more scientists are *taking them seriously* as object of study. Scientific progress is not only caused by adherence to the object of study and to the established method, but also by intuition on *anomalies*. Let us remember Fleming's Petri dish contaminated with *Penicillum*: had Fleming not taken seriously the anomalies, he would have disposed of the Petri dish without observing with curiosity the inhibiting halo. Taking this *anomaly* seriously, realizing that there was *something going on* in the Petri dish, led him to isolate penicillin.

With Kuhn's ideas we can state that the entity of Technopathogenology will be proved through its survival of the generational clash, its historical resistance. The generational clash we had to go through will be described in Chapter IV.

Now, can we pass from one paradigm to another smoothly, without conflict, just by the force of arguments?

Kuhn quotes Planck's autobiography: the substantial changes are not obtained by convincing the advocates of old ideas, but by waiting long enough until, in Einstein's words, the advocates pass away and are substituted by others. It is interesting to add that the blind adhesion to one's own ideas is typical of scientists. It is the *scientist's pride* Eco refers to (Eco, 2000). Therefore, a scientist can recognize the need of change, but when it comes to accepting a paradigm that contradicts the scientist's own paradigm, he or she can offer fierce resistance. This is what happened with

Planck himself, who was Heisenberg's examiner in Heisenberg's doctorate thesis. After arguing with the candidate, Planck finally gave him a very poor *rite* as a mark for his doctorate (which is a 4/10, or a C). Heisenberg even said that: "For new ideas (paradigms) to be accepted, the way of thinking of those who must accept them must be changed." Heisenberg may have received a poor mark, but he had a new paradigm.

To sum up, after dedicating a whole chapter to trying to frame Technopathogeny, we realized that there was something odd in the phenomenon that was preventing us from doing so.

Which was the persistent anomaly?

We could say that in the scientific work sometimes a concern surfaces, a persistent idea that does not leave and continuously returns, whispering that there is something there, something that does not allow the scientist to rest; an almost annoying idea that there is something unexplainable within what is being studied. In our case, and after approaching the two anomalies above cited, by induction and deduction we found that the persistent anomaly of Technique was the apparition of negative effects to health caused by technologies which were thought to be safe – Technopathogeny – and that such phenomenon could not be framed within the existing disciplines, which gave, in the best of cases, partial answers to it.

The first stage of the acceptance of this anomaly was the definition of the phenomenon and then the definition of this phenomenon as immanent to Technique, as we saw in Chapter I.

As we have said, what was left was the inductive and deductive stage, i.e. the data collection stage to verify or reject a theory – which we dealt with in Chapter II. In Chapter III we will focus on the falsification stage.

The first question we can ask ourselves is: is there any case that contradicts the theory elaborated by the induction of the persistent anomalies?

The answer is yes: without a doubt, there are cases of techniques created without defects that can cause technopathogenies. This confirms the theory, and we must add that (as a fact when referring to the attitudes regarding the truth) the absence of technopathogenies is more a consequence of chance than of a precise and preventive investigation of the phenomenon. The phenomenon is not there by chance nor by a conscientious study that had avoided it beforehand.

A second question we will briefly develop is: what is not Technopathogenology?

III. The question on foreseeing

The aim of Technopathogenology is the prevention of Technopathogenies, a phenomenon which, as we have seen in Chapter II, could not be framed within the existing disciplines. Here we must ask ourselves whether we are referring to a phenomenon which is impossible to predict – and, therefore, completely random, which would make it only possible to describe its apparition but leaving no possibility for prevention – or to a predictable phenomenon which the imperfection of our method does not allow yet its prevention. Our guess is that the latter is the most probable. Our hypothesis is that there is a phase lag between the development of the technological product and the application of a method to prevent its collateralities. This phase lag casts an enormous asymmetry in favor of the development of the product to the detriment of the method of prevention of technopathogenies. The technological challenge for this millennium is the development of appropriate prophylaxis methodologies that focus automatically on the germinal technological matrix. The closer the gestation of Technology gets to this ideal matrix, the faster and less expensive the prophylaxis of risks will be (Eguiazu, 1999b) (Eguiazu & Motta, 2001b).

IV. Which is the disciplinary framework?

We thus arrive to a point in which, even though we more or less agree that there is an object of study in Technopathogeny, we are still not sure how to approach it, or rather, where to frame it. That is how the attempts of finding it a disciplinary home begin, first, within the existent and then differentiating little by little a specific framework. The detailed analysis carried out in the previous chapter allowed us to state that the disciplinary orphanage is the last and very little accepted conclusion one must

272

arrive to when there is no other chance whatsoever. As any other orphanage phenomenon (including the orphanage of a human being), we know
the process of finding a new home is a very difficult one. The future characteristics of the orphan will depend on the adopting parents. Similarly,
the future of Technopathogeny will depend on the disciplinary framework in which it is placed. Also, as a child should be ideally raised by its
biological parents – the adopting home is a tolerated substitution but it is
not the most desirable situation – the same happens with the Technopathogeny phenomenon. If this phenomenon can be approached by a specific discipline, the advancement of knowledge will be much more precise and efficient than if it were approached by other disciplines such as
Physics, Chemistry, Biology, etc. These sciences will only orient the
study of such phenomenon from their own perspective which, even
though it is appropriate for the phenomena belonging to their own discipline; it will always be biased when dealing with technopathogenological
questions or problems.

We could say that the study and the search for the truth of the phenomenon will depend on the viewpoint of the observer, that is, on the
approach and the intellectual tools available (Eguiazu & Motta, 2001b).

V. What happens when there is no discipline
for a phenomenon which is not much described?

An interesting experience is the phenomenon of enrichment by sympathy
with the neighboring disciplines. When it comes to investigating a technopathogenological question, there may be several disciplines that help
in part elucidate the phenomenon. Paradoxically, the phenomenon is not
clarified but it enriches the neighboring discipline or disciplines that continue their development enriched with some kind of innovation. This is
what Lakatos (Lakatos, 1982) refers to when he talks of young and ageing research projects. Ageing programs will more likely attempt to integrate a new program to the existent – using them to renovate their own –
rather than accept the entity of the new ones. But in this work in collaboration, an ageing program can hardly be renovated. What it does happen
is that the development of the new program is slowed down or even de-

stroyed. The existent discipline limits the problem to the scope it might provide, which is insufficient to the question that concerns us.

In general, after a long pilgrimage one arrives at the situation in which the new program is incorporated within any of the already existent ones just to obtain some kind of immediate benefit or comply with a requirement. Should the researcher refuse to this illegitimate inclusion, the program will be left without its benefits. In some cases, the evaluation is completely tangential: some statements elaborated by experts are very poor because they are not experts in the evaluated discipline, in spite of the undeniable expertise in their own disciplines.

Ethical reasoning and common sense tell us that it is not possible to do good science within a borrowed theoretical framework. An integration which in fact does not exist is forced and feigned. When the problem is enormously complex, much energy is lost when trying to focus it artificially from a different discipline. The researcher who works in good faith always feels that any attempt of framing the new phenomenon out of the specific, existing or to be created discipline is an unnecessary process that leads to an enormous loss of time and effort.

This proper lack of evaluation can lead, in some cases – if the evaluation system is not flexible – to a *self-willed delirium*. In this case, the fact that evaluators are experts in some already consolidated prestigious science provides them with authority in excess. This necessarily leads them to see that the new program, the new phenomenon, is part of their own science. This only seems a strategy within the system to allow the prestigious evaluator to give his or her opinion notwithstanding the actual suitability to evaluate the specific question. Our conclusion is that prestigious evaluators in consolidated disciplines can provide statements which are completely out of reality by attempting to force a disciplinary framing to complex technopathogenological questions.

As a conclusion, to illustrate this, we can quote these biblical proverbs (Luke):

> No one tears a piece out of a new garment to patch an old one. Otherwise, they will have torn the new garment, and the patch from the new will not match the old. Or: No one pours new wine into old wineskins. Otherwise, the new wine will burst the skins; the wine will run out and the wineskins will be ruined. No, new wine must be poured into new wineskins.

Both proverbs explain the same situation. If we relate them to old and new paradigms, the wineskin proverb suits perfectly well. In the garment proverb, however, the new paradigm would be ruined to suit the old paradigm, which would benefit from the new paradigm.

VI.   Why a Technopathogenology?

The first thing we have to ask ourselves is whether the title: *Why a Technopathogenology?* is adequately phrased. Maybe we should ask ourselves: *What is not Technopathogenology?* This is the criterion we decided to adopt and thus analyze, in a more modest way, the existing disciplines and then study how they adjust to our phenomenon, as we have seen in Chapter II. We can state that the object of study approached by each of the disciplines considered is not the object of Technopathogenology. Searching for *what this discipline is not*, allowed us to work with a maximum depth, with a maximum of intellectual honesty. We were not interested in the fireworks of creating a new discipline or in providing a new name to something that is studied by another discipline. We were never interested in plagiarizing an object of study. What it is important is to track the existing disciplines, that is to say, the track of what Technopathogeny is not and then, very carefully, observe that there is a remnant left, a common remnant that no other science takes into account. This common remnant is Technopathogeny.

Having done such analysis, we can see that another necessity surges: the key question of the discipline. Which is really our question?

The question of our object of study is the most important one. If we define it, paraphrasing Descartes (Descartes, 1945), in a "clara et distincta" way, the rest will be much easier. The basic question is: *Why must this discipline be generated and how is it generated?*

But we could also ask ourselves, as many scientists who have criticized our proposal have done: is this really a discipline or is this a multidiscipline? If this were a discipline, we could also ask ourselves if it should use a natural sciences methodology or a formal sciences methodology, such as Philosophy; if Ethics should be implicit within Technopathogenology, etc. Maybe the big question should be: *Can we make a science out of the study of Technopathogeny?*

If technopathogens include chemical substances, physical factors (electromagnetic fields, for example), or biological factors, such as genetically modified organisms (GMOs), maybe each specific science (Chemistry, Physics, Biology, and others such as Anthropology and Philosophy) could approach the study of this phenomenon. A similar case is the study of the soil phenomenon: *Edaphology.* This science is not defined as a *multiscience* or *multidiscipline*, even though for the study of concrete problems it uses elements or principles from basic sciences. Likewise, we cannot conceive Technopathogenology as a multiscience or multidiscipline.

Let us start with the analysis of this aspect:

VII. Technopathogenology: Multidiscipline or transdiscipline?

Continuing with the example of Edaphology, due to its characteristics, the soil could be observed or studied, as we have said before, by different disciplines: Geology, Chemistry, Entomology, Botany, Microbiology, Physics, etc. But the problem is that each discipline will study it from its own conception. Chemistry will focus on the chemical aspects and Microbiology on its microbiological components (bacteria and soil fungi). But none of these sciences will be able to do it as Edaphology, which has its own criteria and point of view to observe the soil phenomenon. Even though there are different types of soils, this science was able to find a singularity in them which permitted to refer to the soil as a phenomenon which required a specific study. Similarly, the long term damage on health caused by technique (i.e. the singularity) that characterizes the phenomenon we call Technopathogeny allows us to support the need of a new science: Technopathogenology.

When an object is created using different disciplines, we are in the presence of an Interdiscipline. When an object can be observed by different disciplines, we are in the presence of a Multidiscipline. And when the object of study surpasses the existent disciplinary field, we are in the presence of a Transdiscipline (McLoulin, 2002). In a multidiscipline, each science takes a part of an object or phenomenon and studies it. But the phenomenon does not lose its identity.

In the following figures we compare this concept with a jigsaw puzzle. Figure A shows a phenomenon we call ABCD rectangle (studied by eight disciplines). Figure B shows the fraction studied or observed by each of the eight disciplines.

We can separate the part studied by each discipline and bring them together again and the rectangle will be the same. The phenomenon will not lose its identity:

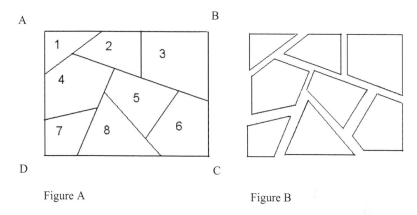

Figure A   Figure B

Figure 8:   Graphic representation of a phenomenon of multidisciplinary study. Figure A: Integrated disciplines. Figure B: Disintegrated disciplines.

We could say that if an object is built by various disciplines, that is, interdisciplinarily, it could be evidently also studied multidisciplinarily. Unlike the soil, cultural technological objects or objects created by technicians are not natural and pre-existent, but developed with the aid of several disciplines. Any natural phenomenon is far more complex than any technological object created by humans. Therefore, this would mean that a technological object could also be observed by a multidiscipline. This would be so if what generates the final technological object is only the addition of each of the parts provided by each discipline. But the problem arises when the technological object generates unthought-of elements. What would happen, then, if we try to apply the multidisciplinary criteria to a phenomenon of transdisciplinary nature as the soil phenomenon or, in our case, a Technopathogeny?

Let us consider now that rectangle ABCD, Figure A, is a technopathogenic phenomenon:

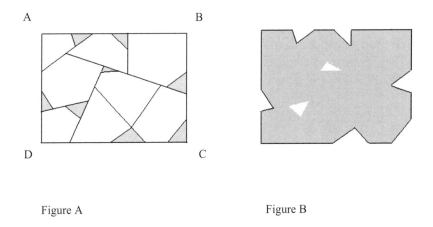

A B

D C

Figure A   Figure B

Figure 9:   Graphic representation of a phenomenon of a transdiscipline study approached with a multidisciplinary criterion. Figure A: Fractions that each discipline takes from the phenomenon. Figure B Graphic representation of the phenomenon integrating the parts observed by each discipline.

Figure A shows how each discipline studies or observes a portion of the complete phenomenon. But there are still voids not contemplated by any of such disciplines (the shaded areas).

If we separated the part studied by each discipline and then, just like the previous case, put together all the observations and contributions of each discipline and saw it as a whole, we would see that the phenomenon is not a perfect rectangle ABCD anymore but an irregular figure with voids inside, just like figure B.

In addition, Technopathogenology observes Technopathogeny as the result of a technological activity, which results in the creation of endless different products. It does not observe each technological object, a pesticide, for example, as an isolated phenomenon. Every technological object can carry a *germ*, and be an object which either individually or along with another technological object or objects can lead to a phenomenon typical of Technology we call Technopathogeny. As we have said before, this is the singularity that can be found in every technique. This is why even if we tried to observe the technopathogenic phenomenon as a multidiscipline – even with the limits and inefficiency mentioned – so many and such diverse disciplines would have to be summoned as each object requires. The holistic vision of the phenomenon as such would not exist.

Technopathogenology is the science of Technology that reflects upon itself and upon its own fallibility.

VIII. Technopathogenology as a science

Having provided supporting grounds for the need of creating Technopathogenology to study Technopathogeny, in order to prove whether this is indeed a science we will analyze if it fits within the criteria or characteristics of the science system.

If we resort to other simple definitions of science, one of them refers to it as "precise knowledge of things by their principles and causes" (Salvat, 1978). This leads us to think that Technopathogenology studies a phenomenon that can be analyzed to its very origin and cause.

Let us analyze it now in the light of scientific knowledge characteristics. Science is described as: a) Rigorous Research, b) Objective, c) Verifiable, d) Systematic, e) Universal and f) Self-Corrective (Colacilli de Muro, 1978).

a) Science equals rigorous research

It is said that in Science one must distinguish the Context of Discovery from the Context of Justification. The former refers to the need of existence of the individual, the scientist that makes it possible. The latter refers to the results, either theoretical or practical, elaborated by the individual. This context specifies that:

> The objective rigor requires to consider methodological prescriptions that refer not only to the accuracy of theoretical formulations but also to the confrontation of such formulations with the facts or objects that each science investigates.

The two first chapters of this book confirm that Technopathogenology complies with this characteristic. Its object of study was soundly supported, theories were formulated and then confronted with facts that had not yet been studied, and then it was found that they were true as well.

b) Science is objective

> Science combines personal research with clear and accurate formulation of the results obtained in the context of discovery, provides information on these results and provides conditions for its verifiability.

Technopathogenology complies with the criterion of objectiveness. In Chapter II we detailed how we got to identify a new phenomenon through induction – using techniques that involved the generation of mycotoxins and the use of pesticides – and how through deduction we were able to verify the manifestation of the very same phenomenon in other techniques. This provides the elements for any scientist who wants to verify the phenomenon using different criteria.

c) Science is verifiable

Let us consider Mario Bunge's words (Colacilli de Muro, 1978):

> In order for a piece of knowledge to be called scientific, it is not enough for it to be – and it does not actually need not be – real. We must know, on the other hand, as we have come to know, or to assume, that the statement in question is real: we must be able to enumerate the operations (both empirical and rational) through which it is verifiable (confirmable or disconfirmable) in an objective manner, at least at the beginning.

We believe that the grounding support provided in Chapter I along with the analysis in Chapter II provide enough elements to prove *how we got to know* about Technopathogeny, how we have identified the phenomenon and how whoever wants to verify or refute our postulation can do so. Technopathogenology is verifiable. We do know, however, that the verification criterion connected with induction is a stage which is not as complete as the falsifying criterion.

d)   Science is systematic

It is said that:

> Scientific formulations are not presented as a mere collection of statements or laws. The theoretical body of a science is integrated by scientific theories connected to one another through logical relationships that provide it with a solid structure. Every scientific theory is also a structure whose statements are connected to one another and which logically support one another.

In Chapter II we have seen that the entire hypotheses in every theory were connected with each other. As we observed in the conclusion of Chapter II, the resulting connection emerged in a natural and unforced manner.

Each hypothesis led to another. Also, each theory was connected to another theory which, in turn, led to the formulation of another one. As we can see, Technopathogenology is also systematic research.

Regarding this characteristic of science, a definition describes it as a "systematized set of knowledge that constitutes a branch of human knowledge." In this case, Technopathogenology deals with real knowledge about an organized and systematized phenomenon, thus constituting a branch of human knowledge. We can also say it involves *methodical and systematic* knowledge and that those of us who have studied this phenomenon can speak of a method to acquire knowledge about it which allows us to advance systematically.

e)   Science is universal

Under this title two statements can be highlighted: scientific objectivity and the degree of generality in its assertions. "One of the essential tasks of science is to establish and convalidate scientific laws or universally valid statements." This allows for explaining single facts, declaring circumstances that make facts possible, predict new facts, etc.

Technopathogenology has enunciated the existence of a new phenomenon that can be applied or researched in any technological field. The knowledge that can be obtained is of a universal nature and transferable. No matter how developed they are, every community uses technology and applies techniques to produce goods and satisfy their needs.

When we dealt with Error, we used as example that the danger associated with contamination was considered to be found in developed countries exclusively and only in some areas of developing countries. There was an erroneous concept that stated that developing countries need not worry about contamination. In connection with this, it is interesting to analyze Prof. Dr. Wassermann's concepts refuting these statements. We recommend the reading of the detailed report on our program, included in the annex. The position disregarding concern was also discarded when, during the 1960s, the advancements in contamination studies allowed us to get to know the causes more thoroughly and thus conclude that contamination does affect all the countries whether they are industrialized or not (FAO, 1982).

Let us not forget the figures we provided in Chapter II showing substances of daily use. Even though such figures show developed countries cases, the risk in developing countries must not be disregarded (PNU-MA, 1987). Let us remember that the United Nations Industrial Development Organization (UNIDO) forecasts a bright future for chemical industries (including highly contaminant fertilizers and pesticides) in developing countries.

In connection to aflatoxins, for example, the enunciation of Technopathogeny allowed to explain it and to declare the circumstances that causes and caused it. It also allows for predicting new technopathogenies by considering the circumstances which can cause it.

Technopathogenology is based on universal principles which contribute to support its scientific nature. Technopathogeny is a universal phenomenon.

f) Science is self-corrective

One of the characteristics of the scientific knowledge is that it is self-corrective. K. Popper says (Collacilli de Muro, 1978):

> Science never pursues the illusory goal of obtaining definite answers, not even of finding probable answers. Nevertheless, its approach pursues an infinite though graspable finality: the unstoppable discovery of new problems, more profound and more general, and of tying our answers (which are always temporary) to contrasts which are continuously renovated and increasingly rigorous.

In the case of Technopathogenology, this self-correction is given by the capacity of receiving fundamental critics. Some of these critics denied the existence of the object of study thus supporting the lack of necessity of the science.

The self-correctiveness will be found if the object of study survives such criticism and increasingly improves the methodological perfection of the science.

As we will say when we speak of methodology, self-correctiveness will allow for the prediction of the phenomenon with more anticipation.

IX. Technopathogenology and its insertion within the science system

Even though Technopathogenology is a new disciplinary proposal to study a phenomenon which could not be framed within the existing sciences, it is not a science emerged out of nowhere. New phenomena that cannot be framed within existing disciplines motivate the need to develop new disciplines. For example, certain phenomena which could not and cannot be studied by Biology or Chemistry motivated the development of Biochemistry. Similarly, Ecotoxicology studies the effect of contaminants on the ecosystem's flora and fauna.

We could represent the examples as follows:

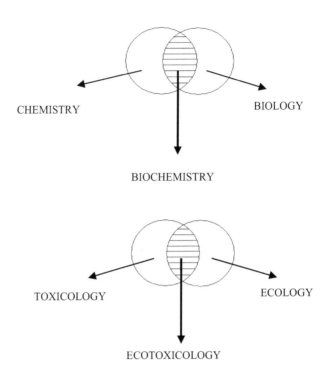

Figure 10:   Graphic representation of two new sciences: Biochemistry and Ecotoxicology.

Likewise, Technopathogenology is created upon the need to study a phenomenon that cannot be framed within the existing disciplines. It cannot be framed within Technology, Medicine or Anthropology, three sciences which are considered highly relevant to this phenomenon and which we will discuss below.

In Chapter II, when we described our attempt to frame our phenomenon, we referred to several disciplines. Because of the characteristics of this phenomenon, we believe that Cultural Anthropology, Technology and Medicine are the ones which are more closely related to it. This does not mean that, as a painter who mixes colors in order to obtain the exact color he or she is trying to obtain, Technopathogenology is taking parts

284

of each of these sciences to obtain its own science. Technopathogenology is an independent science.

Medicine

Since Technopathogeny affects human health, the existence of Preventive Medicine, Epidemiology and Toxicology within Health Sciences would make it very tempting to include the study of Technopathogeny within Medicine.

The reasoning is correct, but there is a new void in this knowledge: Medicine does not contemplate the Technique in particular that caused the unwanted damage – even though it detects such damage and tries to cure it.

That is to say, Medicine can detect the damage (probably unknown) caused by Technique thus unveiling the existence of a technopathogen or the properties of a technopathogen, as a consequence of a flaw of such technique (both factor and flaw unknown at first).

In this context, Medicine must wait until Technique is used and humans have become the last experimental animal. It cannot anticipate the causing technique since each technology in particular has its own methodology. Medicine can only know the flaws of its own technique, which is also a Technopathogeny: Iatrogenesis. In this sense, Iatrogenesis could indeed be the object of study of someone who studies the development of medical technology. One paradigmatic case was the widespread use of estrogen during menopause in the 1960s. During the 1970s a substantial increase in endometrial cancer was detected, which was considered "one of the largest epidemics caused by Iatrogenesis" (Congress of the United States-Office of Technology Assessment, 1981).

But it can say nothing about other techniques.

The paradox here is that even though Medicine can study technopathogenies caused by any technique, it finds it very difficult to accept Iatrogenesis as object of study since in this case it is both judge and party. This is particularly valid for the so-called classic Medicine, which does not easily accept the connection between Iatrogenesis and medicines.

After analyzing Medicine we could ask ourselves whether each technology in particular could correct the flaws of their techniques on the spot and thus solve the problem.

Every technique in particular focuses on a narrow and linear objective (Lenk, 1987) (Mittelstrass, 1986a). For example, the technique of pesticides is focused on obtaining efficient, low-cost substances. The *low environmental risk variable* is incorporated by discovering, later in time, the unwanted effects of these substances on humans or the environment.

Pharmaceutical Technique is focused on the development of specific efficient medicines, for example, an analgesic.

The ideal variable in a medicine about having *no unwanted collateral effect* is implicit in medicines. However, the apparition of serious effects in medicines thought to be innocuous is a fact (Langbein et al, 1989). A more usual alternative is to incorporate a long list of the adverse effects that were detected with its usage, so that anyone who could experience an *unexpected collaterality* knows whether it was produced by the medicine or not. In some cases, there are so many collateralities that it is not uncommon to hear: *if you bear them in mind, you will not take the medicine.* Thus the collateralities are ignored and the medicine is consumed all the same.

In the chemical, veterinarian, etc. industries, examples can be endless (Rose, 1987). At the same time, as we have said in connection to medical technique and the difficulty for self-judgment, the same difficulty is experienced by each of the techniques in particular. The amount of examples is vast.

What we can conclude is the following:

- In spite of the application of scientific technologies and regular trials prior to the commercial launching, in some cases the Technopathogeny phenomenon is nevertheless manifested.
- This phenomenon could not be foreseen by the corresponding technology.
- Another field of knowledge, which differs from the relevant Technology, must be developed to foresee technopathogenies.

It would seem that each particular technology, because they are immersed in the complex world of economic and scientific pressures (to introduce the specific technique in the market and to guarantee its survival against the competition) would be at a greater disadvantage to recognize a technopathogenic phenomenon early enough and prevent it. The difficulty above mentioned emphasizes the necessity of providing technopathological education on technopathogenic prophylaxis to technicians belonging to individual techniques.

In the current state of affairs, it would seem that humans should be the last experimental animal in order to recognize the error or hidden immanent effect in each technique in particular.

Cultural Anthropology

Cultural Anthropology being an already existing discipline that studies humans and their creations (Herskovits, 1964), why not let it study Technopathogeny?

The main objection here is that even though Cultural Anthropology is closely connected to the problem of Technique, it cannot choose among all the creations those which can have an error or a hidden and immanent defect signifying adverse consequences to the health of the very same human that created them. Its object of study is so vast, human creations are so many and so diverse that it could not possibly study this phenomenon thoroughly. In addition, there are other aspects which make the inclusion of this science relevant within the epistemological group of Technopathogenology. When we deal with the methodology, we will refer to a Previous Stage, since any idea for a new Technology is the result of a set of the scientist's previous knowledges. These previous knowledges allow conceiving a new idea. It also depends on the *scientific culture* or values with which the scientist guides his or her work. We will also refer to a *germinal* stage. These aspects are part of the nature of Human culture. What is it that drives humans to develop new techniques? Mercantile utilitarianism? Immediate needs? etc.

Being Cultural Anthropology centered on humans, it can provide the true categorization of human needs not based on denaturalized parameters set by a dehumanized science. In spite of not having experience in the so-called hard sciences, it would help to correctly focus the universe under study.

Out of the three sciences or groups of sciences we can clearly see that Technopathogenology, due to its nature, can be ontologically placed within Technique – its field of application being preventive health.

To illustrate this and to support the idea of how closely linked Technopathogenology is to Technology, let us imagine parachutists who, among all the techniques they have to learn, they must learn the technique of opening the parachute. This *technique* is fundamental and substantial to all the techniques parachutists have to learn. If they ignored this technique, the rest of the techniques learnt would be meaningless.

The prevention of risk which comes from learning how to correctly open a parachute can be compared to the prevention of immanent and hidden risk in technology through Technopathogenology. The agronomist, for example, apart from knowing the techniques to produce raw food materials, must know how to prevent or reduce the possible technopathogenic risks associated with such techniques.

Another analogy would be the analysis fishermen should do when *in spite of* applying all the adequate techniques for obtaining good results (using the proper net, placing the net correctly, time of the year, etc.) they cannot catch as many fish as expected. If the fishermen asked themselves why it happened, they would try different explanations. However, studying this phenomenon seriously would avoid many losses. The fishermen could prove that they did not consider the possibility of there being smaller fish. Technopathogenology would be the science to study the damage that occurred *in spite of* using the apparently adequate net. The actual adequate *net* is provided by Technopathogenology as a science of and parallel to Technology. This contributes to avoiding that some technologies which were considered as safe *escape* for being defective. The small fish are the defects of techniques causing technopathogenies.

Risk Assessment and Risk Management, for example, are *nets* considered adequate to *catch* risk factors. However, there are *fish* that pass through this net and cannot be caught.

X. Possible interactions among the above mentioned sciences

After all the above mentioned, we can conclude that the science that studies Technopathogeny must rise from the last three mentioned sciences (Eguiazu, 1991).

Medicine must provide the knowledge after the technopathogen generated by the immanent and hidden risk of Technique gets in contact with the human being's exposed surfaces: skin, digestive system and respiratory system. This can be studied through Epidemiology, Toxicology, Preventive Medicine, etc. Also in connection to medical techniques, a self-criticism of those which might represent a potential risk of Technopathogeny would be needed. As we have said before, this is hard to obtain with this single science.

Technology must provide the knowledge of each technique and in particular, its circumstances of application and the whole scientific process that allows for the creation of a new technique.

Cultural Anthropology must provide for the essentially human act through which humans begin developing techniques, from the most primitive to the most sophisticated ones. It is a science of the human and therefore would provide to a change of focus by centering Technopathogenology in humans.

Graphically, it could be represented as follows:

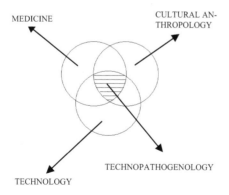

Figure 11: Consolidated discipline fields from which the supporting ground for Technopathogenology was obtained.

In the graph we can observe three circles of equal size. This is for illustration purposes since the participation or contribution to Technopathogenology differs depending on the science. Technopathogenology, in fact, is a science of *that which is not correct in Technique*, which allows a gestation with harmful *germs* to human health. Such germs are symbolic and must be understood as causing damage on health. Even though we call germs that "which give rise to the production or development of something" (Standard Encyclopedic Dictionary), it would not be incorrect to call *harmful germs generated by Technique* to what we have already defined as Technopathogens, given the fact that they also originate long term damage to human health.

If the idea of developing a new science seems too bold, we can but go back to the ancient *mechanical arts*. In fact, new sciences or new specialties are constantly being created – simply by grouping phenomena that are apparently atypical or that have an entity of their own, which cannot be completely framed within the existing parameters. Regarding this, if we go back to *mechanical arts*, we can see that the rough classification by activity was not enough to grasp a series of phenomena which were common to several mechanical arts. For example, *Armatoria* and *Agricultura* had the blacksmith's work in common (the making of swords and ploughs), but the art of working metal was not considered an independent entity, maybe because its importance was not appreciated outside its relationship to the existing arts of agriculture and war.

Also, from the ancient concept of mechanics – rudimentary in itself – it was hard to imagine all the perfectly limited disciplines and subdisciplines that have been surging.

Another example is Biotechnology, which gives shape or independent entity to a series of processes which were used since ancient times.

Technopathogenology is, therefore, the underlying scientific discipline that is necessary to Technology in order to avoid or prevent the creation of techniques with immanent and hidden risks which have negative effects on human health.

To sum up:

- Science knows by reduction of reality and experimentation. This knowledge is inherent only to the reduced reality.
- Another part of the reality or totality of the phenomenon, which was not considered in the experimental reduction, remains unknown.

- The experimental results cannot be extrapolated to reality without certain reservations, since in some cases the nature of the experiment alters the experimented phenomenon.
- The elaborated theory after this reductionist process provides, through induction, a false security. This security is false because of the fact that it can never be considered completely true, since some part of the reality not considered in the initial reduction can always appear to contradict it.
- If Techniques are developed within the known part after the experimental reduction, the unknown part, which also remains underlying but linked to the phenomenon, will manifest itself in an unpredictable manner.
- This unpredicted manifestation can either be neutral, positive or negative to human health.
- The negative manifestation can be either evident or non-evident.
- If the manifestation is negative and non-evident to human health, it is defined as a Technopathogeny.
- The nature of new mechanical arts based on a nuclear phenomenon (atomic or cellular) and the insertion of synthetic substances in nature, stresses the phenomenon of Technopathogeny.
- The existence of a field of knowledge that still does not have a specific science allows us to postulate Technopathogenology to study this phenomenon.

XI.   What is Technopathogenology?

Technopathogenology is then the science that studies the genesis and masking – either voluntary or involuntary – of the causes of technopathogenies and aims at achieving the prevention or prophylaxis of such technopathogenies. A more accurate definition would be: the science that studies the Technopathogeny phenomenon, which includes Technopathogenesis – a group of successive stages or processes that lead to its manifestation – the detection of Technopathogens involved in the phenomenon and which aims for its prevention.

It is the science for Technology to reflect upon itself and its own fallibility.

We have seen that technopathogenies are diseases or harms to human health – either physical or psychic – which do not occur immediately but after many years or generations as a consequence of exposure to non-evident factors generated by Technique (technopathogens) which are present in the human environment and which are caused by immanent and hidden risks present in Technique. Therefore, we can ask ourselves: Is Technopathogenology a *basic science* given that it studies a *clara et distincta* phenomenon, disconnected from a situation of concrete application?

We cannot answer to this question categorically. On the one hand, studying how, by action or omission, a technique can carry the potential germ of a Technopathogeny which cannot be detected until the technique has been applied and the *Technopathogeny comes out of its hiding place and manifests itself* seems to be the core of its essence. But there is also another very important aspect referring to the apparition of concrete phenomena. This phenomenon has two very well defined aspects:

a) Reflection on the essence of this phenomenon.
b) Going from a proved material effect to the essence of the phenomenon.

Case a) would be the most abstract, since Technopathogeny is taken as a phenomenon as such and the aim is to force the materialization of the phenomenon in order to make it visible before the technique has entered the period of no return (application and massive usage).

Case b) could be the applied research, since it involves a concrete phenomenon (the product of an observation). We know that the later a Technopathogeny is manifested, the harder it will be to stop or recall the technique involved. This difficulty will be even greater if the technique entails huge economic benefits.

Therefore, is the systematic study of Technopathogeny useful for prevention to the whole Science and Technique system? The answer is yes. Without a doubt, our problem is that it took us 30 years to discover it and study it thoroughly, and not every mind – without doubting intellectual honesty – admits this study because, as we will see later, it is an issue they will not care to discover, maybe even because they are too proud and deny what they do not understand.

On the other hand, in every science and technique system there are opportunistic people who will accept it, provided they can obtain advantages from its study. In neither case is the actual study and advancement of knowledge in Technopathogenology benefited.

XII. Technopathogenology:
A "light" on the road of technological progress

We use the term *light* borrowing Goblot's concepts in a series of confe-rences given in 1921 (Goblot, 1943), in which he said that: "We are, then, and will always be forced to take decisions feeling our way blindly in the dark, when we lack the lights of science." In order to arrive at such a concept, the author refers to Descartes saying that "...he always had a great desire to learn to distinguish the real from the fake, to find a clear-ing in his attitudes and walk safely through this life".

He continues saying that:

> ...it is necessary for science to be today in conditions of teaching us everything we need to know so that we know how to act. Without a doubt, that will never be. We have to renounce to ask for inaccessible truths – among the ones that can be reached; there are some which will always be denied to us because nobody will come up with the idea of discovering them.

We wanted to underline that last phrase.

Goblot quotes Descartes again saying that "...there are certain ac-tions in life that often do not admit any delay whatsoever."

These interesting concepts were expressed in a time when the non-evident negative aspects of science were not even imagined. If we apply them to our object of study, we arrive to the conclusion that in certain fields of knowledge we cannot afford to feel our way in the dark. If you do so you might trip, fall and hurt yourself. We can compare Technopa-thogeny to tripping when feeling our way in the path of Technology.

Let us now consider Descartes' idea that actions in life do not admit any delay whatsoever. The risk of Technopathogeny shows that there are certain actions that may or may not deserve delay. If we consider Tech-nopathogenology as a proposal of action by humans to avoid technopa-thogenic harm, its study clearly does not admit delay. But if we consider Technopathogeny as a consequence of an ill conceived technology, we can say, in this case, that the technological development does deserve to be delayed. This would mean to allow the time required to at least have the maximum information about the technological development and to have as much certainty as possible about its innocuousness to humans.

Technopathogenology provides light because of its critical spirit. A spirit that discerns scientific knowledge.

In this regard, Goblot said (Goblot, 1943):

> A notion is scientific even when it is obscure and vague, provided the spirit is aware of its lack of perfection and can distinguish between what it knows and what it does not know. A scientific knowledge may not necessarily be a clear knowledge and let doubts survive, provided the spirit conceives such doubts, takes care when formulating them, values them and, whenever possible, measures the degrees of approximation, probability and plausibility.

Let us advance in Technology, but considering what we do know, what we do not know and what we need to know about it.

Knowing what it is and which the aims of Technopathogenology are, we can see it confronts the solid foundation on which the entire Science and Technique system builds the world it calls *modern,* which is the principle of innocuousness of the technological object. The relevance of this issue deserves our attention.

XIII. The scientific-technological work and the stubborn support of the innocuousness of the technological object

Even though we believe we have provided enough elements in Chapter I to support the fact that a technological object can entail a hidden risk to human health, before we continue we would like to further analyze this topic which we referred to at the beginning of this chapter when we mentioned Persistent Anomaly. We will analyze a preconception or postulate adopted by scientists as an unquestionable canon with which they work and which, in the field of technological knowledge, can lead to Technopathogeny.

Many scientists who hold tight to old paradigms and fallacious concepts and imperfect postulates on the idea of progress (coming from Philosophical Schools) do not consider Technopathogeny to be a problem at all. In connection to this, the conception of some scientists are paradigmatic when they say that: "having so many natural contaminants we need not worry about contaminants produced by industry" (Frank, 1980-1983), or as Tomatis, et al say about the criteria of a scientist (Tomatis, et al, 2001), criteria that of course they do not share:

> Synthetic residues on food can be ignored because 99.99% of pesticides humans eat are natural, chemicals in plants are pesticides, and their potential to cause cancer equals that of synthetic pesticides.

We could state then that modern Technique supports the *Innocuousness* of *Technological Object* hypothesis in the long term.

The innocuousness of the technological object –
Hypothesis, theory and dogma

The technological object innocuousness hypothesis –
Falseness – Fundamentals

The Hypotheses, their falseness – Previous cases

Before framing the innocuousness criteria as a hypothesis and proposing its falsification, we will go over the concepts that some thinkers have proffered regarding this subject. We have mentioned criteria and principles coming from different thinkers and doctrines. Even though we have a technological background, we do know that the philosophical in-depth consideration of the problem presented in this work must come from philosophers.

According to Popper, hypotheses that can be taken as theories must not necessarily come from the thorough induction of known cases. The Austrian thinker believes that hypotheses can come from intuition or simply not be based on observation. It is also reasonable to consider hypotheses as coherent anticipations or even the product of "exact fantasy" (Doucet, 1978). Now, Popper implicitly accepts this. But he does impose a condition for these hypotheses, which do not come from induction, in order to be taken seriously. We are saying this because hypotheses coming from induction will not raise a doubt. "Hypotheses must be formulated in such a way that they must be able to be falsified by any researcher."

What is to falsify? It is to have the possibility of carrying out experimental work or another refutation method (when, as we will see with Technopathogenology, experimentation cannot be applied) to contradict them and demonstrate this way their falseness.

Without attempting to get into a field that belongs to other thinkers, maybe Popper's proposal is somewhat extreme when considering that a hypothesis needs only to be based on intuition and be exposed to falsification. Following this criterion, someone can adhere to it and say that a hypothesis is false because he or she feels it is. This would lead to an exchange of opinions between the *defender* and *falsifier* in which the defender must also prove that the falsifier is wrong. As we know, being opinion a trial for which evidence is not necessary, this will surely become a protracted and irresolvable argument. Now, we consider that Popper's criterion is the one that the researcher must adopt. A good researcher must apply to his or her own work the Popperian method of continuous refutation. The researcher formulates his or her hypothesis by intuition, perhaps, doubts about it and then tries to demonstrate its falseness. Veracity will arrive once the hypothesis resists several attempts of destruction carried out by the researcher himself or herself.

Going back to our analysis, if the method fails or if the hypothesis cannot be refuted, the hypothesis that has survived this falsification is closer to becoming a theory, but always remaining a conjectural one and subject to be contrasted against facts. Which are the advantages of this idea? That the hypotheses need not be the consequence of a collection or boring induction of known cases, the fearful enunciation of cases, of everything that has been seen, with the implicit prohibition of ideas and intuitions that go beyond the known facts. Ideas must not be cast into the unknown.

In this case, according to Popper, there can be further progress into the future, towards the unknown, but the idea – which may be intuitive or jotted down – must be able to be destroyed by the facts.

The hypothesis is then considered provisionally valid.

Popper also says that every investigation begins with a problem that someone is trying to solve and that any problem can be well or badly set out. The badly set out problem will be self-dissolved because it will not have the necessary entity to persist. However, if the approach is adequate, it will persist. Maybe we could say that when the research comes from a complex and difficult problem, it spontaneously becomes a program. This program in a way surprises the corporate system of scientific evaluators since it cannot be easily framed through a traditional research project. This is what happened with our case in particular.

So far we presented Popper's concepts. Provided contrasting with the facts can be done and results contradicting the hypothesis are accumulated, this hypothesis can be abandoned by another.

Imre Lakatos refers to the fact that every research program has a more or less solid nucleus *surrounded* by auxiliary hypotheses, and, as the results contradict them the program can be abandoned for another one. This is what the author calls change of a *degenerate* research into a *juvenile* one. In this manner, the advancement of knowledge is given by substituting an old idea with a new one. This substitution is given because the facts are not *naturally* coherent with the theory. Far from supporting the old theory, the facts divert us from what is expected by it.

This, that may seem very simple and rooted in common sense, would then lead to believe that the advancement of knowledge is given in an obvious manner, harmoniously, with cheers among rivals, respecting and nobly abandoning their ideas to accept the opponent's.

But reality from Feyerabend's perspective is completely different. According to this author, acceptance of new ideas is not a "very scientific" process where the personality of the new ideas' advocate is more influential than experimental arguments or facts.

He then quotes the case of Galileo, whom he accuses of not proving his ideas scientifically while defending them vehemently. His ideas prevailed in spite of the poor scientific proof of the time. If Galileo had been just a *mattoide* (madman), who thinks he knows something but in fact does not, his ideas would not have prevailed until our times.

That is, a new program can be imposed because it is defended by an increasing number of researchers, but a degenerative program dies because it is increasingly difficult to be defended by its advocates. Feyerabend says that if any researcher working in a consolidated and known program is ill-treated just like innovators are ill-treated, the program would die. We believe he is making reference to scientific ill-treatment, of plaguing the scientists with questions to see to what extent they can support their theories. There is another type of ill-treatment – scientific, sibylline and wicked – we will see in Chapter IV when we deal with the Ethical Objector. The first is an unintentional ill-treatment generated by the genuine interest in obtaining the truth and it is driven by the scientific vocation. The second, wicked and perverse, is driven by unethical passion.

Feyerabend thus mentions a "healthy anarchism in innovation," in which the real innovator must behave as an anarchist. If the ideas survive, it is because the scientist survives to his or her detractors, but not because the ideas brilliantly fit within the old program. Innovators must have certain psychological qualities and will to persist in order to bear the ill treatment they will receive for being considered *anarchists* because of their innovation.

Heisenberg, quoted by Prof. Hoffmann (Hoffmann, 1997), says in other terms: "in order to be understood, new ideas need other structures of thought, a profound innovation in the way of thinking...," or what Einstein bluntly says in the following two phrases (Piecovich, 2006): "New ideas are accepted if their advocate endures until the detractors have either died or retired." "Problems cannot be solved by those who have caused them."

We wanted to use this second quotation to illustrate the fact that if a problem is generated because of defending an old paradigm, the problem will be very difficult to solve since those who have caused it *will not back out*. They will not acknowledge the fact that they have made a mistake. The investment – either in prestige or in money – can be so high that it can represent another reason for not backing out.

We thus support the need of a unique space to solve technopathogenological problems. The most powerful persons in the Science and Technique system – the advocates of old paradigms or programs – are directly or indirectly responsible for the difficulty or impossibility of solving the technopathogenological problem. This is why they refuse to acknowledge its entity. If the problem *does not exist*, it is not necessary to think of a solution to it.

That is, it seems that innovators must have a personality that endures pressure, inconvenience, indifference, discrimination and persecution in order to allow for innovation in the scientific world.

This means that the psychological nature of innovators should be more important than brilliant demonstrations (Kuhn, 1995).

Broadening Feyerabend's concepts, he does not adhere to any method in particular but follows the "anything goes" motto. He analyzes Carnap's inductivism, Popper's deductivism and Lakatos' research programs' theory. Taking the classical discussion between Copernicanism and Galileo, he arrives to the conclusion that the difference between the *language of observation* and the *language of theory*, as well as the difference between *discovery* and *supporting a concept*, cannot be sustained. Everything is practically the same.

Theories can never be completely falsified, so the facts that contradict them come from previous theories. The most important fact would then be: "Scientific progress does not come from rational discourse but from irrational moments, that is, from the ability of the researcher to convince".

Science is closer to the myth than what many thinkers, advocates of science, want to accept. Even though many *ideologists* of science defend its apparently objective and neutral nature, the facts show that science has behaved in many cases as dogmatic and unprovable ideology. The ideology of science must be limited, since it supports decisions of State and must be limited by people. As former disciple of Popper, Feyerabend proves that disciples can distance themselves from their Master's school once they can support a new paradigm without losing respect for their Master's. Feyerabend's contribution was essential to the skepticism regarding Science and Technique.

> The new in science is not imposed through the great soundness of arguments, neither by its advocates' experimental capacity, but through the endurance and skill, nor through the force of convictions of those who defend the new.

This concept is further supported by Heisenberg's phrase: "...in order to be understood, new ideas need other structures of thought, a profound innovation in the way of thinking...".

The technological object innocuousness hypothesis – Tradition and Technopathogenology

The question is therefore: How is this connected to Technopathogenology?

Interestingly enough, we can see that according to Feyerabend's criteria, Technopathogenology does *work* methodologically. However, we still do not know how. In addition, we have to *convince* that it is necessary. The validation of Technopathogenology will be a matter of time and history.

Technopathogenology is an honest attempt to peacefully solve the growing skepticism in Science and Technique. A science that studies *what goes wrong* is a way to continue believing in Science and Technique. It is also interesting to note that, considering Feyerabend's proposal, this *ideology of State* or *myth*, this traditionalism, as we have called it – meaning "the knowledge, doctrines, customs, practices, etc., transmitted from generation to generation" (Standard Encyclopedic Dictionary) – is what more strongly opposes Technopathogenology. Such attitude of science is understood because its mythical nature would be destroyed with a *science of its fallibility in the technological object,* because science as such is not as *mythifiable* as the technological object obtained from it. It is also understandable because if the scientific system has evolved in such a way that it can make science out of science instead of science out of a phenomenon, it will be more concerned in observing formal structures of the new science rather than of the object of study.

We can then say that, with Technopathogenology, humans' awareness of the actual magnitude of the problem of human environment is thus materialized.

Seeing that Technopathogeny is the result of wrongly accepting the criteria of innocuousness of the technological object, we have three critiques for modern Science and Technique that contribute to falsify hypotheses and that will allow us to understand the phenomenon of Technopathogeny:

a) Criticism of scientists' ethics.
b) Criticism of some doctrines that support modern Science and Technology.
c) Criticism of the production and application of knowledge processes.

a)   Criticism of scientists' ethics

When we analyzed the possibility of Ethics dealing with the study of Technopathogeny (Chapter II) we referred extensively to the scientist's ethics. We can reiterate our conclusion: Scientist's with non-ethical (even proud) attitudes towards Technology will care little or nothing about the innocuousness of the technological object hypothesis. These scientists who lack ethical principles are closer to being plain criminals than to searching for prophylaxis of harmful collateralities caused by technological objects. Such collateralities can even pass inadvertently to scientists acting in good faith.

b) *Criticism of some doctrines that support*
modern Science and Technology

In the Introduction, we made a slight criticism to Positivism when we referred to the fact that, if according to the positivist conception of science, a Technique that emerges spontaneously from the accumulation of positive knowledge should be as perfect as the science it originated from, a Technopathogeny should be non-existent. This disciplinary proposal further advances the discussion on Rationalism, which starts being object of criticism (De Boer, 1984b). Modernism – and its fundamental consequences in the development of the scientific method – is also questioned, along with the mechanicist conception that drove Galileo to say, in order to support modern science: "Measure what is measurable and make measurable what is not".

It would seem that Galileo's belief about the possibility of *becoming the Lord of Nature and tame it through knowledge,* would have become a utopia that precisely will end in our times (Low, 1988).

Under the mechanicist conception, Technopathogenology can be unappreciated because the phenomenon it approaches is very difficult to *measure,* and also due to the fact that Technique cannot be considered a succession of causes and effects. Its teleological aspect must be considered, that is to say, as an order of ends that Technique tends to execute. According to one concept of teleology, one should not confirm in Technique the control of blind need but maintain the need of reason and finality. In addition, this is further materialized by combining Mechanicism with Materialism, according to which it is defined that matter and spirit, the physical and the psychic, do not constitute an irreducible duality; matter is the only reality – there are no spiritual substances which differ from material substances. It is easy to understand why in the cases in which Science sees its innocuousness criteria stumble, it justifies it with the *price of progress* concept.

If it only followed a mechanicist criterion, Technique would fall into an antithesis that is irreducible with the essence of human beings.

We could then say that the concept of Technopathogenology, without establishing it within a determined philosophical doctrine, gets closer to Teleology: it cannot justify the risks entailed by Technique in terms of mere necessity and because Technique is not the product of the accumulation of scientific knowledge, but the result of organized thought towards and end in particular. It could also approach Vitalism, since it sees humans as beings that posses a vital force which is essentially different, instead of as a mere consumer of Techniques. Let us not forget that such vital force is the force that creates Techniques. It can also come closer to Spiritualism because it defends the spiritual essence of humans.

This proves how wrong the mechanicist criterion is, since this doctrine would be leaving aside a phenomenon with relevant entity in humans that is worth being studied.

The experiment, which this conception took as the sole basis of valid knowledge, is also questioned since the absolute separation *experiment-researcher* on the one hand is not possible and, on the other, the necessary reduction that allows for the experiment to be possible impoverishes the real phenomenon. The real phenomenon cannot be described only by the sum of experimental results (Bohme, 1986) (Fetscher, 1988) (Fritsche, 1987) (Heisenberg, 1954) (Saage, 1989).

The apparent soundness of the theory based on reason, experimentation and induction as a basis for science in our times is questioned by Popper, who indicates the impossibility of verification of the formulations (Magge, 1973) (Wild, 1984).

Some prefer passing from an atomistic conception to a holistic one (Schaefer, 1989), which in a way goes back to pre-modern ideas. In some aspects, this phenomenon manifests itself in the so-called postmodernism (Baumgartner, 1988) which pretends to rule in this true Copernican revolution that is happening in the world of ideas. In a word, the apparently solid project of Rationalism and Enlightenment, with its consequences on Science and Technique (De Boer, 1984b, 1987), is insufficient to support, explain and find the solution to the unwanted consequences of Technique. Human reason and Science and Technique seem insufficient, not only to explain but also to prevent the unwanted consequences of Technique (Scheibe, 1987). Thus new movements such as Ecologism arise, which, as Romanticism in the 19th century, calls for a return to Nature and condemns humans as evolution freaks altering this idyllic and primeval state of nature. The action of humans on this idyllic state is considered by ecologist groups as negative since it has damaged such state through the unwanted effects of Technique. Ecologism is also related to the opposition to animal experimentation (Teutsch, 1987).

Certain fundamental ideas of Rationalism, such as *the idea of progress (*Bohme, 1986) (Fritsche, 1987) (Strumpel, 1987), are also questioned. The real or potential consequences of the rational enthusiasm in progress as something unavoidable and its historicist manifestation are also subject to criticism, since the notion that human history is a phenomenon of continuous self-perfection has been challenged.

The magnitude of the damage caused by the uncritical use of Technology during the 20th century has had great repercussions: environmental (global warming, environmental pollution, desertification, accumulation of chemical waste of difficult disposal, Chernobyl, etc.) and social (marginalization, increased incidence of chronic diseases, unethical practices with the testing of medicines, etc.). We must also bear in mind the enormous risks posed by the development of military technology and the refinement of techniques of torture and mass murder, which ethically question the idea of progress, an idea which in some minds can even justify such atrocities.

The method of *Trial and Error* is also questioned, when humans are used as experimental animals without knowing so.

It would seem that the ethical sensibility – generated by the verification that the unwanted consequences of Technique had grown so much – would stop the naive enthusiasm in Science and Technique. This sensibility reaches its climax when one of the modern mechanical arts, genetic engineering, would potentially allow for the creation of hybridomas between animal and human genomes, or because of the *simpler* problem of manipulation and elimination of human embryos. The idea is to provide an ethical answer that is centered in a more human dimension and to stress the principle of responsibility (Ese, 1985) (Hoffner, 1980, 1982) (Jonas, 1984, 1987) (Rolies, 1986). This principle, applied to pesticides, will be described in Chapter IV.

Skeptical on the project of modernity, we began wondering whether human rights include the right not to suffer the unwanted consequences of Technique (Sachsse, 1985) (Schneider-Poetsch, 1987). We found several big voids such as: who must defend the community's diffuse interests? Or rather, who must defend the community's diffuse interests when it comes to the negative collaterality of Technique? Where do the risk and benefit of Technique go to? What right does a human embryo have? What if it has been frozen for a while? That is to say, the nature of the new *mechanical arts* poses a series of difficulties in law that apparently cannot be easily solved through positive law (Guggenberger, 1987).

The hyper-development of Economy and Industry (as a consequence of the application of the new *mechanical arts* that are highly regarded in the *myth of progress*) leads to such consequences as the exhaustion of natural resources (Simonis, 1985, 1989), without considering that part of them belong to *Future Humans* (Brundtland, 1988). This leads to the concept of *Trustee of the Planet Earth*, which means that the planet is lent to the current generation in order to manage it wisely (De Jouvenal, 1971).

The concepts of *finiteness, fragility and supratemporality* of the human habitat or environment are postulated (Eguiazu, 1991). These aspects were proposed as essential postulates, after realizing the need to establish bases or grounds regarding the human habitat that aim globally at its rational use (Brundtland, 1988) (Hoffner, 1980, 1982).

The Langenbruck project tries to prove that an alternative way of life is possible. This new concept proposes that some hard-to-measure needs are taken into account within a strictly mechanicist-rationalist conception of production and commercialization, as well as the internalization of the costs of contamination within the product (Fornallaz, 1986) (Fornallaz, 1988). It also proposes the need of decentralizing the production through a new economy based on social ecology (Fornallaz, 1986) (Fritsch, 1984).

This current panorama allows us to perceive a "crisis of meaning" (used by V. Frankl in Psychiatry regarding contemporary man) in the rationalist project which was considered relatively solid until not long ago (Frankl, 1982).

Finally, the moral crisis of our time is considered as the most worrying aspect of environmental crisis. An utter lack of respect to human life is mentioned – without such fundamental respect to human life, there can be no economic, industrial or scientific progress (Johannes Paulus II, 1990).

It is interesting to quote Pope John Paul II' words: (Johannes Paulus II, 1990)

> Peace will be threatened until the States accept the fact that the earth is a common heritage whose fruits must be managed in the benefit of all, with a management system of resources coordinated internationally.

The United Nations Human Rights declaration must be updated to include the human right to live in a safe human environment (Johannes Paulus II, 1990).

Developed countries have a great responsibility on developing countries. There is an urgent need to consolidate a new global solidarity, since the solution to the environmental crisis also implies tackling the problem of poverty. Today's society must analyze its lifestyle and educate for environmental responsibility (Johannes Paulus II, 1990).

Qualitative growth (Nutzinger, 1986) and its counterpart, the waste of resources and contamination are the result of the avidity of developed societies (Fritsch, 1984) (Leipert, 1986) (Simonis, 1989).

c) *Criticism of the production process and application of knowledge*

It is mentioned that during the 1970s and 1990s the number of scientists in the United States climbed from 12,000 to 2,200,000, having at the time 40 thousand scientific journals publishing more than a million papers per year (Chargaff, 1989). It is also worth mentioning the ephemeral nature of this knowledge, since the results last from 3 to 5 years, until they are substituted by new results.

This forces science to a permanent self-correction. The correction would not have technopathogenic consequences if it was only done on the research paper. It would only entail an economic cost. But the problem arises when the technological application is rushed thus running the risk that the paper that covers the complete phenomenon arrives too late. If this phenomenon has serious consequences on human health, if a large amount of money has already been invested in research and development to apply the first part of knowledge with satisfactory results, it will be very difficult to stop the project. This is so because if a large amount of money is invested based on the first results and a costly technology has been developed, there will be an unwillingness to recall it from the market even though later publications prove that there are negative side effects.

On the other hand, a great trivialization of the object of study can be seen in academic research, which is justified by the so-called advancement of knowledge per se. Although small, such advancements find a place in scientific journals – one wonders whether there really is so much to be investigated and if there really are so many publishable results (Chargaff, 1989).

This is also connected to the pressure scientists have *publish or perish* which, in some cases leads scientists to search for subjects relatively easy to investigate through experimentation. Paradoxically, other more

305

profound questions which would require time to reflect on the importance of the hypothesis under study are left aside.

The pressure for development which was already indicated for Technique also exists for the scientist in his or her "manufacturing of knowledge" (Lakatos, 1982). In this manner, Science is submitted to quantitative production leaving aside the qualitative aspect – thus becoming a *factory of research papers*.

In addition, the trivialization of subjects of study leads to a bitter competition to be the first to present and obtain funds for each subject of study. This leads to many ethical misdemeanors in the academic world, such as: stealing projects, stealing hypotheses, pressure to obtain co-authorships of courtesy, etc. This phenomenon is even more serious in developing countries, where there are no academic ethics courts. In these systems, the scientist is submitted to the arbitrariness of the establishment, which constitutes the only group with real power in the system.

The trivialization and mercantilization of the search for knowledge support the criticism on the modern project of Science and Technique in relation to the quality of what is produced.

The existence of *airtight* divisions for each scientific specialty (Mittelstrass, 1986b) (von Wright, 1988) with their relevant confederacy of experts, makes it easier to obtain subsidies and publish topics and projects only if they are formally well framed within the existent. But the relevance of the object of study is not questioned. On the other hand, there are transdisciplinary topics that call for reflection (such as environmental issues), which are not easily recognized and which do not easily obtain financial aid.

It is not uncommon that environmental projects that require a global or transdisciplinary vision (which cannot be reduced to a Cartesian hypothesis in order to be presented) are not taken into account. Paradoxically, they will only be accepted if they are reduced (thus losing the essence of the project).

The methodological reductionism required to mathematize and quantify natural phenomena impoverishes the actual phenomenon and gives a false certainty of knowledge. In this case, the actual phenomenon is impoverished and substituted by the adequate number.

Science is denounced. Due to such reductionism, in the mechanical model of reality the whole cannot be equaled to the addition of the parts. A consequence of this is that the apparent certainty of knowledge cannot be sustained. Due to methodological reasons, the real phenomenon is devoid of an important part of itself thus leading to its denaturalization. This missing part is fundamental since, if it was a technological application it can carry a potential risk of generating technopathogenies if techniques with methodologically reduced and impoverished knowledge are developed. We could speak of a defective or erroneous knowledge.

Similarly, it could be said that science stimulates the linearity of knowledge in each of its isolated divisions. This hampers the perception of underlying phenomena. Another consequence of this linear conception of knowledge is that in the technical application rigid systems not tolerating errors are developed (von Weizsäcker, 1986).

This rigidity can also be seen as a consequence of programmed research which does not allow for new ideas to be pursued. Rigid systems can be terribly harmful for the application of knowledge, and this makes the *trial and error* method unacceptable, since, in these systems, an error can signify the possibility of no return.

This is also referred to as an industrialization of knowledge along with the professionalization of the scientist. Paradoxically, the ancient myths and beliefs of the most primeval stages of humanity mentioned by Comte (Comte, 1982) are replaced by the mythification of a new type of scientist. Here, the unions of scientific experts, protected by their specific science, justify serious voids of knowledge in the apparently known. For example, if a union of experts approves a pesticide substance or any technological process and after applying it discovers an immanent and hidden error or flaw which has negative consequences on humans, this union will not take the problem into account. This union of experts passes the problem onto the union of doctors for them to discover a method to heal or alleviate the illness produced. The union of doctors, aided by particular sciences, will try to find a way to cure or alleviate the illness produced. The application of medical Technique to cure will probably continue producing other distant effects, maybe also negative. Thus human beings must roam about and adapt themselves to hundreds of *airtight* fields (Wandscheider, 1989).

This situation, which sounds tragicomic, is firmly grounded in the Science and Technique system (De Boer, 1984a, 1984b) (De Boer, 1987). It is argued that even when modern science knowledge has some voids, if due to the hasty application of a Technique there are unwanted collateral effects, science itself will discover the way to correct it. This statement is currently under heavy criticism. We have already mentioned this criterion as the fallacious argument the technologist resorts to in order to justify the risks that Technique can entail. This criterion is used by Science and Technique to support the Hypothesis of Innocuousness: Even though Technique can entail a risk, it will only manifest itself in the long-term, where Science can produce discoveries or knowledge to deal with such damage. Technique will be innocuous in the long run since there will be no permanent damage. *If the damage is corrected, such damage will not exist.* Even though some damage is necessary in order to act as signals to science to correct itself, such damage is minimized as *the price of progress.*

It is interesting to quote now a fruit producer with a university degree: *I do know that the artificial irrigation system I use will eventually salinise the soil, but I trust that science will solve the problem.* Even though in this example the effect of technique is not harmful to health (it only implies turning soil unproductive), this blind faith on science could easily lead some technologists to say: *We know that this technology can be harmful to health, but we trust science will find a cure to it.*

Thinking that Science can solve future potential or real damage to health is completely unacceptable.

This reflection can lead us to think that this erroneous criterion adopted by the modernist project should maybe contain more humble elements from pre-modern times to orient human curiosity. That is to say, human curiosity as a source of knowledge should also be ruled by ethical principles.

It is interesting to observe that in some cases trivial research is defended with the argument that anything that is researched on, however petty, contributes to the advancement of knowledge. But the question is: is everything that can be known worth knowing? (De Boer, 1984a, 1984b, 1987). Should there be not a minimum of self-criticism and self-correction in the human spirit in order to provide high-quality scientific results?

The scientists' education system is also criticized for developing highly risky or destructive techniques (Nutzinger, 1986). We are specifically referring to armament technology (Pauling, 1965). Some *ethically anaesthetized* scientists can be driven by myopia and lack of ethics. An armament technologist, for example, proudly boasted that from the Second World War until today, the destructive capacity of weapons had increased 100,000 times per economic unit invested in the weaponry industry.

These three criticisms to modern Science and Technique allow us to observe serious problems in it when thinking of the innocuousness hypothesis. Such problems are of high technopathogenological relevance since what is at stake here is human life.

Evidently, if we consider:

a) The unethical (even proud) attitude of scientists;
b) The development of the process of knowledge generation based on philosophical doctrines with erroneous conceptions, postulates and paradigms that lead scientists to search for knowledge outside of human goals;
c) The reduction and application of knowledge structured in erroneous norms: trivialization and mercantilization; airtight divisions for each scientific field; utter reductionism; industrialization of knowledge; quantitative criteria; pressure to produce; blind faith in science; etc,

We can ask ourselves how it is possible to be certain that a technological object can be innocuous. If it is, it will be by chance. This confirms that stating that the technological object is innocuous cannot be sustained. The innocuousness hypothesis, sustained through the modern Science and Technique system is a fallacy that is poorly grounded.

To sum up, Technopathogenology is a science that can bring back the faith in scientific work, but with an intrinsic falsification in each technological question that leads us to a kind of falsifiable feedback of its excessive enthusiasm and to focusing more thoroughly on its collateralities.

Feyerabend concludes, as we have said before, that science is much closer to myth than what scientists are willing to accept. In a more irritating way, he says that:

> Just like secularization separated the Church from the State, Science must be secularized from the State; this means liberalizing what is until now a compact ideology of State forcing blind and dogmatic adherence in which there is no room for deviations and, on the contrary, allow for new ideas without the current dogmatic rejection.

We can see that these thinkers' analysis and the conclusions they arrived to regarding the scientific systems are also of interest since they contribute to supporting our proposal.

Going back to the topic analyzed in this title: The technological object innocuousness hypothesis – Tradition and Technopathogenology, and going back to the concept that a good researcher applies to his or her work the Popperian continuous refutation method, with the following case we believe we confirm what we want to prove. In many cases, with new substances, for example, the researcher (lacking intellectual honesty) instead of formulating a hypothesis of potential harmful effects and trying by every possible experimental means to demonstrate that the substance is safe and then, only after having done so for a long period of time launch it to the market, the researcher prefers doing the opposite. The researcher is then formulating the innocuousness hypothesis without submitting it to falsification. Evidently, the first procedure would be enormously costly and the second more economic – which is why it is preferred. The *falsification* of the hypothesis is thus performed by the consumer.

The technological object innocuousness hypothesis:
Its falsification as a result of observation and logic

When we analyzed our attempt of framing Technopathogeny within the framework of the existing system, we established a series of hypotheses and theories. We have said that we find a logical connection between the hypotheses and theories that allowed us to arrive to such conclusion. We have also said that such connection arose in an unforced and natural way. We have also said that we were not obsessed with the idea of creating a new science, but it emerged after several attempts of framing it. The need of this science emerged as an *a posteriori* consequence.

We could say the same with reference to the analysis we are carrying out regarding the falsification of the innocuousness of the technological object, which shows that the history or the facts described by thinkers (concerning the imposition of new paradigms, hypotheses, theories, etc.) also applied to our object of study.

Just like the connection between our hypothesis and theories developed in a natural way, our disciplinary proposal and change of paradigm also emerged in a natural way – instead of applying the criteria of thinkers of *how to* impose a new paradigm to the old one, or how to impose our science. Comparing the road travelled by us to the conclusions that thinkers arrived to, we could say the following:

310

Applying Popper's concepts, we have not only tried to falsify our hypotheses and theories but we have also established our hypotheses and theories (some of which falsify other theories – like the theory of innocuousness of the technological object) in such a way that they can be, in turn, falsified by other researchers. We have received several responses criticizing our proposal (see Annex), we have replied with sound arguments that have yet to be refuted. That is to say, none of them provided convincing elements that would scientifically refute our proposal of the need of a new science.

Following Imre Lakatos concepts, we did not try to *surround* our research program with auxiliary hypotheses and contradict with them the hypotheses of the old program to replace it with ours. We did not attempt to call our program *juvenile* and the existing programs *degenerate*. Neither did we adopt a *stubborn* attitude to impose our ideas. This is proved by our attempts of framing it in the existing disciplines.

According to Feyerabend's criteria, we did not *ex professo* apply *scientifically poor* processes to impose our ideas, leading us to become ethical objectors. We did not try to be *ill treated* to show that our program would not die, or attempt to be *anarchists of innovation*. We did not try to develop the ability to convince, nor thought we should have worried about the soundness of our arguments or about the capacity of experimental demonstration. We did not try to perform *meditation practices* to gain strength in our convictions, nor even *train* as sportsmen to *overcome difficulties*. After 30 years of work we have experienced many of the things described by Feyerabend: ill-treatment, strength of conviction, and endurance. The *soundness of our arguments* or the attempted *capacity of experimental demonstration* – along with the project of developing and setting up an institute – did nothing to convince our Science and Technique System of the validity of our proposal.

Analyzing *a posteriori* the evolution of the events that led to supporting the need of Technopathogenology, we have seen that they did fit within the criteria shown by history and analyzed by thinkers for any new hypothesis, theory or science that managed to be imposed on the system.

As we have said, we can simply confirm that the series of events that were part of our scientific work which concerned worrying about technological risks on human health and that led to supporting the need of creating Technopathogenology – maybe by chance for some, or maybe because history thus proved it – are similar to what any innovating scientist had to go through.

Unfortunately, after all these years of hard work we managed to put the pieces of a puzzle together that includes our entire careers as researchers which allows us to see clearly what we have just described. Until now, we had only collected some isolated pieces – only at the end we could see that there was a logical pattern and that they were part of a whole *landscape*.

In Chapter II we commented on the difficulties of the evaluative system to frame the phenomenon and on the reluctance of the system to accept it as such. We consider that such attitudes indicate a disciplinary void and the need of a new discipline. We could say that in order to arrive at the postulation of a new paradigm and a new science, we had to – without planning it – adopt in our path attitudes that rather than scientific we could call *behavioral*, such as the attitudes described by the above quoted thinkers. Therefore, if such behavior matched the attitudes that are a logical consequence of any innovation, we can think that this supports the idea that Technopathogenology is an innovation. We speak of innovation adopting a positive attitude for ourselves. We could also say that our disciplinary proposal has no sense or entity, as our detractors keep trying to prove. This is open to demonstration by anyone who wants to prove such possibility.

We therefore offer our detractors to apply the falsification criteria to our proposal. We encourage them to try to destroy our proposal.

Going back to the subject matter of this book, just as the grounds used show that Technopathogenology – a science that arose as a result of inductive and deductive observation of concrete facts – has an entity, the falsification of the innocuousness of the technological object hypothesis also emerged as a result of observation and logic. We could therefore say that the falsification of the innocuousness hypothesis is what gave rise to Technopathogenology.

The theory and dogma of innocuousness

Analyzing the modern scientific thought, we can see that in a way it is based on a postulate, a postulate that no one dares to discuss: *the innocuousness of the concrete technological object*. We have established this concept as hypothesis. However, this idea is so much fixed on the scientist's mind that if we resort to the definition of dogma we could define the innocuousness of the technological object as such, since we could say: *this point is so crucial to the science and technique system that it is considered certain and undeniable.*

That is to say, the modern Science and Technique System considers the postulate of innocuousness to be not just an assumption, nor a set of reasoning – i.e. a theory which establishes that the technological object is innocuous – but to be a dogma, since it considers this theory to be – erroneously and falsely – irrefutable. Due to refusing to see the facts or diminishing their value and trying to minimize them with weak arguments, this principle is considered a scientific dogma. This contradicts science itself, which proclaims opposing dogmas. Therefore, even though science must not accept dogmas (Sanguineti, 1977), by defending the principle of innocuousness it ends up accepting a dogma.

Going back to Feyerabend and his comparison between science and religion, we can say that such principle stops being reasoning presented to explain provisionally certain kind of phenomena to become what we would call a *dogma.*

What is this dogma? It is simply the quintessence of what we call science, from Descartes until today. If the technological object is innocuous, we thus validate the *theory of progress.* Being the technological object innocuous, everything is progress, even the tiniest. If, on the other hand, the technological object cannot be innocuous and could, in some cases, even be very harmful, the theory of progress crumbles down. Therefore fallacies surface, such as *the price of progress* concept. They appear as attempts to *repair* the theory of progress.

We thus see that in order to validate the theory of progress we must have a dogmatically innocuous – i.e. safe – technological object. Therefore a program that studies technopathogenies or the harmful effects in the application of technological objects clashes with the innocuousness – or better, with the dogma of innocuousness – of the technological object, and, by analogy, with the perfection of scientific work.

Having classified the principle of innocuousness as a dogma, we will now see its consequence within the framework of the consideration of new postulates for the technological development and in the creation of Techniques.

The innocuousness dogma

The innocuousness dogma within the scientific community

Within the scientific world we find that the following concept is deeply rooted (Bunge, 1988):

> When contrasted with any common knowledge, and the scientific, esoteric, finalist, metaphysical and religious explanations of reality, science, in spite of its mistakes, is the only truth.

This has been accepted by scientists in a more or less general manner; even the most critical accept that given its rigor and contrastable nature, scientific knowledge is the most acceptable. This criterion has been generally accepted and whenever the word *scientific* is applied to any concept, *respectability* is conferred.

The problem arises when, within the scientific community, someone wonders: but do we, scientists, *always* produce true knowledge?

This honest question can be raised by observing the Technopathogeny phenomenon, a phenomenon which should be non-existent within the innocuousness dogma. When we postulated the fourth approximation to Technopathogeny in Chapter I, we provided elements that could easily respond negatively to the question out of which a clear explanation of why this phenomenon manifested itself is obtained.

For example, someone who cures through scientific means should not worry about the collateralities of its methods or medicines. This should apply to shamans or witch doctors, who, because of the lack of scientific method should consider unexpected collateral effects.

Those involved in scientific agriculture should not worry about collateral or harmful effects on the environment or on human health, because this is part of the old methods of natives or of scientific underdevelopment. There are many other examples of expected innocuousness which were contradicted by the facts which showed negative collateralities to human health (such as what happened with thalidomide, for example).

Another paradigmatic example connected to the innocuousness of the technological object as well as to the *trustee of the planet* concept, is nuclear technology and the Chernobyl incident. It provides an example of the fallaciousness of the concept of innocuousness. The probability of a nuclear accident killing more than 100 people was estimated by science to happen once in 100,000 years (Gassen, 1988). Nuclear technology was considered to be practically innocuous: the probability of a disaster equaled a meteorite hitting the earth and killing more than one hundred people. As for the *trustee of the planet* concept and the macro consequences caused by the accident, it is interesting to go back to the opinion of the President of the Federal Office for Radiation Protection (Germany) (König, 2006) in connection to the risks of nuclear energy:

> Chernobyl became a symbol of the loss of trust in politicians and officials responsible as well as on economy, but it was also a symbol of loss of credibility in Science. The explanations that scientists gave lacked enough grounding and showed that such explanations were influenced by political and economic interests.

The author concludes (König, 2006): "The risk is not hypothetical. It is real. This is the teaching Chernobyl has left".

In connection to our disciplinary proposal and paraphrasing this author, we have said that: *Technopathogeny is not a theoretical lucubration lacking connection with the real world. It is not a hypothetical phenomenon but a real one, and as concrete as Technology itself.*

Chernobyl is a typical case that shows the weakness of the pillars on which technological knowledge is built. One of the main components of such pillars is the dogma of innocuousness. Evidently, because of the estimated numbers we have referred to above, the extremely low probability of damage associated with nuclear plants spoke of practically complete innocuousness of such technology. In spite of the accident, there can still be advocates of such technology who could have a point when they say that the accident was not caused by a failure in the technology but by a human error. We of course do not agree with this argument, however, this still could be an argument in favor of nuclear technology. There is another paradigmatic falsifying case of the dogma of innocuousness which cannot be justified at all: the use of DDT.

The discovery of DDT was hailed as a success of human spirit in the war against pests. However, more realistic voices which recommended its careful use were ignored (Cottam, 1946). This product would free humanity from pests, and was even called *the miraculous pesticide*, by Paul Müller. In spite of being a poisonous substance, it was thought that through an adequate use, humans would control all its negative effects. However, Müller did not have in mind negative aspects such as its persistence in the environment for decades, its accumulation in trophic chains and in animal fat, its residual persistence in foodstuffs and finally, its carcinogenicity. These aspects slowly surfaced after the use of DDT, showing that the *Panacea* was not such. Not many relate the negative effects to a failed process in the creation of this *technological object*.

We have also mentioned that apart from the risk of acute intoxication, there is also the technopathogenic risk of damages in long term (which is another proof of the falseness of the innocuousness dogma). DDT was synthesized in 1939. In 1982, IARC included it in the list of substances that show evidence to be carcinogenic on experimental animals – forty-three years after continuous usage. Even though Cottam denounced in 1946 the environmental risks of the product, it was too late: the business was already working (Cottam, 1946) – who would dare make it go back?

Analyzing the situation of this pesticide from the Technopathogenology perspective, we can ask ourselves:

What would have happened if Paul Müller had studied Technopathogenology in his undergraduate course? Would he have developed DDT?

Even though it is known that humans are the only animals who make the same mistake twice, we should use the DDT example to avoid making the same mistake with new technologies.

Technopathogenology and the innocuousness dogma

Evidently, in order to obtain an academic space where to place Technopathogenology, we must first move away from an infallibility program in Science and Technique (and its established method) to a fallibility one. After accepting this program, once the fallibility is accepted, a Technopathogenology could be inserted.

Is this possible? Yes. But it must undergo all the difficulties described by the previous authors, whether by proposing new hypotheses, new programs or new paradigms, or even trying to advance in knowledge through non-orthodox methods.

As we already know, our times are imbued with the concept that science substitutes any other knowledge and, in some cases, it is the only knowledge. This is the accepted opinion.

Even within the scientific community, those who believe in the fallibility of science – even though they accept that science is the closest approach to the truth and any other knowledge would be considered fallible. Some consider that the method is not all, and that there is some kind of uncertainty and fallibility in the scientifically produced knowledge. The problem becomes critical when it comes to technology – i.e. a knowledge applied to the development of a Technique – since we cannot expect for the technological object to be free of immanent flaws that make it fallible. These innovating researchers who question the infallibility of the method are not well regarded in the scientific community. However, even nowadays, conservative thinkers continue supporting the idea of the soundness and infallibility of the scientific knowledge (Bunge, 1988) disregarding the increasing evidence showing the contrary.

Science generates knowledge through published papers. If there is an error in such paper, nothing will happen provided it is not put into practice; moreover, even if the knowledge is materialized in a finished object, nothing will happen provided it is not actually applied. In the light of current knowledge, as long as the hidden errors in the paper are connected only to theory, that is, they remain static, no damage will be caused. This situation is much more critical when the scientific knowledge is applied to the development of a technique. That is to say, the damage will occur when the theory stops being *static* to become *kinetic*, i.e. when it becomes a theory *in motion* – in other words, when it becomes *kinetic* through the technological object. We say *in the light of current knowledge* because the science we have postulated aims at detecting such hidden errors in order to avoid the aforementioned kinetic materialization that makes the error evident when it is too late.

It is highly likely that there are scientists working in good faith, insisting on the idea or question of innocuousness of their activity, who can realize that the theory of innocuousness is wrong. Moreover, they can also realize how difficult or impossible the correction of negative collateralities can be. In such cases, the researchers can accept this new paradigm. They can realize the necessity of a preventive or corrective science generated by voids in knowledge – which leads to technologies with unexpected and unacceptable collateralities – and ask for it. Paradoxically, we could even find large technology multinationals *crying desperately for* a preventive or corrective science. This is so because nobody wants to make mistakes that make them lose prestige or abandon technological developments with the subsequent huge economic losses.

We call this science Technopathogenology, a science that forces to re-evaluate the dogma of innocuousness when tackling a phenomenon supported not only by theories but also by facts – a phenomenon which passed from being a supposition to being a concrete one.

XIV. Technopathogenology: Hard science or soft science, basic science or applied science, empirical science or formal science

This is another aspect we must discuss if we are referring to Technopathogenology as a new science.

We have come to the agreement that any honest scientist can discover the fallibility of science if he or she can think without obstacles. Once such fallibility is recognized, a need arises. This is the need of a preventive science in order to correct this fallibility, because of its serious consequences in the final quality of the technological object. Such scientist should also ask himself or herself: which is the nature of Technopathogenology? Which is the nature among the categories of possible sciences? We know there are two classifications that are very much used.

One of them divides sciences in two categories: Hard Sciences and Soft Sciences.

Hard sciences

Hard Sciences use a strict mathematical language that allows quantifying the phenomenon observed. In this category we can include: Mathematics, Physics, Chemistry, and, although with tolerance to some uncertainties, Biochemistry and Biology. They are usually sciences that take for granted the object of study and do not question themselves on the origin of the object. They are devoted to limit and quantify the *claro et distincto* phenomenon they have in their hands. Hard sciences include careers which require a solid mathematical background. Generally speaking, such sciences would lead the Science and Technique system. They are accused of an unconscious dogmatic authoritarianism which makes them have very little tolerance to criticism. They appear to be rather liberal in connection to the object of study, provided it does not drift apart from the pre-established paradigm. When they receive well grounded criticism, they respond with a disciplinary authoritarianism.

Maybe because it is a new science, Technopathogenology is hard to frame. From the hard sciences perspective, Technopathogenology can be criticized because it cannot establish mathematical models to predict the risk for future prevention.

We have already criticized the methodological reductionism required to mathematize and quantify natural phenomena since it impoverishes the actual phenomenon and gives a false certainty of knowledge. However, this does not invalidate the fact that mathematical models would allow Technopathogenology to quantify the magnitude of the error or defect in science and technique in order to prevent the magnitude of the harm that humans could suffer.

Nevertheless, this could not be possible for Technopathogenology as it is today. In the future, however, hard sciences methodologies could be resorted to and, for example, quantify mathematically the amount of damage to human health that is produced by the existent void in scientific and technological gestation.

A mathematical model to answer this question could take years to develop.

Soft sciences

Soft Sciences include the sciences whose postulates are not mathematically grounded and are open to discussion and criticism. Humanities are included within this group.

The fact that we cannot include Technopathogenology within Hard Sciences does not imply that we can include it within Soft Sciences. Having said that it is ontologically placed within Technology, we cannot definitely consider it a Soft Science. Unlike Humanities or Soft Sciences, Technology can modify nature substantially.

Another classification divides sciences into Basic Sciences and Applied Sciences.

Basic sciences

Basic Sciences would take an object of study without considering its applications. They can be either abstract or concrete. In the first case, they try to contribute to the theoretical framework. In the second case, they try to reduce their object of study to a strictly experimental, reduced problem. For example, the amount of permeability a membrane of a particular cell can have, or the degree of response of a determined gene to certain stimuli. This kind of research can have applications. However, scientists are not interested in it immediately – they are only interested in contributing to the reduced phenomenon and advance in such problem.

Applied sciences

Applied Sciences would, for example, investigate the permeability of the membrane of a cell in particular, having as aim that a toxic substance in particular penetrates it selectively in order to destroy it. Another example would be the study of a gene which, if we manage to insert it in a determined plant, would make the plant resistant to a plague in particular – as we have seen when we described Pusztai's work with potatoes.

As we can see, this classification does not help at all in trying to frame Technopathogenology, since we cannot say that it is a basic science, neither can we say it is applied in the sense we have just described.

However, maybe we should say that it is neither a Basic Science nor an Applied Science in the strict sense. Our long teaching experience allows us to verify that Technopathogenology has, because of its aims, components which are typical of a Basic Science.

We have taught Technopathogenology to undergraduate and post graduate students with different backgrounds: biochemistry, medicine, and technology, among others. The acceptability we have encountered would also support the idea that Technopathogenology is a basic science. Evidently, Technopathogeny is not a phenomenon that can be ascribed or limited to a single Technique, such as Iatrogenesis to Medicine. Technopathogeny manifests itself through the most diverse Techniques and, in some cases, it is the result of the conjoint action of different Techniques. In this manner, Technopathogenology is a science that gathers or integrates all the Techniques within the frame of a phenomenon that had not been described before. As a basic science, Technopathogenology contributes with its principles and postulates to the education of professionals with different backgrounds, giving them a global or holistic vision of a technological problem which is relevant to human health. We can also say that basic research in Technopathogenology can be carried out, since its object of study can be separated from any concrete application.

We can neither deny that it can be an applied science since its application can be studied in thousands of cases whose technopathogenies have been well described, as well as to contribute to other disciplines in risk assessment in order to estimate the possibility of technopathogenic risks and contribute to their elimination or reduction. In the case of aflatoxins, the research of new analytical methodologies for their detection is an example of applied research. Another example is the Intergranular Relative Humidity parameter applied in the storage of grains in order to prevent not only their contamination with aflatoxins but also with mycotoxins in general. In other words: new analytical methods and new parameters created during the search for prevention are clear examples of applied research (Eguiazu, 1993) (Eguiazu & Frank, 1983) (Eguiazu & Motta, 1985) (Motta & Eguiazu, 1991b).

Given all this, and being Technopathogenology a new discipline, if we had to choose one of the alternatives, we would prefer considering Technopathogenology a Basic Science.

Empirical sciences and formal sciences

If we want to use the classification that divides sciences in Empirical Sciences and Formal Sciences we can see here that even though when we started the analysis of Technopathogenology we placed it among empirical sciences because of their object of study, we cannot deny that it can also be considered, in part, an abstract science due to the fact that it uses elements from both. The analysis of the root of the Technopathogeny phenomenon – the last approaches to it – was done in an eminently abstract field.

Our experience allows us to humbly contribute with our opinion to the complex field of Epistemology. We can see that Technopathogenology arises as a consequence of the need of observing a phenomenon in a transdisciplinary manner. This is a complex phenomenon – just like the ones approached by all the sciences – but it is also quite heterogeneous, due to the diversity of elements or factors concurrent in its manifestation.

Maybe, instead of trying to *classify* and frame transdisciplinary sciences in watertight compartments (Basic, Applied, Hard, Soft, etc.), it would be more adequate to *qualify* a science. In this manner, a science born from the need of studying a phenomenon with a transdisciplinary nature may deserve more than a single qualification.

XV. Technopathogenology: Unexpected science for an undesired phenomenon. A caprice or a need?

In order to analyze this alternative we can remember the myth of Proteus: he could change his shape at will in order to get rid of his enemies. Those who do not accept the actual need of Technopathogenology could ask: hasn't Technopathogenology already got a framing? We could be accused of trying to *change the shape* of a science that is already in charge of studying the phenomenon and proclaim contemptuously: maybe its advocates are simply trying to avoid the strict evaluation of their peers – and have enough arguments to accuse the advocates of Technopathogenology of being dilettantes.

Whether this new discipline can be framed within some of the groups already mentioned or not, we can see that only Technopathogenology allows observing the technopathogenological object in three dimensions – something not achieved by the sum of the reductions or projections to each science.

Let us now analyze this through graphic illustrations:

The hole punch example

Reality and experience tell us that phenomena can be compared to a finite plane. As we have seen with the puzzle example, there are phenomena which can be studied as a whole – either by a single discipline or as a multidisciplinary approach. But there are complex problems which a structured and authoritarian scientific system with a unique disciplinary or multidisciplinary framework cannot study as a whole. For its study, we could use the analogy in which every discipline takes, like a hole puncher, a circle, thus leaving behind the plane with holes. This remaining plane is *discarded* since methodologically it cannot be considered by this system, which does not consider an alternative.

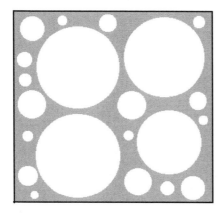

Figure 12: Schematic representation of a phenomenon using the hole puncher example. Every discipline and subdiscipline takes a fraction. The remaining fraction of the plane (phenomenon) – shaded area – is not considered by any of them.

We consider that in this *remaining fraction* not considered by the disciplines – being an unknown part of the phenomenon or object – can lay the cause of a Technopathogeny. The shaded area untouched by the hole puncher would be the area that could not be grasped by the hole punchers during each extraction. In spite of the good will of those who took a section of the plane, this shaded area could not be grasped due to a failure in the methodological tools.

The dimensional ontology example

This is a very interesting graphic analogy applied to support the need of a Technopathogenology.

Going back to the brilliant concept developed in psychiatry by Viktor Frankl called dimensional ontology, which demonstrates how easy the spatiality of a geometrical body can be confused if its projections are analyzed (Frankl, 1988).

The same geometrical example he uses to prove the difficulty in knowing a highly complex object, such as the object of study of Psychiatry, can be applied to other phenomena which require a transdiscipline. He indicates that if the human mind is reduced and simplified excessively, it cannot be grasped as a whole. To illustrate this he used the projection of geometrical bodies (Frankl, 1988).

The same can be applied to illustrate the difficulty in grasping Technopathogeny as an object of study: through *simple projections* in different disciplines.

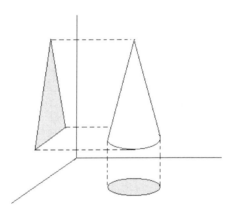

Figure 13: Representation of Dimensional Ontology applied to a three-dimensional object: a cone. In the horizontal projection it looks like a circle; in the vertical projection, like a triangle.

In figure 13, the cone is seen from one projection as a triangle and from another projection as a circle.

In figure 14, the three figures (cylinder, cone and sphere) look similar from the lower plane: like a circle. On that plane only such projection can be reflected.

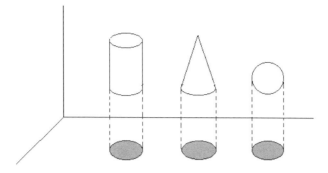

Figure 14: Representation of Dimensional Ontology applied to three different three-dimensional objects: a cone, a cylinder, and a sphere. In the horizontal projection the three bodies look like a circle.

In the same manner, as the author illustrated the need to avoid methodological reductionism to study the human mind, we can also use it for phenomena which are more closely related to Technopathogenology. We could compare, for example, the cylinder with a crime and the cone with a Technopathogeny. The projection of both phenomena on the lower plane gives us, in both cases, a circle which can be, for example, the result of biochemical analyzes. These biochemical studies – neutral in nature – constitute a projection of both complex phenomena which is objective and reduced. For both phenomena the same aim can be considered, for example, the DNA analysis of a sample (represented in the graph by the circle). However, the result of this analysis could be used by the criminologist to identify the victim or the culprit and, by the technopathogenologist, to identify whether a xenobiotic has a genotoxic action. Reciprocally, with the sole consideration of the biochemical analysis results, we cannot infer the complex nature of the phenomenon that caused them. For Biochemistry, the origin of the DNA analysis is irrelevant. It could come from a crime or a routine analysis.

The previous example shows how the reduced abstraction works in every science when it wishes to investigate a complex phenomenon. After this reductionist process, every discipline continues with its own evaluative rules. Analyzing figure 14, we can see that we are only left with a series of circles on the horizontal plane and a triangle, a rectangle and a circle on the vertical plane. This helps to conclude that the reduction of a complex phenomenon in which every single vertical projection is different – although equal on the horizontal plane – does not help to describe it in its totality. In the case of a Technopathogeny, it would be, for example, as if other disciplines attempted to study it, as we will see below.

Going back to figure 14, the most interesting aspect is what we can see in the horizontal plane, in which different complex phenomena are projected or abstracted for the same science as the same phenomenon. This is common where a very powerful or very much developed science expects every new phenomenon to be interpreted through its method. For example, the fact that phenomena associated with a complex agronomic science are observed or analyzed by Plant Physiology. This was our case and we can use it as example. As we have mentioned in Chapter II, the problem with mycotoxins had to be framed as *post-harvest physiology*. Similar cases could be found in new topics that may arise in Medicine and other sciences.

In Chapter I, we referred to the case of a plant species which one researcher wants to study from the medicinal point of view and another researcher from a taxonomic point of view. Each researcher will answer different questions from the same plant species.

Let us now see an example applied to a potential technopathogen causing a Technopathogeny: a pesticide.

In Figure 15 we can see the aspects of the pesticide that are of interest to Agronomy (vertical plane) and to Toxicology (horizontal plane). Agronomy considers it an object to increase production and Toxicology, an object to study its toxic properties – just like it studies any other toxic substance. But it is only Technopathogenology that studies it as a whole and considers it part of a technological process, an object in which a phenomenon which is still unknown (Technopathogeny) can manifest itself.

- Chronic effects: Reproductive, Carcinogenic, Teratogenic, others
- Initiator, promoter, synergism, co-carcinogenic
- Culturing to be used
- Formulation
- Stability, persistence
- Physical properties: Solubility
- Ways of entering the body: Ingestion, respiratory system
- Risk: Occupational, to consumers or both
- In which other techniques is the pesticide included, etc.

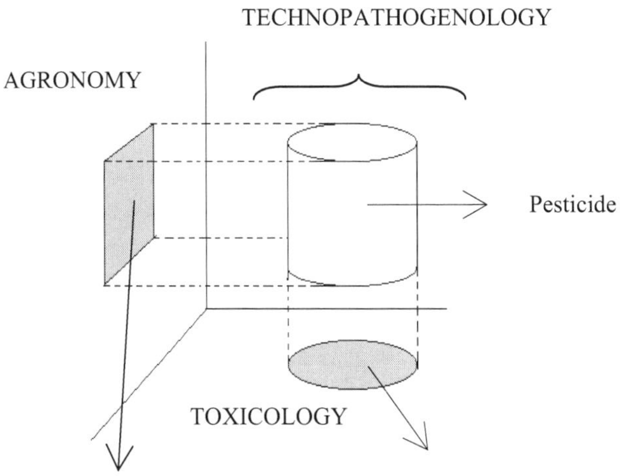

- Pest to control
- Dose
- Formulation
- Restrictions of usage
- Time of usage until harvest
- Cost/benefit ratio
- First aid

Acute effects:
- Extremely dangerous
- Mildly dangerous
- Not dangerous

Chronic effects:
- Carcinogenic
- Non-carcinogenic
- etc.

Figure 15: The phenomenon of a pesticide studied by Agronomy, Toxicology and Technopathogenology, from a dimensional ontology criterion.

Using Popper's concepts we arrived to the conclusion that the *problems* are our real objects of study; that we should pay more attention to such problems rather than to disciplines since what we study are problems, not disciplines. If we were to follow a chronological order, first the problem should be detected and then, after encountering similar problems, the discipline should be developed. But when this procedure is curtailed by disciplinary authoritarianism, the solution to the problems encounters great difficulties. We have found out that our age shows several problems that cannot be evaluated in the light of classic disciplinary evaluation.

The insistence on assigning these problems to certain old and consolidated disciplines is detrimental to their own solution. We may find out that the discipline that is more *powerful* will cut the larger circle from our plane – maybe due to the fact that it has many professional researchers and due to the great accumulation of means of work. This discipline is more interested in appropriating the problem (or what it thinks it is the problem or its reduced version of the problem) than in researching the actual object as such.

Going back to the hole puncher example, this discipline has the biggest instrument – almost the same surface as our plane – and severs such a big circle that there is very little left of it. It then reduces the whole plane to the portion it took from it. The complex problem is wrongly reduced to the discipline that took it over.

From this point forward the problem does not exist as such; the old and consolidated discipline appropriated the problem – in other words, it reduced it to something it could solve. We could compare this to trying to put an object inside a mold with a different shape from the object. The object will have to be *reformed* or *deformed* in order to fit such mold. Designing a new structure to fit the object is not considered an option. The scientific world is reluctant to new molds (Feyerabend, 1986) (Kuhn, 1995) (Lakatos, 1982). Their position is uncompromising. To illustrate this, we can go back to our experience when trying to include our proposal as part of a university program. Not only were we denied a new mold, a new discipline, but also the possibility of including the issue – even if it was reformed – within an existing mold (Post-harvest Grain Handling) (Eguiazu, 1998).

In some aspects this disciplinary reduction could be compared to trying to detect certain bacteria using the biggest magnification of the microscope. Or even better, in the context where bacteria are found – which can be a disease or the elaboration of foodstuff.

This brings about some consequences which are only partly positive, since even though in each discipline it is easier to arrive to a *clara et distincta* division of the reduced phenomenon, in some cases researchers could end up taking what they see (or what they want to see) as central or essential, which is not the case.

We can thus ask ourselves once again about the value of bold conjectures, of addressing the problem as such, maybe in a non-disciplinary manner (i.e. a *whatever works* approach), in the attempt of finding the *core* of the problem. In this case, the advancement in knowledge is done eclectically, going over question over question in a non-orthodox manner. This can unveil a topic or profound question.

Going back to Dimensional Ontology, we can conclude that the characteristics of a phenomenon will depend on the dimensional plane or perspective through which it is observed or studied. Each one will postulate their own conclusions and each conclusion will be adapted to the point of view of their own discipline – unable to extend to another. This is why it is important to declare that in Technopathogeny only the *angle or plane of observation* of Technopathogenology allows to approach the aim so accurately that only then can prevention be considered.

Now, let us analyze our scientific experience with aflatoxins through these three graphic analogies. We found that we could not frame the proper study and prevention of such toxins within Mycology. Now, how did this discipline act?

Using the hole puncher analogy, Mycology took the portion that was relevant to it leaving the rest – the technopathogenic aspects, among others – aside.

Using the puzzle example, when Mycology considered that the aflatoxins phenomenon could be approached multidisciplinary, it provided its fraction. But when Mycology added contributions from other sciences, they *disfigured* their real identity.

As for the Dimensional Ontology analogy, Mycology observed only the aspect concerning Mycology, which was thus subject to study and in-depth analysis.

As we can see through these analogies, Mycology turned the technopathogenic phenomenon we had presented into a mycological phenomenon. Mycology then proceeded to study the phenomenon thoroughly for over thirty years, even providing ground to create a specific program of studies. As the philosopher would say, it never occurred to them ask themselves such question or going into such dimension. Therefore, Mycology perhaps did contribute enormously to getting to know the mycotoxins-producing molds, as well as their anatomy and physiology. However, the problem could never be prevented from such perspective.

It is also worth reflecting on the capacity of the system to take the risk of subsidizing bold conjectures. The facts show that the flexibility and openness of the Science and Technique system are extremely poor.

Let us now analyze the framing problem using another example.

The divers' example

Using the analogy of the submarine archaeological search, we could imagine divers specializing in diving under certain conditions in order to try to find metallic archaeological objects. The divers spend almost all of their lives studying, diving and searching, but getting very little support from the scientific world, which discredits them with formal arguments. These arguments can be: that the divers lack a proper framing, that there is no specific science for what they do, etc. This leads the divers to work with practically no subsidies or formal means – having sometimes even to manufacture their own simple and inexpensive tools.

However, one day, the divers find a strange golden plaque with inscriptions and mysterious drawings. The existing disciplines immediately realize the importance of the discovery. However, they hide the recognition of the work of the divers since, if they did, financial support would have to be given to them.

Seeing the discovery as a *profitable idea*, a myriad of scientists appropriate the idea and frame it within their respective disciplines. Archaeologists would say: *This is an ancient piece and it must be studied with archaeological methods*, thus proceeding to ask for a large amount of funds. Anthropologists would say: *this is the cultural work of humankind, we must study it from the Anthropological point of view*, and, just like the archaeologist, they will obtain funds as well. Metallographers would say: *this is a metallic piece; we must study its composition* – for which they will also obtain funds. Philologists, in turn, would say: *we have to decipher the language and meaning of these strange drawings*, once again, for which they will obtain funds. And then other scientists in turn, will obtain funds from the official research institutions.

Upon seeing all this, the divers say: We have found the piece that was used for anthropological, archaeological, etc. studies. We will ask for funds to continue with our research. However, very much to the divers' surprise, the answer will be: NO, the argument being that the field proposed – diving for archaeological objects – is not scientific because there is no science that can frame it. Upon the divers' complaints regarding the scientific institution's lack of ethics, they will be allowed to *integrate* the work into any of the disciplines studying the discovery and of course choose as director any of the experts from such sciences. The divers might hear from the group that directs their work: we must work as a team because we are working on the same topic. But of course none of the groups will recognize that they need the divers to provide new pieces. The divers would reply: We don't want to become any of those fields which have borrowed our idea; we want to carry on diving for treasures both scientifically and methodically. Plus there is no way we can work under the direction of any of them since they do not understand our question.

To this, the official research institution's reply would be an ominous silence. In addition, if the divers reject the integration proposal, the official institution can offer the divers the possibility of creating an institute of diving suits instead of an institute of archaeological objects. What the corporation is telling the divers is that they either integrate with the ones who are already profiting from their discovery or they will be granted a subsidy to do other things which are not related in any way to what they want to study. The divers will reject both offers thus losing the possibility of obtaining financial support.

Technopathogenology is then the divers' discipline, which brings to the surface problems which are unknown and which are of great importance to other disciplines which only see – according to the concepts of dimensional ontology – a projection of the discovery, each of them using it for their own benefit.

XVI. Technopathogenology: The method

Methodology to prevent the phenomenon

We have seen that Technopathogenology is an unexpected science for an unwanted phenomenon and that it is not a caprice, but a need.

We now go back to the definition of science (Colacilli de Muro, 1978) we have used for this book's purposes: "Science is a complex human enterprise which, through trustworthy methods, can be applied to obtain bodies of formulated knowledge."

We also see that in order to be able to speak of a new science, the methodological rigor pursued or employed as well as the results (to obtain bodies of knowledge) are of utmost importance.

We have said, without pretending to delve ourselves into philosophical discussions regarding whether the criterion is correct or not, that if we can find a logical concatenation among the elements which make up the epistemological group: *Phenomenon, Theories, Methodologies, Results*, we can then assert that Technopathogenology is a new science.

In Chapter I we have provided grounds to support the phenomenon and in Chapter II we have described the Hypotheses and Theories on which this new disciplinary proposal is based upon. It is now the time to deal with the next element on the list: Methodology.

We have found an interesting definition of Method (Aguayo & Martínez Amores, 1958): "Any human activity constitutes a method when it is submitted to a preconceived plan and organization, thus forming a functional unit".

We will see that Technopathogenology is organized according to specific preconceived criteria and plan, thus forming a functional unit. As we have said above, if we follow Feyerabend's criteria, Technopathogenology *works* methodologically.

If Technopathogenology studies the phenomenon of Technopathogeny in order to achieve its prevention, the following questions arise:

Is it possible that by developing a systematic and living knowledge of the phenomenon of Technopathogeny its existence can be incorporated in the very germinal matrix of each new technology thus avoiding its existence? And also: which is its method and which are the tools to achieve such aim, which is the prevention of the technopatogenic phenomenon?

Through the Hypothetical-Deductive method we have seen that Technopathogenology has proved that there was a disciplinary void in the study of Technopathogeny, thus solving the problem of its framing and proving to be the right discipline for its study.

However, given that one of the characteristics of Technopathogeny is its risk on health, it is licit to wonder if we are referring to a phenomenon which is completely unpredictable, therefore random. If this were the case, only the description of its apparition would be possible, making prevention or prediction impossible. If it were merely descriptive, it would be as if medicine only described the illnesses or diseases and would not search for their cure and prevention.

We can then formulate a new theory:

Theory: Technopathogeny is a predictable phenomenon

When we referred to the question on predictability we said that we were inclined to this possibility.

After dedicating Chapter II to demonstrate the disciplinary void to study Technopathogeny, formulate several hypotheses, enunciate theories to support them and postulate the need of a new science for its study, it would seem that what this theory establishes would be logical.

The aim of this theory is to prove that there is in fact a methodology – which might be somewhat imperfect – that can allow for the prevention of the phenomenon. And even though Technopathogeny may not currently be a predictable phenomenon, Technopathogenology would still be the science that could study it more accurately.

We consider that there are certain means and attitudes that scientists and technicians can resort to in order to reduce and prevent Technopathogenies. We have said that the closer to the germinal matrix of a technology such means and attitudes are applied, the faster and less expensive the prophylaxis risk will be (Eguiazu, 1999b).

The question on the method and the tools for prevention

Having said that Technopathogeny is a predictable phenomenon, we must now proceed to explain how this can be achieved.

Without getting into the discussion on whether a science is considered a science only if it incorporates Method, what is actually left to analyze is precisely: what is the method particular to this discipline to study and prevent Technopathogenies? The question could also be: is there really a method which, described as objectively as possible and carried out by other researchers, allows arriving to conclusions which are similar to ours? Or rather, in the line of Popper's falsability: is there a method to try to destroy our theory for those who wish to attempt it?

How would a research on the subject begin?

First and foremost, in connection to the criticism on the methodology of Technopathogenology, in order to refute it we could refer to the following concept: the scientific knowledge is described (Goblot, 1943) as:

> Not being just any knowledge, but a knowledge obtained by certain very strict and safe methods; the spirit of the wise man who holds to very strict rules unseen by the common observer. If such are the characteristics of the sciences, we know scientifically very little.

Technopathogeny is a sign that *the sciences* on which the technological progress is based have also got a false security and also serious methodological problems. It is obvious that the technopathogenies generated by defects in several technological objects indicate that they were not scientifically known.

We will now proceed to describe our methodological proposal.

We have seen that following the methodological structure of empirical sciences and through the hypothetical-deductive method, Technopathogenology has proved to be the most adequate discipline to study the new phenomenon. However, as we have already said, if our hypothesis is that the phenomenon is predictable, the missing answer is: if Technopathogenology is the adequate science for prevention, which are the tools to achieve such prevention?

As a general reflection we could say that this raises the methodical question: how must this be approached? Going from empirical manifestations to levels of higher intellectual abstraction? How can a methodical path be consolidated?

In order to answer these questions we resort to two points we described when we referred to Technopathogenology:

a) From a theoretical question to its ultimate causes.

b) From the moment a fact is observed to its ultimate technological cause.

We will develop these two perspectives – classified as centrifugal (a) and centripetal (b) – below.

a) From a theoretical question to its ultimate causes

The theoretical question regarding a contaminant or a cause of damage that lies within the human environment and, if not stopped, can be harmful to humans requires specific reflections.

The most important questions are: how harmful is a given contaminant? How harmful are contaminants as a group? Or most importantly, how predictable is the effect when attacking the cause? Which is then the *claro et distincto* object of study?

b) From the moment a fact is observed to its ultimate technological cause.

From the empirical point of view, because of its multiplicity, the question requires a considerable amount of common sense for the election of a concrete tool. This question is crucial to be able to turn the abstract or theoretical into efficient prophylaxis, within the intellectual matrix of the creative act. It is the *Eureka*, the deep sense inside a human being that he or she has created or discovered something new.

However, all this could be objected, raising questions such as: but is this not known? Has this not been carried out for a long time? Has empirical work not been done for a long time to detect contaminants? Are there not thinkers who think on how to improve techniques and on their effect on the social aspect – a task which has been largely carried out by the Science, Technology and Society (STS) movement? Are there no people working systematically on risk, trying to prevent it and control it, even through specific consulting companies like the Centre for Disaster Management and Risk Reduction Technology (CEDIM) in Kalsruhe, Germany, which work on understanding risk and, if possible, its early detection, as well as on methods to control such risks quickly? (Universitaet Karlsruhe, 2006). What is new in this concept? What is new in the idea of a techno-patho-geno-logy?

Whatever the question is, there is, above all, the undoubtful existence of the phenomenon. However, we may be unable to answer that question fully and satisfactorily. We can, nevertheless, contribute with the following arguments:

a) The concept may have not been formulated like this before; we simply know we have arrived to it by excluding the known. As technologists, it was our initial road to search for ways of preventing this problem within the frame of the existent. The result of our personal experience was proving the impossibility of such framing. We arrived to our proposal through hard and falsative discussion. Evidently, only a novelty can be expected to decant from the fierce criticism received from the scientific community. Following Popper, the best way to prove that something is unbreakable is by trying to break it as hard as one can and still be unable to do it. The amphora containing a new theory must be willing to stand the hammering of falsification, not break, and only then start to be taken into account.

b) We know this is a summary, that there is plenty done and thought of in the subject, but not in the concept of a "Science of immanent and hidden defect in Technique with negative consequences to human health."

c) We know in our own experience that even though with the Ethics framing Technopathogeny cannot be prevented, the ethical causes of this defect must be included in this discipline since ethical misdemeanors are the cause of the biggest loss of time and effort as well as of the creation of defective technologies. That is to say, technopathogenies are caused both by voids or defects in the knowledge or bodies of knowledge and by its hasty application, but also due to action and omission of the very same actors within the scientific community (Eguiazu et al, 2004).

d) We have behaved in a very programmatic manner since the beginning of our career as researchers, rejecting good offers to work as part of consolidated disciplines. We have rejected forced framings knowing they were good opportunities, but choosing to be faithful to the unconditional search for knowledge. We do not know whether we have succeeded in creating a field that more talented researchers will consolidate, but at least we do know that we have tried to do so with intellectual honesty.

e) Now, how can we respond to the following objection: how can you match natural sciences with ethics, two disciplinary areas which are completely unrelated? Maybe our answer could be: we start with a program and then the discipline's method will emerge from that. So far there is no definite answer to the objection, sensibly backed up by the positive background of our science. It is reasonable that the traditional scientist asks about the method, the laboratory and the instruments, not taking anything for granted.

f) The method for prevention maybe summarized as the adequate choice of tools which, with a minimum investment in time and effort, allow to contribute and advance in the technopathogenological knowledge.

These tools can be, for example, an accurate method to detect aflatoxins through mass spectrometry or high pressure liquid chromatography – accurate but expensive methods – or through less accurate methods (such as thin layer chromatography or field methods as minicolumns or Self-Activated Thin Layer Chamber-Plate).

Nevertheless, we are indeed interested in answering the Technopathogenological question: is this grain correctly stored to avoid the risk of generation or presence of aflatoxins? The best answer to this question on what is correct about this technique might not be the use of a mass spectrometer or high pressure liquid chromatography but a simple technique such as Self-Activated Thin Layer Chamber-Plate. The mass spectrometer is an important device that can provide answers to a basic analytical question or as a contrasting and adjusting technique, but it is of little value to the Technopathogenological question. And, if by the same price of a mass spectrometry one can do hundreds of thin layer chromatographies, the answer as to which is the most adequate technique is clear. A single mass spectrometry test would provide no relevant information to the technopathogenological question, but several Self-Activated Thin Layer Chamber-Plates can provide relevant information as to the evolution or gestation defects of storage technology.

We therefore will be able to observe that the storage technology – one of the elements involved in the manifestation of this technopathogenic phenomenon – does not take into account a simple analysis for controlling intergranular humidity.

The Technopathogenology method

Comparison with other sciences

In order to contribute to the Technopathogenology methodology let us continue by comparing Technopathogenology (c) with Epidemiology (a) and Criminology (b).

We found two distinctive aims of these sciences, (a) and (b), which become connected in Technopathogenology (c).

a) It searches for a material or empirical cause through diagnoses (Epidemiology).
b) It searches for an ethical or moral cause (Criminology).
c) The cause can be a combination of the two: material and ethic or intellectual (Technopathogenology).

What these sciences have in common is the search for empirical evidence. After investigating through this empirical evidence we gradually arrive at the cause. In Epidemiology, the cause can be a pathogen; in Environmental Epidemiology, a chemical. In Criminology, however, the cause will always be a human act, and such act will be driven by a motive resulting from either an ethical or moral cause or from blind passion. Here Criminology and Epidemiology are clearly separated by their ultimate causing agent.

In this sense, Technopathogenology is more closely related to Criminology, since the causing agent in the former is a human mind creating a flawed object, or rather, a human spirit deliberately committing an unethical act – thus even more resembling Criminology (even though most of the preliminary investigation is carried out with methods which are similar to the ones used in Epidemiology).

Technopathogenology. Its method

First and foremost, we will analyze the classic criteria described in connection to the methodology of sciences – empirical sciences in the case of Technopathogenology.

We consider Technopathogenology an empirical science because the phenomenon that it studies and attempts to avoid is concrete: *harm to human health*. However, because of what we have already indicated, it also has characteristics of formal sciences. The fact that it is a science under construction also supports this notion, since concepts, definitions and principles must be abstracted and constantly adjusted.

The following methods are mentioned in relation to empirical sciences:

The hypothetical-deductive method

In Chapter II we referred to the hypothetical-deductive method in order to substantiate the need to create Technopathogenology. We will now refer to the hypothetical-deductive method as a mechanism to detect and prevent Technopathogeny.

According to this method (Colacilli de Muro, 1978),

Empirical sciences are presented as systems of theories, each conformed by a group of initial hypotheses upon which – by logical deduction – other hypotheses are obtained until we arrive, by the same procedure, to hypotheses of a lower level, i.e., less general hypotheses. Once the hypotheses of lower level are obtained, the basic observation premises are inferred, which will be subjected to the verdict of confrontation by facts.

The Technologist will then be able to formulate all the hypotheses required for the development and application of a new technology, so that the theory of innocuousness or risk of such technology can be applied.

We will further analyze this later on.

The experimental method

Another method mentioned in empirical sciences is the Experimental Method.

However, being the human being the victim of Technopathogeny, it is not possible to resort to the experimental method in order to prove whether a factor generated by Technique can be harmful to health since the human being would have to be the actual subject of the experiments – which, in turn, would contradict the reason for the existence of this science.

The observation method

As for the scientific observation, some interesting aspects are mentioned (Colacilli de Muro, 1978):

> The scientific observation requires personal and special aptitudes in the researcher, which are enriched by the constancy, patience, opportunity, precision and clarity in the notes they take and particularly in the critical attitude without concessions for registering, comparing and interpreting the results.

The existing information on this phenomenon provided by auxiliary disciplines to Technopathogenology (Epidemiology, Toxicology, Chemistry, etc.) conform a database that can be compared and interpreted to estimate the technopathogenic risk. If necessary, the interpretation of these results can lead auxiliary disciplines to the need of searching new results in order to obtain, through deduction, prediction of risk.

The statistic method

The statistic method can be useful "to decide how to select the events that will be observed" in case the amount of events to observe is rather large.

The Technopathogenology method

So far, we have mentioned the methodological series applied to Techno-pathogenology as an empirical science. We will now focus on our methodology proposal (Motta & Eguiazu, 2007).

We will first see a graphic representation of Technopathogeny.

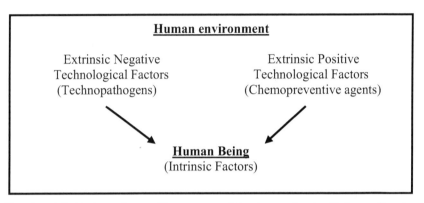

Chart 3:   The Technopathogeny Phenomenon and the elements involved in its manifestation

Just like with any other phenomenon, for a Technopathogeny to occur, different factors are to concur. Such factors can be classified as Extrinsic (belonging to the human environment) and Intrinsic (within the human being).

On the one hand, there must be negative technological factors that cause damage to human health (technopathogens) and positive technological factors or protectors of health (also known as chemopreventors) within the human environment. In both cases, they must be present in a proportion that can cause damage, in the case of technopathogens (in some technopathogens, a level zero must be considered) and that allows for protection, in the case of chemopreventors.

On the other hand, there must be an individual susceptible of being affected by a technopathogen. The variation in susceptibility is known as *host factor*.

Even though Technopathogenology aims at Technique in order to prevent Technopathogenies, studies that attempt to identify host factors are highly relevant too. This would allow the person to avoid exposure to technopathogens that can be harmful to his or her health. The workplace is a very important field of application. The identification of susceptibility biomarkers we have mentioned in Chapter II is then highly relevant.

Nevertheless, what Technopathogenology aims at studying are the Extrinsic Factors present in the human environment, i.e., Technique and its possibility to generate Technopathogens and Chemopreventors.

Regarding Chemopreventors, we have already analyzed the concept of Biological Quality (which we will describe in detail in Chapter IV: Technopathogenology and the new quality criteria).

In this sense, the methodological proposal of Technopathogenology – along with its postulates – aims at fostering the development of techniques that can generate products, foodstuffs or foodstuff complements that provide individuals with chemopreventors in order to protect them from the aggression of technopathogens. In addition, any research that aims at identifying new chemopreventors is highly relevant too.

The other proposal for the prevention of this phenomenon is the study of supporting grounds and the development of postulates. This aims, on the one hand, at identifying possible technopathogens in the techniques already in use, thus establishing regulations to control their exposure. We have called this *a posteriori* control. On the other hand, it aims – as one of its most important goals – at providing grounds for the development of Techniques that do not generate technopathogens, that is, an *a priori* control.

Applied mainly to prevent the generation or exposure of technopathogens, we will see that the methodological criteria and the tools that allow us to avoid or reduce a technopathogenic risk are varied and depend on the chronological stage the development of each concrete science is. This process, as we will mention later on, can be Centrifugal or Centripetal.

The analysis will then consist of confronting Technology in its various stages with a series of variables so that the technopathogenic risk of a technique in particular (both existing or in development) is as close as possible to zero.

Table 27, represents the three evident levels of evolution of a Technique (Motta, 1994): Idea, Development, and Use (The product has been applied).

In the Technopathogenologic method to the prophylaxis of the Technopathogeny, we have identified two other stages in the evolution of a Technique: Previous stage, and Product has been finished but not yet applied.

0) Previous stage
1) Idea
2) Development
3) Product has been finished but not yet applied
4) The product has been applied

0) Previous stage

We make reference to a Previous Stage since any idea is the result of a set of the scientist's previous bodies of knowledge. These previous bodies of knowledge allow the conception of a new idea. It also depends on the *scientific culture* or values with which scientists guide their work. It is a level of reflection.

In the Fifth Approach to Technopathogeny we indicated that the voids in the bodies of knowledge responsible for technopathogenies – if such bodies of knowledge are put into practice – are a consequence of the eager search for knowledge, which would lead us to postulate a *patience criterion* regarding technological progress processes.

Table 27: Levels of evolution of a Technique (Motta, 1994)

Levels of Evolution of a Technique			
	IDEA	**Development**	**Use**
	Pure knowledge level. Planning.	Experimentation Manufacturing	Usage
Cost	Minimum expense or no expense.	The more the state of development is, the bigger the cost.	Return of investment.
Evolution of prophylaxis	Ideal Detection of Technopathogenic risk in this stage will avoid human exposure to the technique.	------------------------------x -----------------------x ------------x ----x x indicates the interruption of the process Even though the interruption of the process means no human exposure, it implies an economic loss, which can be high.	Current -----------x x indicates the interruption of the process Upon detection of damage on humans, the Technique is recalled from the market.

Also, and according to the concepts already mentioned by Prof. Beck, if Technique is a fallible object, *prudence* is a much more important criterion than blind enthusiasm for the new object.

Professor Beck postulates the existence of known or still unknown natural laws, whether they are physical, biological and/or anthropological which can lead to serious consequences if tampered with – including endangering human existence (Beck, 1979a). Professor Beck says:

> Humans are now a lot more committed to respect natural laws than they did in the past. They do not have the freedom to act for or against Nature, but of acting with it or in it, that is to say, acting only provided nature is respected and served.

An interesting phrase we used at the beginning of our work is *leitmotiv*, or recurrent theme. We'd like to bring it to light again, since any leitmotiv that stimulates or rules the work of a scientist would be crucial in the eventual generation of a Technopathogeny.

We can then propose to use an ethical criterion as method. Such criterion must be followed by scientists, and it must comply with the definition of Ethics: "to behave without contravening ones and others' nature" (Colacilli de Muro, 1978).

Let us quote the book of Genesis: *The LORD God then took the man and settled him in the Garden of Eden, to cultivate and care for it.*

We can say that in this stage, the difference between Technopathogenology and other disciplines that focus on the Technological problem is that Technopathogenology becomes a Technique. We have already mentioned that Technopathogenology is the science of Technology that reflects upon itself and upon its own fallibility, its risks and consequences to human health. It is technique seen from the inside, which also allows us to see its imperfections. The other disciplines entail different aspects of the technological problem, but they are not Technique from the inside or from their essence. These other disciplines arise from consolidated disciplines while Technopathogenology arises from Technique.

In short, the method for this stage would be the ethical-reflective: patience and prudence in the progress of knowledge together with ethical confrontation of knowledge.

1) Idea

It is a theoretical level. It is the germinal plane. From the point of view of Technopathogenology, it is the most important stage since it is the moment in which knowledge – Technology – is conceived and generated. If applied, such knowledge will lead to new Techniques. As we have mentioned before, any flaw in this stage will be carried onto the following stages.

In this stage of development of Technique, Socratic Irony can be applied.

The Socratic Method is described as the integration of three stages: Protreptic, Refutation and Maieutics. In the Protreptic stage, Socrates made questions on a certain topic to a person who was supposed to know about such topic; in the Refutation stage Socrates refuted the answer with a series of questions in order to arrive to the Maieutics stage, in which he arrived to the conclusion that nothing is known (Colacilli de Muro, 1978).

Technopathogenology proposes a similar method. Technologists have conceived an idea to solve an existing problem, or an idea that could be applied in a Technique.

Technologists can resort to questions that aim at responding to questions of need: what is the use of this technique? Which benefits will the knowledge bring about if applied? Which risks can it entail? Which are its implications, whether economic or other? Technologists will then refute every single answer or argument and eventually will determine not necessarily that they know nothing, but that there is a need to investigate further in order to avoid the risk of a Technopathogeny.

We can remember the philosopher's quotation (Goblot, 1943):

> We will have a scientific notion of the conceived idea provided we submit it to criticism and that we can distinguish what we know and what we do not know about such idea.

We can go back to the architect example (Motta, 1994). After a previous stage in which they bear in mind the aspects that will define their work (functionality, urban and climatic aspects, comfort, economic aspects, etc.), architects conceive the idea that will be drawn on the plane. So far, we can say it is only knowledge drawn on paper. But this plane will eventually materialize into a building. Should there be any defect on the

344

plane, such defect will be transferred to the building and could eventually even harm people (whether they are usufructuary from the work or not). Now, before the building is materialized, architects can examine the plane and correct eventual errors or flaws. This will avoid not only harming people but also economic loss – especially if the error is connected to miscalculating the structures that support the construction. For example, if the construction of a beam does not observe the correct proportion between Portland cement and sand and stone; or the reinforcing rod used is of a smaller diameter than the one specified by the engineer's calculation.

Technopathogenology proposes a similar attitude: to examine the conceived idea in order to detect possible defects that can cause technopathogenies.

We propose the following method:
- Proposition of a hypothesis on the new idea.
- Confrontation with existing knowledge. By analogy, we can calculate the potential technopathogenological risk.

Auxiliary disciplines such as Physics, Chemistry, Biology and Toxicology have developed knowledge that can be of valuable help to contrast with them the conceived idea and its possible technopathogenic risks. For example, nowadays Toxicology has a database on the effect of several substances in living organisms that allows it to establish a structure-activity relationship, i.e. the relationship between certain structural parts of the molecule of a substance and its effect (for instance, mutagenic). This relationship provides a comparative element for new substances that have the same structural part and thus predict their potential risk.

2) Development

Continuing with the architect example, during this stage the idea begins to be *constructed*.

A series of questions can be formulated, for example:
- Which should the characteristics of the product be?
- How will it be applied?
- Will the people involved in the technique – the users – be workers or consumers? If consumers, is it a large or a restricted group? By restricted we mean, for example, a medicine or a medical treatment. A pesticide, because of its residues, will involve a

large group. A medicine will only involve people with a certain illness that would be treated with it. In addition, in the case of the medicine, people know they are exposed, while in the case of the pesticide, they might not know so.

- Which are the characteristics of the new technique? Does it imply the use of a component that can be a risk factor?
- If the characteristics of the new technique are known, the existent information could be compiled to determine the technopathogenic risk.
- If there is a technopathogenic risk, the required modifications can be made in order to avoid the risk of exposure.

We propose the following method:
- Propose a hypothesis on the new idea.
- Empirical verification.
- Experimentation (auxiliary sciences).

Certain auxiliary disciplines such as Physics, Chemistry, Biology, Toxicology, etc. provide tools that can be used to test a developing technique. For example, short tests or carcinogenicity tests on experimental animals.

3) Product has been finished but not yet applied

As method and tools we propose the same ones we proposed for the previous sections:
- Proposition of a hypothesis on the new idea.
- Empirical verification.
- Experimentation (auxiliary sciences).

If this is a process, certain modifications can be carried out in the technique in order to avoid or decrease its technopathogenic risk. Such modifications may involve a bigger economic cost due to the fact that the technique is already finished. (See point 4 for more details on this aspect.)

If the finished product is a substance (a pesticide, for example), it will be impossible to carry out modifications in the productive or developmental process of the Technique. Then Risk Assessment and Risk Management can be applied with the technopathogenic principles taken into consideration in order to avoid or reduce the risk.

4) The product has been applied

If the technique is already in use in the market, the available toxicological information must be consulted or experiments must be programmed resorting to auxiliary disciplines so that the technopathogenological risk can be evaluated. If, by applying technopathogenic criteria, it is discovered that there is indeed risk, there should be an attempt to replace the technique in question with one which entails lesser risk. If there is no alternative and the use of the technique is crucial, certain management measures should be applied in order to limit its risk.

As we have observed in table 27, if the technique used is proved to be harmful, it is generally recalled from the market. However, this is only valid for acute negative effects or for negative effects that appear in the short-term. Technopathogenic phenomena usually occur in the long term, sometimes, after many years of exposure. Therefore, even if the product is recalled from the market, many people can continue to suffer the negative effects. In addition, given that technological development is costly, it is only natural that the business system tries to avoid recalling the product (a substance, an electronic device, etc.) since that would mean they will not get a return for their investment in research and development. Therefore, technopathogenic analysis and management measures are curcial in these cases to determine the risk – which, in turn, will make the economic cost as low as possible.

As an example of an Applied Technique which carries serious errors, we can mention the use of distilled petrol in seed oil extraction techniques (in soy, corn, peanut, etc.). Regarding this, we have come across a concrete case. The technopathogenological risk can be given by the presence of benzene in the solvent – a substance which is found as a contaminant by-product of the distilment process, even after the oil has gone through the process of separating the oil from the solvent. Benzene being carcinogenic, flawed technologies that even inadvertently allow the benzene to reach exposed human surfaces entail a technopathogenic risk.

Knowing this, the person in charge of using the solvent can ask the manufacturer to provide a different solvent, free of benzene. In this case, the work on technopatogenic risk would focus on distilling techniques. Another possibility is to protect the workers and avoid or limit – with the use of proper devices – exposure to the solvent – thus to benzene. The extraction process can also be improved, for example, by using as little benzene as possible, so that the solvent residues (therefore, benzene in oil) do not reach consumers.

Another case in which we were involved was the technopathogenic risk of high-tension towers. In this case, given the impossibility of moving the location of the towers, it was suggested that people moved or lived as far as possible from such towers.

Another example in the application of technopathogenological criteria to the development of methodologies which aim at preventing or reducing technopathogenic risk is our proposal to include the Intergranular Air Relative Humidity in grain commercialization standards. If this were applied to grain storage, fungal development and formation of mycotoxins would be reduced.

We propose the following methodology for this stage:
- Proposal of hypotheses for the technique in use.
- Empirical verification.
- Experimentation method (auxiliary disciplines).
- Observational method: detecting adverse manifestation in organisms present in the human environment (Ecotoxicology) and technopathogenies in humans (Toxicology and Epidemiology)

Auxiliary disciplines: Toxicology, Genetic Toxicology, Carcinogenesis in experimental animals, Analytical Chemistry, Epidemiology, Jurisprudence, Ecotoxicology: effects in animals and plants that would indicate the manifestation of a risk technopathogen.

The method as centripetal-centrifugal movement

This way of observing the problem emerged from a play on words in German – Begegnung (encounter) and Bewegung (movement) – which we came across through Beck's work.

If we consider technological development a dynamic process, a different approach of analyzing the methodology of Technopathogenology is possible from a centripetal and centrifugal point of view.

The main idea is that the technological creation process is a movement that goes from the inner part to the outer part of a sphere in a centrifugal manner. Now, when technopathogenies connected to any technology are observed, the idea is, although imperfectly, to clarify and undo centripetally the road taken, that is, from the outside to the inside.

In the centre of the sphere there is the process of discovery or realization, the *eureka*, and all the mental processes needed to bring to light a new technique. The material effect of such technique is found in the outer surface of the sphere. The two movements go from one side to the other in a continuous feedback.

There was a case reported by the media involving a medicine used for treating arthrosis which had the technopathogenological side effect of affecting the heart. The company which had manufactured the medicine had to pay several millions of dollars to the widow of the victim. This is a case in which the centrifugal effect was not studied thoroughly enough. The negative effects could not be stopped from appearing on the surface of the sphere, in this case, the medicine. Hence the question: wouldn't the company have benefited more if its researchers had a technopathogenological background? Wouldn't this company have invested in training its researchers and technologists in technopathogenological matters if they had known they would lose so much money?

We believe that Technopathogenology is a need and that companies should be the ones most interested in asking for this kind of training which is very much resisted and rejected by many scientists since for them it only shows a failure in the dogma of infallibility of Science and Technique.

This kind of resistance can be presented in good faith in many cases, because accepting the phenomenon of Technopathogeny can be difficult due to the paradigm in which scientists were educated.

We will now describe this new perspective for analyzing the technopathogenological method:

A. Centripetal

This is done from the outside to the inside of the sphere, once the technique is already in use.

Let us now consider different examples for different steps.

We call it centripetal because we can see unwanted collateral effects and we attempt to search for the causes: first, by determining which technology was used, and second, by analyzing how this technology was created and which were the basic mistakes in the previous centrifugal process. We call it previous centrifugal process because the Technique had to be created, gestated and then *sent* to its usage. The collateralities are detected in the periphery of the symbolic sphere of the Technique we have mentioned.

1. Detection of adverse effects. Observation of microbiological organisms, plants, animals, and humans in order to detect pathological modifications. In this step, the continuous help of Epidemiology, Environmental Medicine, Environmental Sciences, Ecotoxicology, Toxicology, Ecology, Biology, Microbiology, etc., will be required.
2. Determination of the cause.
3. Determination of the exact cause in a multi or interdisciplinary manner. For example, if it is the case of a substance, it should be isolated and identified as well as have its structure and properties, etc. determined.
4. Search for an immediate solution: If it is an everyday use substance, try to substitute it immediately with alternatives which are harmless. In the case of aflatoxins, for example, if a plant variety sensible to them, it should be replaced with a more resistant one. The help of several disciplines will be required: Analytical Chemistry, environmental Chemistry, Measuring Techniques and all the sciences that study the development and application of accurate analytical methods: Spectroscopy, Chromatography, Radiation Measurement, etc.
5. Search for a permanent solution: The aim would be to make the alternatives found in the previous step permanent. For example: ban a risky pesticide, promoting less risky pesticides, ban vegetables that are sensible to aflatoxins, promoting growing more resistant varieties. This step will also require the help of the so-called *sciences of the spirit*, such as Ethics, and more social sciences such as Law and Political Sciences in order to contribute to the integral solution of a complex problem.
6. To promote better ideas for the creation or use of techniques. For example: In the case of a pesticide, it could be considered the search for substances with the same agronomic effect but without technopathogenic risk, as well as the search for practices which do not entail the use of pesticides, and in the case of aflatoxins, the search to varietes resistent to them. Knowledge in alternative agriculture and biological-dynamic agriculture can be implemented as well.

As a complement to the steps described, the multidisciplinary approach and the coordinated work with the sciences above mentioned is rather obvious – without them, Technopathogenology could not be applied and would be very inefficient. It would remain a simple theoretical rambling.

B. Centrifugal

This is done from the inside to the outside and it is done prior to the application of a technique. It corresponds to the Idea stage.

For example, if we are dealing with a substance, we can observe certain aspects of technopathogenic interest: its chemical structure and correspondent expected risk, the available experimental data on risks, which real application the product will have, in which concrete technique it will be used, risks of exposure, etc.

The crucial element here is the relationship between the structure and the activity – or any other method that allows us to see with anticipation if there is any element present within the chemical structure and its biological activity that can cause a negative effect.

It involves the work with Chemistry, Toxicology and Computer Science, which allows comparing an enormous quantity of data in a short period of time.

In connection to the risk of exposure, we can mention, for example, high-tension wires. It is not the same to install them in the desert than in a high populated area, which can cause a technopathogenic risk.

The centrifugal criterion requires the work of Environmental Epidemiology. Existent data is useful if, for example, the technique in question has been approved in one country but it was then proved harmful. If so, it could be analyzed whether there is any proven, innocuous technique it can be replaced with. The question is therefore: which is the least harmful possibility or with less technopathogenic risk that can be used? The principle of the *lesser evil* can therefore be applied.

Ethical criteria must also be observed. This involves attitudes that bring to light all the flaws of technique. There are a set of questions that should always be present: are there alternative techniques that can have the same function? Has there any negative information been hidden? Has the decision been taken under pressure?

In other aspects, the question can be: are there any objections against what is going to be used?

Once the alternative is chosen and fear has been dissipated, a decision can be taken thus allowing the use of the technique.

This would be the ideal criteria: harmful alternatives are discarded during the idea stage. This would avoid human, environmental and economic damage.

The Centrifugal and centripetal criterion and the aflatoxins example

A. The problem started as something centripetal.
  1. An unexpected disease was observed in turkeys in the UK. Also liver cancer was observed in humans in Thailand and Africa.
  2. The relationship between the diseases and the presence of aflatoxins in corn is established.
  3. The *Aspergillus flavus* mold generates a carcinogenic difurocoumarin: aflatoxins.
  4. The causal relation is further investigated. A question arises: why is there mold in the grain? The possible answers could be: the more sensible varieties contain more water in the grain, which is tolerated in the business. An alternative could be to use more resistant varieties where the control of water content is not that relevant. They would be varieties resistant to human errors. Some difficulties to this alternative could be: the old varieties may not exist anymore, the genes may have been eroded or lost; old varieties can mean less turnout; producers might stand against the loss of water in grains since it signifies less weight, therefore, less money.

This can also lead to political questions, or to ones more related to economy or Social Sciences: is there a way in which agriculturists can be attracted to the use of new varieties that carry a certification indicating their produce is free of aflatoxins, even though it means a smaller turnout?

B. From the centrifugal point of view, the question could be: how can I solve the dilemma of having to sacrifice turnout in order to obtain aflatoxins-free produce? Or, for example, how to force the political decision of making the criterion of diminishing water content in grains a compulsory one – therefore avoiding the mold to colonize the grain and contaminate it with aflatoxins?

Another possibility would be, for example, if I decide to use a variety genetically engineered with a genome resistant to fungal attack (which would avoid the generation of aflatoxins), would this pose a new risk on health? Which risk would there be as a consequence of the interaction between the new and the existing genomes? Can events be predicted? If there is no answer, I must either try a different solution or try to find an old variety without attempting to remove its genes. If there is no old variety available, should I reconstruct it using existing genetic material?

If the old variety resistant to aflatoxins still exists, should I investigate if it poses a risk on health or should I assume that being an old genome, used since ancient times, it will pose no risk on health?

If we do not find the answer, or if the old variety is not available, we must resort to preventive measures like, for example, decreasing the water content in varieties sensible to aflatoxins. In this case, we will have to consider that the market will most probably oppose to this unless there is some kind of compensation. For example, if in order to avoid contamination I have to reduce the water content of a grain to an 8% when it is normally allowed to have an 11% humidity content, the 3% of water lost represents a rather major loss in large quantities: 3 tons every 100 tons – that is to say, a great loss compared to the agriculturist who does not dry the grain. This calls upon marketing solutions which can be obtained by resorting to other disciplines such as Economic, Political or Law Sciences.

Every stage must be confronted with ethical considerations in order to avoid superficial solutions.

Similar examples can also be found with other substances such as carcinogenic pesticides, medicines, etc.

To the methodological objection of Technopathogenology:
Criminology as an example for its refutation

We believe we have provided a methodological proposal with which we can study the phenomenon and can manage to either eliminate it or reduce it. However, since there can be objections, we want to draw a comparison with Criminology.

Because it is a developing discipline, the methodology of Technopathogenology may still be not completely able to prevent Technopathogenic risk. Nevertheless, as with every new science, time will give Technopathogenology better, more adequate and more accurate tools to develop better ways of prevention. This would allow not only to prevent the most evident technopathogenies, but also the most subtle and most difficult to detect.

We will now compare Technopathogenology with Criminology. Criminology is described as the study of "Crime, its causes and its repression" (Diccionario Enciclopédico Ilustrado de la Lengua Española), or "the science of crime, its causes and its repression," and if, according to its definition, repression is described as "stopping an action from happening" (Diccionario El Pequeño Larousse Ilustrado), we will find that both Criminology and Technopathogenology are very similar in their definitions and aims.

In the following table we can see the analogy between both sciences:

Table 28:   Similarities between Criminology and Technopathogenology.

Criminology	Technopathogenology
Crime Science: to break the laws enforced by humans	Technopathogeny Science: to break natural laws (either evident or not) by a defective gestation of the technological object.
One of the characteristics of crime is harming human life.	Technopathogeny implies harming human life.
Crime: complex problem	Technopathogeny: complex problem
Studies its causes	Studies its causes
Seeks to contain it, stop it, moderate it, stop it from developing (repression)	Seeks to detect it, contain it, moderate it, stop it from appearing.
Arrives to its cause by observing its evidence.	Arrives to its cause by observing its evidence (illness manifested or to be manifested).
Aims at prevention by studying the causes of the crime.	Aims at prevention by studying the causes of the technopathogeny.
It uses positive sciences to track down the causes of the crime.	It uses positive sciences to track down the causes of the Technopathogeny.
It uses human sciences or sciences of the spirit to dig in the ethical causes or the motive of the crime.	It uses human sciences or sciences of the spirit to dig in the ethical causes that allow the genesis and manifestation of the technopathogenies associated to it.
The most important cause of the crime is moral. On the second plane, we find the auxiliary positive sciences to understand it.	The most important cause of technopathogenies is moral and, the second most important cause is the imperfective nature of positive and technological sciences.

In addition, Technopathogenology also uses several auxiliary disciplines to find out whether certain damage on health to one person or to a group of persons can be considered a Technopathogeny or not. Furthermore, it is also used to detect it and prevent it.

At first, the elements to study crime were coarse. However, even though the resources were limited, Criminology was not daunted by the task of solving a crime.

By collecting cases and begging for help from other sciences to solve subtly hidden crimes and assembling all the results into some kind of logic, it gradually became more accurate and more predictable until the science finally emerged.

At first, the only tool used was a simple magnifier that detected tracks left by criminals. Because the system was so rudimentary, many crimes went unsolved. However, with time, new methods were incorporated into this science, so much that nowadays it is almost impossible to hide a crime. Many sciences have contributed to this method: Genetic Engineering (DNA), Psychology (psychological studies of the criminal), Ballistic Studies, Dactyloscopy, Microscopy, Polarised Light Microscopy, etc. With these and other increasingly accurate fields, certain crimes which could not be solved in the past can be solved nowadays. Similarly, we could say that the only tool that Technopathogenology currently has is a magnifier, but we believe that with time it will develop more accurate methods that will allow it to contribute with elements to achieve the complete prevention of this risk.

We are also drawing the parallelism with Criminology because they are both sciences of diagnosis. Apart from preventing, they use several tools from other disciplines (such as Chemistry or Biology) and accurate research (Human Sciences) in order to investigate cause-effect. Technopathogenology studies the etiological agent (technopathogen) responsible for the Technopathogeny and Criminology, the motive responsible for the Crime.

We understand that the fact that a crime can be solved contributes to avoid it – maybe due to the fear of criminals to be discovered.

As we have shown with Technopathogenology, Criminology also uses many tools belonging to various fields, but it cannot be reduced to any of them.

Another interesting science to use as example is Seismology. Until this day, this science cannot anticipate all the earthquakes, however, such inaccuracy does not mean that the science should not continue research-ing its object of study hoping that one day it can detect earthquakes prior to their occurrence and take preventive measures.

Technopathogeny is a discipline that attempts to complete and im-prove already existing attempts. The idea is to achieve a better technolo-gical gestation. If Technopathogenology had the same object of study as, for instance, Technology Assessment (which is not the case), we should perhaps forget that we ever talked of Technopathogenology.

Our central question actually was: what is missing in the existing disciplines and how can we develop a science that covers the whole phe-nomenon? The aim of Technopathogenology is to apply the prophylaxis during the stages in which the technological invention is still inexistent, that is, during the idea stage. Once the technological invention is mate-rialized, we will encounter resistance to change the already developed object. This implies high risk and damage to health if the object leads to technopathogenies.

Our interest is that Technopathogenology acts prior to the develop-ment and application of a technique in order to avoid damage. This is known in medical sciences as prophylaxis. But such prophylaxis is ap-plied during the causative stage of an illness. Technopathogenology, however, would apply it during the actual gestational matrix of the tech-nique. Medicine or Toxicology, on the other hand, test or observe a tech-nique which is being used, or once it is already developed for its use. When the product shows a real or potential risk, it is recalled from the market. If a real damage is observed, just like what happened with thali-domide, it is also (although late) recalled from the market. Both proce-dures are far behind the development and application of a Technique. All the corrective processes are applied once the technique is in use. Humans then become indirect or informal hamster of the technological process.

Just like Criminology, it is expected that Technopathogenology de-velops into more accurate prevention.

XVII. Some criteria for the prevention of technopathogenic risk

In addition to what we have mentioned as methodology, we will now describe some criteria Technopathogenology adopts in order to prevent or reduce the risk of Technopathogeny.

- The doubt over innocuousness or risk is always in favor of the user of a technique.
- The context in which Technique participates is considered – that is, with which other techniques it can interact. As we have mentioned before, certain technopathogens present in the human environment are initiators, promoters, synergic and co-carcinogenic in terms of their possibility of acting together.
- Upon the possibility of selecting alternatives for a determined aim, always choose the technique which entails no or very little risk.
- A technique can entail a risk both for consumers as well as for people occupationally exposed. Upon the possibility of selecting alternatives for a determined aim, always choose the technique which entails no risk for consumers. Prevention of risk is always easier to apply in the workplace. It is said (PNUMA, 1985b) that:

> The levels and duration of exposure to hazardous chemical products are usually much lower among users than among the workers of the companies in which such products are elaborated. However, serious errors in the handling of chemical products, due to complete ignorance of the acute risk they can entail, have led to many accidents, some even mortal, in the whole world; and this will continue to occur as long as this situation is not corrected.

The report focuses on acute risk; however, we must not disregard long term risks.

- If, according to its carcinogenic risk, a technopathogen (physical, chemical or biological) is classified by important international organisms as having *enough evidence of carcinogenicity, either in humans or animals* it is considered as being a Technopathogenic risk. If, due to the limited or insufficient evidence, the factor is classified as *possibly or probably carcinogenic* or even *cannot be classified as carcinogenic*, it is considered a factor for which preventive measures should be adopted. Only the classification *non-carcinogenic* (IARC, Group 4) permits considering it as presenting *no technopatogenic risk* for cancer.

- The technopathogenic risk is only determined by the entrance of the factor into the human body. For example, a pigment can be considered carcinogenic in experimental animals, which also allows estimating it can be of risk to human beings. However, the risk will not be the same if such colorant is used as colorant in foodstuffs or as paint. In addition, we could add that even if it is used as paint, its risk will not be the same if, depending on its physicochemical composition, it is used as exterior or interior paint.

- If we are dealing with a new substance, its physicochemical properties will allow to determine how long it will need to be degraded until the substance disappears from the environment. The longer it remains in the human environment, the more negative the technopathogenological risk will be. For example: If a problem needs to be urgently solved and there are two substances with potential carcinogenic risk, the one with a faster degradation will be chosen.

- If the factor we are dealing with is physical, for example, the electromagnetic field generated by a high tension wire, we could consider the distance of exposure so that the levels of exposure on people are as small as possible.

- If an innocuous technique must be replaced by another technique because of economic reasons, better properties, etc., for example, a foodstuff colorant replaced by another, the new technique – the new substance in this case – must prove innocuous first.

- The use of chemical or physical agents which were proved to be technopathogenic – such as IARC Group 1 agents: Carcinogenic in humans – will be limited to unavoidable circumstances, for example, medical treatment without alternatives.

- The usage of any technique which involves an agent with technopathogenic risk must be limited to personnel with specific training.

XVIII. Other procedures for the prevention of Technopathogeny

In order to prevent a phenomenon, we can also resort to data on techno-pathogenies that have been already detected by the use of a technique or techniques in particular, e.g. by Epidemiology in humans. We can also resort to data that allows predicting potential Technopathogenies, for example, data provided by Toxicology once the technique is already in use. This data can be used as an alarm signal. As experience shows, only the manifestation of the technopathogenic effect in humans verified by Epidemiology is strong enough.

Knowing the period of time during which the technique was used until it was banned can also be useful since many technopathogenies become manifest due to the accumulation of successive doses.

As for concrete flaws, if we know the technopathogenies that have been already unveiled, the big question would be: How we can take the gestational error responsible for the technopathogenies which should be predicted prior to the application of their techniques?

We must also contribute to the gradual process of analytical-experimental uncovering. Which methodology must we develop in order to uncover the Technopathogenic risk factor?

Another field of knowledge is the evaluation of the investment economic process in a new technological product, regarding which the question is: when is the right time to withdraw the investment? Or rather: when can a process that entails a risk be abandoned without representing a significant loss?

This last point is particularly important since, as we will see later, the economic pressures are highly relevant to ethical misdemeanors.

An early detection of the Technopathogenic risk – while the investment is still small, as we have seen in table 27 – could most probably avoid the majority of ethical misdemeanors since the product would not be uselessly defended, and other alternative development would be aborded.

Another important point Technopathogenology should focus on is the study of Environmental Law. This is particularly important since Law researchers cannot be experts on every single technology. Techno-pathogenology must also contribute to this.

The analysis described in this section could be summarized as follows:

- Accumulation and systematization of data on technopathogenies from either catastrophic accidents or from non-evident manifestations.

  A) In catastrophes: investigate elements in common. For example: what did Chernobyl, Harrisburg, Bophal and Seveso have in common? Which abstractions or general ideas could they have in common?

  B) In long term Technopathogenies: for example, what do the effects of Thalidomide, 2, 4-D, and 2, 4, 5-T pesticides, the work with asbestos or the ingestion of nitrosamines have in common? This is particularly important in the genesis of non-evident effects, such as mutagens, carcinogens or teratogens.

- Induction – with all due reservations of this method – of all this data to build a theoretical framework.

- Uncovering and detection of technopathogenies on the spot. How can successful uncovering methods be obtained in order to reduce the time of action? How can auxiliary sciences contribute to detection and prophylaxis?

- Once the technopathogenic risks have been unveiled, how can this contribute to Environmental law in a way that law specialists understand the great data variation, which must be covered by several sciences in particular? How can prophylaxis legislation be supported?

- Intellectual models that incorporate this paradigm in the creation of technologies must be fostered. How can this gestational matrix be developed so that technologies that have not been created yet are well conceived?

Ethics

Ethics is not mentioned as a method within the Methodology of Empiric Sciences. In Chapter II we have also proved that the technopathogenic problem cannot be prevented by framing its study in Ethics. But we do remember that one definition of Ethics is "to behave without contravening one's and others' nature" (Colacilli de Muro, 1978), hence there are ethical attitudes or criteria that would contribute to prevent this phenomenon (Motta, 1994).

As we have mentioned before, Technopathogenology resorts to these criteria since a technique developed by a human being that causes a Technopathogeny is – following the above mentioned definition – contravening human nature. Technique falls out of human scale (Eguiazu, 2007).

As Ethical criteria we could mention:
a) Ethical criteria in the previous stage
b) Ethical criteria at the level of achieved knowledge and its usage
c) Ethical criteria in the attitude of Science and Technique

a)   Ethical criteria in the previous stage

This refers to the above mentioned Ethical/reflective criteria during the previous stage (i.e., prior to the technological development).

b)   Ethical criteria at the level of achieved knowledge and its usage

1)   At the level of knowledge of the developing Technique

We have described the attitudes regarding truth that represent faults or voids in knowledge or bodies of knowledge that can be the reason for the existence of an immanent or hidden risk, which can lead to the generation of a technopathogen responsible for a Technopathogeny.

This leads to the following questions: which of the described attitudes are ethical? Which attitudes regarding the truth that are responsible for technopathogenies can be avoided? Are there Technopathogenies that can be justified?

Let us suppose a substance in particular can cause adverse effects such as sterility, cancer, be mutagenic or teratogenic, among other effects. Therefore, prior to the usage of a substance all the known adverse effects could be studied. However, in the future other effects which are still not known could be detected. So far, Ignorance cannot be avoided. Another insurmountable attitude is, so far, Error. If a technique in particular is harmful to humans, even though until it was proved harmful the existent knowledge indicated the contrary, it was wrong to accept something as true when in fact it was false. This is also an almost unavoidable aspect.

Ignorance and Error can be considered ethical attitudes since they are unconscious. If a Technopathogeny is the product of ignorance, it is ethical because the negative effect was unknown. If it is the product of an Error, it is ethical because even though the possibility of risk had been evaluated, the absence of risk was erroneously assumed. Knowledge was taken as true when in fact it was false.

Even though Error is considered an ethical attitude – as we stated before when we referred to this attitude in connection to the truth – because it is connected to correctness, being fortuitous, it should be considered whether Science and Technique can progress based on knowledge that only by chance is not harmful to humans. This would mean accepting the *trial and error* criterion.

In connection with this and according to Prof. Beck's analysis of our proposal, it is crucial to recognize certain characteristics or aspects that indicate that the negative effect on human health is not present in a given technique (i.e. that the technique does not carry an immanent and hidden Technopathogeny). However, as Prof. Beck said:

> In some cases, an absolute impossibility cannot be recognized. In such cases, an evaluation of degrees of probability or improbability should be carried out.

Here it is worth going back to the self-correction criterion in Science. Considering that the voids in knowledge can lead to serious consequences to human life, even though we cannot say that *Science makes the mistake of ignoring*, the self-correction criteria – at least in all the fields of knowledge – cannot be universally accepted. In our view, it is not ethical to use humans as hamster for the self-correction to be achieved. This is a controversial issue raising questions such as: is it ethical or not to try a new medicine in a patient who could perhaps be cured by it? As we have already seen, one of the physical factors causing technopathogenies is electromagnetic fields. Nuclear Magnetic Resonance used for medical diagnosis exposes the patient to much higher levels of radiation than what is considered safe, but it is said that the results and diagnosis obtained by this study justify the risk (IPCS, 1987).

Those technopathogenies resulting from attitudes other than the two we have just described can indeed be avoided since they are conscious attitudes.

In our opinion, Doubt, Uncertainty, Opinion and, especially, Mendacity are unacceptable causes of technopathogenies. They are unethical attitudes because they are, as we have said before, conscious attitudes. If there is Doubt, Uncertainty or just an Opinion of the lack of risk of a technique in particular, it is irresponsible to use such technique. In all these cases, the possibility of risk is known but it is disregarded. It is not ethical to use a technique because *until now adverse effects on humans have not been detected and were such effects detected, the product would be retrieved from the market.* This concept, which is very much used, has been criticized by some scholars. In some cases, as with some medicines, perhaps a technique could be accepted if its use is crucial.

As we have said before, all the possible known adverse effects of a technique must be studied in every single new Technique. Doubts, uncertainties, or just opinions about their lack of risk cannot be accepted. As the phrase goes, it is better to *"err on the side of caution"* (PNUMA, 1985b).

Mendacity, apart from being an unethical attitude, is a shameful attitude. In this case, the risk is indeed known, but it is hidden.

2) *Doubt always in favor of consumers*

As we have said before, this is a criterion Technopathogenology uses in order to prevent Technopathogenies.

With reference to this point – which we can make extensive to the whole point b) – *Ethical criteria at the level of achieved knowledge and its usage,* we can give as an example the criteria used by certain International Organizations and Institutions in connection to the risk of exposure to electromagnetic fields (NIEHS-DOE, 1995):

Advisory Panel to Australian Minister of Health (1992)

> It has not been scientifically established that magnetic fields of extremely low frequency initiate or promote cancer or have any other harmful effects on humans. However, it has not been scientifically established that such fields are not harmful.

Swedish National Electrical Safety Board (1994)

> We suspect that magnetic fields may pose certain risks to health, but we cannot be certain ... There is good reason to exercise a certain amount of caution.

French National Institute of Health and Medical Research (1993)

> The epidemiologic results presently available do not permit the exclusion of a role for magnetic fields in the incidence of leukemia, particularly in children. New investigations are necessary to confirm or deny this role

It is interesting to note that all these institutions bear in mind the possibility of a potential risk on health. It is also shocking to note the lack of information on the actual risk and how the regular use of the technique is promoted until the risk actually appears. This situation exists in spite of the attitude of precaution indicated by all these institutions. Although such precautions seem reasonable, they are ignored until the economic system finds epidemiological results in order to withdraw the technology in use.

c) *Ethical criteria in the attitude of Science and Technique*

In the first two points, especially *a) Ethical criteria in the previous stage,* we made reference to the ethics of the individual (the person generating or using the knowledge). In this point, we make reference to the ethics in the system in which the person participates.

Ethical misdemeanors in the system can be associated with the development of knowledge and its application – which we have seen in the previous point. Such misdemeanors can lead to generating knowledge with voids which can potentially cause technopathogenies.

These ethical misdemeanors refer specifically to the ones incurred by some scientists. They are so common and universal that some of the ones quoted below were taken to the Swedish Parliament (Westerholm, 1999). Among the most important ethical misses we can mention:

- Stealing of ideas.
- Frivolity in the choice of the object or subject of study. Total or partial plagiarism.
- Exploitation of young researchers.
- Lobbyism in order to obtain subsidies excluding other projects which are of good quality without scientific reasons or arguments. This is supported by an administrative system that continuously derides *target persons.*
- Modifying experimental results by taking or adding data so that the hypothesis is not contradicted.
- Lack of suitability of the peer review. Referee boards conformed by prestigious professionals from various disciplines who, in order not to see their prestige reduced, give wrong opinions on questions or programs which are alien to their field of expertise.
- Power abuse from referees, who use their position to exclude the best qualified from obtaining funds. This ensured by impunity and the so-called *blind peer review.*
- Pressure to constitute a courtesy team, through which co-authorship is asked in exchange for granting resources or subsidies, even if there is no real intervention in the actual work.

364

- Exclusion of publishing critical work with fallacious or tangential arguments notwithstanding their objective value (Pusztai, 2000).
- Scientists' ethical misdemeanors when generating knowledge, for example, by setting up data in order to justify a publication, to remain in the system, to attend a congress and justify the travelling expenses, etc.
- Stealing authorship: taking texts written by other authors without quoting their origin, or doing it in an ambiguous manner in order to make an idea or authorship appear as their own.
- Hasty, mediocre publications, simply to comply with the *publish or perish* motto.
- The lack of application of the Jonas principle. This means that it is not compulsory to demonstrate new technologies are innocuous prior to their mass usage. The responsibility of those who invent and develop the new technology finishes when the product is on the market (Eguiazu, 1996).
- Hasty application of phenomena linked to profitability, without the necessary knowledge of collateral effects (Bultmann, 1996).
- Trying new technologies in the third world without a previous consent.
- Excluding ethical objectors from the Science and Technique System – part of the institution's selfishness is to stand against ethically engaged persons (Deiserot, 1997) (Schraeder et al 1995) (Westerholm, 1999).
- Hushing up collateralities by sending products of economic interest to the third world (FAO, 1986, 1990).

In order to illustrate this last point, the following table shows pesticides imported in Argentina in 1986 (Eguiazu, 1987, 1988):

Table 29: Levels of active principles in different pesticides with high risk or moderate risk of carcinogenesis that were imported to Argentina in 1986.

Active Ingredient in Pesticides of High Risk of Carcinogenesis	Active Ingredient in Pesticides (kg)
Alachlor (Lasso)	559,902
Captafol (also teratogenic)	12,220
Captan	134,036
Chlorothalonil	20,373
Folpet (also teratogenic)	11,500
Aldrin	29,825
Active Ingredient in Pesticides of Moderate Risk of Carcinogenesis	**Active Ingredient in Pesticides (kg)**
Chlordane	16,747
24-D	284,852
Maneb (also teratogenic)	26,995
Mancozeb (also teratogenic)	1,123,670
Zineb	238,068
Heptachlor	133,925

These products were considered highly risky and restricted or banned in California. However, they continued to be exported to Argentina (Eguiazu, 1996) (Jonas, 1984). Even though these products were eventually recalled from the Argentine market, the damage had already been done. This data is from 1986; by the time the present book was under revision, there were some endemic areas that presented concrete technopathogenic manifestations with cases of neoplasms higher than the expected, which is attributed to the continuous use of such pesticides for twenty-five years.

The ethical misdemeanors described – so important that they were even taken to the Swedish Parliament – are just the beginning of a great movement of self-criticism in Science and Technique (San Martín, 1987, 1990). It begins by the simple verification that, paraphrasing Shakespeare's *Hamlet*, "something is rotten in the State of Denmark" (Shakespeare); in the same manner we can say that *something is rotten in the State of Science and Technique*

Nobel Prize winner Luis F. Leloir (Leloir, 1983) says, in connection to fairness in the distribution of resources for research:

Those who act as judges are also the ones who use the resources, they are interested parties. This situation is not very satisfactory, since those who hold the power can keep the biggest piece of the pie for themselves.

To which he adds in connection to the efficient use of resources:

> It is not convenient that funds increase abruptly, since this may lead to the setting up of structures or work groups based on people with little training....

Leloir describes the abuse of power of some evaluators who exclude qualified candidates to give themselves or their disciples the biggest subsidies. He also doubts whether the subsidies obtained in such manner are efficiently used (Eguiazu, 1991).

People with ethical commitment resist these practices and they normally end up being left aside and excluded by the system. Because subsidies represent the tools required to carry out the experiments, their lack would signify shutting up target researchers.

This has led universities from developed countries to create a space to protect Ethical Objectors through a specific Ombudsman (Universität Karlsruhe, 2000). (See Chapter IV)

Following the ethical criteria proposed, technopathogenies could be prevented or their incidence decreased. Even though some cases could be caused by Ignorance or Error, in the case of chemical substances and because of the level of knowledge reached by Toxicology, we believe that those two attitudes should not cause technopathogenies.

XIX.   A utopian proposal

Apart from the measures described, there would be another possibility of reducing the risk of technopathogenies (Motta, 1994). Considering that technopathogenies are a consequence of faults regarding truth or of voids in the knowledge used for the development of Technique, the possibility, evidently utopian, would be of limiting the diffusion of scientific knowledge. This would assure that incomplete knowledge about an object is not taken by parties interested in profiting by the object. Even though the system would say that peer review is quite rigorous and a thorough evaluation of knowledge is always done before such knowledge is sent out to the public, facts show that the quality or thoroughness of such evaluation is not good enough. This is why many journals state that the authors of the articles are entirely responsible for the content of the publications.

Let us consider that "there is no scientific knowledge that has not been subjected to criticism" (Goblot, 1943). In other words, the fact that a knowledge in particular has been criticized makes it scientific. If the knowledge has not been submitted to criticism, it is not scientific. The ideal situation is that every knowledge is severely criticized by its own author first. This attitude is avoided by some scientists who fear having to discard their theories. If they find their theories are *incomplete* they will attempt to do what we have described in Chapter II: to *repair* their theories. Reparation of theories is a mechanism very much used when an *old* paradigm (Kuhn, 1995) or a degenerate program (Lakatos, 1982) is defended against evidence that totally refutes it. In this case, additional justification that explains this strong evidence as an exception is resorted to. Submitting every new technological knowledge to criticism can contribute to decreasing technopathogenic risk – provided such criticism is substantially different from what is currently done.

Of course the system will say: *but we are already doing this*, in this case, we can reply: *then you are not doing it right.*

The idea proposed is utopian because Science has surpassed the boundaries of ethics, being now in the hands of honest, humanists and philanthropists but also sometimes in the hands of unscrupulous and materialistic persons.

Four levels of objects are described (Colacilli de Muro, 1978):

Ontic level: constituted by everything there is, exists or happens in the universe.

Gnoseologic level: constituted by the processes of knowledge and their still unexpressed results. This level is circumscribed to the subject that elaborates the knowledge.

Ontological level: constituted by all the objects (things or facts) from the Ontic level that are known (whether well or poorly known). They are cultural objects if they were created by humans or cultures if humans have adapted them for their own benefit.

Expressional level: constituted by everything the subject of knowledge uses as resource or instrument to express what he or she knows. This is part of the ontological level and it includes the spoken and written word, signs, etc.

The utopian idea would be to create a fifth level included in the Expressional level and which we could call *Scientific-Expressional level* (Motta, 1994). Here, the ideas or knowledge generated and already spread (either through oral, written or recorded, etc. means) can only be taken by other scientists with a strict ethical commitment – practically whistle-blowers – who would evaluate the work before it is sent to the Expressional level, thus stopping a knowledge which can potentially generate a Technopathogeny from being inadvertently taken by a technologist to produce techniques. Such knowledge can only be spread once it can be used by other individuals knowing there is no risk of Technopathogeny. A field of application of this proposal could be the development of new chemical substances. Needless to say, this team of incorruptible evaluators with an unconditional commitment towards the truth must be carefully selected.

To summaries everything we have said in connection to the contribution of Technopathogenology to prevent non-evident damage on health connected to Technique, we can finally say that Technopathogenology as a basic science contributes to training people linked to Technology who, just like meteorologists who can predict or forecast the occurrence of rain, will recognize the conditions for the manifestation of a Technopathogeny in order to avoid it.

Such people can be connected with:

- The generation or development of new technologies: Physicists, Chemists and Biologists – to mention three sciences that include several fields of expertise. After considering the criteria or technopathogenological canons, they would identify whether the technique entails a potential flaw that can eventually generate a technopathogen.
- Its use: Technicians. The technopathogenological training would allow them to reduce the risks as much as possible both in people occupationally involved and in consumers.
- Risk Assessment: doctors, toxicologists, epidemiologists.
- Management tasks: lawyers, law makers, etc.

XX.   Technopathogenology: The results

Following the criterion on the need of a logical concatenation between Phenomenon, Theories, Methodology and Results in order to give support to the idea that a new discipline can be considered as such, we have now to discuss the results.

Technopathogenological results are the knowledge that this new discipline has generated, which has been expressed in the articles we have published. However, since the aim of this science is the prevention of damages on health which do not manifest themselves immediately but after several years or even generations, and that are produced by the exposure to environmental factors generated by Technique, the results that could be expected from this discipline are formulated in questions such as: how many Technopathogenies were prevented? How many Technopathogenies could be prevented?

The first question is, for the time being, impossible to answer. Since the damages on health that Technopathogenology aims to prevent are non-evident and long-term, the results of prevention are very difficult to measure. They will also be observed in the long term. Regarding the risk of cancer, for example, it is said that (US DHHS-PHS-NTP, 1985):

> It is reasonable and sensible to accept that the reduction of exposure to substances – particularly those showing carcinogenicity activity in experimental animals – will also impact on a reduction in the incidence of cancer.

Therefore, applying the same criterion, which we could describe as logical, we can also consider the following technopathogenological example: a person is occupationally exposed to a factor that can cause sterility. Although the person may be never affected, a logical analysis allows us to estimate that developing a technique that avoids the generation of such factor would avoid the person from suffering such condition. We could conclude that *If you avoid the risk, you would avoid the possibility of harm.*

By following this criterion, the prevention of aflatoxins in stored corn was achieved, and in a very simple manner. The criterion was: since aflatoxins are generated by a mold, if the apparition of such mold is actually avoided, the generation of the toxin would be avoided as well (Eguiazu, 1983). This means that by controlling the conditions in which mold is generated through early indicators (that appear way before the toxin itself), the apparition of the toxin is avoided. Therefore, by avoiding the generation of the toxin in foodstuffs, the foodstuff will not be contaminated thus not threaten the consumer with hepatic cancer.

XXI.   Technopathogenology – A summary

Putting together the concepts we have already seen and the concepts we will mention later, we could say that Technopathogenology is the science that:

- Studies the phenomenon of Technopathogeny (which includes Technopathogenesis – a group of successive phases or processes that lead to manifestation of the phenomenon), the detection of the Technopathogens involved in the phenomenon and the measures for its prevention.
- Studies the causes of the genesis and masking – either voluntary or involuntary – of technopathogenies and aims at achieving their prevention.
- Studies Technopathogenesis, which involves a set of processes that, due to their complex nature, cannot be fragmented, since they integrate elements from Natural and Abstract Sciences (especially Ethics).
- Not only studies the existence of technopathogens in Technique, but also their genesis and prevention. Technopathogens are also generated by concrete techniques which were ill created from their very beginning.
- Aims at identifying potential risks to health in apparently safe techniques (which can be called *apparently healthy carriers*).
- Is a consistent tool of technology. A science that aims at solving and preventing a problem that another science has *disregarded*.
- Aims at understanding and interpreting the reality of technology as it is. That is to say, knowing technology in an authentic manner by pointing out aspects undescribed or even deliberately disregarded because being considered not very *nice*, such as the non-evident negative collateralities of such technology.

- Does not pretend to completely cover or to give a complete answer to the technological problem, even less to substitute a discipline or multidiscipline already focused on solving the problem.
- Can be called upon to participate in a multidiscipline environment in order to evaluate, in a comprehensive manner, any problem associated with technology. *To protect future Humans* so that the risks that may come along with the undeniable benefits of technology do not need to be justified as *the price of progress*, aiming instead to achieve *a progress without a price*.
- Is at the forefront of the technopathogenic problem.
- Aims at providing a proposal so that any technological change or advancement is actually safe and not random and that its risks are gradually and progressively reduced. A technological change, whose search and accomplishments undoubtedly beneficial for human beings do not drift apart from the responsibility assigned to humans ever since their creation. A change that does not *spoil* the environment or the fellow living creatures, who are many times not the direct beneficiaries of the work created by the Technical Man.
- Aims at contributing to the establishment of *canons* which Technology should respect, so that the generated change does not lead to adverse effects of late manifestation in human health.
- Covers a transdisciplinary phenomenon which is essentially human (Eguiazu & Motta, 2000) and whose utmost aim is that within the proper conception of technique – within the knowledge used for its development – the potential voids that might cause technopathogenies can be discovered (Motta & Eguiazu, 2005).
- Has as object, in its broadest sense, the unconditional search for knowledge without any limit that would stop it from reaching the uttermost causes of the phenomenon (Eguiazu & Motta, 2000).
- Ontologically lies within Technique – its field of application lies within preventive health.
- Evaluates the creative process and the risks on human health.
- Investigates and proposes criteria to prevent possible technopathogenies when facing a Technique already developed. It also aims at reaching the process of creation of a new Technique.
- Does not curb development since it analyzes objects which do not yet exist. It *tackles* Technique before it becomes a concrete object. It does not tell Technology *I am going to evaluate your*

technique, but rather, *let us build Technique together*. It does not criticize but *accompanies* the technological development.

- Is necessary to bring prophylaxis to provable facts which imply damage on health after the application of new technologies which were thought to be innocuous.
- Considers Technopathogeny as the result of a technological activity, which results in the creation of endless different products. It does not observe each technological object, a pesticide, for example, as an isolated phenomenon. Every technological object can carry the germ and – either individually or along with another technological object or objects – can lead to a Technopathogeny.
- Studies a phenomenon that can be investigated to its very origin and cause.
- Is, in fact, a science of that *which is not correct in Technique*, which allows a gestation with harmful *germs* to human health. Such germs are symbolic and must be understood as causing damage on health.
- Is a science that can bring back the faith in the human scientific and technological work, but with an intrinsic falsification in each technological question that leads us to a kind of falsifiable feedback of its excessive enthusiasm and to focusing more thoroughly on its collateralities.
- Emerges as a consequence of the need of observing a phenomenon transdisciplinarily.
- Allows observing the technopathogenological object in three dimensions – which does not happen by adding up the reductions or projections to each science.
- Is unexpected for an unwanted phenomenon, and that is not a caprice but a necessity.
- Does not study the illness but the possibility that a technological flaw causes an illness, or the technological causes that predispose to it. In other words, it studies the non-evident etiological causes that can engender a morbid state in order to achieve its prevention. It does not study the patient, it studies the Technique.
- It contributes to cover, in Beck's words (Beck, 1970):

> The lack of an adequate sensibility and receptivity regarding the original essence of things and their ontic dignity – both of humans themselves and of the structures of the living entity and nature.

and the need to "renovate humans and society in their receptive and respectful capacity towards the being" (Beck, 1970) in order to avoid serious repercussions.

- It is the science for Technology to reflect upon itself and its own fallibility.
- It is a science that diagnoses and provides basic information to take decisions. The other sciences are to Technopathogenology what Biochemistry, Diagnosis through Imaging, etc., are to Medicine.
- Fills up, as a science, the disciplinary void in the field applied to studies of technological risks, since it focuses on the causes of technological gestation of the phenomenon and not on its consequences.
- Technopathogenology is the underlying scientific discipline inherent to Technology whose aim is to avoid or prevent the creation of techniques with immanent and hidden risks which have negative effects on human health.

XXII. Conclusion

Having supported in Chapter I the existence of a phenomenon still undescribed and, in Chapter II, the disciplinary void for its study, we believe that in this Chapter we have provided the grounds that substantiate the hypothesis of the need of a new discipline we call Technopathogenology and which we have defined as the science that studies the phenomenon of Technopathogeny. We have also provided elements regarding both the proposed methodology and results.

We have seen that technopathogenies are diseases or harms on human health – both physical and psychical – which do not occur immediately after but after many years or generations as a consequence of exposure to non-evident factors generated by Technique (technopathogens) which are present in the human environment and which are caused by immanent and hidden flaws.

The characteristics of this Science are:

- It covers areas of Technique still not taken into account by other disciplines or multidisciplines.
- It provides the proper framework to study the phenomenon.
- It proposes a methodology that allows for prevention.
- It has its own foundations and criteria.

In this Chapter we have briefly presented the criticism to some philosophical conceptions. We have stated that the phenomenon we are studying could be caused by the blind adherence to some of such conceptions.

For example, in connection to Positivism, it is interesting to note an author's concept (Sanguineti, 1977):

> In Comte's work – a document which is still relevant – certain problems which today have become universal and that are closely related to the sense and application of an important fraction of the contemporary scientific development are first discussed.

Paraphrasing this author, we could say that: *Technopathogeny is a phenomenon that today has become universal and that is closely related to the sense and application of an important fraction of the contemporary scientific development, such as the technological knowledge/development.*

We could even state that Technopathogeny is a consequence of Positivism. As for Technopathogenology, we could say that it is the science that emerges as a consequence of the failure of positivist thought, to repair the errors it has committed. Positivist thought may perhaps be justified in purely materialistic objects which can be explained with physical-chemical laws. But it starts tumbling down when it affects a living matter – even if it is a mere cell. It falls apart when the object of study are human beings in their most intimate aspects, the ones that define them.

The enormous investments industries make in order to develop new techniques and the fear of economic loss generated by new criteria applied to productive processes – allows understanding a reasonable attitude of self-protection that denies any possibility of long-term risk in its technological developments. We can illustrate this with the following case: a European professor, advocate or representative of industry, when confronted by a researcher from a developing country who was committed to the need to tackle questions of great significance to protect human health, replied: *Don't pursue this – it can be very dangerous.* Evidently, if the professor recommends *not to go against the system*, there must lay the key to this question. The developing country researcher had interviewed dozens of important European researchers to discuss the risk of technological errors and, surprisingly, they all replied: *don't worry, that is not a problem.* The researcher felt humiliated and insulted in his intelligence.

Even though this attitude is rooted in Industry, we must also bear in mind the problem brought about by Science not letting go old programs or paradigms. Going back to the Chernobyl problem and applying what we have seen in this chapter in connection with nuclear technology, we can say that the old paradigm (Kuhn) or degenerate program (Lakatos) which states: *Nuclear energy is innocuous and useful,* must be substituted by a new paradigm or young program which states *Nuclear energy/risks are higher than nuclear energy/benefits.*

It is very difficult to go back once a Technique is being used and even more if such Technique has just been finished and is ready to start recovering the investments made. The solution must be sought before big investments have been made, by searching for prophylaxis of the conditions that allow for the apparition in a concrete part of the human environment of any particular contaminant. With this awareness, we arrive to the concept of Technopathogeny and to the concept of a specific science. If renowned professors do not want to *meddle*, thus giving very superficial arguments to solve the problem superficially (Frank, 1980-1983), or, better still, get rid of the problem altogether, perhaps it is due to the lack of a science. Surely with this science Industry will be less reluctant when facing committed scientists since it will see that such scientists are not trying to harm the industry but rather aim at *doing a technological good.* For example, when we showed a company our work on Intergranular Relative Humidity, instead of being *scared*, the company sent our articles to its branches saying: *look at this interesting work on grain storage.* Why then, can't this attitude be imitated by other multinational corporations developing technologies?

If those who supposedly know must look away because they do know that investigating the problem goes against the interests of the industry that already develops and obtains revenues with technologies, it is because they are dealing with a problem when it is too late to go back. We must try to solve it much before any big investment has been made, that is to say, in its genesis. This was the origin of Technopathogenology.

The development of other disciplines we used as example, which came out of the necessity to study particular phenomena, support the need to develop new disciplines for new phenomena. This is a precedent that supports the need of creating Technopathogenology.

As every new discipline – even traditional ones – it can be improved, but what we cannot deny is the need for its existence.

As we have said in the Introduction, we do not want to fall in an almost obsessive *methodical doubt*, that is, in thinking that every single technological object will have an undetermined and unknown part that could represent the cause of a Technopathogeny. We would fall into a kind of immobility that would stop any type of technological change. The most correct attitude would be to speak of a *Methodical Rational Skepticism* which we could define as doubting the innocuousness of any technological object already existent or to exist until – through the application of the criteria postulated by Technopathogenology and its tools – the opposite can be proved.

CHAPTER IV

Technopathogenology and its impact on society

'Science in the service of humankind'

In this Chapter we include eight readings we consider of interest because they belong to different areas of Society (Science, Economy, Education, Consumers) where Technopathogenology can contribute to the prevention of Technopathogenies.

This includes:

I. Technopathogenology and the Cultural Clash in the Scientific system
II. Technopathogenology and Protection to Consumers
III. Technopathogenology and its Economic Implication
IV. Technopathogenology and new Quality Criteria
V. Technopathogenology and Education.
VI. Technopathogenology and its Contribution towards a Stricter Regulation in the International Commerce of Hazardous Substances. The Case of Pesticides.
VII. Avoiding War and Technopathogenic Risk as a Global Responsibility – Two Initiatives with one Goal in Common: The Protection of Humans.
VIII. Technopathogenology and the need of an ethical objector in Science and Technique.

The fact that a discipline can include in its internal logic readings and knowledge coming from such diverse fields but with one common element – Technopathogenological risk – further supports the enormous need of the existence of a consolidated science to study such phenomenon. Without such unifying science, all the knowledge would be scattered. It would be a collection of apparently unconnected knowledge.

I. Technopathogenology and the cultural clash in the scientific system

'In good Science ignorance and errors can be expected.
In bad Science, even lies are found'
Alberto Motta

Difficulties of intercultural communication in Science and Technique and its consequences on scientific progress – Technopathogenological consequences

> Creation is a disturbing force in society because it is a constructive one. It upsets the old order in the act of building a new one. This activity is salutary for society. It is, indeed essential for the maintenance of society's health.
>
> Arnold Toynbee

Introduction

In 2003 we were invited to a Congress on cultural differences, specifically focused on how to achieve intercultural communication. The experience obtained in thirty years of work on the development of a new field of knowledge we call Technopathogenology led us to participate in the congress with a paper called Dificultades en el Diálogo Interculural en Ciencia y Técnica y sus Consecuencias en el Avance Científico (Difficulties of Intercultural Communication in Science and Technique and its Consequences on Scientific Progress) (Eguiazu & Motta, 2003).

In order to show how communication difficulties manifest themselves among the members of Science and Technique system and the consequences it entails, first we have to speak of the concept of *culture.* In its broadest sense, what is generally understood by the concept of culture or cultural differences are different races, religions, habits, etc. (Beck, 1979a).

The dictionary definition refers to "People who are more or less cultivated, or who are more or less learned as a result of having engaged in developing human knowledge" (Diccionario Enciclopédico Ilustrado de la Lengua Española).

But there is another concept applied to culture, which is the *value* given to an object whether it is material or immaterial. This is the meaning we will consider in this reading.

We can speak of the human produce as culture in a broader sense and include Technique in culture, which has extraordinary consequences in the concept of Technique and Technology (Beck, 1999a, 1999b) (Eguiazu, 1999b).

As we have seen, we speak of *cultural objects* when we refer to objects humans have built and *culturized objects* when we refer to those objects humans have not built, but nevertheless use (either as such or modified) (Colacilli de Muro, 1978). In both cases such objects constitute goods that humans use in order to satisfy their needs (Motta, 1994), using the concept of goods to things that have value or that have value attributed to it (Colacilli de Muro, 1978). We will base our work on this last criterion.

Which are the values in Science and Technique?

Following the criterion of value, difficulties in communication which lead to make the progress of knowledge more difficult are not necessarily the result of ethnic differences. Such differences, if there is good will, could even favor progress. Neither could cultural differences – following the dictionary definition – necessarily lead to difficulties in the progress of knowledge. However, according to the criterion of value, there can be difficulties in communication which may take place in the workplace itself (Eguiazu & Motta, 2003).

Any object can be assigned different values: Moral, Economic, Religious, Ethic, Spiritual, etc. We can then ask ourselves two questions: Which values can be assigned to the search for knowledge as an object? When the difficulties in communication manifest themselves?

As for the first question, just like other objects, knowledge can also be assigned Moral, Economic, Ethic, Vital, etc. values.

As for the second question, we have to bear in mind that in the Science and Technique system there are two individuals: the researcher – focused on generating knowledge – and the decision-maker or authority, who determines which project or question will be chosen to be researched.

The cultural differences between the researcher and the authority – that is, between the values that a researcher or creator of the project and the decision-maker assign to an object of study – will determine that if the two parties do not communicate properly in order to clarify their differences, the object of study might be left aside and with it every single knowledge it could generate. The difficulties or lack of communication can lead to unexpected situations in which the decision-maker, after taking an adverse measure, might say *I didn't know* in reference to what he or she had already decided (Eguiazu & Motta, 2003). This is because many statements do not focus on the core of the proposal but on secondary arguments and, in some cases, on trivialities and even on personal hostilities or rivalries.

Cultures in Science and Technique

Culture in Science and Technique can be divided in two ways of seeing Science and its progress. One of them is the classical way in which growth is achieved by accumulation of increasing knowledge and by learning methodologies. Here, the rigorous application of a method is more predominant than the substantial innovation. We could define it as values of *pure knowledge, accumulation, erudition and method.* These values, among others, are typical of the culture of the scientific system we will define as Aloentic.

The other culture is based on the researcher's realization of a void, and knowledge is obtained by filling its internal contradictions. In order to achieve this, researchers resort to the tools they have nearby, which in some cases can be formal and, in other cases, informal. The most important aspect of this culture is the commitment of not parting from the path, even if methodical and material difficulties – or even *anomalies* – are encountered which might lead to destabilize the hypothesis or previous theories. Here we can speak of the values of *Intuition* (Doucet, 1978), *Innovation* and *Progress through risky hypotheses*. This is the culture of the scientific system we will define as *Authentic*.

Apart from the differences of values each researcher assigns to his or her object of study, there is also the culture of authorities in which the obvious value of progress in knowledge must be usually shared with the value of the exercise of power and authority. Such values, in an Aloentic system, usually foster formal research and, in some cases, can drift apart completely from reality. This leads to placing the exercise of power and administration over the motivation to generate new knowledge. It is with this culture with which the difficulties in dialogue lead to impediments in the progress of knowledge. Such impediments emerge when the researcher gets into unknown areas which are out of the boundaries expected by authorities, areas which, when discovered, provoke a reaction from authorities. Authorities then, want either to hide them or to participate in their discovery.

The culture of authority might not understand the culture of those who fight passionately to progress in a new field of knowledge, consolidate a new object of study and perhaps generate and develop a new discipline which they see clearer and clearer as time goes by. This creative culture can hardly be subjected to the culture of authority which, when encountering this kind of researcher, reacts with authoritarianism and incomprehension and tries to subject it by making it normalize or compromise.

We bring into focus cultural differences because they manifest themselves in the way evaluation is carried out and in the way knowledge is promoted. In the culture we call *Aloentic*, which could also be called *formal* if more importance is given to the researcher's background and to the way in which the question is put. In extreme cases, the formality of the proposal is more important than the entity of the question. In general, there are no cultural differences between these types of researchers and decision-makers. However, in the culture of more genuine researchers who really commit to their research, more stress is laid on the question itself than in the researcher's background or qualifications. What is required in this case is a complete adherence to the question. However, pursuing the question in a complete manner might sometimes lead to unknown fields and *thorny fields* of knowledge. This does not happen on the safe ship of the obvious. That is why Westerholm considers the concept of "the unconditional search for knowledge" as crucial (Westerholm, 1999). If the word *unconditional* is taken seriously, not many innovations could be framed under the *conditions* that cheer certain evaluators. The difficulties that arise from the existence of these two cultures and the difficulties of communication among them were manifested in our country in a recent document published by an association

(ADUIC) which criticizes the imperfections of the evaluative method and the resulting inequity.

In our case in particular, we know how hard the evaluation in our Science and Technique system is for research topics such as the one described in this book. Here we see that more importance is given to the culture of form and method rather than to the culture of essence and the intuition of new paths taken.

Form and Method are two values used by Authority to discredit projects. These values are usually used to disguise the real motive of the rejection – the value which the researcher does not share with the system. The real interest is to discredit the object of study which is very complex and not much reducible and many times even critical and a source of uneasiness.

Such attitudes are adopted consciously by the authority to avoid dialogue and to not allow bringing to light the essential or nuclear question of a problem. Its real interest is for researchers to change their object of study. The researcher who resists changing his or her object of study out of ethical commitment or out of respect for the transcendence of the question or its intellectual relevance must suffer the consequences. Tangential evaluations are therefore not unusual, with special emphasis on irrelevant form and method issues, leaving aside or ignoring the entity of the actual question. A method which is very much used when a denouncing or irritating question is presented is simply to ignore it. In this manner, the evaluation board severs the essence of the question and evaluates trivialities.

No research work can resist or survive like this, to the hard test of its decreed *lack of existence* in any evaluation. Any possibility of appeal or discussion is forbidden. There is no possible dialogue. This way, a problem that does not exist cannot be discussed. Any formal evaluator can disqualify vital projects ignoring the researcher's question and answering what was not asked. This is done because these projects are expressed with simplicity. The new cannot be framed within the existent and consolidated framework because it is new, and therefore, *it formally does not exist.* Hence, new and original paths are aborted and there is no chance of finishing their gestation. On the other hand, old questions which do not contribute any longer much to the advancement of knowledge always receive the heavy and obvious positive evaluation and the subsequent increases in subsidies, promotions, etc. In this manner, *more of the same* gets funded: poor in innovation but rich in form and methodology. As we will see, the system improves quantitatively but not qualitatively.

This way, disciplines which grow quantitatively but not qualitatively are given support.

How many doctoral theses in biological disciplines – for example, in a plant species – are repeated endlessly, proving the same phenomenon over and over again in new species or subspecies with results which are poor in innovation but obvious, expected and safe? What would have happened if the researcher had formulated a more daring question that went beyond repeating the same but with little variations? What would happen if the daring question lay outside the biological field by including, for example, an ethical question? And if, in addition, this question affected certain interests, could this researcher do a *brilliant* career in the system?

It is highly likely that due to the complexity of the question the researcher will not be able to publish as many papers he or she would if he or she followed the expected path. This is because complex questions are not easily classified and quantified. Intellectual honesty conspires against success. The researcher might suffer a real *disciplinary tyranny* and, if the question is not reduced to a more *authoritarian discipline,* the project might remain without real evaluation. Using the analogy we will also use when we refer to the issue of quality in the fourth reading, we can say that between Scylla (*simplification and disciplinary subjection*) and Charybdis *(unconditional search for knowledge),* the ship of scientific progress might get damaged and sometimes even capsize.

Maybe these two cultures could also be established, with some correlations, in the psychological field – in which we do not want to enter – (Ulmann, 1974), or be classified as Divergent and Convergent Thinking (Guilford, 1977) or as different types of intelligences (Ulmann, 1974). Maybe there could be a correlation between these two cultures and the people who adhere to them. It would also be too simplistic to classify one as not creative and convergent and the other one as creative and divergent since the problem is much more complex. The difficulty inherent to the changes of research programs, paradigms or methods (Feyerabend, 1986) (Kuhn, 1995) (Lakatos, 1982) is also obvious and here the two cultures could also be established. One culture is related to conservation and the other one, to change. We are neither interested in further analyzing this since we only wish to establish the result of our observation and also of the experience of other researchers. This observation led us to establish the existence of two cultures in Science and Technique and the impossibility of dialogue between them.

We could also comment on the unfairness of the evaluative process when one of the cultures tries to impose its criterion on the other. This brings as unwanted consequence discrimination as well as demoralization for the researcher, which we will analyze in the eighth reading.

The values that the Science and Technique system attribute to the way in which the objects of study must be addressed (for example, technological risks) – framing them within a pre-established disciplinary framework – led to difficulties in evaluation because of which we had to face enormous difficulties in our work. Had we accepted such values, we could not have developed and supported this new discipline since we would have had to frame it within Ecology, Environmental Sciences, or any of the disciplines we have already discussed.

It would be tedious to describe each of the reports each of our presentations received, but they all concluded in rejection of our work.

The rigidity of the disciplinary structure – to which every proposal must be framed – implies that certain topics, like our field of study – protection of human health from non-evident technological risks – are excluded.

There may be no interest in promoting or developing certain projects or questions, however, in the case of Technopathogenology, the evaluation difficulties we have observed show that the system did not agree to the development of a new disciplinary field because – among several reasons or *excuses* – we did not find a discipline in which to frame our proposal of study.

Among the most difficult aspects of the Science and Technique system intimately connected to a lack of respect of our work, we can include the attempts of quick and superficial framing without evaluating the actual relevance of the projects. Apart from the manifest arbitrariness, we believe that perhaps the essence of our work was not understood. The confirmation of this hypothesis contributes then, as we have seen in Chapter II, to prove that there is a disciplinary void in the Science and Technique system to frame questions such as the ones asked by Technopathogenology.

We have already referred to some values humans assign to different objects. We have mentioned: religious, economic, moral, etc., and also values applied to Science and Technique: erudition, innovation, intuition, etc. Below we will refer specifically to the latter group.

Cultural values in the scientific system

The different values which are part of different groups or scientific communities allow us to classify them into two categories: *Authentic* and *Aloentic*. Below we list a set of values we believe, thanks to our experience in the system, apply to an Aloentic Scientific system, and their opposites, which apply to an Authentic Scientific system. We will describe them with arguments that, also according to our experience, we have been able to observe. Others, with their own experiences, will surely be able to improve the description of each value incorporating more aspects to each of them or even incorporating other values.

The word *system* refers to the environment in which the researcher develops his or her activity. It is not a general concept; on the contrary, it refers to a specific environment. Therefore, both Aloentic and Authentic systems can be found within a national research or academic organism.

Below we describe such values and, even though they are described separately, it is obvious that some of them, maybe some more than others, will be interrelated.

Table 30:   Values assigned to Aloentic and Authentic scientific systems

Cultural values in the scientific system		
Aloentic		**Authentic**
1	Obviousness	Vs.	Creativity
2	Erudition	Vs.	Intelligence
3	Authoritarianism	Vs.	Freedom
4	Formalism	Vs.	Essence
5	Method	Vs.	Innovation
6	Requirements	Vs.	Education
7	Mediocrity	Vs.	Excellence
8	Quantitative	Vs.	Qualitative
9	The superfluous	Vs.	The necessary
10	Collectivism	Vs.	Individualism
11	Superficiality	Vs.	Entity
12	The written text	Vs.	The person
13	Disciplinary tyranny	Vs.	Disciplinary flexibility
14	The pre-existent	Vs.	The new
15	Growth	Vs.	Development
16	Inductive	Vs.	Falsifiable
17	Structured	Vs.	Non-structured
18	Mercantile utilitarianism	Vs.	Ethical utilitarianism

Cultural values in the scientific system		
Aloentic		**Authentic**
19	Squandering	Vs.	Economizing
20	Grant holder	Vs.	Disciple
21	Director	Vs.	Tutor
22	Harasser – Harassed	Vs.	Demand – Progress
23	The tool	Vs.	The work
24	Credit: Formality	Vs.	Credit: Merit
25	Tidiness	Vs.	Limited untidiness
26	Copy	Vs.	Original Idea
27	Intellectual opportunism	Vs.	Intellectual honesty
28	Inopportune anomaly	Vs.	Innovative anomaly
29	Extortive political manipulation	Vs.	Honest recognition of merit
30	Collective thinking	Vs.	Autonomous thinking
31	Conformist	Vs.	Transgressor
32	Group of opportunists	Vs.	Solidarity group

1. Obviousness vs. creativity

The structure of an Aloentic system, characterized by all the values described, determines that a creative researcher who proposes a new topic or a new idea has enormous difficulties or maybe finds it impossible to develop it. The lack of suitability of the evaluators and the fact that this system lacks an intellectual openness that allows, at least, to give the candidate the opportunity to test his or her new idea, determines that only that which can be contemplated by regulations can be evaluated. Regulations, in the broad sense, not only refer to the administrative way in which a science must work (evaluations, scientists promotions, etc.), but also to establishing which are the accepted scientific disciplines and in which cases a problem deserves to be promoted in the scientific world.

The Aloentic Scientific system is structured, as we have seen, over old and degenerate paradigms, unlike the Authentic Scientific system, where the possibility of conceiving young and new paradigms opens the door to creativity. This openness and freedom are what allow a researcher of an Authentic system to substantiate and create a new academic discipline in the university environment, while in an Aloentic system every proposal will be rejected and merged into the existent. This is due to the fact that every new academic field is created by authority and many times, due to political reasons. This new creation is not the addition of new systematized knowledge which almost inadvertently cries desperately for a new discipline, all this mediated by researchers, but something completely different. The creation of new disciplines in an Aloentic system is done only by directions of the political authority that must make *academic room* for the representatives of their own corporation.

It is interesting to quote A. Toynbee's (Toynbee), Is America neglecting her creative talents?:

> To give a fair chance to potential creativity is a matter of life and death to any society. This is all-important, because the outstanding creative ability of a fairly small percentage of the population is mankind's ultimate capital asset.

2. Erudition vs. intelligence

It was once mentioned that *some replace with erudition what others achieve with intelligence.* This is true. In the Aloentic system, a researcher tries to accumulate a large amount of knowledge which, consciously or unconsciously, hides his or her lack of creativity. For example, a large book can contain many bibliographical quotes but no original ideas from the author – which does not necessarily weaken the documentary or informative value of the book.

This is something that happens by default in an Aloentic system. That is to say, if evaluators are not intelligent people with an intellectual broadness of mind, they will not be able to evaluate intelligence. Erudition, on the other hand, is easier to evaluate. There is a story in which a teacher was testing his student in a Math exam. The student could not remember the expected formulation; however, he could solve the problem using different means. Instead of failing him, the teacher congratulated him. He was an authentic professor. An Aloentic professor would only have tested the student's memory and would have most probably failed him.

3. Authoritarianism vs. freedom

These values make reference to the subject matter chosen by the researcher.

Interestingly enough, Popper considers authoritarianism as the worst of evils of Science and the scientist's attitude. This is why he considers that criticizing or falsifying theories is more enriching than consolidating it with more and more data that confirms it. Therefore, Popper says that every new idea or theory must be submitted to criticism or falsification (Popper, 1973).

If the scientific community is asked about this, everyone will agree and will condemn any kind of authoritarianism throwing up their hands in horror. Now, many authoritarians believe that if their theories are submitted to criticism or if they even partly accept the opposite theories, they may lose authority.

In an Aloentic system there is authoritarianism but, in order to avoid confusions with the Tyranny vs. Openness values we will describe below, control does not necessarily apply to subjects which do not fit within the existent disciplinary field but also to subjects that lie within existent disciplines.

Hence the question, how do authoritarians then manage to avoid Popper's proposal of enriching criticism? The mechanism is very simple. There are two institutions in charge of this: tangential report and anonymous peer review.

A) Tangential verdict

We use the term *verdict* because it refers to a "conclusion expressed, to judgment" (Standard Encyclopedic Dictionary). In this case, the report determines whether a project can be funded or not, whether a researcher should be expelled or not, etc.

During this stage, the researcher takes the new ideas to the evaluation board whether as a report, publication or request of subsidies.

If it is a report to obtain the approval of its scientific activity, the new idea is ignored or disregarded. Therefore, what has been done is always less than the minimum required to be approved.

If it is a manuscript to be published, a thorough statement on superficial formal points is made (extension, style, etc.) ignoring the essence or the leit motiv of the project. The answer is an utter NO that does not even leave room for formal modifications. This way, the publication is excluded, thus avoiding the discussion or criticism – if a work with new ideas is not published, it will never be submitted to a scientific discussion.

The fear of researchers to have their work criticized reveals insecurity in their arguments. On the other hand, researchers who are self-confident about their arguments do not fear being criticized, on the contrary, they ask for it since they have elements to defend their ideas. If evaluators fear the truths expressed in a manuscript that could attack the old paradigm they support, the easiest way to defend themselves is by obstructing the publication of the new ideas.

If it is a request for subsidies, the previous strategy is applied, denying the access to tools so to obstruct the realization of an experiment, a study, the direction of an institute, etc. The system sometimes resorts to subtle moves. In some cases, such moves are rather coarse, like, for example, not telling the researcher that an electronic version had to be attached to the application. The statement is very simple: The electronic version was not included. The request is therefore not considered. The new idea cannot be made known to the general public.

B) Anonymous assessor and anonymous evaluated

This is another institution that conspires against criticism. What the anonymous evaluator or peer review system aims at is to avoid retaliation from spiteful authors. It also aims at avoiding favoritism. This is how an Authentic system should work. But in an Aloentic system, the effect can be completely the opposite. In fact, the anonymous peer review goes against new ideas since they can be formally rejected and without reply. On the other hand, if the referee is not honest and the origin of the manuscript does not remain anonymous, he or she can, knowing the idea comes from an important researcher, copy it or part of it and incorporate it to his or her own work, or even give it to some other researcher. This is what happened with two not very well-known researchers whose work was rejected by an evaluation board but later found, when the work was presented in a congress, that a suspiciously similar work had been presented by another researcher who was friends with one of the members of the evaluation board.

In addition, being the report tangential, the evaluator can deny the fact that such idea ever came across him or her.

Even though we believe that mutual anonymity in an Authentic system would be ideal, we consider that in this system, ruled by ethical principles, mutual anonymity would be unnecessary. This would even allow for the evaluator to call the evaluee to openly discuss the different criteria. In the case of new ideas which are too new or irritating, in an Authentic system the evaluator should be able to call the evaluee and tell him or her: I have to reject your proposal and declare it unacceptable. Please prove why I should not.

The authoritarian nature of an Aloentic system alienates the researcher, who is constantly trying to comply with administrative requirements, to hand out reports in time, i.e. to do everything in order to obtain a favorable statement. In the Authentic system, however, the value of freedom is crucial; it will enable the researcher to focus on the progress of knowledge. We could say that researchers could experience creative joy. They would not live with fear of the phrase *publish or perish.*

Authoritarianism is so strong in Aloentic systems that when researchers are at their prime, instead of having their own opinion, freedom and creativity, they still speak of their director as a *demi-god* with childish fear and still refer to him or her as *my director,* whose point of view is not questioned but blindly accepted. What can be expected of an authoritarian system that, instead of celebrating the researcher's own opinion, innovation and creativity, is almost military? Blind adherence to a director, generally leaving aside the researcher's own opinion, provides order and rules, but is the complete opposite to a healthy scientific production. In an Authentic system, however, where even though every Institute would have a Director, such Director would always be a professional whose prestige would support his or her designation; the Director would never lose the real concept of team work. It would be a person who is willing to share and argue ideas with other researchers while respecting every researcher's intellectual property and freedom. Such person would have authority but will not be authoritarian, conducting the activities of the institute using cooperative work as the main tool to reach its goals.

4. Formalism vs. essence

The Aloentic system values the object of study for its apparent scientific complexity, which is why the topics of basic research are apparently more important. The Aloentic system is based on Formalism: "Scrupulous observance of prescribed forms, as in religious worship, social life, arts, etc." (Standard Encyclopedic Dictionary). In general, discoveries made in other countries are repeated, leaving aside the essential motivation the researcher should have. This can be expressed in the following question: *Have I become a researcher in order to do more of the same, or to answer an essential question, significant enough so as to fill a substantial void of knowledge?*

Answering an essential question is what motivates authentic researchers. The apparent simplicity of the question demands a prior enormous intellectual work to reach to the bottom of a phenomenon that will later be formalized by the experiment. If such intellectual work is not done, if the essence in the object of study is not sought for and researchers copy forms already developed in other countries and repeat them more or less accurately, valuable results are not obtained. It is obvious that the most valuable and essential work is the one that was done first and not the second copy.

As we will see later, Authentic systems have researchers who identify problems and researchers who solve them. It is hard for an Aloentic system to identify complex problems. It simply studies more thoroughly issues already discovered by others or tackles issues supported by variables of little scientific value. This may lead to the extreme of making experiments on almost anything just for the sake of making them, even if they have no relation to anything, just to have a paper published. The concept of *let's try, describe and publish* substitutes the concept of *let's keep moving in this direction even if it gets harder and harder.*

5. Method vs. innovation

In the Aloentic system, the search for knowledge is ruled by Norm, by Methodological Rigor; only this way can the generated knowledge be considered true. Therefore, in this system, the researcher can see anything that drifts apart from the established method as a complex, dark, uncertain or complicated field; the same happens when thinking of topics that represent an innovation.

In the Authentic system the search for knowledge is not conditioned by well-defined preconceptions. The Authentic system is like an annoying and cheeky child pestering with embarrassing questions which are difficult to answer. It is curiosity taken to the extreme; there is openness and Methodological Eclecticism. We consider this to be the only way to innovation. If a norm or *recipe* could be established for innovating or discovering, how easy would it be to make discoveries or inventions! An Aloentic system could go to the extreme of establishing *invention regulations*!

6.   Requirements vs. education

Regarding the researcher's development, the value of requirements structures the person, telling him or her what to do in order to be a researcher. We could say that with time, a person could come to realize that he or she is not truly a researcher, which would be a tragedy. Access to knowledge happens through a pre-established model. A model structured in administrative parameters.

Proper education with the participation of a tutor provides, on the other hand, the opportunity for the person to discover his or her own capacity and potential of research. The person discovers and develops in a harmonious manner his or her own potential or ways of achieving knowledge.

The Authentic system aims to encourage a researcher through Vocation; we could say that *initiative, enthusiasm, dedication and persistence are the four pillars that support vocation.*

7.   Mediocrity vs. excellence

In the Aloentic system, the pressure for administrative requirements and the search for quantity determine the impossibility of the search for excellence in knowledge. The requirements increase as the amount of subsidies increase or the higher the position the researcher has, which leads to the researcher's negative self-correction in order to avoid drifting apart from certain requirements or in order to be *politically correct.* The substantial innovation is sacrificed. The work published is perfect from the formal point of view, but poor in innovative quality.

In the Authentic system, the only pressure is given by new ideas, crucial questions, new inventions, etc. The pressure is given by the essential, never by the formal. All this contributes to the search for excellence.

In the Authentic system it is the wise man who evaluates. In the Aloentic system, however, it is the stubborn man, who is always linked to the decision-making group of power.

8.   Quantitative vs. qualitative

In the Aloentic system what matters is the amount produced: how many works were published, how many congresses, meetings, symposiums, etc. the researcher has attended to. The researcher is more focused on producing than in searching for quality. In the Aloentic system, the more pages a book has the more scientific value it has. The value of an article depends on whether the journal was published abroad or not and on the language it was published. The importance of an Institute depends on its size, personnel and instruments. In the Authentic system, quantity is irrelevant. Content is more important than volume.

Then there is the value of prizes and distinctions. In an Aloentic system, prize giving is circular. That is to say, a committee of evaluators awards a prize to a person of a group and then, that same person can be a member of the evaluation committee thus awarding the prize to a person of the first group who had already been nominated. Therefore, a researcher can have prizes given by the corporation but may be less creative than an authentic novel researcher.

9. The superfluous vs. the necessary

These values are linked to the ones described in the previous point and can be applied to the question the researcher is trying to answer, or to the questions or aims the system is trying to evaluate or encourage. Among the elements that will be considered by both the Authentic and Aloentic systems we find: the question itself, the number of variables and repetitions or trials expected for its answer, accuracy in measurements, means required, personnel required, arguments or antecedents presented for it, way of presenting it, way of publication, etc.

An Authentic system aims at the quality of knowledge; among the aspects above mentioned, it will only take into account those which are necessary in the investigation process.

For example, and in connection with the means required, in an Authentic system a simple and economic measuring device to calculate relative humidity can be more useful to investigate how to prevent the apparition of potentially carcinogenic mycotoxins than a very expensive device to measure how such mycotoxins are metabolized by a rat's liver. An Aloentic system would consider a greater scientific value to answer this second question.

An Aloentic system values more a researcher who can publish in a renowned international journal than the ideas a researcher can develop to find the solution of, for example, problems in his or her own region. International stands for prestige whilst *local* sounds, perhaps, not as important. Therefore, a formal article – even if it is basic science dealing with an irrelevant issue – is more important because it is published through politically correct means, especially if it is in an international journal. This is more valuable than a crucial question of high regional value, both human and social, published out of the main stream.

We have published works in popular publications to connect to technicians who surely do not have access to *prestigious journals* about technopathogenic risks associated with their activities in order to protect users and consumers of the techniques. One of the evaluators in our evaluative system said that *those articles are of no value because the publication is not prestigious*. This means that the prestige of the publication is more important than the content of the work. Many works of high social, regional, etc. relevance are rejected because they cannot be framed within the *prestigious* publication's aim and not because they do not contribute substantially to knowledge.

In an Aloentic system, more importance is given to the apparent complexity of an article than the problems it can actually solve, or its applicability. There was a case in which a researcher, when considering two articles dealing with damaged stored grain – one referring to the damage caused by poor storage and the need to take measures of prevention and therefore of great practical value, the other referring to the damage caused in an enzyme due to poor storage – gave more scientific relevance to the latter saying that *that was indeed scientific work* simply because it spoke of enzymes, a subject which, in addition, was of his competence. We believe this is also a case of Erudition vs. Intelligence. This also leads us to the problem of the evaluator who speaks only of the part he or she understands or of the apparent scientific complexity. Other projects which can, in spite of this, have real entity, are disregarded.

10. Collectivism vs. individualism

We have once heard that the biggest productivity in a workplace has been always generated by a small percentage of people. Maybe it is due to this concept that in an Aloentic system *integration* is sought for, so that there are not only people providing new ideas, but also so that what is produced by the few enthusiasts or capable people looks as it was produced by the whole group.

By referring to Individualism we mean "personal independence in action, thought, etc." (Standard Encyclopedic Dictionary) we do not mean to say that the researcher must be selfish or "self-interest egoistic" (Standard Encyclopedic Dictionary). In the Aloentic system it is common that a large number of researchers group to work in a project. If the project has an original idea, a single person's idea, it is diluted among the many authors signing the work. This is very common and it usually aims at *fattening* the researchers' Curriculum Vitae. This is rather obvious: If ten researchers develop one project each, each of them will have one publication in their CVs, but if ten researchers share ten projects, they will have ten publications in their CVs. Interestingly enough, the Intellectual Property Law in Argentina (Law 11723) defines collaborative work (Ley 11.723) as follows: "The mere plurality of authors is not considered collaboration, unless the property cannot be divided without altering the nature of the work."

We can see that the conditions for considering the participation of two or more authors a work in collaboration are very clear.

Now, in the Aloentic system a number of situations can arise. One of them could be the authors agreeing mutual co-authorship of their works – even though neither do any actual contributions. Today you co-author my work, tomorrow I'll co-author yours. This is not scientifically ethical, but at least it is a mutual agreement. The worst cases are when a young researcher is the author and the Director includes himself or herself as co-author without having contributed at all, that is, just because he or she is a Director. The Director might also feel he or she has the right to include himself or herself simply because he or she has corrected the work or suggested bibliography. Another serious situation is when the Director includes, without having participated, a *friend* of his or her along with the young researcher so that the publication can be included in the friend's CV.

In an Authentic system co-authorship is not devalued. In fact, there are many works in which many researchers participate, but the ethical principle of intellectual property is respected. There must therefore be a real contribution from each researcher in the final quality of the published work, a contribution that, if non-existent, *would alter the nature of the work.*

As for collectivism, there is an aspect that can also be connected to what we will describe on point 19 about Economy. Such aspect can present two forms:

A. We have described the situation of including in publications people with very little or no merit at all. One of the reasons is, as we have already said, fattening the Curriculum Vitae. But another reason is to increase the list of publications of the team, which is many times required for the Institute to receive subsidies as we will see in the eighth reading. The same happens when in statistics, countries use family income instead of per capita income to hide inequities between rich and poor people. A rich family may have the same income as a poor family, but in the rich family only one member of the family works (for example, as a business executive), and in the poor family all the members work for very long hours and contribute with their meager salaries to the total family income. The difference surfaces when analyzing what each member earns. In the case of the rich family, one member can earn as much as the sum of all the salaries of the poor family. Similarly, in order to strengthen Aloentic research teams, instead of considering the number of publications per capita, the group is considered as a whole. As we have seen, this only works if all the members agree, but if it is a group in which the *core engine* is powered by a researcher who supports the whole group, the situation is rather different. If the number of works were considered individually, the fact that this researcher had done most of the work would come to light. Just like the two families, there can be two groups with the same amount of publications but it is not the same if the whole group participated in the whole production or if it was the produce of a single researcher. If such situation came to light, the subsidies would be destined to the researcher who powered the project and not to the whole team. In an Aloentic system, this situation is hidden by the team director for fear the funds might be assigned to a group with a more balanced production. An authentic researcher would see that, not only others are improving their backgrounds thanks to his or her work, but also that the subsidies received thanks to his or her merits are diluted in a team that is wasting them. We are not referring to a selfish attitude but to the need of respecting the author's intellectual property and to a more productive use of the funds.

B. Another way is to include in the list of published works by the team or institution articles published by authors persecuted by the very same institution. Having several publications, the institution will ensure that it will be granted a subsidy or insertion within a program. However, the authors of the publications are ignored when it comes to distributing the subsidies received.

11. Superficiality vs. entity

As we have seen in point 7 (Mediocrity vs. Excellence), production in an Aloentic system is superficial. The works published, congresses attended to, meetings organized, etc., generally only aim at complying with administrative requirements. There is no real interest in a thorough analysis of the real motive for a publication or a meeting.

We can quote a phrase from a researcher: We have to prepare a paper to present in the congress. This phrase came from the researcher when she found out that the congress was being held in a beautiful tourist place. The most important reason to attend the congress was to include one more item in the CV and, in addition, do some *scientific tourism*.

12. The written text vs. the person

In the Aloentic system, given the characteristics or idiosyncrasy of the evaluative system, the researcher is only a file number; the Authority generally does not know the researcher's background. For example, the work of a researcher with over twenty years of experience can be rejected by an Evaluator who will only base his or her decision on the actual writing presented by the researcher – a researcher whose background is, many times, not known by the evaluator. This can be tragic for the researcher since his or her permanence on the system might be conditioned by the Evaluator's conclusion on the report. This is why (as described in point 3 – Authoritarianism vs. Freedom) every time the researcher submits a report, he or she is fearful and worried, feeling under a lot of pressure. Given the restrictions of space imposed for the writings, it is more vital for the researcher to know how to adhere to form rather than describe the new discoveries. In order to remain in the system, it is more important to know how to inform than what to inform.

If the researcher does not have the adequate writing skills or the adequate skills to write politically correct reports, he or she can see his or her permanence on the system seriously jeopardized. We can also add that the written text paper seizes of the reality.

Writing reports is another administrative aspect of the researcher's activity. In an Aloentic system, these reports or periodic *writings* are the *sword of Damocles* hanging over the researcher's head over his or her entire active life, constantly threatening his or her permanence in the system. That is the reason why the researcher must be obsessively careful in the correct presentation of these writings. In an Authentic system, however, since what is valuable is the person, these reports – which will enable the system to recognize the value of the researcher – are only taken into account at the beginning of his or her career. After a strict evaluation at the beginning (a strict selection of the person based on his or her vocation and talent, as well as on some kind of concentration and commitment to the question he or she is trying to answer), the written text becomes increasingly flexible, only maintaining the requirement that the publication must be innovative. In an Aloentic system, the written text is a tyrant; it is always as if the researcher is writing for the first time. It can be as absurd as making a researcher who has published in many prestigious journals to type out or write all his or her published articles in a formal text in order to comply with the requisite that a report must be voluminous. This attitude is a form of moral harassment, as we will see in point 22, since it ends up deteriorating the neurological and psychiatric aptitudes of the researcher. This is not even a form of harassment to test the researcher in his or her beginnings which will not be repeated later, once the researcher has shown the capacities required. On the contrary, this is continuously repeated until the researcher's retirement.

13. Disciplinary tyranny vs. disciplinary flexibility

Associated to the values of Authoritarianism vs. Freedom by which, as we have seen, the system permits or limits the subject of study (which can or cannot be framed in an existent disciplinary system), these values only make reference to the disciplinary system.

In the Aloentic system, the disciplinary tyranny makes the researcher adjust to the existent. The researcher must frame his or her study within existing disciplines if he or she wants to be a researcher. The disciplinary openness in the Authentic system, however, would even let the researcher develop a transdiscipline if necessary, to frame his or her studies.

This is how, for example, researchers with a background in Chemistry will have enormous difficulties if they have focused their studies on Toxicology or Technology, for example. Their reports will be systematically evaluated by Chemists who, not being experts in Toxicology or Technology, will systematically declare the reports unacceptable. The problem with the corporate nature of the system is that if, for example, a researcher asks for his or her reports to be evaluated by a Health Commission (if it deals with toxicology) or by a Technology Commission (if it deals with technology) even though his or her requests are granted, such commissions will invariably redirect the report to the Chemistry Commission. This leads to an *eternal return* to the same evaluators and, therefore, to the same statements.

In an Authentic system, the lack of comprehension of a new field of study is something that the system itself does not permit. An idea cannot be rejected if its advocate is an honest researcher who is passionate about it. In many similar situations, this led to great discoveries. However, the disciplinary tyranny that characterizes an Aloentic system does not comprehend certain research topics which are therefore rejected thus leaving potential important achievements aborted.

14. The pre-existent vs. the new

In the Aloentic system, a researcher's view is only considered valuable if it has been proved or supported by another researcher of higher rank, especially if such researcher is a foreigner. It disregards any view that does not comply with the above described, no matter how valuable the view is, or the fact that it has been proved by the researcher.

The Authentic system, however, allows for new hypotheses and theories which the researcher can prove or falsify. This can lead to open new fields of knowledge.

15. Growth vs. development

These values are very similar to the ones described in point 8 (Quantitative vs. Qualitative). In the Aloentic system, scientific growth is based on quantity. Scientific growth is measured in terms of the published works or the length of the CV. Likewise, the growth of an Institute is measured in terms of the number of researchers it has incorporated, the amount of instruments it has added, the expansion of the building, etc.

However, the Authentic system aims at development. That is to say, the more and more original progresses a researcher achieves in his or her field of study, the bigger his or her development is. Ortega y Gasset, in reference to universities, said that in underdeveloped systems, it is more important for a university to plan the building, construct it and then do whatever they can do with it. However, in developed countries the most important thing for a university or institute is the people; they can always start *in a little room.*

This thinker considers that the humbleness of the resources is no impediment to make great intellectual achievement. The only requirement is to choose and promote the right people.

16. *Inductive vs. falsifiable*

The Aloentic system is based on Inductivism, that is to say, the results of an experiment are corroborated by more experiments and new theories are built with difficulty and fear by apposition of data. Such theories end up being extremely inertial. Criticism is almost never accepted. Here Einstein's phrase would apply: the advocates of a theory are so much against changing it that they die with the theory rather than accepting its change. Researchers are usually against modifying their theories. There is then a mechanism to repair theories in which each mistake or incoherence with the expected results can be explained with a subtheory that supports it.

The only requirement the Authentic system has is that each theory can be falsified. That is to say, that it can be destroyed through experimental work or intellectual criticism, leaving the possibility for anyone who desires it to destroy it. In the Authentic system, every theory is a work hypothesis, fallible and capable of receiving criticism.

17. *Structured vs. non-structured*

These values can summarize the characteristics of both systems divided into the different values already seen. It is believed that production is more efficient with the application of a structure criterion. In connection to this we could say that we have heard a researcher say that in his Institute the researchers *synchronize their watches with the Director's.* We can go back to what we have mentioned in point 3 (Authoritarianism vs. Freedom), where researchers, even those who are at the prime of their careers refer to their director as if he or she were a *demi-god*, refer to him or her as my director whose criteria are not argued but blindly accepted.

We then ask ourselves: Can a researcher know when he or she will have a question? When the new idea will emerge? Can a researcher say: I am a researcher from 8 to 12 am and from 4 to 8 pm? Can the brain of a researcher behave as a shop that opens and closes to customers at specified times? The answer could appear to be obvious; our experience has proved it to be emphatically negative.

In an Aloentic system, in some cases so much detail is required to obtain a subsidy – where the tools will be employed, how the subsidy will be used and the results expected – that there is no actual room for creative uncertainty. This is why one can wonder whether the subsidy required will be used to obtain new knowledge or to justify these expected, known results following a road which has already been taken.

In the Authentic system, the lack of structure gives the researcher freedom. The researcher will be free to think of his or her idea and develop it, to choose the right moment to write a book, etc. Nevertheless, this system imposes certain conditions. Researchers must have ideas, must write a book and develop a significant experiment, that is to say, they must generate quality knowledge. We consider that any authentic researcher whose vocation is supported by the four principles quoted in item 6 imposes upon him or herself certain exigencies. Sometimes even on the verge of paroxysm, being careless with his or her own health.

Regarding the administrative aspect in connection to the request of subsidies, in an Authentic system the researcher will of course expect results – results coherent with the hypotheses obtained by intuition. But, as we have said, creative uncertainty is valued. Every unexpected new result is not rejected – which is the contrary to what happens with Aloentic researchers, who fear being criticized or the interruption of their projects.

18. Mercantile utilitarianism vs. ethical utilitarianism

The Aloentic system is based on Mercantile Utilitarianism. We include the adjective *mercantile* to make reference to the motive of profit and to differentiate it with the concept of Utilitarianism, which refers to (Standard Encyclopedic Dictionary):

> (a) The doctrine that actions derive their moral quality from their usefulness as mean to some end, as happiness. (b) The ethical theory, held by Jeremy Bentham and John Stuart Mill, that the greatest human happiness determines the highest moral good.

According to this last criterion, every research must aim at achieving useful knowledge.

We can exemplify a paradigmatic example of Mercantile Utilitarianism with the research developed by some companies. This is the case of the research of new substances used in human medicine, agriculture, chemical industry, new foodstuffs or raw materials, etc. Because of the economic pressure of the investment applied to the search for profit and in order to avoid economic loss, the companies determine which ethical values should be left aside – in some cases, even risking human health. For some other companies, the pressure of this Utilitarianism leads to leaving aside ethical principles.

This mercantile utilitarianism implies that certain organizations focus on the freedom of the creator and manufacturer of risky technologies, chemical substances, etc. to send the technologies anywhere in the world where they can be used freely, until the country that receives them shows that such technology implies a damage on health.

We believe that the Authentic system, however, aims at an Ethical Utilitarianism, that is, the search for utility but distinguishing good from evil. In this kind of system, it may happen that the situations described above are avoided; countries with little scientific production, unable perhaps to show the negative side effects of a technology, banned it simply because it had been banned in developed countries (as we will see later in this chapter).

Mercantile utilitarianism will also be present in official organisms of Aloentic systems: researchers aiming at obtaining subsidies or increasing their income seek for *lucrative ideas.* Also, agreements with companies are signed, or projects that can be useful for such companies are developed. This leads to leaving aside ethical aspects thus leaving room for the attitudes we have mentioned when we referred to Ethical Criteria in the attitude in Science and Technique.

Even so, there is something even worse than mercantile utilitarianism, which is wasting, as we will see in point 19.

In other cases, with the justification of *providing knowledge,* certain topics that have very little or no usefulness at all are researched.

In an Authentic system, on the other hand, Ethics is the leading principle: ethical respect must always be present. In Technology, and because of the consequences it can entail for humans, it is a *sine qua non* condition.

19. Squandering vs. economizing

Why are we saying this? It is rather obvious. Based on the values described, in an Aloentic system the scientist would be more concerned about publishing than about creating. Scientists' survival in the field will depend on their papers, which is why they spend large amounts of money on reagents, equipment, etc. We have heard a researcher say: *whatever we research, it will always be a contribution to knowledge.* The question is not important; what's important is to publish something, even if the study does not prove anything at all. Having an ethical criterion, this cannot happen – especially in developing systems where funds tend to be scarce and handled by closed corporate groups. The criterion of researching just for the sake of it will perhaps leave without funds those who, even though they might have a good question that has been thoroughly developed, did not manage to enter the closed corporate group. The waste of having granted funds to questions that, though frivolous, have been posed by people within the corporate circle who comply with the formalities required is justified by saying that it did contribute to the advancement of knowledge all the same. Such researchers even disguise or justify their question by saying that it contributes to the advancement of knowledge when in fact, in many cases, they are just trying to remain in the system, which they could not do had their questions been required to have a previous entity – which is what an Authentic system requires. That is to say, in these cases they are simply trying to cover their incapacity to research in depth questions.

Another attitude – which could be called misappropriation of funds rather than wasting – is the use of official funds for projects whose results will benefit certain companies, like, for example, those companies which want to give scientific form to the sale of their chemical products.

In the Aloentic system, waste can many times be caused by pointless discussions among powerful researchers who fight for unethical reasons, such as a space of power.

In the Authentic system the scientist will only carry out an experience after having supported its need and after a thorough analysis on whether it is worth developing or not. We could also add that researching *what is that is really worth investigating* may have more entity than research itself. As we have said, if Aloentic system researchers asked themselves this question to focus their work, it would be hard for them to remain in the system, since they would not know what is worth investigating.

We could say that there are two types of researchers: a) researchers who *retain and manage* and b) researchers who *invent and discover*. The former are typical of an Aloentic system and the latter, typical of an Authentic system. The former are interested in receiving more and more funds to manage and grant – thus growing their power within the system. The latter are often seen as *mad scientists*, focused on their question, forgetting about themselves and the world around them.

It is also interesting to bear in mind that in the Aloentic system the official funds for research are intrinsically wasted; because of the heavy and bureaucratic ways through which they are granted, they are never granted to those who have the ideas or enthusiasm to carry them out. The funds are granted to the Director who acts as administrator and guarantor. The waste lies in the fact that many times these funds arrive when they are no longer required and many other times, the Directors or Guarantors use them to cover other needs. Even in the cases in which the funds apply to projects that can be framed within consolidated disciplines, this system has the disadvantage of excluding young scientists with new ideas that might have been taken into account within an Authentic system framework. In this system, even ideas that seem *crazy* and that of course could by no means be considered in an Aloentic system could at least deserve a minimum initial support so that the one who brings the idea has an opportunity to prove its value.

Having referred to the possibility of wasting subsidies, we can say that the concept of efficiency is completely applicable to the use of resources or subsidies for the generation of knowledge. This is true, obviously, if by efficiency we understand: "The relationship between the work done, the time invested, the investment done in carrying something out and the result achieved" (Diccionario El Pequeño Larousse Ilustrado). In this case, efficiency would be given by the quotient between production and the money invested. In Production, the following can be included: basic discoveries, technological developments, patents or inventions, works published, congresses organized, number of courses and conferences given, etc. All these aspects are common to both Aloentic and Authentic systems. The difference is given by what we mentioned in point 8: An Aloentic system is only interested in quantity, whilst for an Authentic researcher, quality is essential. Therefore, we could add as production in an Authentic system, answering recurrently and cyclically a question and making in depth discoveries, among other things.

Then the calculation of efficiency would be:

$$\frac{\text{Production}}{\text{Expenses}}$$

The efficiency will increase by increasing the production at a constant expense or reducing the expense at a constant production.

The critical point is not the expense but the real definition and evaluation of production. How can production be assigned a number?

Generally, in an Aloentic system expenses are not a problem, which is why a large quantitative production is required. In this system, this might not be a problem, but because of what we have mentioned in point 8, what can be dubious is the quality and even the veracity of what is produced. In some Aloentic systems expenses are so large that if they had been used in an Authentic system they would have produced a Nobel prize. Being the aim quantity, assigning a number to production is not difficult: It is easy to talk about two congresses, ten published articles, attending four courses, etc., to quantify production.

In an Aloentic system we can find two situations. In one of them, inefficiency is produced by a small production; in the other one, even though the production is high, the quality is low. Therefore, if we measure efficiency in terms of amount produced, we would say that it is high, but if we measure efficiency in terms of quality, we would say that the quotient is very low.

That is to say, in an hypothetical example, if in an Aloentic system a researcher produces 100 articles with US$ 10,000 and in an Authentic system the researcher produces one article with US$ 100, the quantitative efficiency would be the same but the quality of the single article that the authentic researcher wrote, who studied thoroughly what was worth researching before spending the money, could be of a much better quality than the Aloentic researcher articles.

Another frequent case in Authentic systems is that researchers sometimes produce articles without official expenditures since they may receive funds from donations. In this case, the efficiency in official expenditure would be enormous since the denominator would be zero.

An almost funny case is when in the Aloentic system the researcher spends large amounts of money but the production is nil, in conclusion, efficiency is zero. When the number is zero, the quotient is always zero. The tragedy is when the denominator is dramatically high since large amounts would have been spent in producing nothing.

Aloentic researchers are almost paranoid when, after having spent large amounts of money see that their efficiency equals zero because there is no production and they find they cannot justify their expenses. Then, they can start adopting a desperate and harassing attitude against lower members to try to obtain some kind of production. To justify the lack of results, they can even destroy experiments and accuse of that to third parties.

Another example of inefficiency is connected to point 6 (Requirements vs. Education). We have mentioned that an Aloentic system does not let researchers discover their own qualities and that some can discover too late that they are not qualified for such activity. As we have said, this is tragic for the person, but also an economic waste since the funds that the system invested in the researcher's education were completely unproductive. Just like an Aloentic system justifies any research topic, because everything contributes to the advancement of knowledge, in this case it can also justify this attitude, saying that it is necessary because *it is the only way of detecting true vocation*. This is tolerated by the highest authorities in the system who care very little about detecting and promoting true vocation, their only concern being to remain high on the pyramid supported by a large number of grant holders and researchers who, even though they come and go, constitute the labor force of their work. Being it an Aloentic system there is no Tutor, and the Director does not worry about the people under his or her direction. The Director is much more interested in his or her plans than in taking care of each of his or her subordinates so that they develop harmoniously. If after ten years of being a grant holder, the Director does not renew the grant, it will be the holder's problem. The Director will not worry about it. In addition, the Director will always have ways to justify this decision. Even if *lack of suitability* to be a researcher is a reasonable justification, the grant holder should have been told so after a year and not after ten years of research.

In an Aloentic system one can hear some say that: If in order to sustain a project or program I need to ask for ten grant holders, I will ask for them – they are paid by the State anyway. It does not matter whether they remain on the program or not (i.e. if they are any good or if they have a true vocation or not).

Moreover, a Director will not be interested in leaving disciples to continue his or her work – for he or she will most probably not have an original work or relevant subject of study. In an Aloentic system, a researcher is generally interested in making a living out of Science, not in dedicating his or her life to it. You can hear people saying: When I retire I will only work on my hobby. For this researcher the investigation was only a day job.

Inefficiency is obvious. We could illustrate this example with another equation:

$$\frac{\text{Number of resulting researchers}}{\text{Number of new grant holders}}$$

In an Aloentic system the result is very small. If, hypothetically, in a ten year span, out of ten grant holders only one becomes a researcher, the result would be 0,1. If after ten years none of the grant holders becomes a researcher, then the result is zero, that is to say, inefficiency is complete. In the Authentic system, since the disciples generally remain in the system, the result is a bigger number. The ideal result would be 1 (one). We could even say that the result could be even bigger than 1 – there can be researchers who decide to tackle the researcher's subject after reading his or her articles that were not necessarily formal disciples.

Another consequence of Waste in an Aloentic system is that it makes many authentic researchers that are disregarded by the system to act as Science's *cartoneros*. The term *cartoneros*, (or cardboard collectors) is used in Argentina to refer to people who pick up recycling material from the street (bottles, cans, plastic, paper, etc.) which they then sell to make a living. Similarly, some researchers act as *cartoneros*: having been denied financial aid by the State, they must resort to various institutions and companies to ask for the donation of material (usually discarded) they can use for their research. Such donations are more closely connected to charity than to scientific subsidies. These elements, after being repaired, enable researchers to work on their projects. Some examples are: office furniture, computers, obsolete lab equipment, etc. In spite of the simplicity of such recycled equipment, if the scientific question is adequately put and if it is a relevant question, the answer can be found with the help of it. In order to find answers to initial hypotheses complex equipment is usually not important. Paradoxically, many discoveries made by *Science's cartoneros* who were denied a minimum financial aid from the system were later used by the powerful members of the scientific corporation; they did have the means to carry out further research on the discoveries made by the humble researcher with more vision and ideas than means. This is very similar to the diver's example we presented above.

Wasting vs. saving and the Grameen system

It is easy to observe the differences found in society and the different classes that can be found within one single society. To illustrate our analysis, we consider a society in which two well distinct extremes can be differentiated. On the one hand, we have the very rich, who do not know what to do with their money and spend it lavishly. On the other hand we have the very poor; actually living below the poverty line, surviving with very little money but making the most of it. These differences are also found in scientific research and academic life.

Aiming at both equality of opportunities and economy for the system, we propose a system similar to that created by Dr. Muhammad Yunus for small enterprising projects. Dr. Yunus created the Grameen system (Yunus, 1999) of small loans that are granted to the person requesting it without the need of third parties or guarantors. If this system was applied in Science, it would allow saving a large amount of money thus avoiding, like in the Grameen system, the over wasting of funds, and most importantly, that good ideas are not frustrated or aborted by the system.

Even though we did not know the Grameen system, our work, which is now materialized in this book, could be carried out thanks to the support of the Rosario Stock Exchange, especially in the beginnings and, paradoxically, towards the last stages of our Program – two stages in which we were denied formal scientific subsidies.

In order to analyze our proposal, let us observe two crucial issues: *research funds do not get to the people who have the ideas and vocation to develop them,* and *there are ideas which can be valuable but cannot be framed within an existing framework and can therefore end up being aborted.*

We believe that in an Authentic system the Grameen system could be applied, especially for the second issue.

We even ask ourselves – even assert – whether scientific research could not work like the Grameen system.

Dr. Yunus describes this loan to the poor as follows:

> The problem with loans is that banks require so many guarantees that those who have such guarantees are not precisely the poor, who are the ones who actually need the loans.
>
> The ones who do have guarantees, the rich, keep the money and use it badly because they lack both the enthusiasm and the sense of economizing the poor have.

Similarly, the promotion of science, especially in developing countries, is based on the same principle as commercial loans: *The more you have, the more they lend you.* This is really so. When asking for certain subsidies, we have been told by official research organisms: *It cannot be granted due to the lack of infrastructure in the Institute.* This creates a kind of *vicious circle of denial.* That is to say, because one does not have the means, one does not receive financial aid and because one does not receive financial aid, one cannot have access to the means to do research projects. The scientist's activity is thus completely nullified. The Aloentic system proposes an alternative – completely unethical, of course. If somebody who does not have money asks for a loan, he or she must do it *through someone powerful, who applies for it for him or herself and then sponsors the poor one.* If the *powerful* wants to take advantage of this situation, he or she can ask the poor to *associate* with him or her and receive credit for part of the work done. In short: they ask to pay back with co-authorship. It would be as if a person asked for a credit at a bank but the bank grants the credit provided the person associates the bank's manager to develop his or her business. Another alternative – bordering corruption – is that the scientific system can grant the researcher's request but, in exchange, asks the recipient to sign a receipt for a larger amount of money.

These situations are in some cases very oppressive. The ones who suffer most from this are honest and sincere researchers. In an Aloentic system, the upstarts that simply want a grant or some funds do not generally suffer. They accept the figure of the Director and if they suggest an idea maybe it is not such an important one, so they do not really mind *sharing* it. Anyway, if they get to be directors, they will apply the same law to their disciples and will recover what they have lost at the beginning.

Which would be an authentic solution to get out of this situation? The Grameen loan.

What is the characteristic of the Grameen loan?

That it loans a minimum sum without requesting for guarantee. It has been proved that there is an outstanding rate of return in this system.

What would be the characteristic of a Grameen loan in research?

A minimum sum would be lent to a young researcher with an idea. After some time, the results would be asked. This is how the Rosario Stock Exchange loan worked for us when we were beginning. It worked as the Grameen Bank, without us knowing so. And it did not even ask for results.

We managed to demonstrate the presence of aflatoxins with a loan that this institution granted us without even asking how we had spent the money. But they did see the results and the publications. Paradoxically, the *Bank*, that is, the Science and Technique system, granted large sums to research programs which had originated from our proposal, and that covered aspects which were important for the researchers, not for the common people. We were not even credited. That would have been only possible had we accepted the figure of Director/Guarantor. What is extraordinary is that the Director must not necessarily know much of the subject he or she is to direct.

In an Authentic system, our case would be like the poor Dr. Yunus refers to, forsaken by the system and not getting the minimum they need to survive. Or is it that young, enthusiastic researchers with new ideas are not one of Dr. Yunus' *poor*? Or is it that if such young researchers are granted a research loan (i.e. a subsidy), they would not produce a return in the investment expressed in production of 100/1 based solely on their enthusiasm? Why we not eliminate the oppressive figures of the *Director* or *Guarantor* and see what happens? We are not speaking of eliminating the Tutor who, as we will see in the following point, is a person who endorses the qualities of the young researcher but does not obtain co-authorship or funds in exchange. The irritating relationship in which a powerful Director must share co-authorship in order to grant subsidies must be eliminated.

Let us not forget that the young researcher with ideas can only count on his or her ideas. Like the man in the Bible who "had nothing, save one little ewe lamb" (Samuel), the example that prophet Nathan used as a parable to make King David note his lack of ethics. It is interesting to see that David's furious response in a situation in which a person takes from another person the only sheep that he had is the normal response anyone would have if taking ideas from a young person. It is terribly unfair that a poor researcher who has spent long hours researching *what is worth researching* when he or she finds it, is obliged by the system to hand it in to a *Director* who is very busy and is not very much concerned about the young person's problem or his or her previous sacrifice. In addition, even though the *Director* has already got many sheep, he or she wants to keep the young man's sheep as well. The Aloentic system is greedy and is managed by greedy people who want not just the money but also the credit and undeserved honors. This is how authorships are stolen and fake directions are established. The poor man who owns the one and only sheep must give it away in exchange for a piece of stale bread.

This is what happens with research in many parts of the world.

The Grameen system applied to young researchers would eliminate this irritating injustice. The tutor will receive the young researcher's thank you for having helped him, but not money or co-authorship.

20. Grant holder vs. disciple

21. Director vs. tutor

In the Aloentic system, the young researcher is the Grant holder and the person in charge of his or her work is the Director. That is to say, they are both administrative and not scientific figures, which is why the Director's position does not necessarily guarantee suitability or aptitude to detect, support, promote and respect creativity. The post of Grant holder does not guarantee a vocation for research work. The entrance of the Grant holder to the system is not conditioned by scientific aptitudes but by formal administrative reasons, given basically by certain characteristics such as good grades at university. Grant holders can remain in the system as researchers provided they comply satisfactorily with administrative requirements already mentioned in some of the values above described: Erudition, Form, Method, Mercantile Utilitarianism, etc. In the case of some grant holders with no vocation, the activity generally continues until the person gets a better post outside the system, for example, in the private sector. That is, they use the scientific system as unemployment insurance. If they do not have the possibility of a change, they continue in the system, sometimes unhappy about it, which is what many times leads them to realize that they have no vocation or aptitude for what they are doing and, in addition, because of the demands of the system, become harassers, as we will see in the following section. Other grant holders are led by the Aloentic system itself to the drama of understanding that they are working in an environment for which they have no aptitude or vocation. The Aloentic system makes them believe that because they are university graduates they can also be researchers. This is what we heard from a university graduate in microbiology: *every university graduate can be a researcher.*

If the student has aptitudes typical of an Authentic system and wants to work in an Aloentic system, at first his or her enthusiasm might blind him or her and not let him or her see how negative the system is. Soon the student will see that he or she is expected to *share* his or her ideas with the person who directs his or her work and, eventually, will realize that the researcher is actually carrying the Director on his or her shoulders and, intellectually, that he or she is being part of an aged program (Lakatos, 1982). Any intellectual product, publication, invention or the intellectual property is retained or appropriated by the Director, that is to say, by the *elder*, thus leaving the youth with a feeling of having been left with nothing. Because the young is considered almost an apprentice, he or she can be denied the totality of his or her merits, such as appearing as collaborator in a project in which he or she had actively participated. This situation is even more extreme when the denial of merit is accompanied by the transference of such merit to a person who had not even participated in the project. There was a case in which a researcher was suggested by his Director not to include his collaborator because the collaborator was learning; he suggested instead including somebody else who turned out to be his friend. Even though such person had not participated in the project at all, he proposed him because he needed the credit.

Upon seeing the researcher's quality and vocation for science, the Director had told him: *You have an inner engine.* This, which can be flattering for the young researcher, is actually adulation in the Aloentic system but will eventually become a tragedy (see the eighth reading).

We can see that Merit and Credit do not necessarily involve the same person. The Director's job, as we have said before, is purely administrative. The Director can be an expert in a field in particular, but may not be very creative to develop new concepts. This would not be important if the Director bore in mind the concept of equity in credit and merit. This unfortunately is not always handled in this manner. A young researcher who had recently started researching on a topic he had proposed was told by an authority that he had to work for a certain Director because this Director needed to improve his credentials. Such *Director* is the one who, in turn, proposed including somebody else's name as co-author (which eventually did not happen).

We have also heard from this kind of Directors – whose only merit is managing a project they can profit from – that if the grant holder wants to leave the system and this attitude can harm the Director, the Director can tell him or her: *You cannot leave the project because you have gotten me involved in it.* This situation ends up in what we describe in the next section: Harasser – Harassed. Some directors use the power they have been given to grant initiation grants to simply make young researchers work for them. Such work is not aimed towards the researcher training as in an Authentic system, but to fulfill the director's personal ambitions. In extreme cases, the young researcher even has to work for his or her director to obtain prizes and recognition. A director once told his young researcher: *We could enter a competition with this work.* The young researcher feels that in spite of having worked intensely and far beyond the regulations, his or her work was absorbed by the director's ambitions. The young researcher is then left with nothing, for when he or she asks for recognition he or she is simply replied with the regulations. In other words: young researchers are stripped off of their enthusiasm and vital energy to serve the director's personal interests. A professor once told a very creative and enthusiastic student who had built technological objects which could even be patented and who had written excellent articles: *I myself will present your article in a congress because you are not known and you will be rejected given the high level of the congress.*

In his work Cuatro Gigantes del Alma, Mira y López includes among professional jealousy the hatred of the old to the youth (Mira y López, 1950). This can be very common in an Aloentic system, especially if the youth is enthusiastic, capable, creative and innovative.

This way of working is, for an enthusiastic youth who is respectful of authority, a safe passage to mental exhaustion first and to burnout later. If, because of the topic the young researcher has chosen he or she is turned into an ethical objector, this hatred can end up in extreme cases of perversion, such as moral harassment, which we will develop more thoroughly in the eighth reading.

On the contrary, in an Authentic system, young researchers are Disciples that far from being used are respected. Their enthusiasm and idealism are driven towards their own intellectual and scientific growth. In this system, the Tutor acts accordingly to the definition in the academic field: "(1) One who instructs another in one or more branches of knowledge. (2) A college official entrusted with the tutelage and care of undergraduates assigned to him" (Standard Encyclopedic Dictionary).

This definition can be fully applied to the scientific field.

The tutor, the *elder*, leads the youth, believing in his intellectual property when developing a creative product. If in doubt he decides in benefit of the young. We can see that in this case, Merit and Credit do involve the same person.

In the Aloentic system, Directors may sometimes also be the administrators of the subsidies. Even if they do not participate in the research itself, they will of course receive credit for the projects. Directors can be skillful administrators of the system. The most important point is the administrative work. However, in the Authentic system, the Tutor will work side by side with the disciple. The passion for advancing in knowledge through questions is most important.

In some cases, in the Aloentic scientific research, before asking the young researcher which the subject of study is, he or she is asked: *who do you work for?* (i.e. who his or her director is.) It is more important to work with a known director than to work with dignity or quality of work, or even than the value of its object of study. This is how *powerful* research *work groups* proliferate but where the dignity of the researcher is not respected. That is to say, the potential of a young researcher, his or her psychological capacity of doing research is less important than the fact of being accepted by a director in particular or being part of a group in particular.

Some young researchers are so impressed by this brilliant corporate style of science that they renounce their own field simply to call themselves specialists in the field of the corporate group.

In an Aloentic system, the young researcher would be more focused on entering a research group directed by a powerful researcher than by choosing a question originated in his or her scientific vocation. This is why Authentic researchers with a special ethical or human vocation avoid a corporate inclusion that does not question the object of study. Researchers with such sensibility usually first choose an object of study that goes in keeping their ethical and human interests and then go from group to group seeking for support and recognition. This support will of course always be denied and these researchers will be left to work on their own.

The pressure in the Aloentic system that constantly generates a fear of exclusion leads to a situation which, in order *not to be left outside* of the system, researchers accept positions – directions and integrations of teams – even though they are not connected to the initial question. The person who in such a way integrates, artificially, without a real question in common and with the sole interest of developing his or her own question, will soon see his or her own mistake materialized. The figure of the perverse harasser described by Dr. Hirigoyen can be frequently seen among these research directors. According to Dr. Hirigoyen (Le Nouvel Observateur, 2006):

> Because of the kind of training they receive, directors do not bear in mind the sensibility or feelings of persons (...). Finally, it is important to bear in mind that the perverse generally acts in the name of morality, which gives him or her position of practically indisputable authority.

Others try to cheat the evaluative system by presenting a topic and then attempting to develop another topic which is what really interests them. Like in the previous case, in no time the researcher will see the mistake materialized, which can be manifested through health problems or through the rage of the system if it discovers the researcher's real intentions. Even when we did not have such intentions, we have once been victims of the rage of the system when we were denied a subsidy by being told that our real intentions were the development of an Institute. The rage of the evaluator due to the actual existence of the institute – which, in spite of his efforts, does exist and cannot be eliminated – is manifested through the denial of granting a minimum subsidy because it was going to be used to develop a project within the institute.

As we have seen in point 6 (Requirements vs. Education), the Authentic system *educates* the young researcher, which is why we can refer to him or her as a *Disciple*. Disciples can recognize by themselves their own research aptitudes, their vocation, the feeling that *something within themselves fights to be materialized* – an expression by Ortega y Gasset we will repeat later. Tutors simply give their disciples the tools to develop themselves as researchers. The criteria of strictness and evaluation are scientific. On the other hand, the Aloentic system *perverts* the student. We could say that the system forces students to be researchers and maybe deceives them. The strictness and evaluation criteria are administrative.

In the Aloentic system it is common to initiate people in research through a grant because they comply with all the formal requirements (good grades, etc.), but without inquiring on a true vocation on research. Such people receive the grant but use it as a provisional contract, as we have already said, as an unemployment insurance, waiting to obtain a more convenient contract in a different job. What actually happens is that not long after, such people stop being involved in the scientific community. The Aloentic system spends tremendous amounts of money initiating in research people who do not value this opportunity and squander it to no avail. Such people usually know an authority in the system who offered them the grant because he or she needed people to develop his or her work, or simply because he or she has the money and prefers giving it to someone he or she knows – even though somebody else might have more potential. Paradoxically, people with a strong vocation for research, proven by their work and dedication, have been left aside for formal reasons. Time can show that some of these people keep researching in spite of personal economic loss. Who is responsible for this mistake? Why wasn't a better decision taken? Why wasn't true vocation taken into account, which would have differentiated the opportunist from the true researcher?

In an Authentic system opportunity of initiation is only given to people with a true vocation and a great potential of perseverance in research, qualities we have mentioned in point 6 (Requirements vs. Education). The Aloentic system, however, does not take into account any of such qualities.

The consequences of such criterion adopted by the Aloentic system are: Economic, since they imply a waste of time and money on a person without vocation. Human, since a person with a true vocation is disregarded for administrative reasons which have no connection whatsoever with his research potential. In addition, if the person without vocation or aptitude remains in the Aloentic system, he or she will also end up being harmed because after advancing in the researching ladder, he or she will realize that he or she is not apt and will become a bureaucrat of science.

We can quote the American writer and journalist Ambrose Bierce (Bierce): "Politics is the conduct of public affairs for private advantage." We can also quote the French contemporary writer L. Dumur (Dumur): "Politics is the art of making Men believe they are being served when in fact they are the ones who are serving." Paraphrasing both quotes we could say that in an Aloentic system: *Directors apply a policy of conduction in a way that they use the capacity of their grant holders for their own personal interests.*

In the eighth reading we will illustrate the stealing of ideas with *the case of the plane and the photocopying machine.* The grant holder draws the plane in pencil and the director photocopies it and then destroys the original. That is to say, in an Aloentic system, where the Director has the privilege of managing the subsidies, what he or she actually does is to pay a minimum wage to carry on copying the grant holder. This could be defined as an Aloentic scientific scheming.

In the Authentic system, however, the Tutor is seen as a person who is not only experienced but is also good hearted, honorable, and has a strong sense of morality and integrity. The Tutor is seen as a human being who wants to teach the *art* to his or her disciple. By *art* we understand the type of work in which altruism is the biggest motif. It is the satisfaction of the craftsman transmitting knowledge to the apprentice. We can say that an authentic researcher is a *craftsman* seeking for knowledge, a person who feels love for his or her work. An Aloentic system Director, however, lacks an *art,* at least on the scientific level, since his or her *art* is to remain and grow in the administrative system. There is no altruism but selfish utilitarianism.

Following the analogy of the physician we used in the Conclusion of Chapter II, we can say that although the Tutor is a specialist of a scientific field, he or she will have, just like any specialized physician, a previous education that will enable him or her to counsel the disciple if the problem the disciple presents cannot be included in his or her field of studies. The Tutor will tell his or her disciple which field to resort to in order to develop his or her project. The Aloentic system Director, however, would act as an unscrupulous specialist physician who, in order not to lose the patient, treats the problem as if it belonged to his or her field knowing it does not. In this case, the patient will either not get better or will actually get worse. Similarly, the young researcher will not improve in obtaining answers to the question that he or she is investigating or will perhaps get disappointed and lose the will to research.

22. Harasser – harassed vs. demand – progress

Harassment in the workplace is an issue that, because of its relevance, has been studied by psychologists, psychiatrists and jurists, among others. Because this issue is of great relevance to the ethical objector question, we will thoroughly develop it in the relevant reading. Nevertheless, we would like to refer briefly to it.

In the Aloentic system, we could say that the members of the corporate group (as well as its authorities) are characterized by the following (which are the same characteristics the harasser has):

- They lack sense of guilt.
- They are inefficient at work.
- They are compulsive controllers and liars.
- They hide under the position of director.
- They are cowards if confronted.
- They use unfounded excuses to harassment (Treviño Ghioldi, 2005).
- They say the harassed is a masochist (Le Nouvel Observateur, 2006).

And, we could also add:
- They are great pretenders and liars.

Therefore, these people frequently act as harassers, being responsible of moral harassment, and both psychological and moral harassment. Such attitudes can be used either against people from the Aloentic system or against people with an Authentic system nature. When used against Aloentic system people, harassment is grounded on administrative or non-scientific reasons. But when used against a person from an Authentic system, the administrative or non-scientific arguments are false accusations that hide the real motivation: not wanting to share an idea, a credit, etc. Since moral harassers are inefficient, they usually want to appropriate the achievements of people with a profile typical of an Authentic system. Harassed persons can suffer various conditions.

Usually, a harassed person could, as a cathartic attitude, harass in turn the people below him or her. However, an Authentic system person, because of his or her morale, will never be an harasser; he or she will repress the pain inflicted by harassment in such a way that it will lead him or her to suffer serious health problems – which, in addition, will make such person become inefficient at work. We can thus conclude that if a person with an Authentic nature must work in an Aloentic system, he or she will go through hell.

This happens because the harassed have the following qualities:

- Strong sense of ethics and justice.
- An excellent capacity for work.
- Strong sense of comradeship.
- Work well in teams; they are independent and have initiative.
- They are valued by their team. They abhor using people to accomplish their own aims (Treviño Ghioldi, 2005).

We can also add:

- They abhor plotting in the dark to make a person be substituted for him or her.

In addition, Dr. Hirigoyen (Le Nouvel Observateur, 2006) describes other characteristics of the harassed:

> One would expect it to be a weak person. To a certain extent! But, on the contrary, the harassed are generally very honest or at least have strong personalities. They are very frequently people who would listen to the other: personnel delegates, nurses, doctors, people of communication. The victim is usually the one who resists his or her colleagues, even his or her superior, but also, although less frequently, his or her subordinate.

What we could define as *the logics of the harassed* is completely different from *the logics of the harasser*. The harassed does not usually recognize or finds it difficult to recognize the harassment, since this cannot be included within the cannon of decency. In order to protect himself or herself from moral harassment, the harassed aims to distance himself or herself from the abusing environment, but the system criticizes this saying that the person *does not want to be part of the group*. It is a cat and mouse game, in which the mouse, knowing the risk it runs, refuses to play with the cat and the cat accuses it of not wanting be friends. The system leaves him or her aside first and then expels them. The harassed can even be accused of *not respecting the authority*, of *troublemaking* and even called *anarchist* – which, according to Feyerabend would be a compliment rather than an accusation. Maybe we could include here Cardinal de Retz's (1613-1679) concept (De Gondi): "When the rulers lose their shame, the ruled lose respect."

This criterion is totally understandable or acceptable if we also consider Benito Gerónimo Feijoo's words (Feijoo): "The fact that there are many of them does not make them less ignorant. What can be expected of their resolutions?"

If the authority treacherously manages to convince the corporate group – which it belongs to – of a lie presented as truth, the wrong conclusions might be drawn, thus harming innocent people. The corporation constituted by ignorant people, fearful of the fact that they indeed might be taken as ignorant, and in order not to doubt the decision of the corporation member who asked for the measure, will never revert the measure taken notwithstanding the number of reasons that prove that such decision was wrong. The impunity of the injustice system is assured.

At first, this type of harassment is hard to recognize. The victim will tend to think that he or she is to blame for this situation. This characteristic is something already recognized by those who have been working on the protection of ethical objectors.

The choice of the ethical objector and the detection of moral harassment must be left in the hands of experts in this field. Not anyone can do it, and certainly not the party involved.

We could say that the Aloentic system aims to transform the authentic researcher into what the system actually is. That is to say: a pretender who avoids or protects himself or herself of harassment, or a seeker of the superfluous or the vain.

In the Authentic system, as we have said, there are also certain requirements, but they are constructive. Such requirements seek for a harmonious and gradual development in the group and in the person, respecting him or her and seeking to distinguish the person's conditions, aptitudes and intellectual capacity – as we have said, his or her virtues and vocation.

When the young researcher has characteristics of an Authentic system, we could qualify these values as: Harasser-Harassed vs. Requirements-Progress; Parasitism vs. Constructivist Pressure.

Moral harassment and its implications in the ethical objector will be specifically detailed later.

23. The tool vs. the work

We have said that in the Aloentic system erudition is used to replace what cannot be obtained with intelligence or creativity. We can say the same in connection with resources. In this system, resources are given a fair amount of weight. Using a state-of-the-art equipment generates great enthusiasm, but it does not necessarily mean that such equipment will be used to develop questions of real entity. In the Aloentic system, some research groups are more interested in the equipments than in the relevance of the question.

The lack of tools is often used as an excuse to justify a small production or the lack of creativity.

However, in the Aloentic system, what is important is the person and his or her work. Equipments are simply useful devices or tools, which, of course, when necessary, can be highly complex. But let us not forget that Shakespeare did not use any state-of-the-art computer. He just needed pen and paper.

24. Credit: formality vs. credit: merit

In the Aloentic system, the credit within the scientific system that allows to get a better position, obtain subsidies, obtain promotions, directing and managing scientific personnel, etc., is obtained by complying with corporate formalities. It is essential to *go by the book* and *be tidy* with the regulations. In the Authentic system, however, credit is given exclusively for inventiveness and proven capacity of discovery. Form is secondary and it is left in the hands of administrative personnel.

The Aloentic system permits that wise managers with little capacity of invention, creativity and vocation of research *suck* credits simply because they know how to duly comply with form.

25. Tidiness vs. limited untidiness

In the previous point we said that in the Aloentic system going by the book and being tidy with the regulations are taken as *commandments*. Young researchers are commonly harassed by evaluators, who disqualify the reports sent arguing that they have a series of unacceptable untidiness, thus producing a moral damage in the evaluated researcher. We can mention a case in which a researcher had applied for a grant, but the evaluator criticized that the bibliography was badly presented. Nevertheless, because of his merits, he did get the grant, but he obtained the penultimate position. So far the moral damage for the evaluee does not seem that serious. But it does increase enormously when those who criticize or disqualify the reports are in fact extremely interested in pursuing the innovation of *the untidy* and, whatever it takes, copy the innovation and incorporate it to their own projects which are developed with extreme tidiness and all the resources required. The moral damage for *the untidy* is double. First, he or she is disqualified for trivialities and then, his work is copied. A researcher studied the influence of tidiness and untidiness in research works (Abrahamson, 2007). According to this researcher, what used to be considered negative in the past cannot be considered like this any longer. As this researcher says, science is starting to incorporate the principle of *limited untidiness.* In addition, in connection to companies, he says: *let us suppose that a company has found an <u>unexpected niche </u>and is growing considerably. Stopping to get reorganized is not necessary, they can carry on even if stumbling. When the market slows down, then they will have the time to get organized.* The unexpected niche mentioned by this author equals the new idea or discovery of the scientific world.

Now, is this innovation or simply untidiness? The argument can be clearly seen here, innovators can say: You do not innovate, you are just untidy. They can even be disregarded with phrases like: Who do you think you are? Einstein? As we have mentioned before, only History, a consequence of persistence in the time of the researchers who are supposedly innovators, can solve the dilemma. The acceptance of limited untidiness by researchers of elite universities can make the creative activity of future innovators easier. This will avoid the typical degrading statement based on an obsessive tidiness required from researchers, and which gives tidiness an excessive weight in the final decision.

26. Copy vs. original idea

In an Aloentic system, copy and plagiarism are tolerated. We could say that in this system, the successful person is he or she who makes the first photocopy of an original project, erases or crosses out the author's name and writes his or her name instead. The real origin of the ideas is never mentioned. In the case of a book or an article, sometimes fragments (either long or short) can be copied without mentioning the author, or doing it in an indirect manner, incorporating it with the rest of the bibliography but without indicating the quotation in the text. In the Authentic system, the original idea and the respect to it and its authors are the most important points. Whether it is an important or a small idea, it will always be attributed to its actual author or authors. The original idea is always mentioned and respected. The origin of any idea is always mentioned and, apart from the proper bibliographical reference, there is an adequate marking within the text.

27. Intellectual opportunism vs. intellectual honesty

In an Aloentic system, it is fairly common that researchers pursue *profitable ideas*. This concept is used to define any idea that, because it is new, or current or adequate to the taste of researchers, will enable to obtain generous research subsidies. This could be called *intellectual opportunism*. The possibility of these researchers arriving to substantial discoveries is very low. On the other hand, in this system, researchers who remain faithful to a question – with the subsequent intellectual honesty – many times do not have either the success or support others do have. The researcher who focuses on developing a single idea is too busy and concentrated to spend time seeking for other profitable ideas. This opposition between intellectual honesty and intellectual opportunism can be seen by comparing the position achieved in the system by the researchers after many decades of work. So, having as starting point the same – or even less – education, opportunist researchers can be *more successful administratively* speaking than others with a higher academic and scientific level.

28. Inopportune anomaly vs. innovative anomaly

In Chapter III we referred to the concept Kuhn uses to describe the general process of innovation or discovery. We have said that, according to this author, any innovation or discovery needs previously that the researcher or discoverer feels that an anomaly is constantly returning as an *ostinato* in his or her field. We have said that perhaps, at first, the researcher will try to eliminate it so that it does not obstruct what he or she is trying to investigate. But because such element keeps surfacing, thus altering the expected theory, it ends up being recognized as a phenomenon in itself. The persistent anomaly is but the manifestation of a phenomenon which is not very much known appearing within one which is known. Time, the persistence of this anomaly, and the intuitive capacity of the innovator to recognize in such anomaly something more than an annoyance, make him change focus towards such anomaly. The discovery is thus produced.

Because the Aloentic system is a structured system, even the results of the studies seem to be predictable beforehand. So when the researcher observes that some data diverts from the *expected,* he or she eliminates them so that his or her report leaves no traces that will later lead to criticism that cannot be refuted. If an Aloentic researcher was in the same situation as Fleming, he or she would probably throw away all the contaminated dishes in order to avoid being punished for not keeping the adequate sterility conditions in his or her lab. The Aloentic researcher sees such anomalies as something annoying that obstructs his or her work. In more extreme cases, he or she can even destroy his research and then make up some justification. In a system that appeals to the logic of the expected and repels every indetermination for not understanding it, what kind of innovation can be expected?

In the Authentic system, however, the researcher can feel inclined to get rid of the annoying anomaly, but it will later drive him or her to a discovery. Like an unexpected call, at an inadequate time, that can mean a satisfactory piece of news.

29. Extortive political manipulation vs. honest recognition of merit

Even though we will deal with this topic more thoroughly in the eighth reading because of the relevance of this situation in the ethical objector issue, we can now mention this question since political manipulation of an authentic researcher can take place in an Aloentic system. For example, resorting to political manipulation to grant a subsidy, position or promotion, i.e., granting it only after obtaining the political interest motivating it (for example, some kind of support, or a signature), notwithstanding the merit the researcher may have.

30. Collective thinking vs. autonomous thinking

This point, related to the nature of thought in each system, is connected to point 3 (Authoritarianism vs. Freedom). In an Authentic system, autonomous thinking is possible and desirable. This kind of thinking – free of influences, with free will, free of conditioning pressures but with a healthy pressure typical of the development of an idea, etc. – allows the person to be more creative. But in an Aloentic system, mediocrity leads to a single possibility of thought: Collective Thinking. Dissidence is not allowed. In an Aloentic system, that who is stubborn enough to sustain his or her autonomous thinking will last in the system the time that the psychopathic process takes to deteriorate his or her mental health – as we will see in the eighth reading.

31. Conformist vs. transgressor

Transgression is generally seen as a negative attitude, since it defines the act of breaking a law, for example. However, this attitude can also be seen as positive, if the transgression results in breaking the impediments that check the progress of an idea.

If we apply these concepts to our present concern, we can see that an Authentic researcher many times will have to become a transgressor in order to advance in knowledge. This attitude will be more obvious and painful if the researcher is working within an Aloentic system in which, according to its definition, will have to make an effort to break the impediments that curb his or her freedom of work. If the researcher tries a conformist attitude, the only thing that he or she will gain is to damage his psychic health. The researcher will have a sense of failure in the long term because he or she will realize that the biggest calamity was not having tried hard enough. This sense of failure cannot be replaced by generous subsidies or important material achievements.

In an Authentic system, however, transgressors might clash first, but, in the long term, they will be accepted for their contributions. Sometimes, these researchers are supported and promoted during their lifetime, but the majority of times their contributions are recognized after their death through their lasting work. As we have said before, it takes a transgressor to achieve innovation.

In an Aloentic system, if the researcher is also Aloentic, he or she will adopt a Conformist attitude. He or she will comply with the director's orders without problems.

This point, which is related to points 10 and 27, refers to the work in teams.

It is very common to accuse researchers who complain that they cannot achieve their work by saying that they do not want to be part of a group.

We have already referred to the fact that the system had attempted to include us in already consolidated groups so that we could carry out our project.

The problem is that when one speaks of a Group in an Aloentic system, one is making reference to a group of Opportunists. According to its definition, an opportunist is "One who uses every opportunity to contribute to the achievement of some end, and who is relatively uninfluenced by moral principles or sentiments" (Standard Encyclopedic Dictionary*)*. In some cases, we can even find social climbers, who simply want to be credited.

However, in an Authentic system, team work means solidarity group. According to its definition, *solidarity* refers to the coherence and oneness in nature, relations, or interests, as a class (Standard Encyclopedic Dictionary). We can also add that this group is characterized by:

1. Equally understanding the aims and the work to be done. Equally understanding the importance of the task.
2. Being willing to equal sacrifice, self-denial and dedication to accomplish the aims.
3. Not claiming for a merit that is not the merit earned in A and B.

It is obvious that any researcher with a solidarity nature working with a group of opportunists will be exploited.

Other characteristics of the systems

We will now describe other characteristics we have observed in the Authentic and Aloentic systems. Some, in the case of the Aloentic system, are questionable from the ethical point of view:

- There are two types of researchers: those who usually discover problems but do not generally find a solution to them and those who find solutions even though they were not the discoverers. In an Authentic system, both types of researchers are respected and supported. In an Aloentic system, however, the researcher who has the idea is not given support by the one to solve the problem. This researcher will have to join a consolidated group in order to solve the problem. The innovation capacity of these researchers is minimized especially if they are young researchers. Therefore, young researchers who discover a problem are only supported if they are credited as solving a problem detected and assigned by the Director. A fake situation is created: that the topic was assigned by a director, a *fake discoverer*, who always positions him or herself as the author of an idea or a problem. The frivolity of this procedure, in which he or she who appropriates an idea detected by someone else assumes not only the capacity to solve it but also to direct whoever has detected it, leads to deviations. It is not known whether the problems are solved correctly – this fiction leads to an appropriation of the problem or the idea, without bearing in mind the existing limitations to solve it. The solution of problems from those who appropriate the idea or the problem thinking they have the capacity to solve it will always be done half way through, without arriving to the nucleus of the problem. In an Aloentic system, stealing ideas from researchers who detect the problems is very common. The detection of problems requires creativity which, due to the fact that Aloentic researchers do not have it, is underestimated.

- If a researcher from the Authentic system wants to develop his or her question within an Aloentic system framework, such researcher must have a *high resistance to punishment and demoralization.* Only later such researcher is recognized. Or, perhaps, how many talented researchers who cannot endure punishment are lost on the way? Would it not have been more convenient for the system to be more tolerant? It is said that a scientific authority in Argentina, at the beginning of the Research Council meetings, said that a bit of ill treatment of good researchers should not be harmful, because good researchers endure, even if they are punished. Does this not sound a bit authoritative? Would it not be better to respect the researcher?

- The Aloentic system pretends it cannot see a new phenomenon that it does not want to clarify, because they surely do not understand it. But the phenomenon does exist and it deserves to be the object of study of a science. The Authentic system, on the contrary, sees the phenomenon as a problem and a challenge and tries to contribute to its solution.

- Going back to the hole puncher example, an accurate evaluation of reality implies including the part that is left from the punched circles.
- In the Aloentic system, recognition is built simply by using bricks from the bottom to the top. In the Authentic system, however, the vertex is recognized first and then the foundations are built.
- In the Aloentic system, your work is no good, but if I am co-author and, better still, if I direct it, it will be good.
- In the Aloentic system, the authority can tell a researcher: I will plagiarize your idea; if you *want to* we can work together. I will be co-author and direct the project. If you do not agree I do not care. I will have the jurisdiction and all the resources to work on it.
- In developed countries, aloenticity in a scientific system is also seen by hiding the unexpected side effects of a technology. Especially private companies send the products to countries (especially third world countries) where such side effects cannot be observed thus enabling the product to remain in the market.
- In developing countries, on the other hand, Aloenticity is seen in the inequality with which the subsidies are given, how intellectual property is dealt with and the system's general efficiency.
- Aloenticity in developed countries is also seen in the attitude of certain important professors and scholars who, when asked about the collateral phenomenon of a technology, seek to distract those who ask with trivial arguments.
- Aloenticity seems to be less dangerous for the general population in developing countries than in developed countries. This is because the Aloentic science in developing countries will hardly yield a marketable risky product.

Example: Technopathogenology

The incomprehension between both systems is especially seen when a researcher has detected a void in knowledge and, at the same time, an orphanage that requires proposing a new scientific discipline. This is the case of Technopathogenology.

In an Authentic system, when a problem is detected in a researcher's context, instead of reducing it to the existing disciplines, it is taken as it is and then it is tried to be solved. This is what led us to Technopathogenology.

By adopting such criterion, which we consider the only valid way to advance in true science, we found the cultural differences between the system in which we developed our activity and ourselves. The differences are such that we could not even get to know what the Science and Technique system felt about our proposal. Every note, letter, email we sent with scientific grounds was responded by the authorities with administrative issues. The insurmountable amount of administrative arguments – as we will also see in the eighth reading – constituted a barrier we could not surpass. The conservative nature of the Aloentic system prefers ignoring or denying new knowledge if it cannot include it within the existent – which is what happened with Technopathogenology. It would rather impede the production that could generate the new disciplinary proposal – or even its destruction, if it has already started showing its productive potentiality – rather than giving the benefit of the doubt to the new if it does not fit within the already regulated and consolidated. The argument of saving a possible waste of funds if using it on the wrong ideas or paths leading to dead ends is fallacious. This argument is very poor, since the large amounts of money spent in Science and Technique are not spent for supporting risky hypotheses but for investing on promoting more of the same, more of which does not really contribute to relevant knowledge. This leads us back to point 19 (Economy vs. Wasting).

We hardly had any official support for the development of Technopathogenology – neither did we in our initial research that led to the discovery of aflatoxins in local corn in 1976. If the initial risky hypothesis was real and the development was of relevance and the concept lasts, we simply had to investigate it, check it and prove it, in spite of the absurd negative responses that prevented us from receiving the subsidies that would have, perhaps, allowed for the development of a better work. We did not spend much because we were denied of support. However, after more than thirty years, we have had a decent and, why not, efficient production.

Conclusion

We have identified cultural differences in the Science and Technique system. Differences of values that lead to difficulties in communication (or even to the lack of it) which tamper with the work of the researcher and the advancement of knowledge.

Such considerations lead to inequities in the evaluation process, to enormous amounts of money spent and to attitudes or situations that will be more thoroughly described in the reading that deals with the need of an ethical objector in Science and Technique. Apart from being supported by the Aloentic system values, great expenditures are also caused by ethical misdemeanors of the administrators – such as keeping part of the sum granted for a subsidy. Therefore, rejecting an Authentic project on the grounds of avoiding economic risk is a fallacious argument.

Cultural differences are also adopted by the system as a *right of admission reserved* sign. By resorting to administrative arguments, the system creates an insuperable barrier for any researcher who the system wants to control, leave aside or even eliminate (target person). Administrative arguments can make reference to reasons or justifications included in any of the values listed in the table: Obviousness, Erudition, Authoritarianism, Form, Method, Requirements, the Quantitative, the Superfluous, Collectivism, Superficiality, the Written Text, the Discipline, the Pre-Existent, Growth, Inductivism, Structure, Utilitarian Mercantilism, the Director, the Tool, Formality, Tidiness, etc.

We repeat the list of values in an almost tedious manner to show that it is almost impossible for Authentic researchers to avoid the system not finding in their presentation some detail that could be a reason to exclude their work. Any detail will do. The system works at full discretion, this is "the freedom or power to make one's own judgment" (Standard Encyclopedic Dictionary) and without any possibility of arguing or appealing to another administrative instance. The autonomy that big scientific academic corporations have, leads to the fact that any application of resources or any appeal to revise negative statements are generally rejected and the original statement is always corroborated. Researchers can naively request a revision of negative statements reaching the last instance of administrative right. But the result will always be the same: negative, without arguments, logics, or reason – pure and simple authoritarianism.

In an Aloentic system giving more importance to administrative arguments rather than scientific arguments is an easy way to hide the incapacity to evaluate or to hide the interest in marginalizing a research project. This would avoid the open scientific discussion where the poor arguments to oppose to the researcher's proposal would come to light. Being the system totally discretional, when the administrative arguments are used by the corporation's lawyers, they can be easily used to punish or expel whoever presents the innovation. This is attributed to causes other than the innovation itself. The aim is to save the image of the institution which has committed such an obvious injustice.

It is known, however, that a democratic system is a system in which minorities are respected. Any innovative knowledge in Science and Technique will obviously be part of the minority group. Our question is therefore: Are new ideas and innovators treated with *democratic* respect in the Science and Technique system? The answer is that in the Science and Technique Corporation there is very little room for innovators and they are often treated with authoritarianism, they are discriminated and they are eliminated from the system.

In the power and decision-making structures not all the cultures are represented.

The scientist's responsibility is to aim at the establishment of authentic scientific systems. Maybe this is why an ethical objector is required in the Science and Technique system – which we will deal with in one of our readings.

Only by implementing creative dialogue is that equity is achieved in the system. In the same way, the unconditional search for knowledge is favored.

We believe that the values adopted in an Aloentic system and their *strict requirements* only aim at *pretending a scientific level* which is far or even completely out of its reach. This is hidden by a high dose of authoritarianism. The characteristics that define the Aloentic system will allow us to define it as a *ritual and cult of the absurd* system.

The Aloentic system can only lead to a *bad science*. We can quote the Italian historian Cesar Cantú (Cantú):

> False science is worse than ignorance. Ignorance is a virgin field which can be toiled and soiled; but false science is an infected field with bad weed which is difficult to pluck out.

We can summarize the key objectives of both systems: The Aloentic system aims to control and restrict the researcher in such a way that, as we will see later on, it can lead to serious persecuting attitudes against him or her. The Authentic system, on the other hand, within the frame of respect to a person, to his or her ideas and vocation, out of respect for the *Freedom of Thought,* which we underline because we consider it a *sine qua non* condition in the scientific work, aims for the unconditional search for knowledge thus achieving intellectual growth and development as well as academic quality.

There are cultural differences in the Science and Technique system both between the researcher and the authority and in the way research work is carried out. The evaluation system is criticized because it focuses more on the form and method than in the substantial progress of knowledge. If an honest dialogue between both cultures cannot be obtained, the differences will eventually lead to more inequality within the system which, affecting the process of generation of knowledge, can lead to being responsible for damages on health.

Going back to the objectives of this book and considering that the consequences of the voids in knowledge applied in the development of techniques can be harmful to human health, we can conclude, going back to the phrase that opened this reading: *The aim must be to achieve good science and, should a technopathogeny appear, it should be due to ethical causes and not due to the unethical reasons that are typical of a bad science.*

II.   Technopathogenology and protection to consumers

Introduction

A specific situation brings to light a general problem

In our experience, Technopathogenology would be of high relevance in the protection to consumers.

A problem internationally known is the one regarding the risks of exposure to cell phones antennas. The damage to health they cause can be included among Technopathogenies. One case involving these antennas occurred in our city and it made us think that Technopathogenology could protect consumers in other senses.

We could exemplify this with the case of mycotoxins and its relevance in protection to consumers (Eguiazu & Motta, 2006). Even though it was done from a different perspective, the theories and hypotheses were described thoroughly in Chapter II.

The study of such contaminants is an important example since it shows the logic of a search within narrowing boundaries or aims. The reason for narrowing the aim was to define the relevance of the issue, i.e., to ask: what is relevant and what is substantial? or rather, beyond the apparent multiplicity: What are the underlying elements? What is the unifying factor? These questions helped to leave aside the secondary elements and focus on the most relevant point: protection to consumers. The search is done with the elements at hand, whether they are big or small tools. When there are no more tools left, everything is left to thinking; the only tool left is the logical intellectual relation.

On the layperson eyes the search can seem chaotic; for the researcher, however, it has a great intellectual harmony and rigor since it can see the bottom, not just the surface.

Nevertheless, as we will see below, there are many aspects connected to Technology that can represent a Technopathogenic risk. For this reading, as we have already mentioned, we will use the example of the cell phones antennas, since it is an issue which is widely known by consumers.

Protection to consumers: Its relevance

Several countries have established legislation for the protection of consumers, as well as created organisms that work for their protection. In the United States, for example, the Consumer Product Safety Act was passed in 1972 to protect the population from damages to health and deaths associated to the consumption of products. Under such Act, the U.S. Consumer Product Safety Commission was created in 1973 (US CPSC, 1992), which regulates an enormous amount of aspects associated to the risks to consumers, among them: Medicines, materials for artists, chemical products, combustible substances, cosmetics, foodstuffs, household products, toys, etc. – just to name a few of the 250 products that have been regulated, according to a 1992 report (US CPSC, 1992). We can also quote the case of European Communities which have created a special directorate, the Directorate-General XXIV, to protect the rights of consumers in four crucial aspects: health and safety, economic interests, comparative information and right to compensation. In connection to health, which is our area of interest, this Directorate is responsible for controlling the application of laws elaborated by other Directorates. In addition, it guarantees giving information on the decisions taken and the results of the controls. We can also mention the creation of an Office for Product Quality Control (former Office for Veterinary and Phytosanitary Inspection) and the creation of a special group of inspectors responsible for the evaluation of health risks and control of foodstuffs (European Commission, 1997).

It is interesting to point out that in Germany there is a group which studies risks connected to healthy environment in the households; there is also a group that studies consumer protection quality management. Both groups are considered of interest by the German Society for Environmental and Human Toxicology (DGUHT) (DGUHT, 2007).

In our country we can mention the Argentine Law no. 24240 (Consumer protection Law) and different organisms, such as: Defensoría del Pueblo de la Nación (National People's Protection Office); Defensoría del Pueblo Provincial (Provincial People's Protection Office) and the Dirección de Defensa del Consumidor (Consumer's Protection Directorate). Each organism is in charge of different aspects involving human rights. We wanted to know whether technopathogenic risks associated to consumer products were being contemplated by any of those organisms, so we contacted the Consumer's Protection Directorate of Santa Fe since we considered Technopathogeny problems would be addressed to such entity.

We were told that the type of queries varied depending on the period of administration (Gomez, 2004) as listed in table 31 below.

Table 31: Types of queries addressed to the Consumer's Protection Directorate of Santa Fe (Argentina) from 1993 to 2001.

Year	1993	1995	1999	2001
Query	Guarantee of imported household appliances: washing machines, refrigerators, TV sets, etc.	People disappointed due to aggressive marketing techniques. Time-sharing modality: rented houses for holidays.	Purchase of products with fake identity. Fast signing which is then attempted to be cancelled.	Quantity and quality of packaged products. Two-thousand queries are mentioned.

We can see that queries or complaints on technopathogenological issues were non-existent (for example, long term risks of substances handling, consumption of medicines, foodstuffs additives, residues of pesticides in vegetables, handling of electronic devices, exposure to electromagnetic fields, chemical products of household use, cosmetics, etc.).

The table shows a large amount of evident issues. This is not surprising, since non-evident issues require a specific methodology for their study, as well as qualified people, i.e., scientific evaluators.

The need of consumer protection from technopathogenic risks:
Two examples

Before referring to the problem of cell phones antennas we will exemplify the question of Technopathogenies and consumer protection with mycotoxins and pesticides. We have already discussed this problem in previous works. In one of them (Eguiazu & Motta, 2006), we used the problem of aflatoxins (which, as we have seen in previous chapters, initiated our scientific work) as example of consumer protection issues.

The description of the problem of framing this discipline within existing disciplines in Chapter II allowed us to understand the risk these substances posed to consumers. This is proved by their carcinogenicity and the possibility of being present in foodstuffs. In addition, and due to their relevance to consumer protection, we can also mention other factors we discussed in Chapter II which contribute to risk: Imperfections of the analytical methodology that was applied commercially is the bright greenish-yellow fluorescent (BGYF) or *black light test*, presumptive text for aflatoxin in corn (Shotwell, 1983), and the masking of the BGYF in grains. We have mentioned that when observing commercial samples of corn many of them did not show the BGYF fluorescence indicating fungi attack and possible presence of aflatoxins. However, through mechanically cracked grain we observed that the fluorescence was found inside them: some grains that tested positive for aflatoxins had not shown the fluorescence on the outer part. We thus proved that the widely advertised commercial system was inefficient since it did not indicate that grains should be cracked to show the fluorescence masked inside the grains. This aspect constituted a potential risk for consumers since a detection technique that could actually disguise the presence of aflatoxins was relied upon. After our discovery we postulated that the grain be analyzed before and after being cracked. If after being cracked fluorescent grains could be observed, a chemical analysis for aflatoxins should be carried out.

We must also mention that the difficulty in framing our discipline was also related to the fact that we were trying to tackle the problem of these contaminants within a *protection to human health* framework. We must also remember the hypothesis postulated in Chapter II in connection to such substances: Can prevention be achieved within a Jurisprudence framework? – A hypothesis which clearly aims at consumer protection.

In the Reading VI we will prove that in order to efficiently protect consumers, technopathogenological aspects associated to pesticides must also be considered.

In Chapter II we have described the technopathogenic risk of such substances. We have also seen the limitations that analytical chemistry finds in identifying raw materials or products that are contaminated with these substances – difficulties we have also observed both for mycotoxins and for chemical technopathogenies in general. Therefore, measures that aim at avoiding the use of active principles of technopathogenic risk are crucial for consumer protection considering that even in developed countries the most accurate methodologies only detect part of the large amount of products that can be used in a determined crop. In connection to this, the editorial section of a publication by the International Register of Potentially Toxic Chemicals (IRPTC) commented on the importance of education of consumers and the crucial function specialists have in such education: "Have they ever explained that there is no chemical product either natural or artificial which is totally free of risks in every possible condition?" (PNUMA, 1985a).

Another editorial (PNUMA, 1985b) mentioned that:

> The director of an important factory of chemical products in Switzerland said that ignorance, misinterpretations and the lack of information were the most important risk factors for his employees. Such statement should be taken very seriously not only by the chemical industry but also by all the authorities and users of chemical products, whether they are agriculturists, craftsmen, housewives or hobbyists.

Our work spreading knowledge regarding the high relevance of the long exposure to (not one, but several) substances led a group of occupationally exposed people to become interested in what we had to say. They worked in the storehouse of a laboratory in a university. They asked us to evaluate the technopathogenic risk associated to their work (Motta & Eguiazu, 1990).

Another interesting aspect in consumer protection (which is given high relevance in the report on pesticides mentioned in Chapter II), apart from the difficulty Analytical Chemistry has in identifying residues, is the fact that out of the five active principles most frequently used in lettuce (Mevinphos, Endosulfan, Permethrin, Dimethoate y Methomyl) only one (Permethrin) can be eliminated by washing because its residues remain on the surface of the leaf. The other four, however, are systemic (they are absorbed by the plant) and can therefore not be washed out (Mott & Snyder, 1987). The five active principles present a technopathogenic risk.

If this is a complex problem in developed countries, it is much worse in developing countries. A research showed that approximately 50% of the active principles that entered Argentina without restrictions were either prohibited or severely restricted in stringent States such as California (Eguiazu, 1988). In 1994 in a Symposium organized by FAO we showed how permissive the Code of Conduct of FAO was in allowing the entrance of risky pesticides to developing countries. This code defended more the industry of pesticides than the health of population. The code of FAO (FAO, 1986) was not efficient in excluding what was harmful to the population. We can also ask ourselves, what is the point of being an expert in the analysis of pesticides if we are not going to be able to detect all the existing residues, or their quantities below the limit of detection? It would seem that we are trapped in a dynamic in which, on the one hand, we continuously receive substances that pose a high risk on humans for which methods to detect are laboriously developed, but when this is achieved, the active principle is probably replaced with a new one, having to start over from the very beginning. Exposure on humans can thus never be avoided. Analysis can only be used as a late indicator to show that there are risky substances at work.

The large sums invested to develop new active principles determine the *understandable* attitude of the industry trying to commercialize a product until it obtains the expected revenue. This is why commercial interests and government policies work in unison. For example, once a candidate to president said in his candidacy speech that if he won, he *would flood the country with agrochemicals.* In 1986, approximately half of the active principles that entered the country were carcinogenic or had mutagenic, teratogenic, or fetal damage effects (Eguiazu, 1988). This was shown in a congress on Ecotoxicology in which, ironically, a professor on Ecotoxicology from a developed country said that even if pesticides were carcinogenic, they were the only choice for developing countries because the only alternative they had without the pesticides was to starve to death.

This shows how influential corporate economic interests can be on politicians, especially on those who are ignorant in technologies such as the ones applied in agricultural industry but who will then have the lives of consumers in their hands.

A recent research carried out in a hospital in our city showed a clear relationship between the use of pesticides in our country and the effects we have mentioned in previous articles.

Such pesticides may be recalled from the market (as DDT was), but it will be too late. They will be probably replaced with other pesticides until, many years later, it will be proven whether they were harmful or not. In this vicious circle, consumers are always the ones who suffer the consequences.

It would be much more effective to ban the use of risky pesticides. This is why a preventive science is important: Technopathogenology.

In order to protect consumers – who are defenseless, unaware of the risk posed by pesticides – it is essential that legislation both local and international (FAO, WHO, etc.) be improved by developing more programs and stricter codes of control.

An example that illustrates the lightness with which potentially risky technologies are used

As we have mentioned at the beginning of this reading, we will describe the case of cell phones antennas in Rosario (Zinna, 2004). Even though the case we are most experienced with is mycotoxins, we will describe the case of the antennas because it is more widely known by consumers and therefore more illustrative for this reading. In this case in particular, instead of speaking of *consumers* we will speak of *exposed citizens*, since many of these people are exposed even though they are not consumers.

A timely technopathogenological statement would avoid future difficulties

The installation of these antennas began long ago all over the city. In 1996 one of them was installed in a downtown school. This antenna had, as all antennas surely had, all the relevant municipal permissions to be installed since at the time the authorities did not know of any possible side effects (International Conference on Cell Tower Sitting, 2000). Eventually, thanks to the information that described the possible damages on health and to the pressure of people informed, a restrictive legislation was slowly developed which called for the disassembling of the antenna installed at the school.

However, the company that had installed the antenna (and which had invested large sums on the project) lodged an appeal in court on the grounds that when they were given permission there was no restrictive law. This delayed the disassembling of the antenna for several years. Meanwhile:

A. The company can keep on recovering the investment since the authority is usually tolerant and does not investigate the possibility of other risks apart from the evident one being present. Interestingly enough, PROCABIE already existed (we had created it in 1984) and had been declared of interest by the Rosario City Council in 1991 (Decree 8270) (Concejo Municipal de la Ciudad de Rosario, 1991). INCABIE also existed (also created by us in 1984), a foundation which, on our petition, was formalized by the University of Rosario in December 1985 (Resolution 744/85), and which worked until this university dissolved it in

August, 2002 without any academic or scientific grounds. This means that both institutions existed well before the installation of the school antenna.

B. The possible victims, the school children, among others, had to continue attending the school and being exposed to the emissions, unless their parents decided to transfer them to another school (which also implied some kind of damage, since the children would most surely suffer from the uprooting).

Even though the school finally removed the antenna in 2004, there was a long period of exposure which could have been avoided.

A common mechanism

With this simple example we can see that the mechanism described can be applied to any case presenting a side effect in Technique that is related to pesticides, medicines, natural contaminants, etc. The procedure is always as follows:

a) The high cost of investment forces the causer to minimize the risk, be it of a biological, chemical or electromagnetic nature. In some cases the causer can actually not be aware of the damage. The authority is tolerant or claims ignorance when approving the proposal.

b) When the risk is known, it goes public and the pressure of the possible victims mounts. The causer uses the law as protection managing to maintain the project (i.e. whatever is causing the damage) working as long as it is possible.

c) When the investment has been recovered, or when the pressure of the victims is too high and cannot be resisted any longer, the causer might give in to the requirements, substituting the technology that causes the damage by an innocuous one or by a lesser risk technology which is probably widely used in Europe and the USA.

Why nobody was ever consulted?

It is important that the official institution gathers all the possible information on risks. It is not enough to analyze the adequate construction of an antenna from the structural point of view and leave aside the possible technopathogenies which can come as consequence of its continuous operation. No permission for the installation should have been granted without a specific statement that proved there were no risks. Once done, it is very difficult to undo it. Even though the antenna was eventually disassembled, people have already been exposed.

Discussion

We could summarize the detailed description we made in Chapter II – our original research proposal that started with the problem of mycotoxins and gave way to a Journey that has lasted for more than 30 years, in which we encountered increasingly deepening questions until we arrived to the postulation of Technopathogenology and its relevance in the protection of consumers – in the following facts, which are linked to one another by a search logic:

- We started with a concrete contaminant, Aflatoxins, given its relevance in human health and the need for the consumer to be protected against the risks and damages to health produced by these substances. It was the first job of this type in our region.
- With the information we had gathered from around the world, we attempted to convince authorities of the urgent need to protect consumers while trying to find financial support for our research.
- We performed the first tests in corn batches from our region.
- New attempts of convincing authorities of the urgent need to protect consumers while trying to find financial support for our research.
- We evaluated commercial analytical techniques of routine application for such contaminants. We proposed improvements to such techniques in order to reduce the error margins in the results they cast. This contributed to reduce the risk of exposure of consumers to these substances.
- The studies continued in Europe. The analyzing techniques were improved and the environmental conditions that predisposed the fungal attack were studied.
- We proposed the theory that the study of mycotoxins under the perspective of consumer protection did not fit within the Science and Technique system.

- Finding we could not frame our research within the existing entities, we created PROCABIE – i.e. a new research program suitable to the question.
- We searched for the prophylaxis of these contaminants through the control of the environmental conditions that favored the existence of the causing agent.
- We proposed the following Anthropo-Ecological or Technopathogenologic Hypothesis: The loss of resistance comes as an unexpected consequence to technological modification.
- We presented proposals to prevent or reduce the risk to consumers: New Analysis techniques were developed (Minicolumns and Self Activated Thin Layer Chamber-Plates); use of microbiological and chemical techniques: first visible mycelium, propagules count, determination of acidity (Eguiazu & Frank, 1984); adoption of new criteria applied to selection and genetic improvement of cultivated species; proposal of new parameters for storage and commercialization of grains, HRAI and the development of a new technique for its measurement.
- New, more accurate techniques were developed – they eliminated the false negatives and were more adequate to the conditions in underdeveloped regions. The possibility of analyzing samples with minimum lab requirements allowed to identify contaminated samples that could have otherwise been used for human consumption.
- We proposed a Prophylaxis and Control of Aflatoxins for the Agricultural products Law.
- We considered that such contaminants only represent a minimum portion of the Technopathogenic problem associated to chemical factors since aflatoxins are simply a few out of the vast number of existing substances – whether they are natural or synthetic – that either have a commercial application or that are generated as waste (such as by-products of industrial activity).
- The hypothesis of the existence of non-evident risks that was relevant to mycotoxins – which are natural substances – was extended to other groups of substances of anthropogenic origin, such as pesticides.
- Articles on pesticides were published on different types of publications – one of them on jurisprudence – stressing the need to

bear in mind the long term risks such substances can have in order to establish a more effective protection to consumers.

- We postulate the existence of a phenomenon still undescribed we defined as Technopathogeny.
- We extended this concept to other substances and contaminants in use (both natural and anthropogenic). Through a deductive analysis the manifestation of Technopathogeny in these substances was proved.
- We tried a general prophylaxis with an early detection test of mutagenic effects (Ames test). The idea with this test (which is to be applied to global samples instead of to a substance in particular) is that, supposing the actual substance that provokes the mutation cannot be identified, if the test is nevertheless positive, it can be stated that the human environment is potentially mutagenic for consumers. That is, bacteria can reach what the chemical analysis cannot reach.
- We postulated that Technopathogeny is a global and additive phenomenon.
- We asked the question on prophylaxis. A disciplinary void was found to study this phenomenon.
- We postulated the need of a new discipline, Technopathogenology, to study accurately and efficiently the genesis, detection and prophylaxis of this phenomenon.
- We proposed a specific legislation to deal with this problem in order to provide an adequate protection to consumers: the Technogeny Law (Motta & Eguiazu, 1989).
- Because of the relevance in the safety to consumers we proposed the need of an ethical objector in Science and Technique in order to guarantee the transparency in the genesis and application of technologies and the protection of researchers who see their work jeopardized in the cases in which dealing with certain issues can affect interests.

The observations, demonstrations and results obtained in each of these stages are highly relevant for the protection of consumers. They allowed advancing on this road for more than 30 years and eventually led to the development of Technopathogenology. They can be summarized in the following points:

445

1. In our region, the object of study, mycotoxins, is highly relevant for the consumer's health. We provided grounds that supported its risk.

2. We proved the contamination in batches of corn in our region – therefore, the risk to consumers. The results of regional tests showed that 4.9% of corn of exporting quality was contaminated – which led us to think that such value would be higher in grains destined to local consumption.

3. We observed that bringing to light the degree of contamination in our country would signify financial loss for some of the actors, for corn batches that should have been used for human consumption would have to be used for animal consumption. This would mean a lower market price. We also observed that trying to study issues that dealt with a topic that could not be framed within an existing disciplinary frame generated reticence in the Science and Technique system.

4. The fact that our studies would bring to light such situations allowed us to see clearly that the system was unwilling to unveil the facts. The position of private entities, however, was completely different.

5. We proved that commercial tests were a source of errors since they could lead to false positive and false negative results. The deficiencies in the analysis contribute to the risk of consumers in case of false negative results.

6. Environmental factors cannot always be controlled: favorable conditions for the attack and formation of toxins during storage – where several microenvironments can be generated – are easily developed. If we want a grain system that is *tolerant to errors* (von Weizsäcker, 1986), in which the environmental storage conditions can vary without causing the apparition of mycotoxins, we believe that instead of aiming to an environmental prophylaxis, we should aim to a resistant substrate prophylaxis. We would like to stress the modifying effect of technique, which is fundamental still in apparently natural contaminants such as aflatoxins. We make evident how difficult it is to undo genetic modification if it is related to an unexpected negative characteristic. There is great resistance to modify the substrate if such modifications alter favorable genetic characteristics which make

the product profitable (turnout, for example) and which were sought for decades, even though technopathogenies of late manifestation had been detected.

7. The mycotoxins problem is closely connected to Technique (Production of cultivated varieties, manipulation of grains, commercialization) in the genesis and higher incidence grains contaminated with such substances. Therefore the mycotoxins can be framed within the Technopathogenic phenomenon.

8. The problem can be reduced significantly by using adequate techniques of analysis, manipulation of grains, commercialization and legislative control.

9. The phenomenon of Technopathogeny can manifest itself in other techniques, for example, the use of pesticides. The circumstances of risk and concrete damage to consumers were indeed caused by action or omission of the technical human.

10. We finally verified the inanity of the effort of trying to avoid (if such thing is possible) a contaminant since there is a large number of them and they are continuously generated, making us run always behind the problem. We have also proved the difficulty of developing a relevant and useful legislation (Eguiazu, 1990).

11. The phenomenon affects Technique in general. Technopathogeny is a global and additive phenomenon.

12. There is a need to tackle studies aiming at its prevention. We contribute to this aim with contributions to the evaluation of environmental mutagens and proposals of new Quality Criteria. All these contributions to the problem were possible thanks to the technopathogenological approach. Had the approach been different, it would have been very difficult for us to contribute with such elements.

13. During our research we encountered several difficulties, especially in the attempt of framing our work within known and consolidated disciplines within the Science and Technique system. All these projects in consolidated sciences received funds, but our proposal did not. The evaluators did not understand that the detection and prophylaxis of risks to consumers could be of enough interest to receive financial support. That is to say, that it was a program with individual entity.

14. The reticence of the Science and Technique system to investigate this type of phenomena implies that there are in fact difficulties in their study. It was a problem that resisted to be reduced to disciplines which the system proposed as the only alternative. A question like: Why is the Science and Technique system reticent? One can find many answers but we believe that the answer with most weight is that the Science and Technique system has a conservative attitude. Going back to the analogy we have already used, any piece that does not have exactly the same shape of a mold in particular has to be *reformed or deformed* in order to be able to fit in it. The idea of *proposing a new mold for the new piece* is not even considered. The scientific establishment is reluctant to new molds (Feyerabend, 1986) (Kuhn, 1995) (Lakatos, 1982). It would seem that the Science and Technique system, when facing a complex, new and critical question would react addressing the researcher in the following manner: If you want your work to be promoted or subsidized *in order to evaluate your question we need persons with a background in the subject and specialized in it, i.e., a person suitable to do the evaluation. However, this argument on the search of someone specialized is in fact hiding an interest in seeking somebody from the establishment who, even if such person is no expert, can give an opinion about the new subject.* The Science and Technique system rejects the final sentence: *There is no evaluator for this question.*

15. As for suitability, which is crucial in order to give the right approach to new phenomena, it is very difficult to obtain. Another difficulty is thus found to study new phenomena. It is not uncommon that evaluators who are highly skilled in an area wrongly believe they are qualified to give their opinion in other areas. This leads to a situation in which if evaluators are no specialists on a subject in particular, they analyze such subjects from their field's point of view thus reducing the evaluation only to the aspects that are relevant to their field disregarding the rest which they do not understand. Therefore, it is common to hear, for example, *from the agronomic point of view the project falls short of expectations, or no useful results can be expected from it.* This is endlessly replicated with other disciplines. *Your question must be reduced to the existing disciplines where we already have spe-*

cialized people with important background that are suitable to work on the subject. To sum up, the disappointing conclusion is: *The proposal must be reduced to something the system can understand for the project to be accepted.* If the researcher accepts this requirement, he or she would have failed in intellectual honesty. This attitude is seen when evaluators consider original reports unacceptable stating that not enough information was included in the presentation. This can hide the lack of knowledge of the question sent since if evaluators were experts on the subject they would not need further information, only what is new to the subject. It is as if a writer was asked to include the conjugation of the verb *to write* or if his or her handwriting was evaluated instead of the content – which is quite likely if the evaluators are not writers. In a group of writers the presentation would be reduced to the very essentials or to the new contribution of the writer.

16. The procedure described in the previous point – even though it contributes to the disciplinary formality – does not contribute to the actual progress of knowledge. It is common sense that being a specialist in one discipline does not grant universal wisdom to evaluate every single presentation or project simply based on formal suppositions. The essential original proposal can therefore not be evaluated and is disregarded in the evaluation. *Form* is therefore given more weight than *essence*, as we have seen in the previous reading.

17. The original research on aflatoxins could not be framed with our approach within any consolidated discipline. If we had accepted a partial or reductive approach of it taking it as totality, we would have become specialists in some of those disciplines, but we would have not answered the question on prevention and protection of consumers since further analyzing it would have been substituted by the consolidation of experimental achievements. This is something – a group of substances (aflatoxins) – that harms human beings but we do not know why they are there. The disciplinary inclusion classified by some as corporative (Pengue) is not good to pursue the question with complete freedom. Through subsidies and promotions, the researcher gets tempted to abandon the original question. As for the corporate nature of the system, we are not really sure if it is this way – maybe an ex-

pert in Social Sciences, not us, should analyze this thoroughly – but what we are sure of is that this is a very slow system for changes of paradigm. It is fast to accept innovations within paradigms and existing programs and slow to accept changes in consolidated programs and paradigms. According to Heisenberg as quoted by Hoffmann (Hoffmann, 1997) such changes should also be accompanied by changes of mentality or in the schemes of thought of scientists; if not, they will neither be understood nor accepted. In his famous lecture of 1943 which opened the conferences on *Was ist leben?* (What is life?), Schrödinger said that scientists should not fear to present risky theories even if it meant being the laughing stock of their colleagues (Hoffman, 1997). A change of paradigm or program usually comes along with collegiate moral harassment which turns whoever proposes it into a laughing stock. When the system recognizes the entity of an idea that will enrich the existing programs and paradigms, it accepts the changes but it does not accept the programs or paradigms from which the new ideas originate. The system is open to enrich and continue with the innovations taken as their own innovations and closed to accept where the changes or innovations come from. On the other hand, in many cases there is the temptation of plagiarizing new ideas. In other words, the idea or work of the creator is accepted, but the intellectual property is not.

18. What we described in items 15 through 18 clearly shows the inefficiency of the Science and Technique system within which the future environmental jurists who will be responsible for the protection of consumers work. Thus there is a void that must be filled.

19. The consumer protection system is so far incomplete and does not thoroughly analyze complex risks questions. If, due to what we have observed in the previous item lawyers and jurists are not aware of Technopathogenies; they are unlikely to legislate on a phenomenon they do not know.

20. Just like the aflatoxins process (from their genesis until they reach consumers) is of an enormous complexity, which determines the enormous difficulty in the prevention of such contaminant, the processes involving the apparition of other factors with a potential technopathogenic risk are also very complex. This leads us to think that without a specific science, attempting to

450

approach the prevention of such risks in a multidisciplinary manner (Analytical Chemistry, Jurisprudence, Medicine, Toxicology, etc.) will not have the expected efficiency.

21. Some risks are minimized by the institutions and then it is late (sometimes too late) when they are recognized and, if at all possible, eventually neutralized.

22. We have provided the grounds for the Technopathogeny phenomenon.

23. We have developed the methodological bases for Technopathogenology.

24. As a Science, Technopathogenology fills in the void in the disciplinary field applied to the study of technological risks, since it focuses on the causes of the technological gestation and not on the consequences.

25. It promotes educating professional technologists about the existence of the phenomenon and its causes so that they can detect potential causes of technopathogenic risk in the early stages of its development – both for consumers and for people occupationally exposed – before it becomes unavoidable.

26. We proposed a change of paradigm: instead of: *Create, apply, wait to see if there are unexpected side effects, correct the errors on the way*, we propose to change it for: *Prevent in the technological matrix*. In other words, the old paradigm: *Technology is almost innocuous since the Science that has originated is almost infallible. The few exceptions are unimportant, so let us continue with this as we have it*, should be changed by the following paradigm: *Technology brings about Technopathogenies, let us keep on progressing but with the incorporation of a specific science: Technopathogenology*.

27. In this whole process, from mycotoxins to Technopathogenology, we find what we could define as: *The same intellectual leit motif: Protection of humans, consumers or citizens*. Such *leit motif* was neither understood nor accepted by evaluators. The scientific/academic/administrative system kept sending our question to evaluators who were not experts in our field, and we therefore obtained negative results.

28. It was necessary to begin another line of investigation related to it: Quality of the evaluative act in questions that imply substan-

tial changes of approach and method and proposals of change in ethical paradigms.

29. Technopathogenology would provide ethical objectors with several valuable elements to aid their crucial participation in Science and Technique. When we speak of Technopathogenology we are speaking of a scientific discipline which has ethical analysis as one of its pillars – along the entire risk process under study. Creating a discipline that includes ethics within its framework makes it very difficult to hush what ethical objectors have to say. In other words, we could say that ethical objectors stand on solid ground since there is a scientific discipline that provides them with clear elements of knowledge with which they will soundly report the problems encountered. This avoids that other researchers who are not that committed *hide* the problem, and work leaving it aside.

We have described the participation of the ethical objector in consumer protection in an article that dealt with The Quality of Foodstuffs and the Protection of Consumers (Eguiazu & Motta, 2004b). Our proposal focused on the fact that problems involving service to consumers are very delicate since consumers generally do not have the knowledge required to know what they are consuming. Therefore, an easy solution would be that the ethical objector detects everything that damages consumer's health, but he or she must know what to focus on and therefore there must be a science which specifically studies such phenomenon. Without a Science for ethical objectors to learn to find the critical points in Science and Technique, their activity will be highly restricted, since there will be critical points they will not detect simply for not knowing they exist.

We therefore believe that the best contribution to ethical objectors in Science and Technique is to teach them about the object of study through a science thus providing consumers with elements to defend their rights against the ones who deceive them with false scientific information. Given the lack of a specific science to study this phenomenon, the problem is disregarded and therefore unsolved. Just like in other disciplines in which the scientist who is ethically committed to the search for knowledge, the technopathogenologist is, in essence, an ethical objector. Maybe this is one of the reasons why this discipline is so much rejected in the traditional Science and Technique system. Nevertheless, the ethical objector must be someone specialized and have the administrative and legal support needed to comply with his or her hard task.

Conclusion

In this reading we have demonstrated that consumers are exposed to non-evident risks we call technopathogenic. Precisely because they are not evident, such risks are not given the necessary relevance both by consumers and by protection policies. Such policies focus on more evident, concrete and short-term problems. Technopathogenology focuses on the part of the risk phenomenon which is not contemplated by these policies.

We have supported the fact that consumers must be protected from technopathogenic risks. Now, if consumers we call *Active Consumers* (because they are the direct beneficiaries of a technique) must be protected, much more should *Passive Consumers* be protected. Practically everybody knows the figure of the Passive Smoker, a person exposed to the smoke (residue) of a product that he or she does not consume. A great effort is made to protect these persons. In the same way, we can call *Passive Consumers* those persons exposed to the *residues* of a Technique which he or she does not benefit of. Therefore, such persons should have more right to be protected (Motta, 2011).

Just like with mycotoxins, there are several other cases of technopathogenic risk which are not considered and to which consumers can be exposed for decades without any measures being taken.

As described in the last summary of point 20, the problem with mycotoxins shows that if such enormous complexity is found in a single problem associated to technique, what can we expect then of other technological risks?

The current preventive elements are not adequate. The technique is corrected once the damage has manifested itself. Until this day, the period of exposure on consumers cannot be avoided until the technological noxa is recognized and inactivated.

We believe the inclusion of Technopathogenology is necessary for it aims at detecting subtle differences in Technique which can lead to defects in them. Such potential defects can be responsible for damages on human health. Technopathogenology is a science that detects subtle differences in technique – just as a botanist can detect differences between two plants that could be regarded as the same species by other botanists who were not interested in showing such differences.

It is necessary to adopt the Technopathogenological criterion which states that, when in doubt about the innocuousness of a Technique, precautions which favor consumers and not the businessman must be adopted.

The uneasiness suffered by the researcher to investigate the areas described should be shared by consumers. Consumers should not be passive and wait for scientists to solve problems. Consumers must be aware and participate actively asking for adequate reports if they suspect any kind of risk – which would also contribute to avoid or lessen the difficulties in the study of this type of phenomena within the Science and Technique framework. The ethical objector would represent such associations of consumers. In the scientific system, this would encourage the training of evaluators – since it would demonstrate the existence of an evaluative void. Let us not forget that Technopathogenology was systematically rejected by scientific evaluators simply because it did not fit within the existing disciplines. A discipline in gestation is systematically denied or oppressed for a long time. This should be avoided, even though History shows that this is what happens with any new scientific proposal.

We therefore provided grounds for the necessity of Technopathogenology as a discipline to achieve an efficient protection of human health from technological risks. This is of paramount importance because it is mentioned that technology first *captures, seizes the consumer who then becomes dependent* or *captive,* or *handcuffed* to the necessity of such technology and must inevitably accept its risks as a price of progress. About this dependence it is very interesting to comment on the case of cellular phones. It is mentioned that the dependence can be such that it can lead to *nomophobia* (no-mobile-phone phobia): a total dependence of the cellular phone – the person cannot conceive or imagine life without it. According to information (Alfred, 2011), 53 % of cellular telephone system users suffer this psychic disorder. In relation with the consumer's health, we can see that this technological devise is related to two technopathogenies: a somatic technopathogeny (epidemiological studies performed by the International Agency for Research on Cancer, demonstrate that the cellular phones can favor certain tumors in the head (Dubois, 2009)) and a psychic technopathogeny, because it can lead to nomophobia.

Our findings throughout thirty years of investigations were neither perfect nor irrefutable, but they allowed us to develop a theory.

III. Technopathogenology and its economic implications

Introduction

The economic implications of the short and long term risks associated to technologies are known worldwide. This is proved by the development of disciplines or multidisciplines such as: Technological Evaluation, Environmental Impact Evaluation, Cycle of Life Evaluation, Risk Management, etc.

Throughout this reading, we will try to describe the short, mid and long term economic implications, the training of a modern technologist in Technopathogenology would have and then contribute to the idea of its utility and applicability in modern technology (Eguiazu & Motta, 2001a).

Which economic implications do technopathogenological risks have?

In order to answer this question, we had to approach it from two different viewpoints:
a. The human being as a victim of technopathogenies and
b. The consequence on the technique itself when finding a defect in it.

From the point of view of a), the long term economic implications are the consequences on human health. Analyzing a disease from an exclusively economic aspect, it is important to do calculations and ask ourselves:

How much does the treatment of the Non-Hodgkin lymphoma cost to workers spraying 2,4-D?

How much does the treatment of beriberi cost?

How much does the treatment of mesothelioma caused by asbestos cost?

How much does the treatment of Thalidomide children cost?

How much do orthopedic devices or accompanying persons (who will be needed throughout the patients' lives) cost to them?

How much does a treatment for leukemia caused by electromagnetic fields or power lines cost?

How much does a treatment for primary liver cancer caused by aflatoxins cost?

All these cases can be considered damage by action. We can also ask ourselves:

How much do medical treatment for diseases associated to the lack of vitamins and other essential nutrients – caused by the intake of poor biological quality foodstuffs – cost? The relevance of the damages we have called *by omission* is already being considered by developed countries. This is proved by the growth of biological or organic agriculture.

From the point of view of b), a technique with a potential defect that can cause a Technopathogeny (for instance, raw materials used for human consumption). In order to see the economic implications of technopathogenies in the short or medium term we can ask ourselves, for example:

How much does it cost to incinerate cows suspected to suffer from encephalopathy?

How much does it cost to destroy grains contaminated with aflatoxins? Or, which is the economic loss if they have to be used for animal consumption?

How much does it cost to reject grains contaminated with carcinogen pesticides residues?

The answers to these questions – both in relation to humans and to raw materials – would constitute a paper in itself, however, for the present work's sake, we believe it is not necessary to measure the economic losses in order to prove that Technopathogeny has economic implications.

Were these facts avoidable prior to their appearance?

The big question the technologist asks is whether technopathogenies and their consequent economic losses could be foreseen before their actual manifestation. The signals did exist. Let us analyze, for example, the following questions:

Were such signals not heard by the manufacturers or people involved because their conscience was numbed by the enthusiasm generated by the positive aspects of the technique in question?

456

Can we think that Technopathogenies were simply inevitable due to the imperfection of the scientific tools used?

Which hints or suspicions of risk were there before the massive liberation of such technologies?

Which degree of knowledge was there about their potential risk?

Was the damage justified for economic reasons only for the corporation or both for the corporation and consumers?

Did consumers accept it because of the immediate benefit obtained?

Would a technopathogenological training of the technologist have had positive consequences in the economy?

What we are also interested in here, in our role as educators, is that Technopathogenology be included in the career programs in careers that study the use and creation of technologies that can cause technopathogenies.

Going back to the case of DDT, what would have happened if Paul Müller had studied Technopathogenology as an undergraduate? Would he have developed DDT?

Even though Cottam denounced in 1946 the environmental risks of the product, it was too late and the business was already working (Cottam, 1946). Who would dare to make it go back?

Even though it is known that humans are the only animals who make the same mistake twice, we must use the DDT example to avoid making the same mistake with new technologies.

Provable and proven facts of modern technology praxis

It is common place that the application of technologies believed to be safe not only do not always bring about the expected results but also bring about unexpected results. When such unexpected results are negative to human health, they are called *technogeny* or *technopathogeny.* The effects can be of such magnitude that in some cases they can astonish the Science and Technique system and, in other cases, cause the collapse of the possibilities of avoiding negative effects. This would happen when the negative effect on human health has become evident. For instance, people living near a nuclear plant can suffer the consequences of the inadvertent leakage of nuclear material by showing a significant increase of cancer in the population. Once this disease appears, only palliative measures can be applied; the damage has already been done. Sometimes, if there are great interests at stake to defend the technological product – which is already finished and is massively sold in the market – some scientists of doubtful ethics deny or minimize the side effects in order to defend the business' interests.

In some cases, if the situation cannot be sustained, evaluators of doubtful ethics are sought to minimize the risk if the product or technology is exported to other countries. This is what happened with the systematic export of pesticides. It is cheaper to invest in evaluators who are tolerant to the product than to substitute the product based on non-evident unacceptable damage to humans.

Another example referred to biological technology is the denial of the effects of the so-called genetic erosion found in crops which are prone to the apparition of aflatoxins – and, more recently, to the potential or actual side effects of some transgenic crops – in order to defend their massive use.

It seems that it is less costly to attend to the possible lawsuits for damages. Such damages must be proved and, like any damage either to a human being or to the environment, it is more difficult to prove its causality than to invest in the experimental verification of its safety for consumers. In other words, even though potential side effects of a product are suspected, in some cases it is left anyway in the market. Cold economic calculations can demonstrate that not all the victims will sue the company and that not all of those who do sue will win the case. Even though the company will lose some cases and pay large amounts of money, the sum will always be less than the investment in backing out a development. Even leaving aside the human aspect, we believe that it is not a good business for the company since nowadays this kind of speculations is rapidly known and spread, thus damaging the image of a company.

It is also less costly to invest in tolerant evaluators, who may or may be not part of government institutions, who minimize the risks or contribute to the indetermination, uncertainty or lack of cause of the risk phenomenon – or even attribute it to a false cause – than to invest in research on safety before the technology has been developed.

This denial of risks causes that, in general, it takes a while from the moment a technopathogenic harm is detected until it is attributed to the technology that caused it and even more until the technology is stopped and recalled from the market.

This means that real damage will necessarily occur since the relatively long time of usage is a fact. Once the damage appears – sometimes in humans, such as the bovine spongiform encephalopathy – the system slowly starts to recall or substitute the technology. If there is a high pressure of voters, the measures are taken faster, at a pace that make the ensuing economic losses worse, as happened with the cremation of livestock in England. Had consumers not been well informed and had not pressured the government through efficient mechanisms they would have most likely eaten the livestock with the knowledge of the governmental control institutions. The existence of informed consumers guarantees an adequate conduct on the part of the institutions.

In order to focus more on the essence of this paper, we will now further explore the economic implications Technopathogenies might have in addition to the damages to human health.

Our experience with a natural contaminant Aflatoxin:
A complex technopathogenological example with economic implications

Because of our personal experience, in our analysis we will discuss agricultural technology, especially in connection with grain handling and production and its contamination with aflatoxins.

We have seen that the phenomenon called *technogeny* or *technopathogeny* associated to aflatoxins can be recognized in agricultural technology. Not only must this be recognized in the most evident – i.e. common practices in agriculture such as cultivation, harvesting, genetic selection, etc., but it must also be extended to the post-harvest handling and finally, to the elaboration of foodstuffs. It is very important that this phenomenon be associated with the need of a specific science that responds to the ordinary citizen's constitutional right to have environmental information (Eguiazu & Motta, 2001a). If the technopathogenic phenomenon can be recognized in the agronomic practice, the analysis can be extended to other practices of interest; therefore, we may find long term immanent and hidden consequences to human health in several techniques (for example, a dam, an industrial residues combustion plant or a high voltage power line, etc.).

Let us go back to our work and experience with mycotoxins and focus on the aspects that are most relevant for this reading. In 1974, an official from the former Junta Nacional de Granos in Argentina suggested that we should initiate our research on the presence of a carcinogenic contaminant in grains (aflatoxins). The reason for this was that he had information of contaminated corn batches and peanuts that were rejected by importing countries. We never imagined that this was just the beginning of a long journey. The first thing that caught our attention was the fact that we received a prize from the Rosario Stock Exchange (Eguiazu, 1976), which showed interest in our work and decided to support it. Sadly, the interest shown by this institution, which groups several commercial entities, was not replicated by academic/scientific institutions. The scientific community disregarded the problem, arguing that the fact that it was not adequately framed gave it little entity to any relevant scientific discipline. This meant that for an Analyst Chemist, our work hardly meant any progress in knowledge; for a Plant Physiologist, there was nothing new on it; for a Traditional Economist, it was a problem of market quality.

A question arose which remained unanswered: Which is the science that contributes to our question in a strict and thorough manner? The research on the causes of the contaminant continued, as we have said, with the environmental aspects that are involved in the generation of such contaminant and other similar substances from the same family.

For this research we used sunflower cultivars, since the presence of mycotoxins in them was by far less known than in corn.

For such studies and because we were working with a wide variety of samples (in chemical composition and in physical constitution) we found that some cultivars were more sensitive to the attack of the causing agent and to get contaminated with the carcinogenic substance (Eguiazu, 1983).

Trying to find the causes of this, we found a strong connection between it and the technological changes made on the primeval or original species. Such technologic changes had been carried out by geneticists to incorporate desirable economic and agronomic characteristics to the crop. This led inadvertently to a reduction in the natural resistance of the crop to the attack of aflatoxins producing molds. Thus the question: What is more important, to study the characteristics of the producing mold and of the contaminant's chemical composition or to focus on the circumstances that favored their apparition? If we add to this the technological characteristics of the storage and industrialization of grains –

which also favor the apparition of mycotoxins – we can see that the technological phenomenon involved in the apparition of these contaminants is undeniable.

At first we called it the *Anthropo-ecological Hypothesis of the apparition of mycotoxins*, but now we can call it the *Technopathogenological Hypothesis*, which helps to explain the apparition of mycotoxins in almost any profitable grain (Eguiazu & Motta, 1997).

This hypothesis contradicts an old argument that minimizes the apparition of contaminants of industrial origin and which is worth going back to: that aflatoxins (and mycotoxins in general) have always existed in nature and, just like Humanity survived them in the past, it will also survive other contaminants.

This is an opinion supported by many scientists who choose to ignore that even though these are natural contaminants, the way they enter humans and the damage they cause are of a technological nature. The little support we received to continue our research on these contaminants in order to contribute to their prophylaxis led us to ask ourselves: Is it because there is not a science to study this phenomenon?

The lack of a specific science is closely connected to the lack of suitable evaluators, that is, people with a solid background and who thoroughly know the subject because they have worked on the issue or similar issues for many years but with the same approach, with the same question. This systematic doubt on where to frame the problem has led us to frame it, as we described in Chapter II, within several different disciplines: Agricultural Chemistry, Mycology, Foodstuffs Technology, Analytical Chemistry, Climatology and Grain Post-harvest handling. We have seen that even though this approach partially answered certain questions, it made it increasingly more difficult to answer the basic question; it only kept us drifting apart from the original question: the connection between technology and the presence of carcinogenic contaminants. This is the reason why even if there was in our country, and for many years, a specific program to study mycotoxins, it did not solve the actual problem of the systematic apparition of such contaminant in grain batches that were detected by the quality control offices in strict international markets. It neither solved the problem of economic losses. Even though researchers who were experts in different aspects of the problem were supported, and even though there was a progress in knowledge, the basic problem was barely solved.

The experience we have just described proved that apart from the risk on health – which is what led us to begin our research – mycotoxins implied economic implications. Therefore, any work aiming at the prevention of their apparition and contact with humans will not only mean a reduction in risk on health but also in economic losses.

The economic implications of these contaminants might be related to various reasons:

a) *Associated to the technopathogenic effect*

The medical treatments and other damages applied to or suffered by victims of intoxications with such substances.

b) *Associated to the presence of the contaminant*

The presence of mycotoxins in grains implies an economic loss due to the downgrade in quality or, in extreme cases, due the compulsory destruction of the product. This is what happens when the product, given its high level of contamination, not only should not be used for human consumption, but it should neither be used for animal consumption. In connection to the reduction of economic loss, an analytical technique and a technique to stop the development of the aflatoxins producing molds were developed.

The first contribution came up when we asked ourselves this question: Why can't a simple and easy to obtain technique be developed, a technique that detects the contaminated grain thus avoiding risk and economic loss? By being able to detect incipient levels of contamination, measures can be adopted: Grain can be stopped from reaching human consumption, and measures in the grain handling stage can be adopted in order to avoid further contamination so that the product can at least be used for animal consumption.

Other losses can be caused, for example, by mixing contaminant-free batches with contaminated batches. For instance, 1 kg of highly contaminated grain can affect the value of a whole hectare of grain. However, the presence of the contaminant is very difficult to avoid since the kilogram of contaminated grain can be present in only a few corncobs which are not recognized and separated by the harvesting machine, making contamination by contact inevitable. The application of an analytical technique could therefore avoid the risk of contaminated batches ruining large quantities of uncontaminated batches.

As for the second contribution, it is supported by the following concept: Even though mycotoxins can be developed in the field, the main form of their apparition in grains is during storage. Producing molds are known as storage molds, since, during this stage, the Intergranular Relative Air Humidity is, together with temperature, a determining factor in the development of molds. This is why we resorted to a prophylaxis method in order to preventively measure the Intergranular Relative Air Humidity: Its application would provide more safety than by using only the value of grain humidity currently in use – as we have already explained when we referred to aflatoxins.

c) *Associated to marketing criteria*

The use of the HRAI parameter has an economic connotation, since the usage of the Relative Humidity Parameter instead of the Humidity Content parameter could make producers sell their grain with less levels of humidity than those commercially accepted. That is to say, with the usage of the Relative Humidity parameter, the agriculturist will have less kilograms to sell. Let us not forget that, for example, if the commercialization humidity is of 15% and producers sell their grain with a 12% of humidity (because they stored with such humidity content in order to avoid molding), it means that they will lose 30 kilograms per ton. The persons responsible for the stockpile might very well ask: who will pay for the 30 kg of grain lost per ton? The question is ethical, since those grains which are commercialized and/or stored with the levels of humidity indicated by the commercialization regulations can represent a risk of fungal activity and therefore the generation of mycotoxins. This is what happens with the sunflower grain in which cultivars with a high level of oil (a parameter aimed at by genetic selection) have a high humidity level for commercialization, and therefore, there is water in the grain available for the development of molds (Motta, 1985).

So we asked ourselves: Is this a posteriori effort worth it? Isn't it better to focus the effort on the origin of the problem? And if the origin of the problem is the Technique, why wasn't it thought of before the development of the technological object? (In this case, grains and the so-called post-harvest handling.) Why wasn't the prophylaxis against all risks – even the non-evident and non-acceptable – first adopted? What went wrong in the creation of the actual technology? Why was this problem not tackled? However, these questions led to another situation that has an economic implication, which we describe in the point below.

d)   Associated to the technologies of genetic improvement

This is another paradigmatic example of late economic implications since, as we have seen, basing the genetic selection to obtain cultivars resistant on fungal attack can signify economic loss. This is so because such cultivars may produce a lower turnout as an unwanted agronomic and industrial effect (in quantity of grain, for example, or amount of oil obtained). Measures should be adopted or analyzed in order to compensate the producer or businessman for the inevitable quantitative losses that would come as a result of sowing grains that are resistant to contamination with mycotoxins. It would also be interesting to investigate what happens with the implementation of every new transgenic crop. Apart from the expected benefits, are there any unexpected negative effects?

This is why an economic problem connected to these contaminants is also present in the prevention attempts. It is evident that the Science and Technique system can be unwilling to include research of these contaminants from the technopathogenological point of view. This approach is not accepted since it could affect the development of other consolidated research issues – whether governmental or private or both – aiming at the production of agricultural products responding to the conventional parameters of quality thus affecting their economic interests.

We therefore postulate the need of *Technopathogenology* which, as a preventive and systematic study applied to the development of any technique (agricultural, livestock, chemical, electronic productions, etc.) would not only avoid the damage of human health but also the economic loss due to the lower quality of the products obtained, due to the cost of having to recall from the market dangerous products, due to the loosing of strict markets, etc.

The Ecological Knapsack and the Technopathogenological Knapsack

The concept of the Ecological Knapsack is an interesting concept proposed by Dr. Schmidt-Bleek (Schmidt-Bleek, 2007) which aimed at reducing the ecological damage or waste of resources. This concept praises efficient production in terms of saving matter and energy which produces long-lasting technological products.

According to Dr. Schmith-Bleek, for any technological development there is a waste of matter and energy from having developed the product, that is, a kind of *Ecological Knapsack* which is inherent to every technological product.

For example, he says that such waste is not only found in the concrete material that was used, but also in the material that was discarded for this development and also in the waste during transport of the raw materials from one place of the Earth to another. Dr. Schmith-Bleek states that the costs which are part of this Ecological Knapsack are not currently borne in mind – at least not all of them – in the economic analysis performed for the production of any given product. That is to say, the Industry is only interested in the economic cost of the materials that are used or wasted, not in its ecological cost. For example, in the paper production industry, only the cost of the wood is of concern, but not its ecological impact, such as cutting down trees and reducing forests, which includes the desertification of lands, the loss of landscapes, etc. The consideration of an ecologic cost would include, for example, the cost of reconstituting an area to its original state after extracting coal.

The concept of the Ecological Knapsack is also interesting from the immediate damage on health that a product could eventually cause.

Another interesting aspect is the life span of a product. A long lasting product without failures would have less Ecological Knapsack than a product with a short life span which would have to be discarded, thus promoting the use and waste of more resources. This is an interesting concept.

We can therefore apply this whole concept to Technopathogenology and, paraphrasing Dr. Schmith-Bleek speak of a *Technopathogenological Knapsack.* This concept does not contemplate the ecological costs but the long-term health costs on human health – which would be a contribution to Dr. Schmith-Bleek's concept.

If the ecological economic implications involved in the development of a product were born in mind, the development of such product would have a minimum damage of the ecosystem and a minimum damage of human health in the short-term. If the Technopathogenological Knapsack was born in mind in the development of new products, the least possible long-term risk would be aimed at.

In addition, a technique conceived with a technopathogenological perspective in mind would have a smaller Knapsack, since in the application stage the measures to fix a risk would be much less than in a technique conceived without technopathogenological concepts.

Prospective and conclusion

Using as example the praxis in Agronomy and conservation, storage and foodstuff preparation, a series of critical points can be recognized which, if ignored, can lead to defects in the final product, that is to say, bad biological and biopathological quality which can cause Technopathogenies.

In addition, this phenomenon also has an impact on the economic side.

It is interesting to verify, then, that there is a phenomenon which is completely an orphan of a specific science (*Technopathogenology*), which explains the poverty of traditional, reductionist evaluations that cannot grasp the essence of the phenomenon: non-evident and hidden risks in technology which manifest in the long term.

Another aspect that proves this *orphanage*, apart from the lack of a specific science and evaluators specifically trained is the orphanage for citizens who want to make use of their right to have environmental information. This right has been established in Argentina by Art. 41 in the Constitution.

The Nordic Council of Ministers considers the right to what they call *Environmental Information* as important as basic human rights. This would include information on any side effects of any process or technology.

How can citizens make use of their right to have environmental information if there are no specialists who can generate trustworthy information? Every contribution in this regard is a product of other disciplines; we could say that it was taken by other approaches or other objects of study which contribute with part of what is necessary, but fragmentarily and with little efficacy. A strict scientific hermeneutic work (of interpretation) is required in order to allow interpreting and getting from

466

every work what is of interest to the citizen. That is, comprehension and interpretation are also crucial in the scientific-technological work because, if interpretations are taken for granted, they can lead to serious mistakes, among them, the technopathogeny phenomenon.

We speak of a hermeneutic/scientific approach following Gadamer's postulate (Dutt, 1993) coming from the sciences of the spirit:

> ... from Thomas Kuhn onwards, it is believed that there also a hermeneutics of the natural sciences, since a reasonable application of natural scientific results to the life's praxis cannot be obtained only by natural scientific methods.

The author speaks of the need of an independent and specific method in natural sciences to develop techniques and the application of knowledge.

According to this author, the Natural Sciences methodology is not enough to apply accurately its own results. In order to be passed on to humans – the ultimate recipient of any scientific effort – such accurate application should be accompanied by a specific hermeneutics.

We can therefore understand the enormous lack of environmental information and, more specifically, the lack of information on the side effects of technique, since the scientific-technological world is only awakening from its long lethargy.

The goal companies have of obtaining short-sighted benefits cannot be accepted any longer.

The Hannover World Exposition 2000, which resembled the 1933 Chicago World Fair, had an interesting motto to quote as conclusion: Humankind-Nature-Technology.

Its aims are also interesting to reproduce here:

> The Expo's aims are not to show competitiveness but rather how humankind, with the aid of Technique, can achieve a new balance with nature following the postulates of the Agenda 21 of sustainable development.

This is substantially different from the Chicago World Fair, which privileged Technique over humans. The paradigm has clearly changed – the aim has stopped being adjusting Human and Nature to Technique, but has shifted to a harmonious and intelligent coexistence among the three. The motto and aims are much more reasonable than those back in 1933.

This approach had already been under work by the Langenbruck project, created and directed by Prof. Fornallaz, founder of the Swiss

Academic Society for Environmental Research and Ecology (SAGUF). This group proposed and followed a new kind of Economics called *Ecological Economics* (Fornallaz, 1986).

This reading can lead to a new research line on the subject so as to quantify the magnitude of the losses for not bearing in mind technopathogenies and also the possible profits for bearing them in mind.

There have been similar studies to address the problem of the consumption of tobacco and lung cancer. Having determined the millions of dollars that would be saved if consumption were reduced, it is our wish that the same is done with the prophylaxis of technopathogenies: it would save pain, diseases and expensive treatment as well as economic losses for not being able to export products whose technopathogeny cannot be excluded by a solid previous study.

As we will see in the following reading, the contribution of Technopathogenology to the development of new quality criteria will allow obtaining products which meet the need of consumers. This concept is worth mentioning since the development of products of a higher quality than traditional massive consumption products can mean that certain products can be classified as *unconventional* in the market thus allowing a higher price for them, i.e., another positive implication of Technopathogenology to Economy.

The great challenge for experts in Economy is to have a technopathogenological training in order to be able to say how much a technopathogeny costs. And, just as with Industrial Engineering, whose contributions to reduce evident risks provide companies with measures to avoid loss, economists should be able to prove how much money they can actually save if technopathogenological criteria are applied to any technological development for prophylaxis.

IV. Technopathogenology and new quality criteria

Introduction

In this sense, Technopathogenology is a contribution for both the consumer and the company and it is closely related to the previous reading.

In Chapter I, we mentioned that apart from the positive aspects, Technique has several negative ones which can be either evident or non-evident – the latter being of technopathogenological relevance. We have also said that negative aspects affect the relationship between Humans/Human Environment due to the alteration in the correspondence and proportion of the components of both the Human Environment and Humans – an alteration that can occur by either action or omission. We then classified risks as risks by action and risks by omission.

If technique takes or incorporates components from the human environment and if we consider that Quality is defined as "The group of qualities (features) of a person or thing" (Diccionario Enciclopédico Ilustrado de la Lengua Española), we can say that Technique alters the quality of the human environment.

There are no known parameters of quality applied to the Human Environment. The usual procedure is to make reference to pollution by a substance or radiation, for example, in cases of impoverishment of the quality of the air, water, etc. In general, quality parameters are applied to goods that have been already produced. We therefore developed the concepts of Biological and Biopathological Quality so that we could apply them to the Human Environment. Evidently, if the human environment is responsible for damages of human health, we consider that quality criteria parameters must be established.

This led us to propose quality criteria for the Human Environment, which we supported using the criteria used by the agricultural and livestock industry.

The difficulty in making the different quality criteria compatible allows us to use an ancient sailors' problem as analogy:

Passing between Scylla and Charybdis:
the dilemma of modern agricultural and livestock production

In the Strait of Messina, in Sicily, there is a famous rock shoal called Scylla and, by it, a famous whirlpool called Charybdis. Whoever has read the classics knows that sailors in the Antiquity had to be careful of not falling on one or the other. Thus, in European languages, the phrase *passing between Scylla and Charybdis* is used as a symbol of impartiality and measure, in order to avoid two major risks or as an example of avoiding to falling in a risk attempting to escape another.

The situation of Scylla and Charybdis is repeated in various analogies in connection to the modern agricultural and livestock production.

Quantity and quality: The first analogy

Since Ancient Times, agricultural and livestock production has been motivated by two very clear aims: to produce enough to feed local population and to use the rest to exchange with neighbors. All this produce had to respond to certain quality parameters. Agriculturists would take their produce to the market and profit from good sales and for responding to the buyers' quality standards – who would do their best to find something in the product that would give them a reason to request to lower the price of the product (i.e. find aspects that lowered the quality of the product).

Therefore, from the primitive ancient markets to Medieval markets (of which, in some European cities, we can still find the squares where the markets were held), to modern virtual electronic operations, the essence has not changed. Quantity and Quality are the same concepts as were in ancestral cultures but some fundamental aspects have actually changed.

Quantity and quality: Past and present

We can say that the essential that has changed in these concepts is not *how* but *what,* which we can explain as follows:

Quantity

This point is simple, since the aim of the agricultural and livestock production paradigm has always been the same.

But there is an essential difference. In the past, it was known that in order to increase the output quantitatively, both the area sown and the number of working hands had to be increased.

However, modern agricultural and livestock production show us the contrary: with less hands – i.e. people dedicated to agriculture – more is produced for the same or even less productive surface.

In order for this to be possible, the ancient human work and surface sown are substituted by making profound changes in the species to be sown and, if possible, also on the soil where they will be grown. Other examples are: mechanization, fertilization, agro chemistry, irrigation and genetic modification of the species.

Quality

Let us imagine two grain buyers: one in Medieval Times and one in Modern Times. We can imagine someone in a medieval market inspecting the grains, observing and checking there is no mold or insects, that is, visual characteristics, and also organoleptic characteristics such as smell and flavor, etc. We imagine someone who is trying to establish the price of what he or she will purchase only using his or her senses. Today, however, a buyer will probably demand complex chemical analysis to guarantee the presence of certain factors and check the absence of undesired ones.

That is, from the old medieval market in which buyers could base their decision on rudimentary parameters, we moved to modern times in which the parameters on which buyers base their decisions *cannot be seen*, i.e., they require more than the old organoleptic evaluation. This new evaluation goes from simple analyses – such as water content – to complex genetic material evaluations. In spite of the increasing complexity of the requirements, they are, in essence, always *what the client wants*.

And what the client wants is increasingly *what consumers want*. But what consumers want is not always the same. They always want more and what they want sometimes lies on scientific knowledge or grounds and sometimes on momentary trends.

There was then a revolution in the concept of quality. Quality stopped being a market concept to become a demand of consumers. The purchaser and salesman do not set the rules alone anymore: they must comply with the demands of consumers. Therefore, purchasers and salesmen have to model their decision upon what consumers want. In the revolution of quality, purchasers and consumers merge into one single criterion.

Technology must therefore listen to other requirements generated by the final user of a product – a user who, if rightly informed on the quality of a product will not be easily convinced by purely commercial arguments. For example, trying to impose aspects that make a product visually appealing instead of offering or stressing the nutritional values of the product. Such characteristics go beyond those generated by the *internal mechanisms* of the Science and Technique and Management systems. Informed consumers want biological and biopathological quality, which is proved by the widespread growth of organic agriculture. This situation was unexpected half a century ago. Consumers passively accepted the industry and management criteria. There was a blind faith in Science and Technique supported by more or less naive publicity on the wellness of products. In table 32 we summarize the evolution of quality criteria from 1933 to 1995 (Eguiazu, 1998).

Table 32: Evolution of criteria according to quality criteria for consumers from 1933 to 1995.

Science, Technology and Industry System	Consumer or citizen
1933 Establishes consuming patterns. Classical criterion, based solely on profit. Economy = higher profit. Same patterns in industry and consumer.	Passively accepted the science, technology and industry and management criteria (including advertising).[1]
1995 Must adapt criteria to those demanded by citizens or informed consumers.	Establishes the rules and proposes science, technology, industry and management the quality parameters in foodstuffs based on health care.

Why use the Scylla and Charybdis analogy?

We can see then that, on the one hand, there is an accelerated and essential change in the methods that allow for an increasing production. On the other, an increasing and essential change in connection to what is required and who is the one who requires it – i.e. quality for consumers.

The researcher's question is therefore: Are these two processes in harmony or is there a phase lag or lack of coordination between them?

Or rather: Is the productive process continuously fed by consumers' demands or is it that quantitative production only imperfectly, and more than once belatedly gives consumers what they want?

Does the dilemma we used for the title of this reading actually exist or is it only an intellectual exaggeration?

---

1   *Science Finds, Industry Applies, Man Adapts* was the motto of the Chicago World Fair (quoted by José Sanmartín) (San Martín, 1987).

Below we will try to answer this question.

We have seen that the evolution of foodstuff and raw material quality has always worried humankind.

Grains, the most basic foodstuff, have had commercial relevance since Antiquity and since immemorial times. Its commerce has always been regulated by quality criteria that ensured its value as foodstuff. It was known that the grain quality could be altered by both external and internal factors – among the latter, the loss of germination capacity of the seed.

Among external factors we can mention physical factors that can lead to the loss of quality, such as humidity and temperature or insects and other animals, their parts or feces, certain microorganisms such as molds (biological factors), etc.

Nowadays other factors appear: human errors in the gestation and application of technologies or in the interpretation of market requirements – which is why many products are rejected by consumers who find the product does not satisfy their needs. Nowadays new market requirements motivate the incorporation of new concepts such as Total Quality, which we will refer to later.

The dynamics of commercial exchanges among countries lead to, among other aspects, the unification of quality criteria both for buying and selling countries. Such criteria must be constantly revised.

Bearing in mind the Total Quality Criteria, any new member wanting to integrate a block must thoroughly analyze each of the parameters of the product it wants to buy or sell in order to respond to the market requirements.

Consumers are more and more informed about food quality in connection to health; they establish market trends in the strictest countries and are willing to pay overpriced products if they respond to their needs.

This phenomenon is verified by the growth of *organic production*, which follows biologic and biopathological criteria. By organic production we refer to non-chemointensive production, as the following table shows (Eguiazu, 1994). It is not related to green production or the so-called Green Revolution – which was motivated by turnout criteria rather than by biological and biopathological criteria. There are even specific parameters to differentiate and evaluate products cultivated with organic agriculture from those cultivated with conventional agriculture (FIBL, 2006).

Table 33:   Production schemes for the three models

A – Organic	B – Intermediate	C– Chemointensive
• Production must be done without any chemical products. • Only ancient cultivars must be used and only combining crops obtains better production. • The final product quality aims by consumers. • Biological and Biopathological Quality. The aim is not to leave any chemical residue in the production, even the so called *allowed*. • Low or no environmental and/or intoxication risk for the worker or producer. • The final product does not have chemical residues. • This type of agriculture is called *organic.* • Low to high mechanization.	• The use of pesticides must be rational, based on the thorough knowledge of the biological cycle of each plague. • High genetic potential hybrids must be used and in some cases cultivars (varieties). • Turnout is important, but consumables must be reduced to the bare minimum so that the producer can obtain a reasonable profit. • Average turnout in good and bad years for production. • Stability agriculture. • Pesticides must be those reasonably allowed in central countries. • Respect for the principle of automatic exclusion. • Risk Management. • High Mechanization.	• Production must be done with a high quantity of chemical resources, with high turnout hybrids and chemical fertilization. • Intensive use of transgenic cultivars. • Consumers' qualitative aspects are not borne in mind. • Only a high turn out that ensures paying for costly consumables and obtaining a high profit is important. • The final product parameters are commercial and industrial quality. • Quality for consumers only interests if it has become a recognized parameter for commerce and industry. • If a limited amount of residues is established it must be respected (for example) only for export and not for domestic market. • This scheme is only of interest if the buyer requests it. • High risk due to the use of biocides barely clarified and understood. • Use of germoplasm of a low variability potential, with a little adaptability to change and, in some cases, with a high adaptation and dependence of biocides. • The principle of automatic exclusion is not accepted. • High Mechanization.

Evidently, the production scheme in our country is the Chemointensive one (C) but, as in some cases high unwanted side effects have been observed in areas where this scheme was applied indiscriminately, we see the emergence of concepts such as sustainable agriculture that try to obtain a more balanced position – which in the table is defined as Intermediate (B).

The organic scheme (A), called Organic Agriculture, is growing fast in central countries in Europe and the USA, having started as a kind of concretion of the old agriculturist dream of self-sustainable agriculture. In some cases, the European producer's self-esteem – that in a way resists to be considered an appendix of the industry because they have been completely subsidized – has been the motor of this change (Anonymous, 1993).

The organic scheme started as a game of alternative groups – in some cases with strong ideological or religious connotations – but little by little it grew until it became a relatively profitable activity with international and national organizations that support it institutionally. Paradoxically, this scheme grows especially fast in countries where big corporations developing the chemointensive agricultural scheme work.

Consumers in developed countries want a quality based on scientific parameters of conservation of health which go beyond purely organoleptic parameters such as color, flavor, size, etc.

Exporting countries which are not sensible to these new demands will find their income from exportations reduced.

This is why it is crucial to understand the importing markets demands – demands that have become part of actual regulations. Not knowing them might lead to significant economic loss.

We have observed that any attempt to improve the turnout in agricultural and livestock production leads to a loss of quality. We can therefore see that Food Technologists are to know how to pass through that narrow path between Scylla (Quality) and Charybdis (Quantity). That is, to find a balance between both extremes and not fall in a very good quality but with small turnout or in a very low quality but high turnout.

Technopathogenology and organic production

As we have seen in Reading II, our work is directly linked to protection to consumers since their protection is prevention from technopathogenic risks. In connection to the topic we are developing in this reading, Quality, the so-called Organic Production is the type of production that addresses more closely consumer protection. This quality aims at obtaining foodstuffs which are proportionate for consumers. Organic production contributes both to an optimum biopathological and biological production – two concepts we will develop later. In the former, this is achieved by not using agrochemicals and in the latter, by using varieties of high biological value.

In connection to this and with mycotoxins and its risk for consumers as an example, a document was prepared for the Schweisfurth Foundation. This foundation is entirely devoted to promote projects connected to the organic quality of foodstuffs (Eguiazu & Motta, 2004b, 2006).

Quality criteria and its impact on commerce

We have dealt with the problem of mycotoxins. It is interesting to mention a paper (Whitaker, 1993) that shows the importance of the sampling of batches methodology to analyze the commercialization processes. According to this paper, there is a difficulty in the international commerce of substances prone to be contaminated with aflatoxins – both for importers and exporters – in connection to whether the concentrations are higher or not than international guidelines. The batches rejected in the port of entry by the importer, can represent a major economic loss for the exporter.

An analysis prior to the exportation would reduce the possibilities of rejection. The number of rejected batches depends on the methodological differences in sampling – such as the levels of acceptability of a sample agreed by the importer and the exporter.

We can see here how a defect in the commercialization procedure, in this case, a sampling technique, can mean that the carcinogenic contaminant is not detected on time and be consumed. The final product can contain a mycotoxin which may have not been detected because of an error in the sampling technique. The final effect will be, as a consequence, the manifestation of a technopathogeny.

As for commerce, the application of criteria and procedures also allows us to speak of Commercialization techniques. They can also be responsible for technopathogenies. For example, and going back to the example of aflatoxins, a country can lower the level of acceptability of contaminated batches. Lowering the allowed concentration will lead to a bigger rejection of batches but also to less contamination of raw materials or foodstuffs with this substance – thus less incidence of technopathogenies caused by it.

The search for quality

The FAO system

If we take a period of more or less twenty years of publications of FAO – between 1971 and 1993 – we can see that the quality criteria become increasingly more accurate and oriented towards the consumer. The qualitative aspect in connection to consumers is given more relevance now than what it did back in the early 1970s – when they were practically unknown (Eguiazu, 1998).

Knowing the relevance of the quality of agricultural products in connection to consumers, FAO, through CODEX Alimentarius, underlines the necessary hygiene controls in each stage of the food chain. It recommends the application of the system of Hazard Analysis Critical Control Point (HACCP) in order to obtain as much innocuousness as possible.

HACCP (Whitehead & Orris, 1995) is described as a system that allows determining concrete risks and adopting preventive measures. It is a system that aims at the innocuousness of foodstuffs based on the control of critical points in its manipulation in order to prevent problems, detecting them on time and providing more accurate answers. Their progressive adoption will eventually lead to a harmonized approach to the innocuousness of foodstuffs throughout the world.

The Total Quality Criterion

This criterion was originally developed for the Japanese automobile industry by Ishiwaka (Ishikawa, 1985) but can be applied to any business enterprise. Therefore, it can also be applied to the Technopathogenology criteria.

Back to the case of foodstuffs, grain production and commercialization is similar to a modern industry. This is so because it continuously improves the most uncertain aspects of the most primitive and ancestral production of humanity.

Hishikawa's Total Quality criterion proposes three fundamental elements to apply to quality control:
1. Which are the actual quality characteristics?
2. How are they measured?
3. Are there any substitutes?

We can see that in many cases the real and basic quality variables not only are not measured but they cannot be substituted.

Hishikawa also states that the hardest part is to determine what is *important* and what is *complementary* to Total Quality. Therefore, applying this concept to our case, the color of a fruit, for example, may not be important, but the content of certain vitamins is.

Finally, another point is how *latent flaws* are revealed. For example, in our analysis, the content of hazardous substances or the lack of a basic element for health.

The concept of Total Strategic Quality

Other authors speak of a *Total Strategic Quality* (Ricco, 1993).
Some aspects of such criterion are:
1. *Learning to hear what the client wants,* an important aspect to consider when offering a product, for example, to a new market.
2. Another aspect emphatically given weight to is *the society of no quality is over*, which states that only organizations that focus primarily on quality will survive. This refers both to the need of classic quality indicators as well as to no quality indicators.
3. Variables that need to be measured. According to the author, in his experience, *we continue to ignore variables that need to be measured.* This is a very interesting aspect in connection to commercial parameters. Now, what are essential variables? Why do we keep ignoring them? In the case of aflatoxins, before their detection they were *invisible* essential variables. After their discovery, the requirements of demanding consumers made them *visible* essential variables when developing the corresponding analytical techniques and their regular analysis. When we referred to the Relative Humidity parameter in the prophylaxis of fungal attack and the presence of mycotoxins (Chapter II), this parameter was also an invisible variable until its importance in

prevention was given weight to. It is essential, then, that the researcher states which are the essential variables and which are not.

4. *Quality not only requires values but also systems, processes and consistent tools.* Regarding this, the search for consistent tools, that is, parameters for the consumer who wants total quality, is the utmost aim of Technopathogenology.

Towards a total nutritional quality: The second analogy

Even though the concept of Total Quality is interesting because its orientation towards obtaining good quality products, for certain products quality defined as *total* can be ambiguous and can lead to erroneous interpretations.

From the point of view of automobile manufacturing – from which the Total Quality concept was developed - good quality is possible through a system of control of stages and critical points in the manufacturing of intermediate products. In this case, Total Quality is relatively simple and predictable and the term *Total Quality* perfectly defines the object sought for. If Total Quality is achieved in every single stage, then the final quality will also be total. Every single positive addition in the quality of each stage can lead to amazing results in the final quality of the finished product.

This is different in the agro-alimentary industry where cereal or oleaginous grains are treated, for which no unified quality criteria can be applied (as it is with a mechanical object, such as an automobile). In spite of the high degree of complexity of an electromechanical object, it will never be as complex as a living organism such as a grain, which is enormously complex and indeterminate.

When it comes to grains, quality criteria are not unified. But other criteria can be applied, such as *Commercial Quality* and *Industrial Quality*, as well as the ones we proposed: *Biological Quality* and *Biopathological Quality*. Each of them refers to a specific aspect of quality, that is to say, the presence of different qualities in the product.

Commercial quality

This is used for grain commercialization. It is ruled by usually simple and measurable parameters, such as the presence of living insects or parts of insects, broken grains, fermented grains, stained grains, grains with ripeness defects, seeds of strange forms, grains damaged by drying, etc. Such qualities determine that the more the quantity of them, the poorer the quality.

Industrial quality

It includes parameters of interest to the industry that will buy the grain for its elaboration. They are more complex, as well as the lab instruments used to measure them. For example, parameters applied to oil (if an oleaginous crop), such as: its composition of fatty acids, its acidity, etc. In the case of wheat, parameters that define its aptitude for bread, for example, in the flours obtained from milling: gluten content, elasticity of the dough, etc.

Biological quality

By this we define the presence of vital components for human health. Not only for the nutrition but also for health protection. The substances with this ability are grouped within the wide concept of chemopreventive agents. There are substances such as saponins, and other commonly called salvestrols, for example, that exhibit the important pharmacological effects of anticancer activity.

Biological Quality includes components that are typical of each product be it fruits, vegetables or grains. For example: Vitamins, amino acids, minerals, pigments, fatty acids, phytoalexins, isoflavones, polyphenols, etc.

Biopathological quality

This type of quality defines the presence of elements in the product that damage health in the long term, for example, xenobiotics, whether natural such as mycotoxins for example, or anthropogenic such as pesticide residues.

Having defined the four quality criteria, the concept Total Quality can lead to an erroneous idea about the product, since it would mean that it has simultaneously the four qualities described (Eguiazu & Motta, 1996).

In practice, it is very unlikely to obtain these four qualities simultaneously and, in some cases, they can even be contradictory.

In order to illustrate this, let us consider the following cases (Motta & Eguiazu, 2004):

Table 34:   The four Quality criteria applied to agricultural production.

Case	Commercial Quality	Industrial Quality	Biological Quality	Biopathological Quality
1	Yes	No	No	No
2	Yes	Yes	No	No
3	No	No	Yes	No
4	No	No	Yes	Yes
5	No	No	No	Yes

Case 1: Could be a wheat batch that conforms to the quality criteria necessary to be classified as Grade 1 (best commercial quality level) but because it has undergone a mild process of self-heating it may lack an adequate baking quality, or may have a very low Vitamin E content, or have residues of pesticides, etc.

Case 2: Could also be a wheat batch that could be classified as Grade 1 quality and because of its variety characteristics and adequate post-harvest handling can have a good baking quality. However, it may have a low Vitamin E content and contain pesticide residues.

Case 3: Could be a sunflower batch which could have, for example, a strange aspect (grains gnawed by insects, for example) and cannot therefore be classified as Grade 1 or 2. It can have a low oil turnout but can have a fatty acids composition with a high nutritional value. It can also contain pesticides residues.

Case 4: Could also be a sunflower batch with strange matter, damaged by insects, with low oil content but fatty acid composition with a high nutritional value and free of contaminating substances.

Case 5: Could be a wheat batch of bad commercial quality because it has broken grains due to an inadequate post-harvest handling, and it can also have strange matters. Due to its low quantity and bad quality of gluten cannot be used for baking. It may have a low content of Vitamin E. However, compared with batches of similar characteristics, it has no pesticide residues, which gives it a better biopathological quality.

Here is another dilemma on the foodstuff production, which is why the Scylla and Charybdis analogy is useful. Depending on the quality criteria adopted, be it for the consumer or for the industry, it would represent obtaining a higher or lower profit. A grain of high oil content would have a high quality for the industry but not necessarily for consumers.

For example, we could say that a grain that is damaged by insects would have a poor commercial quality, but if it does not have pesticide residues it will have a good biopathological quality. Conversely, if in order to avoid insects damaging grains pesticides are incorporated and their residues reach consumers, such grains would have a good commercial quality (no insect damage) but a poor biopathological quality. From the point of view of Technopathogenology, the first case is preferred.

Therefore, as for foodstuff products, a closer approximation to the concept of total quality would be obtained with a concept that would unite the two qualities of interest for consumers: biological and biopathological. We can therefore speak of: The Total Nutritional Quality.

The total nutritional quality

We propose the concept of *Total Nutritional Quality* which is defined specifically for foodstuff as: *The harmonious combination of nutrients that a person needs (vitamins, minerals, etc.) and that foodstuff can provide, as well as the absence of contaminant components (especially of long term effect), whether they are natural or anthropogenic.*

We consider this is the most precise criterion for the prophylaxis of Technopathogeny. The concepts of Commercial Quality and Industrial Quality are not enough anymore (Eguiazu & Motta, 1992, 1996).

From food to human environment

We have referred to the attempts to develop criteria that aim to obtain foodstuff that respond to consumers' needs. However, as we have said in the definition, since foodstuff is only part of the human environment we must make sure the whole human environment complies with human needs.

It is obvious that the aim of the agricultural and livestock production is mostly a foodstuff to be consumed. What is not that obvious and, in many cases is not taken into account, is that such foodstuff must comply with the consumer's requirements. In addition, such requirements must be based on certain parameters, whether subjective or objective, of the same consumer. Thus, paradoxically, a fruit might be considered a high quality product by uninformed consumers if it has a nice color and shape when in fact it could be of low quality in other more important parameters (vitamins, enzyme complexes, antioxidants, etc.).

There is currently a shift in the quality criteria of foodstuff, which focuses more and more on *quality of life* parameters for consumers. Through organizations – especially in developed countries – informed consumers establish requirements and see they are complied with. For example, the European Community protects the rights of consumers in Europe in four crucial aspects: health and safety, economic interests, comparative information and right to compensation. As we have mentioned before on the reading on Consumer Protection, the European Union has created the Directorate General XXIV which defends the interests of consumers through the development of an UE consumer policy, thus guaranteeing the transparency of the market and improving the safety of products and services in the EU market (European Commission, 1997).

Agriculture and livestock production, post-harvest handling, the industrialization of raw materials and, finally, the product to be consumed, must follow these guidelines. An example of this is the development of biological or organic agriculture.

In some aspects, it is much easier to change consumer criteria through publicity than to change fixed regulations of the agriculture and livestock production system.

It is known how much time it takes to develop a classic phytogenetic creation and the subsequent need of return of the investment. Therefore, consumer criteria can be left aside if their immediate incorporation implies leaving aside other guidelines that are related to high turnout or massive usage of resources.

This is why the motto (San Martín, 1990) "Science Finds, Industry Applies, Man Conforms," is paradigmatic. It is a model of progress that today only a few, even in the scientific-technological world could defend tooth and nail.

This change of criterion was not produced by the quiet acceptance of more solid theoretical arguments but due to the evidence of facts, especially the apparition of a phenomenon, the inherent and hidden side effects in technology.

A phenomenon for which its more severe an coarse aspects can be illustrated with the example of the Thalidomide Children or with less evident diseases connected with technological processes taken as innocuous, as, for example, working with asbestos or certain pesticides. In the less evident aspects of this phenomenon, apart from the human health problems we have already mentioned we can also include the Bovine Spongiform Encephalopathy (BSE). It is currently being discussed whether the prion or virus particle that is the apparent causing agent is what actually caused this disease or should it be attributed to a massive modification of the animal environment, including the quality of their feeding habits. Here the consumer would be at risk due to an unexpected side effect of feeding and cattle raising technology. The food of a strict herbivore cannot be modified without expecting consequences. There must be a reason why Nature has made some animals herbivores and other animals carnivores. Their digestive functions cannot be exchanged.

What would have British consumers thought if asked whether they were willing to take the risk of a serious disease as a consequence of livestock production techniques in exchange for lowering the meat price a little which, in a biologically acceptable system would have been more expensive?

What would British meat producers have thought if asked the same question and been warned of the high risk of their animals being put down?

Maybe the answer would have been, please do not sacrifice real quality for consumers for a doubtful business!

In spite of what we have said in connection to the difficulty of modern Science and Technique accepting this realistic paradigm, modern businesses do try to do so through the *Total Quality* concept, which it tries to incorporate in order to be competitive and acceptable for consumers.

What leads to this reasoning is not a humanitarian concept but the clear commercial vision that quality and loyalty rules will be increasingly necessary in order to respond to consumers who are more and more informed. Offering the product to a consumer who is not easily misled by advertising can be risky if the product has hidden flaws. This is further stressed in the criteria for exporting to developed countries.

Quality for consumers: Guarantee of respect to concrete human beings?

As we can see, from the Chicago World Fair in 1933 to this day, the criteria and regulations for consumers have changed many times. Now, who is that consumer who must carry the weight of deciding on the quality of the food that makes his or her quality of life better? Is consumer a synonym of citizen? Is it that they cannot trust scientists, industry or agriculture experts – whether they are connected or not to politics – to decide for them? (Eguiazu, 1998) (Zip, 2001).

Let us analyze in detail the Nordic Council of Ministers (Bingman, 1993) resolution on Environmental Information as a basic Human Right. We know that Scandinavia is the universal example regarding human rights. They stress Environmental Information as a basic human right through the following questions: How good is the quality of the environment in which humans live and feed? How safe is the technology being used and how much information is there available on its inherent side effects? Is the right to be informed on the quality of the human environment a basic right?

Informed consumers could therefore decide and be a part on the decisions that are taken on the quality of their foodstuff. They must be able to influence the requirements and criteria for their foodstuff and must be able to request that they are as good as in the strictest countries. This ensures a real use of the freedom of the basic right to a healthy environment. Nevertheless, there is an objection: that the basic environmental information cannot be reached by everybody – it is not only not easy to generate but also, those who have it (if they are an interested party) would hide it in order to protect a business of doubtful ethics.

Consumers are therefore practically defenseless, facing a stream of data generated by interested parties and unable to tell the validity of the experts' statements.

Quality of human environment for consumers: Research and control – Total quality of human environment

We thus arrive to the need to define the criteria that aims at a *Total Quality of the Human Environment*. This would be the sum of all the qualities put together (total nutrition in the case of foodstuff), for each of the components of the human environment: air, water, household, foodstuff, medicine, etc.

Environmental researchers would then be necessary; we could describe them as scientific researchers of environmental immanent and hidden side effects of technology that have negative consequences on human health, or better yet, *technopathogenologists.*

Such researchers must study only the quality aspects of each technology and the alteration they may cause of the human environment as well as the fact that the results of such alteration can be transmitted to exposed human surfaces thus causing damage. Consumers are therefore protected.

This group of risks associated to technique lacks of a specific science that is slowly being developed throughout the world. Different proposals are being developed – either disciplinary or multidisciplinary, such as the already mentioned Technological Assessment – through a slow process of exclusion of these phenomena within the existing disciplines. Given that such disciplines cannot be used to lodge this phenomenon, a specific discipline is developed. This discipline must include the ethical analysis of the causes of quality deterioration for consumers. As we have shown in this book, regardless of the different proposals there are still certain voids, among others, the ones connected to ethical analyses which are highly important for consumers – voids that are approached by Technopathogenology.

Putting together the concepts from the reading on Protection to consumers with the concepts in this reading on quality criteria, maybe the best way to guarantee that a citizen can exercise his constitutional rights to a healthy human environment is the acceptance within the scientific community of the systematic study of this phenomenon of technological side effects. This would require the training of scientific researchers in detection and prophylaxis of problems of quality for consumers. Specific evaluators will also be required. All this supports the urgent need to develop Technopathogenology.

The aim of service to the Science and Technique community would then have a concrete immediate area to perform.

Below we will see two areas in which Technopathogenology can contribute to Quality.

A. *Technopathogenology and its contribution to food science*

Technopathogenology provides new quality concepts for human environment in general. Let us go back to foodstuffs and their relation to the human environment.

What is the relationship with Technopathogenology and Food Science?

Food Science deals with the process of production of food and its control of quality. Why is a science necessary for something that appears to be complete in itself? This question might seem obvious, but let us get back to it.

Because of what we have said in connection to quality criteria, we can see that there is a *clara et distincta* relationship between both disciplines. The objects of study in both are different, but we will see how they can be complemented.

Has everything been said about the quality of food?

Here we must stop to comment on a very common phenomenon: the deterioration of quality that cannot be foreseen. Here is where Technopathogenology can be of help.

Let us go back to the following cases: DDT, Aflatoxins, and Pusztai potatoes.

DDT is a harmful residue in foodstuff, but few people associate this with a failed process of creation of this technological object that was called *miraculous pesticide* by Paul Müller. Much is said about its negative effect, but very little is known about the previous mistakes that led to its creation and use as technology.

Aflatoxins appear in foodstuff deteriorating its quality, but not many relate it to a weakening of the genome produced by geneticists that wanted to improve turnout. For example, yellow corn or *indentata* (because the grain resembles a horse tooth) has a great turnout and, therefore, from the agricultural and livestock production company point of view, very good industrial quality – in this case, agronomic quality. However, these cultivars are very sensible to the *Aspergillus flavus* causing mold and therefore, to the apparition of aflatoxins. Other ancestral corns, or the so-called *indurata* are much more resistant but since their turnout is lower, they are replaced by the former. We can therefore see that a technological mistake and an error in the choice of genetic material – led by an incorrect adoption of quality criteria, i.e. preferring a better industrial quality (Quantity) rather than a better biopathological quality, leads to a negative aspect on health.

The third case is the case of the Pusztai potatoes. They showed the presence of the *Galanthus nivalis* lectin, which had a good pesticide effect but was unhealthy for humans if such lectins appeared in potatoes and its by-products since they can cause serious intestine damage. The civil courage of the researcher who detected this on time and assumed the loss of prestige and the aggression of his colleagues for publishing the results, saved consumers from suffering the consequences. By defending the truth against a system that tried to shut him down, Professor Pusztai became, without realizing it, a whistleblower.

One important point we would like to stress is that in the three cases, the harmful side effects on human health caused by expensive technologies were discovered at the end of the development or while in use. But nothing is said about the previous steps or small previous errors – almost imperceptible – which, had they been detected on the right moment, would have avoided the creation of an ill-conceived or even harmful product. We know about harmful substances that can be found in foodstuff, but we do not know much of the technological process which, by action or omission, originated them.

It would seem that at times Food Science is concerned about quality control but not about the process that originated the damage on quality.

They act as watertight compartments. This is natural since, as we know, Science and Technique do act with some kind of water tightness. They consider it is unnecessary to revise the safety of a previous process. It is a unidirectional vector which, once it is shot, has no return. This unidirectionality is understandable since it ensures the flow of processes without many interruptions. This is crucial to ensure profit. However, the idea that there must be some kind of parallel process of control that is also scientific but different from the normal processes is gaining little by little theoretical space. What is difficult is to incorporate this concept in every concrete process and consider it as a whole in an efficient prospective manner.

From the previous examples – to which we could add many others – we could ask ourselves:

How does the technopathogenological analysis contribute to the quality of food?

488

This analysis refers to the whole process of gestation of a technique which could avoid several future problems. The aim of such analysis is to save time and effort or to early detect risks.

The case of Pusztai's potatoes is paradigmatic. Had he not detected the problem, the potatoes would have been consumed since pesticide lectin was not searched for in quality control. From the biopathological quality perspective, this product was therefore of bad quality. However, these potatoes were of a good agronomic quality, that is, of a good industrial quality. This was considered a great achievement, since lectin stopped pests from attacking potatoes, which would have given the product an excellent quality. If potatoes are attacked by pests, they lose commercial quality. The use of lectin would have protected potatoes from pests thus achieving the *quality control* desired. Nothing had been said, however, in connection to whether lectin was positive or negative for the digestive system of those who consumed it.

Something similar could be said about aflatoxins-sensible corn. Genetic tests for resistance or sensibility to fungi attacking the plant and making it sick were made. Fungi that could attack the seed causing its death were also investigated. These tests were performed with turnout in mind. In order to avoid the seed or plant being attacked by fungi, there are fungicides that are applied either to the seed before it is sown or to the plant already developed in the crop. But if mycotoxins producing fungi attack the grain already formed, the damage in terms of turnout may not be important. Aflatoxins producing molds do not influence significantly the turnout. They do affect the grain, attacking it and generating the toxin, but since it appears when the grain is already formed, it has no agronomic consequences. In general, only a few grains of the spike are attacked. In some cases, they are associated with the damage caused by some insect in the spike. The *Aspergillus flavus* attack is not of interest in relation to the high turnout expected since it does not influence it directly.

The sensibility of the grains would let them be attacked by fungal mycelium or spores which, in their first stages would be practically invisible. This would mean high chances of permanent existence of the contaminant (although in small quantity).

How does Technopathogenology contribute to prevention in these cases?

As a preventive science, Technopathogenology allows to incorporate the concept of prophylaxis by the technologist, that is, the concept that a technique must comply with some kind of *Hypocratic oath* from the technologist, just like the principle of a physician's activity should be *primum non nocere* (first do not to harm). A technopathogenolist should therefore thoroughly study the grounds for innocuousness connected to the food development process, aiming at avoiding voids in their gestation that might be harmful to health.

Conclusion

With the examples of two consumption products and/or raw materials, such as potatoes and corn, we have seen the importance of Technopathogenology in the prevention of latent risks in food for consumers. Just as it is during the production stages, this discipline is also important in the complex world of foodstuff production and elaboration. We can mention in connection to this the over 8,600 foodstuff additives (see table 13) of which, and as we will see in a reading on pesticides, according to the data by IARC, only a few of them show enough experimental evidence that prove their innocuousness. Not only such products represent a risk in themselves, but also chemical reactions they produce can generate substances of high technopathogenic risk.

Technopathogenological training for Food Technicians would help to prevent circumstances that might jeopardize quality – circumstance that are, so far, hidden within the very germinal matrix of a given foodstuff and which, without the proper methodology, cannot be foreseen.

B.   *Quality of agricultural and livestock products.*
     Technopathogenology and its contribution
     to post-harvest grain handling

We have seen the contribution of Technopathogenology regarding Quality.

In connection with the quality of foodstuff or the raw materials used for their elaboration we will see below how Technopathogenology can contribute to the post-harvest grain handling process. This stage is crucial for the many crucial points involved that define the quality of raw materials. We will see why the participation of Technopathogenology is necessary along with the disciplines currently applied to the grain production process (Mechanics, Chemistry, Agronomy and Marketing, among others).

Knowing then the concepts of Technopathogenology and of the qualities described, we will see some post-harvest grain process points where we can apply technopathogenological aspects. For those who work in this crucial stage in the grain production process, these points may be critical regarding the conservation of quality. This would contribute to improve the workplace environment thus avoiding risks on people who work on post-harvest grain handling. This could also provide quality to the product thus protecting consumer health.

Post-harvest is evidently an intermediate stage in the grain production process. Even though this is evident, it is important to stress it since if we study the qualitative problems in the post-harvest process, we find that some of these problems originated in that stage. For example: combustion products for artificial drying, overheating problems and the damage it produces to industrial quality (for example, baking quality of wheat), grain cracking during handling operations, etc. Some of these problems are of technopathogenological relevance, as we will see later.

Other problems, however – such as those generated by mycotoxins with their subsequent qualitative damage, or the pesticide residues in grains that causes its rejection from strict markets, or also the storage ability or natural resistance to deterioration of fruits and seeds – cannot be easily catalogued as post-harvest in the classical sense because although they are found during the post-harvest stage, they were gestated much before the product was harvested and stored. For example, in connection to pesticides, residues of some active principle could be found in stored grains. This happens because the pesticide was necessary, because a plant had been developed following economic/productive criteria that made it sensible and dependent on it.

Their detection in the post-harvest stage does not imply that they were actually generated in that time and place, but much before that. This is why such problems cannot be catalogued as post-harvest in the classical sense. They were generated much before such stage – in many cases, as we have said before, with the genetic selection of the grains. The choice of certain pesticides used during the whole production process is also an example of this – products that can even be forbidden or restricted in the international market but appear in the final stage as unwanted residues.

In this case, post-harvest is an area of detection of problems, but their origin must be sought for prior to post-harvest. That is to say, according to what we have seen in this reading, the critical points of control which are responsible for these problems must be sought for outside post-harvest. However, we must also underline that small problems prior to this stage can become more serious during the post-harvest, for example, the biological damage by fungal attack and formation of mycotoxins.

The following table (Eguiazu, 1998) summarizes what we have just discussed:

Table 35: Problems that are strictly Post-harvest and others which, although detected during this stage, are generated before it.

Strictly Post-harvest	Detectable in post-harvest but not necessarily generated during post-harvest
• Drying. • Storage. • Transport. • Pest Control. • Commercialization. • Commercial Quality. • Industrial Quality.	• Mycotoxins. • Low storage ability. • Pesticide residues. • Biological Quality. • Biopathological Quality.

Critical points in post-harvest grain handling that are of technopathogenological relevance

Below we will see critical points which are relevant to Technopathogenology in the post-harvest process (Motta & Eguiazu, 2004).

1) The material to be handled: Grains

This is an aspect that grain post-handling technicians cannot modify. However, they must recognize that according to the criteria adopted for genetic improvement, the characteristics that make grains more resistant to fungal development and contamination with mycotoxins among other things get lost in the selection process (Eguiazu, 1999a). Since such resistance characteristics are not present in the grains anymore, they are susceptible to the attack of these microorganisms. After the attack, contamination with mycotoxins appears. As we know, some of such substances are potentially carcinogenic, which is why they are controlled in the international market. The resistance to mycotoxins – as well as to the presence of other substances associated with them – has been detected in corn (Brown *et al.*, 2001). Another example is the content of linolenic acid in corn oil, also related to the resistance to mycotoxins (Santurio, 2003).

Genetic modification of grains can make them more sensible to rehydration – which also contributes to fungal attack, as it has been proved in sunflower seeds.

To sum up, post-harvest handling technicians cannot modify the products they receive to store. However, knowing their characteristics – for example sensibility to fungal attack – they can adopt control measures in order to prevent contamination that can avoid a potential techno-pathogenic risk.

2) Mycotoxins

In the previous point we mentioned the grain as a possible element responsible for the susceptibility to fungal attack. However, in grain storage, the Intergranular Air Relative Humidity is the key factor that leads to the gestation of spores and the development of mycelium and then the apparition of mycotoxigenic fungi. It is important to stress that due to the ubiquitous nature of the propagules, they are already present in the harvested grains ready to be stored without modifying their aspect – thus the importance of controlling the environmental conditions of storage (in order to avoid their development).

It is therefore crucial that technicians control stored grain. When we referred to mycotoxins in Chapter II, we supported why measuring the relative humidity content was more important than measuring the water content of the grain as a measure to prevent the development of fungi and contamination with mycotoxins (Motta, 1987). It was also proposed as parameter in grain commercialization and storage (Motta & Eguiazu, 1991b). In addition, we have also developed a simple method for its control (Eguiazu & Motta, 1985)

As we have also seen in Chapter II, modern storage techniques can have defects that may favor the fungal development in grains and the contamination with mycotoxins. We would like to stress the fact that we refer to post-harvest grain handling in general and not to storage only. Apart from the different storage techniques, various other techniques are used in the transfer between silos, between silos and transport, etc. Such operations may harm the grains, such as cracking or fissuring them, and must be born in mind since they constitute the doorway to propagules and therefore favor the development of such pathogens.

Mycotoxins also constitute a risk of exposure for people who work with grain handling. Even though the risk of exposure through breathing has been less studied than the risk of mycotoxins by intake, it cannot be disregarded. The risk of mycotoxins by respiratory exposure can occur by breathing spores, mycelium or other particles of the fungi substrate (Knutti & Kullman, 1994).

Early fungi forms (propagules) can become more dangerous if the conditions allow them to.

3) Pesticides

Pest control is fundamental during post-harvest grain handling; apart from the above mentioned fungi it includes insects, rodents, etc. They constitute an important reason for losses. For pest control, pesticides are used.

From the point of view of Technopathogenology, it is important to show the potential long-term risk of some active principles, even for products that can be considered of no acute toxicity for being practically non-toxic. This means that products with a high LD50 level can still present technopathogenic risk due to their potential carcinogenicity (Eguiazu, 1987a, 1988).

In order to reduce technopathogenic risks, technicians will have to get informed on the products to be used – not only in terms of their acute toxicological risk, stated by LD50, but also in terms of their potential carcinogenic, mutagenic, reproductive, etc. effects. Such information is usually not available, or is insufficient or inadequate, which is why Technopathogenology believes it is crucial to adopt precaution measures not only for the workers handling the product but also in order to reduce the residues to the bare minimum.

4) Combustion products

The adequate storage of grains implies that they must encounter certain levels of humidity. This is why grain drying is a common practice in post-harvest handling. In general, hot air produced by direct combustion is what passes through the grain mass. The air then gets mixed with incomplete combustion products, whose relevance depends on the fuel used. It is not the same to use propane gas or gas oil. In this sense, the combustion issue is crucial. In a complete combustion of hydrocarbon the final products are carbon anhydride and water. However, other accompanying substances and impurities may be present, and in the case of the occurrence of an inadequate combustion, it will mean the apparition of polynuclear aromatic hydrocarbons. This family of products already described includes various substances, such as Benzo(a)pyrene, which present carcinogenic risks in the long term.

Such compounds are not only dangerous as residues in grains but can also be present in the air (IARC, 1983) and therefore represent a technopathogenic risk both for people occupationally exposed in the drying plants and for people living near such plants.

Technopathogenological training would provide the technician in charge of such plant resources to avoid or lessen such technopathogenic risk. And, in the case of driers, ensure that combustion is as complete as possible. Also, even though it might represent a higher cost, use fuel that does not form risky combustion products.

5) Dust

The technopathogenic risks described can be hazardous both for people occupationally exposed and for consumers.

In this section, we will mention another risk: Dust. Dust presents a higher risk to people occupationally exposed to it as to people living in the neighboring areas. For example, acute lung hemorrhage was found in children exposed to dust contaminated with fungi (Sorenson *et al.*, 1995).

Grain manipulation generates dust whose evident risk can be manifested by fires and explosions that, apart from the material damage, imply a risk on people. But from the technopathogenic point of view, we are interested in chronic respiratory diseases caused by this factor. Chronic bronchitis is one of the respiratory problems most commonly found in people working with grain handling. Other adverse effects are pneumonitis and Organic Dust Toxic Syndrome (Knutti & Kullman, 1994). The relationship between the exposure to organic dusts (and to endotoxins associated to them) and chronic respiratory diseases such as byssinosis has been proved (Olenchock *et al., 1989*) (Olenchoch, 1990a, 1990b, 1994).

6) Other

Other substances associated with the prevention of the problem of dust are Mineral Oils, which can constitute another technopathogenic risk both for people occupationally exposed and for consumers. Some companies have developed white mineral oils which can diminish the development of dust significantly. Some of the advantages mentioned are: less risk of explosions, reduction of environmental pollution, improvement of working conditions, less wear of facilities and more shininess of grains (which gives them better commercial value) (EMCA, 2003). However, the characteristics of the manufacturing processes, production and synthesis of chemical products determine that the substances required bring along impurities and other substances derived from the elaboration process. As for the mineral oils, IARC's classification groups them as follows: untreated or mildly treated, Group 1 (i.e. carcinogenic to humans); refined oils, Group 3 (IARC, 1987b). (Let us remember that Group 3 includes the non-classifiable agents regarding carcinogenicity on humans due to limited evidence on humans or limited or inadequate experimental evidence on animals.)

The different substances included in the mineral oils family is classified by IARC in 8 different groups: Group 5 includes white oils and petrolatums suitable for food and/or medicinal use. Two qualities are distinguished within this group (IARC, 1984):

Medicinal quality: includes highly refined oils, colorless, free of unsaturated compounds, aromatic and other compounds that alter their color, smell, flavor and acceptability for feeding or medicinal use.

Technical degree: this quality includes less refined oils of variable viscosity.

According to the definition of Medicinal White Oils and Technical-grade White Oils, (IARC 1984):

Medicinal White Oils are highly refined, colorless oils free of all unsaturated compounds, aromatic compounds and other constituents that influence color, odor, taste and acceptability as a pharmaceutical and food-grade material. They can be made from paraffinic or naphthenic crudes with comparable yields; paraffinic medicinal oils generally have lower specific gravity and volatility than naphthenic oils of the

496

same viscosity and contain hydrocarbons predominantly with carbon numbers in the range 10-50. Technical-grade White Oils are less refined than medicinal oils; they are colorless oils and are made in several viscosity grades. They can be made from naphthenic or paraffinic crudes.

Substances included within the medicinal quality are expected to have an optimum quality for what risks on health is concerned. This is why alimentary quality control specifications and regulations have been established. Interestingly enough, polynuclear aromatic compounds have been found in oil samples of this level of quality used for medicinal or cosmetic purposes (among them Benzo(a)pyrene, which is, as we have observed, carcinogenic). In this case, it is presented as an impurity of the distillation process. According to the two above definitions, if the Medicinal White Oils are contaminated with polynuclear aromatic compounds, we can expect less refined Technical-grade white oils.

Therefore, not only must long term risks be known in oils and ensure they are of feeding quality, but also in the substances that are found in such oils. Technicians could, in addition, consider adopting different technical measures to prevent the risk associated to dust.

Conclusion

We have seen how Technopathogenology can contribute with new elements to consider during post-harvest grain handling. This leads to adopting control measures in certain relevant aspects:
1. To achieve quality in the workplace environment.
2. To obtain optimum quality products for consumers thus providing protection against risks on health. But also:
3. To avoid economic loss (Eguiazu & Motta, 2001a).

Unlike the parameters considered in reference to workplace safety (for example: risk of electroshock, noise, mechanical injuries by transport equipment and grain movement, risks of suffocation or explosions, etc.) or the parameters considered by traditional quality criteria in grains (for example: cracked grains by transport equipment, grains gnawed by insects, self-burnt grains by overheating caused by high levels of humidity, etc.), the parameters considered by new quality criteria are not that evident, which does not make them less important. We should rather say they are more important since they can affect human health.

It is crucial to consider them so that relevant management and/or safety measures can be adopted in order to prevent technopathogenic risks (both for people occupationally exposed and for consumers in general).

V.   Technopathogenology and education

Introduction

In this Chapter we have referred to the contribution of Technopathogenology to prevent technopathogenies in different areas of society. We have included, among others, the importance of consumer protection, the importance of consumers in the factors determining quality criteria and, as we will deal in the Reading VIII, the need of an ethical objector. In order to achieve these three aspects, an adequate training is important. As we have seen in one of the previous readings, an informed consumer will have tools to defend him or herself. We have taught Environmental Technopathogeny to undergraduate and graduate students, but we consider that this kind of training must start in the early stages of school education (Motta & Eguiazu, 2003).

In a pedagogical work, knowledge was analyzed as a challenge under the complex thought perspective – a new epistemic model whose main representative is E. Morin (García de Ceretto, 2001).

Its reading led us to think that it would also be of interest to educators teaching Technology in secondary school to receive Technopathogenic training.

The teaching of technology includes several issues. We believe non-evident risks associated to technologies – more precisely, to the techniques derived from them – should be included among such issues.

Our teaching experience

Given the need to make the knowledge on this new phenomenon known and to train human resources for this new problem, as a result of our research program PROCABIE we created in 1987 the chair Environmental Technogeny at Universidad Nacional de Rosario (UNR) (Tecnogenia Ambiental-Resoluciones).

Even though the course was optional, it was attended by a large number of both graduate and undergraduate students.

Although the course was open to students of UNR and other universities, until 1995 it was mainly attended by students of the UNR School of Agricultural Sciences. We believe that this was due to the lack of information about the course, since from 1996 on, the course started having massive participation of students from the School of Biochemistry and Pharmaceutics, thanks to the actions of a Student Union member, Miss Carmina Cuaranta. This included students from Biochemistry, Biotechnology, Pharmacy and Chemistry. The course was also attended by students of Medicine, Industrial Engineering, as well as students from many branches of the Universidad Tecnológica Nacional (UTN). We stress the attitude of Miss Cuaranta who, by her own initiative, made the course known to students of other schools. This clearly shows that students – i.e. the ones who want to receive the training – show an interest that authorities, who should value the contribution to knowledge, did not show. Contrasting the students' enthusiasm, the response of authorities and colleagues, as we will deal in the Reading VIII was indifferent or even hostile. This type of reaction was not due to ignorance but because they knew that this was a critical and dangerous issue – even more so when approached by the researchers who had discovered it and whom they could not control.

Technopathogenology was also included in the university training of Humanities' programs (Kobila, 2001). Students found it very interesting that a course can involve students from different fields. This supports the fact that Technopathogenology should be a discipline in itself.

Even though it only happened twice, another interesting experience was the talks given in our city, Rosario, to seventh grade students (12 and 13 years old) and to fourth year secondary students (15 and 16 years old). In both cases, students showed interest and acknowledged the importance of technological risks. This is why we believe that primary and secondary school teachers with technopathogenological training could work with students on these issues more thoroughly than what we did in one talk.

It is also interesting to comment on the fact that Technopathogeny was included in a Technology course in the last year of a secondary school in Rosario (Esquivel & Masteloni).

The ongoing growth in the contents of this subject since its creation – both qualitatively and quantitatively – led this course to go from being a one-semester course into being a two-semester course. Given that this was an optional course, our teaching experience showed us that it was hard for students to focus on new extracurricular issues while, at the same time, complying with their curricular subjects. This is why we decided to offer the course in two semesters and worked in collaboration with the chair of Curriculum and Didactics of the School of Higher Education (School of Humanities, UNR) to divide the contents in two semesters.

In addition, even though the course was oriented mainly to train undergraduate students, the possibility of offering this course to Technology professors was also contemplated (McLouglin, 2002).

Why teaching Technopathogenology?

Considering what we have said in the conclusion of the paper that led to this reading (García de Ceretto, 2001):

> Educational Institutions are summoned to the challenges in the times we are living, which is why it is important to generate knowledge that prioritizes the ends and goals of education aiming at the best that the system can give.

We believe we have provided with enough grounds to prove how positive it is to include the study of Technopathogenology in education. Including this kind of knowledge in university training would provide a useful tool to build a criterion to adopt managing measures aiming at diminishing risks.

Even though our experience is related to the training of undergraduate and graduate students, we consider it is important to train Technology teachers since their training in this new phenomenon will raise awareness of risks in technology not only in professional technologists but also in future citizens and consumers.

The authors of a pedagogical work (Aguayo & Martínez Amores, 1958) have stated: "A conscientious and intentional education is living life according to a system of human values." We can say that teaching Technopathogenology not only provides knowledge on immanent risks in technique but also teaches students values oriented towards a progress based on respect to human values: *valuing life*. It is interesting to analyze here the concept developed by Prof. Barbro Westerholm, Coordinator of the Swedish Parliament Scientific Ethics Committee, in her work Good Conduct in Research (Westerholm, 1999):

> The ethos of science must be oriented towards the creation of new knowledge, a knowledge required to interpret and understand reality and which is needed to make the world a better place to live in.

Teaching students the human and life values provided by Technopathogenology builds informed consumers. As we have said, through organizations – especially in developed countries – informed consumers establish requirements and see they are complied with. One example of this is the already mentioned Directorate General XXIV, created by the EU to protect consumers' rights in Europe (European Commission, 1997).

Any informed citizen would reject the old Chicago World Fair motto (San Martín, 1990): "Science Finds, Industry Applies, Man Conforms."

In those times, only the positive aspects of technique were considered. Technopathogenology was unthought of.

Now this attitude has changed and nobody questions the fact that the right to environmental information and the right to know the side effects of techniques are basic human rights, and this, in Argentina, is implicit in article 41 of the National Constitution (Constitución de la Nación Argentina). We do not know, however, whether this is observed or not.

As for the safety of chemical substances, according to a newsletter of the United Nations Environment Program (PNUMA, 1985b):

> All the persons assuming a responsibility in the manufacturing, handling, use and disposal of chemical products should be aware of the importance of the education and training programs for all the groups of the population – most importantly children – that should be permanently organized and carried out. It is equally necessary to fill the voids in information, which is the responsibility of manufactures and authorities. Safety is a serious issue, since while management operations remain insuf-

ficient, the chemical products that are present in the environment will keep being many people's nightmare; worse yet, they will keep causing damages and victims, and in some cases, true disasters.

This reading shows that our proposal of bringing Technopathogenology into education contributes to recognizing the crucial importance of education programs aimed to the whole population and attempting to bridge the information gaps – in our case in particular, concerning the non-evident risks of Technology.

The great challenge is then the development of an adequate knowledge in the different levels of education. Due to the nature of this work we focus not only on training graduate and undergraduate students but also in training Technology teachers and teachers of disciplines that involve technology. This will enable to bring Technopathogenology to all the educational levels leading to the university. Only in this manner will the training of students in Technology be complete.

VI. Technopathogenology and its contribution towards a stricter regulation in the international commerce of hazardous substances: The case of pesticides

Introduction

As we have seen, chemical substances – whether natural or synthetic, with commercial application, or waste (sub products of industrial activity) – play an important role in technopathogenic risks.

When certain substances of use or waste are proven to be risky for humans, whether in the long or the short term, certain measures are adopted to limit or to stop the risk of exposure in humans. The huge economic investments make companies reluctant to abandon the production of these substances, stop the commercialization of the excess, or abandon or modify technological processes that generate hazardous waste material. This, in turn, leads to unethical commercial practices such as: trying to continue with the elaboration and sale of such substances, selling the excess, or trying to find a place where to dispose of the waste material from factories. Distancing from human values and prioritizing avoiding economic damage, the health and life of people is thus jeopardized.

This is why international organizations, becoming aware of the magnitude of the problem, have started elaborate programs, agreements and codes in order to stop or reduce the damage in countries that are unaware of such risks.

This is evident in the case of pesticides. We will use these substances to illustrate how important it is to develop principles that limit or stop the risk for consumers – especially technopathogenic risks – and to support the need to extend these principles to all the substances and to all the techniques that carry such risk. A typical case could be the dismantling of nuclear energy plants in developed countries: taking either the plant or the technology to third world countries should be stopped. These kinds of attitudes show the lack of ethics of developed countries scientists, who issue reports that minimize the risks if such a technology is exported to third world countries. Let us remember the case we used to illustrate Mendacity, in Chapter I: risky pesticides in developed countries are not necessarily so risky in underdeveloped countries since a higher temperature will grant a higher degradation. If a scientist with this criterion was asked to establish whether the technology used in his or her own country is harmful or not, the risk parameters will most probably be very different. In developed countries there is the common practice of *buying* reports from scientists if behind such statement enormous economic interests are involved. Going back to the nuclear power plants, it is interesting to see, as we have mentioned, that the very same scientific community that hailed the use of nuclear energy, today – after the Chernobyl incident and then after the incident of Fukushima – is reverting its criterion and concepts to developing new safer ways of generating energy. About the last incident it is interesting to mention that the Japan Scientists' Association (JSA) appeals to the Japanese Government for a basic change of energy and nuclear power policy (INES, 2011).

In order to postulate the need to apply technopathogenological principles to the commerce of pesticides we will use a paper we wrote (Eguiazu, 1996) based on a presentation on the FAO Seminar and Workshop: Code of Conduct Application on the Use and Application of Pesticides (Rosario, Argentina, 1994) where the contribution of Technopathogenology to the commercialization of pesticides was presented.

The FAO code

The negative side effects of pesticides on humans have been known for a long time. This encouraged activities that aim to an increasingly careful use of them.

Due to this initiative, in 1985 FAO developed an International Code of Conduct which aims at decreasing some negative effects (FAO, 1986).

Within this code, a Prior Informed Consent procedure (PIC) was incorporated in Article 9 in 1989 (FAO, 1990). This was presented, on the one hand, as great progress and on the other, also criticized as permissive.

In this reading we will try to establish grounds of strict and universal regulations that allow to increase the efficacy of the code in order to avoid unacceptable risks on humans.

The incoherence in the commercialization flow of pesticides

The lack of coherence in the commercialization flow of pesticides has been known for a long time: some pesticides are banned in some regions whilst there is no legislation whatsoever on them in other regions, or their use is even allowed (Eguiazu, 1987a, 1988).

The questions that arise on this problem are: Why are they banned? Upon what grounds? In some cases, the reasons are purely administrative or commercial; there is no real unacceptable risk on humans. But in most cases, the ban responds to increasing evidence based on scientific experimentation. Such experimentation shows the increasing degree of risk on humans derived from the continuous use of such products.

Another crucial question is: Can this flow be stopped in case there is scientific proof of non-acceptable risk for humans? Here is where we find no answer, since there is no universal regulation and no unification in the criteria of the scientific entities that establish which is the risk and the acceptability of each substance.

Criticism to the code

The FAO code was adopted by the XXIII FAO session in 1985, RES. 10/85. The first formal criticism to it, in which the lack of existence of a universal regulation that banned unacceptable risks was pointed out, was raised at the first International Congress of Ecotoxicology in Buenos Aires (1988). Only one paper was presented on the technopathogenological principles and criteria applied to pesticides and their long term risks on human health (Eguiazu, 1988). Such paper exposed the purely guiding nature of the Code and proposed the inclusion of a Principle of Automatic Cancellation as the only way to achieve maximum protection to humans against non-evident and non-acceptable risks of pesticides (Eguiazu, 1987a, 1988).

Six years after that, during a FAO workshop, the modified version of the Code was analyzed (which included the PIC principle) (FAO, 1994).

In spite of the inclusion of this principle, the lack of a strict and universal regulation was still self-evident. As a result, new modifications that called for the maximum protection of human beings – either as exposed workers or as consumers of agricultural products – were proposed (FAO, 1994).

Evident and non-evident risks of pesticides

The core of the problem in using chemical substances lays in the fact that there are no clear or sufficiently thorough definitions, formalization and application of the concept of risk. Following modern criteria, *Risk* goes beyond the simple enunciation of the arguable figures of Medium Lethal Dose (LD 50), no observable adverse effect level (NOAEL) and the acceptable daily intake (ADI).

The concept of risk on humans exposed can be more adequately described as follows (Eguiazu, 1987a, 1988, 1994):

Evident risks

Evident Risks are any negative effects on health that can be caused by normal operations of handling a substance, also considering the possible errors of the operator.

This includes cases of serious intoxication with immediate symptoms and acute effects.

Non-evident risks

Non-Evident Risks are any negative effects on health that can be caused in spite of handling a product with the normal precautions. They are usually long term effects and in low doses, with complex symptoms.

Evident risks are usually handled thoroughly by producing and/or importing companies. The aim is to avoid them with good agronomic measures.

Unlike evident risks, non-evident risks are not really well handled by importers and appliers, which constitute in some cases the so-called grey information. Grey information includes contradictory scientific information, which requires an in-depth knowledge of all the current opinions. Let us remember the case of Maneb, which we mentioned when we discussed how Doubt is adopted in favor of the company instead of in favor of consumers in Chapter I. The advancement of knowledge is based on a scientific discipline with the final presentation of hypotheses. One thus arrives to a wider panorama than the reduced information available in the commercial and industrial environment. Within non-evident risks we can include:

Acceptable evident risks

1. High Medium Lethal Dose.
2. Low risk of intoxication without evident negligence in normal use, liquid transfer, etc.
3. Low risk of fire, explosion, etc.

Non-acceptable evident risks

4. Low Medium Lethal Dose.
5. High risk of intoxication without evident negligence in normal use, liquid transfer, etc.
6. High risk of fire, explosion, etc.

Non-evident acceptable risks

1. Risks of carcinogenicity, mutagenicity, teratogenicity, effects in reproduction, fertility, etc. Only accepted when:
   1.1. There is a very low scientific evidence of their occurrence or they manifest themselves at very high doses.
   1.2. Their use is essential and there are no alternatives.
   1.3. Their active principles are of low durability. Risk is practically limited to the operator and does not reach consumers.

2. Risks can be prevented with the application of technopathogeno-logical criteria.

Non-acceptable non-evident risks

1. Risks of carcinogenicity, mutagenicity, teratogenicity, effects in reproduction, among other technopathogenic risks with a high scientific evidence and in very low doses.
2. Carcinogenicity – notwithstanding the doses.
3. Even with the application of certain technopathogenological criteria, risks cannot be avoided.
4. When it is known that whoever will manipulate the product will not bear in mind the principles to avoid the risk.

This categorization allows us to clarify the degree of evidence and acceptability of the risk. Even though it is subjected to be improved or completed, we believe that the essential is present and it allows us to establish the most important risks: non-evident, non-acceptable risks. The others can be managed with a good agronomic practice.

The Code: Analysis of its critical points

If we analyze the Code thoroughly – both its original version and its amendment – a series of critical or weak points can be found, especially in Art. 5 (Reducing Health and Environmental Risks). In this article we can see that a series of general recommendations are made but none of them define the essential risk of pesticides. Neither do they categorize the risks or mention concrete biological effects. Article 5.4 mentions "unjustified confusion and alarm among the public." What this means is that consumers or citizens may exaggerate when they require more safety – which clearly shows a defense of the product.

Article 9 (Information Exchange Among Countries and Prior Informed Consent Principle) mentions a mechanism of negotiation between governments. It is expected that through this mechanism, the country home of a company wanting to export a forbidden product should inform the importing country the reasons for the prohibition. If the importing country rejects the product in question, the import of such product would be cancelled.

There is no mention of a universal regulation clearly establishing a principle of use or exclusion for each product according to its toxicological properties. Article 9.2 even seems to disregard this issue when they give economic and administrative reasons to accept or reject a product in particular. Public health issues are seen as less important.

Even though the inclusion of PIC in 1989 is considered a progress in comparison to the 1986 code, it still leaves some problems unattended. It is still unclear what to do with the products that have been banned in some part of the world due to unacceptable risk on human health.

The problem is that the PIC procedure seems to allow the operation to take place anyway if authorities come to an export/import agreement. The fact that the product might be banned on sound scientific grounds in a more developed country seems unimportant.

The negotiations are made between governments – NGOs would have a very little say. Agricultural workers organizations (who are in contact with the products), university associations (especially agricultural technologists) and, finally, consumers organizations, are not explicitly included in the Article 9 of the code. It is evident that import decisions are made by a small number of people. This decision is thus left to the ethics of these people and their individual knowledge of the product to import.

The regulations established in the 1989 amended version imply that a banned pesticide can be imported and then presented as a consummated act. NGOs might then learn too late about this without having had the chance to intervene.

On the other hand, going back to the classification of risks, we can see that the most important risks are the non-evident and non-acceptable risks given their difficulty to be recognized. But it is not specified how they would be controlled. Nothing is said about the effects that do not depend on the dose size, since they could be additive.

In order to achieve the ultimate aim of protecting humans from technopathogenic effects, the Code must include a clear statement oriented towards a delay in the use of non-acceptable substances which are of risk to humans. The inclusion of such clear statement is rejected on the grounds that there is no total evidence of the risk. Therefore, what is used as an argument to decide for or against the use of a determined substance is opinion.

This clearly shows that either the decision is taken in favor of the product (i.e, of its most possible unrestricted use) or in favor of the human being by a cautious exclusion of products of proven risk.

The principle of cancellation or automatic exclusion

This principle was proposed in the first criticism to the FAO Code during the First International Congress of Ecotoxicology (April, 1988) (Eguiazu, 1988). This showed that there was no principle of cancellation or automatic exclusion for pesticides, not just for those who had shown a technopathogenic effect but also for any other effect to human health. The lack of this principle in the case of pesticides with non-evident and non-acceptable risks enables a relatively unobstructed and free of restrictions transport, commercialization and storage in the rest of the world. This paper showed that almost a 50% of the total volume of pesticides imported to Argentina in 1986 were included in the list of pesticides causing mutagenicity, carcinogenicity, teratogenicity and fetal damage by the State of California.

The principle of Automatic Cancellation was then proposed to give a stricter nature to the code, a consequence of which would be the immobilization and handling of such pesticides as risky substances or hazardous residues.

Updating the principle of cancellation or automatic exclusion

The cancellation or automatic exclusion of a non-acceptable risky substance is not enough in itself to attack the problem. The core of the problem is that it is a badly gestated technological product that is sent to the market probably in good faith, hoping that no technopathogeny appears as a hidden problem (Eguiazu, 1992). Measures are taken only when humans, as if they were inadvertent laboratory animals, unveil the problem. Nothing is said, however, about the responsibility of the technologist, or rather, the whole Science and Technique system that backed the use of a product with an immanent and hidden risk. On the other hand, the principle referred originally solely to carcinogenic substances, disregarding the possibility of applying it to other risks which, in some cases, could be more serious than cancer.

FAO's Code of Principle of Information and Previous Consent: Efficient tool or open door to the commercial flow of non-acceptable hazardous substances?

Let us take Kant's categorical imperative (Kant, 1781): "Act only according to that maxim whereby you can, at the same time, will that it should become a universal law," and its consequence:

> Act in such a way that you treat humanity, whether in your own person or in the person of any other, never merely as a means to an end, but always at the same time as an end.

Can this principle be found to be implicit in the basic ethical considerations that support PIC? Or is this put in such a way that it can be avoided?

Can a pesticide be banned in one region and used in another at the same time? If so, who must decide on its use? The State? A democratic consensus of citizens? Consumers organizations? Associations of exporters or importers of pesticides? Associations of agricultural technologists? Associations of agricultural workers? or Associations of producers? Or FAO?

Does the procedure implicit in PIC involve all the interested parties? Or is it simply a deliberation of governments or intermediate officials?

What reasons are given in favor of a flexible prohibition which is not automatically universal?

In this case, a product which is banned in a region can be used, transported and commercialized in another region.

This means that even though the country of origin bans the product, such product can be exported to another country. There would be no strict law or universal regulation of exclusion.

What we understand by this is that the reasons given to ban a product are never related solely to human health. Some examples show administrative reasons or a commercial war between different companies. In this case, the prohibition would be based on political reasons and not on human health.

As we have already said, it is fallaciously mentioned that the humid and warm weather of the Southern Hemisphere would fasten the degradation of the products when applied. The faster natural degradation in some regions would notably decrease the risks that would be more serious in the colder Northern Hemisphere (Korte, 1988).

Another argument used is that environmental regulations in underdeveloped countries should not be as strict as in developed countries. The argument used here is that since people are in such bad nutritional and social conditions in those countries, the most important aim should be to feed them. We do not agree to this point. Regulations should actually be stricter in underdeveloped countries considering that the lesser level of instruction may lead to a thoughtless consumption, to the inexistence of legislation or, if such legislation does exist, to the lack of observance, all of which leads to risk the lives of consumers. According to the advocates of the use of pesticides without restriction: *Worrying about the additive adverse effects on health caused by low doses of substances which are highly useful such as pesticides only contributes to make the production and distribution of foodstuff harder.*

This argument shows that underdeveloped countries are expected to be thankful for being allowed to participate – even if it is in an imperfect manner – in the advantages of progress. No matter if for such progress' sake pesticides which might be banned or limited in developed countries are used, because in underdeveloped countries the benefits are higher than the risks.

These advocates also state that even if there might be a hypothesis that speaks of an additive or irreversible effect of risky substances where we cannot speak of a *no effect dose* this argument could be used for banning a product only in developed countries.

Humans in underdeveloped countries must first reach the level of development of first world countries and only then worry about these risks, which are also minimized. This position can then be summarized as follows: *Even though there are hypotheses showing additive and irreversible risks at sub chronic doses of determined pesticides that recommend their prohibition in some cases, such hypotheses have not been completely demonstrated yet. We therefore recommend the use of these substances in underdeveloped countries since in this case, the practical benefit is much higher than the hypothetical risk.*

In underdeveloped countries the alternative would be then to be at the mercy of pests since in Southern hemisphere countries insects would have a higher rate of reproduction than in colder areas.

It is also usually said that in the risk and benefit analysis the cost of reduction of certain substances would not really show an increase in the general health of the affected population. This is usually argued in, for example, the discussion on the reduction of nitrates and nitrites of phreatic stratums by advocates of nitrogen fertilization (Jenkinson, 1995).

In general, this discussion tends to relativize the importance of arguments that propose a universal regulation based on the risk on humans that leads to the prohibition of products.

The question here is how much each environmental factor actually influences the preservation or diminution of human life, and whether the concrete incidence of the *pesticide factor* is quantifiable in the context of other possible environmental agents affecting health as an additive factor that act on a concrete individual. In the cases when the information is contradictory in terms of safety or lack of safety of a product, deciding whether a product should be used or not becomes a question of deciding in favor of the consumer or in favor of the company.

Similarly, the argument stating that natural substances having a negative effect similar to the one attributed to banned pesticides are more relevant in terms of health is not sound. It is argued that there are in nature many more natural carcinogens than the few synthetic substances with such effect to which the human would be exposed (Frank, 1980-1983). It is very interesting to remember the comments of Dr. Tomatis *et al* (Tomatis *et al.*, 2001) that we mentioned in Chapter III in reference to a criterion of a scientist in connection to the risk of synthetic pesticides, a criterion that of course they do not share:

> Synthetic residues on food can be ignored because 99.99% of pesticides humans eat are natural, chemicals in plants are pesticides, and their potential to cause cancer equals that of synthetic pesticides.

All this is like thinking that because of the risks that traffic represents to passers-by, it would be irrelevant to make sure the street signs are secured in order to avoid that they fall on their heads.

All the arguments used only aim at thinking of the problem as less relevant than it really is and at minimizing the possibility of applying a universal norm.

What reasons are given in favor of an automatically universal strict prohibition?

Following the hypothesis of addition of effects at low doses, it is reasonable to reduce the exposure of a substance – if identified – to a bare minimum.

If we apply the categorical imperative and the principles of basic teachings from important religions, we can see the harm caused by the lack of a prohibition or universal exclusion regulation: on the one hand, to the categorical imperative and, on the other, to humanity (since the human beings of developing countries are the object of a doubtful business). The developing country person is not treated as an aim but as the object of a business that would benefit principally developed countries producers and exporters of substances as well as developing countries importers and distributors.

The problem of the experts' statements based on contradictory evidence

Maybe the core difficulty for a universal regulation based on scientific evidence is that such evidence is contradictory, insufficient or even non-existent. Taking advantage of this situation, each group of experts can argue according to their choice or preference. As an example, we can mention the work published by IARC in 1987 which included the tests done until that year (IARC, 1987b). As we mentioned in Chapter I, by that year about 70,000 substances were of daily use. Contaminants were not included. The work included 618 agents (substances: of use or contaminant; Mixtures and occupational exposure).

Out of the total amount of agents evaluated, 50 are classified as carcinogenic to humans (Group 1), 37 as probably carcinogenic to humans (Group 2a), 149 as possibly carcinogenic to humans (Group 2b), 381 as non-classifiable as carcinogenic to humans (Group 3) and 1 as non-carcinogenic to humans (Group 4) (IARC, 1987b).

We can see then that for a bit more than an 8 percent there is enough evidence to classify the agent as carcinogenic to humans and for almost a 92 percent the evidence on humans or experimental animals is insufficient, inadequate or non-existent. What we can see here is that whether it is pesticides or any other agent, the evaluators still give a confusing statement since it is highly likely that the weight of the evidence does not allow a categorical classification of risk and therefore, the agent is very much likely to be approved for use. This is worsened considering the ethical component – or of utter corruption – present in the defense of a product in order to protect a profitable business.

It would seem that even if there is enough scientific evidence to ban a chemical product – even if the product is banned in developed countries, it would not be enough to exclude it from the market. Some evidence would be found to counter the developed country prohibition thus generating uncertainty. Therefore, the decision taken in the first world – which was at the time soundly supported – is dampened with real but out of context arguments, or with a clearly sophistic argument. What was originally a clear decision is not a clear decision anymore. All this is done to support the enormous exporting business.

This leaves the door open to export the product to developing countries.

The principle ruling these North-South transactions can be described as follows: *If there is no clear evidence in favor of the prohibition of a product, we shall keep on using it until the evidence appears.*

What's more: *Even if there is clear evidence in favor of the prohibition of a product and even if such product has already been banned somewhere in the world, this would never be universally valid.*

The benefit of the doubt *In dubio pro reo* should be called here *In dubio pro chimia.*

This is about defending an unrestricted sale of substances unless the evidence on its risk is irrefutable.

This is very dangerous since the late effects can appear after many people have suffered irreversible damage.

Humanity – the human being – is turned into a means that ensures a commercial transaction since if in doubt, it is decided against the person and in favor of the product.

However, reason and common sense – which popular wisdom calls the *least common* of the senses – indicate us that something is not right in this principle, that it is necessary to develop a strict regulation which must be based on the fact that can be put as follows: *If the product in question was banned, there must have been clear evidence in that sense. Any new discussion is simply a sophistic attempt to relativize the evidence in order to defend a suspicious business.*

*Three suggested principles to include in the code oriented
towards strict norms against non-acceptable risks*

1.   The principle of automatic exclusion

This principle was presented in a paper in 1996 (Eguiazu, 1996) and it
was described as follows: *If an agrochemical product has manifested in
experimental conditions or with enough scientific grounds its carcinogenic effect, anywhere in the world, it must be automatically banned and
excluded from the market in all the countries adhering to the code.*

This is the principle we called *automatic cancellation* back in 1988.
After this, it was suggested that the product in question be handled according to regulations on residues and toxic substances. Their use should
be completely forbidden.

Another way of expressing this would be: *If a product is banned
somewhere in the world with enough scientific grounds, this prohibition
should be automatically accepted in all the countries adhering to the code.*

In the light of the progress in the field of Technopathogenology, especially in connection to ethical commitment, this principle could be
modified and expressed as follows: *If an agrochemical product has manifested its carcinogenic effect and other effects of technopathogenic relevance in experimental animals or has shown epidemiological evidence
in humans, with enough scientific support, backed by prestigious international organizations, it must be automatically banned and excluded
from the market – both locally and internationally.*

Or rather: *If a product is banned somewhere in the world and there
is enough scientific evidence, this prohibition should be automatically
accepted by all the countries.*

These principles, that include other risks apart from carcinogenic
risks, are the only way of protecting humans from the doubtful business
that allows the migration and import of highly hazardous substances.

Applying the technopathogenological criteria we have already mentioned, we can include another principle: *Technopathogenological criteria (described in Chapter III) must be applied for the handling of agrochemical products whose technopathogenic effect, especially if carcinogenic, has not been proved due to insufficient, inadequate or inexistent
studies.*

It is interesting to mention here the criterion adopted in Ecuador for pesticides 2, 4, 5-T, Aldrin, Chlordane, Chlorobenzilate, DDT, Dieldrin, Lindane, Mirex, Parathion and Toxaphene. A Ministry Regulation (0242) was passed in 1985 stating that it "Forbids their registry due to being health hazard products and because their elaboration, commercialization and use was banned in several countries" (IRPTC, 1987a, 1987b, 1987c, 1987d, 1987e, 1987f, 1987g, 1987h, 1987i, 1987j, 1987k). We can see here that the decision of banning a product simply because it has already been banned in other countries is reasonable, simple, practical and economic.

2. The principle of conditioned exclusion

This principle was developed to be a bit more tolerant for the chemical product: *If an agrochemical product has manifested in experimental conditions or by epidemiological evidence a mutagenic, teratogenic, fetal damage or other effects (enzymatic disruption, allergy, etc.) with enough scientific evidence, it must be banned and automatically excluded from the market in all the countries which adhere to the code, unless there are reasons serious enough in each region that indicate the contrary.*

Just like what we have indicated in the previous principles, in the light of the new technopathogenological concepts, we could modify this and present it as follows: *If an agrochemical product has manifested in experimental conditions or by epidemiological evidence a technopathogenic effect with enough scientific evidence, it must be banned and automatically excluded from the market – both for the commercialization in the manufacturing country and for exportation. In addition, its use as pesticide or any other use that entails a technopathogenic risk must also be banned, unless there are very serious scientifically proved reasons indicating the contrary and making its temporary use inevitable, provided technopathogenological criteria are respected.*

This principle would leave open the possibility that some product of non-evident but acceptable risk be tolerated if there is no other possibility of being substituted by another one of a lesser risk but with a similar agronomic effect.

These two principles disregard completely the traditional toxicological parameters, such as LD50, ADI and NOAEL.

516

These parameters are rather imperfect in the face of those effects which do not depend completely on them. Among these effects we find: carcinogenic, mutagenic, teratogenic, or fetal damage, whose manifestation can be found after the use of the substance during a long period of time, even though in the short term no symptom is manifested.

3. The principle of responsibility

The previous discussion – whether to exclude or not a substance of proven risk – is only the consequence of a phenomenon which is more profound: The existence of imperfections or defects immanent in the Science and Technique system that allow that products with unpredictable risks are created and sent to the market. The system sends the market a technological product – in this case, a pesticide. This product is expected to be innocuous, but if there is new evidence that proves the opposite, the product is banned or recalled from the market.

This also calls for a strict regulation, since the immediate consequence of this proceeding is the need of an *inadvertent laboratory animal*, which is the human being exposed. This was explored by Hans Jonas in his Imperative of Responsibility of the technologist (Jonas, 1984) which, modified and applied to pesticides could be expressed as follows: *The responsibility of the producer sending an agrochemical to the market must ensure that after the commercial application of the product no side effects appear on humans. If late side effects appear, they will still be the responsibility of the original producer.*

This would maintain the responsibility of the producer of risky technologies for much longer, after they were accepted. This acceptance comes after the formal tests of the Science and Technique system. In this manner, the undesired side effect, not evident and not acceptable – in technopathogenological terms, the immanent error or defect with negative consequences to humans, which was a hidden error in the technological product – has a culprit: its creator, producer and marketer.

Conclusion

As far as pesticides are concerned, even if the Prior Informed Consent principle (PIC) leaves the door open to a negotiation between countries (prior to the commercial operation) it does not establish any real regulation to which the member States must adhere in concrete cases. If there is consensus among the relevant officials, the operation becomes effective. The Code is a valuable contribution to the attempt to fix healthy regulations for all the operations connected with pesticides. The most interesting part of the Code from the point of view of protection to citizens or consumers is, without doubt, the PIC principle. However, the inclusion of Automatic Exclusion or Cancellation and Conditioned Exclusion would provide the Code with a greater credibility. With these two new principles, the parties would have to adhere to PIC as a universal regulation and not depend on the people who participate in the process, neither on political or commercial pressures. This would ensure a higher credibility.

Today, there is a global consensus as to the risk entailed by chemical substances. This is shown by the development of the PIC principle, to which we can add (WHO-UNEP-FAO):

- The Rotterdam Convention on the PIC procedure for certain pesticides and hazardous chemicals in International Trade which: a) provides early alarm signals for hazardous chemical substances and b) Prevents the International Trade of certain chemical substances.
- The Stockholm Convention, which aims at controlling and eliminating the production and use of certain persistent organic pollutants (POPs), and
- The Basel Convention, which aims at: a) Limiting the toxic Commerce of hazardous wastes and b) Ensuring the adequate disposal of waste.

However, in order to prevent non-evident risks on human health, we believe it would be interesting to apply technopathogenological criteria to the international trade or management of chemicals, whether they are of use or residues. And, why not, to any technology, whether it is a chemical substance or not.

In the case of pesticides, we have seen that even with the application of technopathogenological criteria, the idea of establishing the Principle of Responsibility – perhaps we could call it the *Principle of Technopathogenological Responsibility* (PTR) – would not entirely avoid the use of products carrying technopathogens. The human being continues to be an inadvertent experimentation animal and will never be completely compensated for an unexpected technopathogeny. However, a PTR would make the Science and Technique system analyze the product much more thoroughly than what it does until now. This would enable a significant reduction of technopathogenic risks. In addition, the responsibility for hidden errors or side effects would not end when the product enters the market. This responsibility would begin when considering technopathogeny as part of the prior responsibility. This principle which we are proposing constitutes a sword of Damocles and, at the same time, a challenge to the Science and Technique system for *doing things well*, to create technological products more and more proportionate to the human being. It is our wish that these musings inspire those who have this delicate process of international trade of substances and risk technologies in their hands. Many years have passed after the publication of these principles and it would be a nice surprise that our postulates are now taken into account to improve this process.

VII. Avoiding war and technopathogenic risk as a global responsibility – Two initiatives with one goal in common: The protection of humans

In October 2005 the INES Council 2005 was held in Vaquerias, Argentina. Its subject matter was research on Peace in South America.

The value of ethical objectors is undeniable – as it is the activity of any organism that aims at searching for peace, that is to say, at protecting humans from the risk of wars. Interestingly enough, we have come to realize that Technique too, even though in a less evident, noisy and destructive manner – with the exception of cases like Chernobyl or Bophal – can also kill. We believe that we have proved it beyond doubt in this book. This is why we dared to include this short article (Eguiazu & Motta, 2005a). We think the reader will agree on the importance of this reading.

Introduction

As a general principle, INES/INESPE speaks of the global responsibility of scientists and engineers as keepers of peace.

We scientists and engineers manifest together as a group when we have to oppose to wars, to the massive use of nuclear weapons, etc.

In spite of our global manifestations and accusations, the political power always acts with impunity, even basing its actions on lies. We can exemplify this with cases like those of A. Nikitin, M. Vanunu, D. Kelly, etc.

Political power turns a deaf ear to this and even though things can end up in a war, politicians recognize later this mistake apologizing, saying that *they did not know* or that *they were wrong*, or that *the threat was not real after all*.

There are many other cases – G. Emde, A. Pusztai, M. Herbst – where, even though the actions or indifference of the political power is not manifested with the dimension or rumbling of a war, a technology can also be harmful or even jeopardize the lives of many people.

It would seem that power always acts from power itself or following its own internal logic. The arguments based on the truth and human rights are of very little interest. Human rights follow the rules of political correctness.

Power is pragmatic and its members do whatever they will. When power is exercised there are no arguments against it that can stop it. If justice acts, it can do it after the deed is done, but it will be difficult for it to stop the power's machinery once it has been activated. The perversion of power is such that those who have power are very unlikely to recognize they are wrong and back down. On the contrary, they keep moving forward destroying any evidence of their mistake.

Technopathogenic risk as a global responsibility and technopathogenologists as ethical objectors

What we express in this title is basically supported by our work for over 30 years, which we have devoted to the study of the technological development process. As we have already mentioned, our work was inspired by the Stockholm Conference in 1972, which had as leitmotiv the protection of consumers from non-evident and immanent risks in Technique.

We have postulated that – just like in the search of the prevention of war – technopathogenological risks should be framed as Global Responsibility given the fact that, as we already know, we use the term Technopathogeny to define illnesses or damage on human health – both physical and psychological – which are not manifested immediately after exposure but after several years or generations as a consequence of exposure to non-evident factors generated by Technique, or Technopathogens present in the Human Environment by immanent errors or flaws hidden within it.

As we have seen in the first reading, one of the values that can be attributed to the search for knowledge is the mercantile utilitarianism, an expression we use to describe craving for profit. This can lead to the use of knowledge with voids in the development of technical objects (whether they are built or adapted). Such voids are responsible for potential technopathogenies. As we have seen, mercantile utilitarianism is an attitude commonly seen in private companies. These companies – going back to the central concept of this reading – are in a *market war*. This *war* consists of trying to get rid of the competence, of trying to be the first to launch a new product in the market, etc., which leads inevitably to serious consequences. As we have seen, the eagerness to produce new goods and launch them in the market before the competence can lead to frivolous and hasty applications of knowledge which is not sufficiently proved thus leading to certain negative consequences – among them, Technopathogenies. This is why we believe not to be wrong when we state that Technopathogenies can be the result of a *war*. Perhaps one section of this reading could also be: *Technopathogenology: a consequence of commercial war*. The compliance with the criteria implied in Technopathogenology would contribute to prevent such wars. No sensible businessman would develop a new product without the prior technopathogenic studies simply to be the first to launch it to the market. If the competence had done the studies required, it could use the proved safety of a product as a commercial strategy. Being the first in the market would then be less important.

We support the need to consider these risks as a single phenomenon or object of study because of their complexity and logical connection with their causal elements. This is why we have postulated the need of a specific discipline – Technopathogenology – for its study.

We believe that the Technopathogenologist, sooner or later, will be forced to become an ethical objector as we refer in the next reading. The

Science and Technique system, with its continuous hostility and opposition, can break down the scientist's work. And this is what happened to us. One of us was dismissed and the other one suffered such serious health deterioration that he was imposed an early retirement.

In the conference held in Vaquerias we also referred to other similar cases like Emde, Pusztai and Herbst.

We can then ask ourselves:

Are there not similarities between these extreme actions in politics – i.e. war – and the exercise of *power* in the corporate Scientific/Technological field?

Are there not similarities when voices that denounce ethical misdemeanors within the Science and Technique system are shut down?

Isn't the political power within the Science and Technique system harassing the denouncer until he or she becomes an ethical objector, even harassing the denouncer until he or she is expelled from the system?

How many times is a scientist who finds a risk or a questionable circumstance of application of a technique (like Dr. Emde) pressured to minimize the risk because the corporation where he works wants to carry on developing the project?

Doesn't this lead denouncers slowly but systematically to their resignation, illness, retirement or even death?

This thesis is very much resisted since, naturally, many scientists do not accept it. However, those very same scientists who resist such thesis could paradoxically commit to altruistic attitudes such as advocating for peace and opposing to war and nuclear weapons. Human good will is immediately stimulated in evident and horrid cases, as we have exemplified. But in spite of the good will, it is not always easy to recognize the subtle connection of ethical misdemeanors that lead to tragedies such as Thalidomide.

This paradox can occur due to the fact that for some scientists it is easier to recognize the external crime of war or massive destruction than the small ethical misdemeanors and even ignorance in their own trade.

Our thesis is that ethical objectors in Science and Technique might exist, but they may easily go unnoticed. Now, which are the similarities and differences of an ethical objector of the everyday life and one of Science and Technique?

Even though we will refer to this when we speak of Acute and chronic ethical objector, the main difference could be exemplified here by the analogy of the frog and the frying pan. As we have said before, when a frog is thrown into a boiling pan, it will jump immediately and run to safety. This would be the case of a quick or acute ethical objector: When facing an irritating situation, an immediate reaction is produced. On the other hand, when the frog is put in cold water and we slowly heat up the pan, the frog will not notice the danger and will eventually die. This is the case of the chronic (or patient) ethical objector.

This is the most common case of ethical objectors in Science and Technique, especially in public corporate systems. Therefore, just like a frog dies because it does not realize what is causing its death, the ethical objector will suffer a slow and subtle harassment, a myriad of indirect accusations that will undermine his or her health while, at the same time, being denied of the most essential equipment to work. This has been described by French Psychiatrist M. Hirigoyen. Given the subtlety of the persecution, it takes a long time to come to realize the harassment and its causes. In this case, the ethical objector will not denounce the risk.

But, which is the core of our dissertation?

We are interested in the fact that, just like the harassment by state power managed to hush some ethical objectors, ethical objectors in Science and Technique can also be hushed by harassment.

Which is the final consequence of this silence? It is simply a technical object of low quality. Now, when is a scientific or technological product of low quality? Not just when it falls short of the expectations for which it was created but when it carries potential flaws responsible for the phenomenon we have already described as Technopathogeny.

This phenomenon is a potential damage to health that goes unnoticed at first but that manifests itself after the application of a technological product.

The most paradigmatic case is that of the Thalidomide children.

Our belief is that in order for a Thalidomide child to exist there must have been a technopathogenic error in the creation of the product.

In order for this error to manifest itself there must have been a series of errors or ethical and scientific defects adding up and finally leading to human damage, overflowing the safeties of the Science and Technique system.

The human being is then turned into the inadvertent laboratory animal of technological innovation. *Accepting the risk to allow for technological progress* – apparent and fallacious inevitable condition – leads us to the following question: Human as inadvertent laboratory animal as a residual risk of technological progress: Is this really unavoidable?

Human as inadvertent laboratory animal as a residual risk of technological progress: Is this really unavoidable?

In the case of Thalidomide, had there been a specialized ethical objector, the critical points would have been brought to light as well as the willingness of the system to support its investigation.

Had there been a control of the causing factors of this Technopathogeny, there would have been no Thalidomide children (that is, if a technopathogenological research had been done parallel to the technological development or if the technological development of this medicine had applied the methodology of Technopathogenology).

We thus arrive to the conclusion that if Technopathogenology is applied to any development, we can avoid using humans as inadvertent laboratory animal – even if this science is new and methodically in formation.

This science aims at solving or investigating the dark points in the scientific technological development. If Technopathogenology becomes a standard practice, we will see that both ethical objectors in Science and Technique and people harassed by the system because they will not look the other way when they detect evident flaws will gradually disappear. But most importantly, there will be less and less ill-gestated technological objects. The human, inadvertent laboratory animal will then belong to the past.

We believe that Technopathogenology is a science that far from trying to find esoteric or metaphysical solutions – as it was accused of – aims at obtaining scientific solutions to a concrete problem.

We like the analogy of Criminalistics as a science to solve concrete crimes and its theoretical companion, Criminology.

With the development of Technopathogenology we discovered that apart from detecting and preventing technological risks, we found and proved the need of the existence of a mechanism to protect ethical objectors in Science and Technique.

Criminalistics, for example, evolved from an empirical and basic activity to a sophisticated science that involves specialized scientists so that not many crimes go unsolved nowadays.

A similar evolution is expected for Technopathogenology. This would avoid using humans as inadvertent laboratory animal to unveil latent technopathogenies. Technopathogenology could also avoid the harassment on researchers since, in order to be able to harass, power will need to know or at least be able to defend this attitude, i.e. its ignorance. Technopathogenological research can bring to light most unethical attitudes which cause corporate power harassment.

Indirect, hidden moral harassment to ethical objectors of Science and Technique will be harder to apply. Just like Criminology and Criminalistics can prevent normal crimes in society, Technopathogenology could prevent the *crime* of harassing ethical objectors in Science and Technique, just like the *crime* of using humans as inadvertent laboratory animal.

Just like ethical objectors are ignored in wars, what can an ethical objector do in Science and Technique against organized political power? Is what ethically committed scientists can do against the corporation similar to what ethical objectors do in wars?

As we will refer in the next reading, our personal and general experience shows us that the ethical objector in Science and Technique will face similar attitudes. These go from an initial disappointment to discriminatory acts and end with persecutory acts. If the ethical objector works in a private corporation, he or she will be immediately dismissed. If it is a public corporation and the person cannot be dismissed due to administrative reasons, the process will be slower, more insidious and therefore worse for the person's health, as we will describe in the last reading.

The ethical objector will have to be warned about the critical scientific points, but must also be trained in a discipline that includes not only the scientific research of the technological process including its weaknesses but also an ethical analysis of the whole process.

Conclusion

Just as we agreed on the need to protect ethical objectors that oppose to war and fight for peace, we hope we have contributed to raise awareness on the need, by analogy, to protect and promote ethical objectors in Science and Technique. Any ill-gestated technology which lacked ethical objectors to denounce its flaws during the scientific-technological and management processes implies a risk. Even if such risk does not involve the magnitude and commotion of a war, it can constitute a silent war which, just like common wars, leaves a myriad of victims and cripples.

This is why it is essential that technologists have a sound ethical training, in order to rectify the potential damage of their own developments. Once this kind of training is included, we could speak of the need of an *Ethics Guardian* (Vertrauensperson), already suggested by Günter Emde. An Ethics Guardian should exist in every workplace, especially in scientific academic environments. He could also be called *Person of Trust*, someone who can be told about any inappropriate behavior in the corporation that can jeopardize the health of many persons or, in the case of intellectual work, the lack of honesty in the distribution of merits and credits.

This is what we believe we are contributing with the technopathogenological training of technologists.

Where do we consider an Ethics Guardian necessary? When we referred to Ethics among the proceedings for the prevention of Technopathogeny in Chapter III, we mentioned ethical misdemeanors in Science and Technique. In order to support the need of an Ethics Guardian we can reiterate the following:

- In all the cases in which intellectual property (projects, ideas, etc.) is stolen or plagiarized, or when researchers out of work are pressured to exchange co-authorship for work.
- When a hugely profitable technological development is defended, ignoring, hiding or lying about its weak points. Some examples are: pesticides, genetic engineering, nuclear engineering, etc.
- When an innovator or discoverer is persecuted, avoiding a discussion about the entity of his or her invention or discovery and attacking people (persecution of colleagues). For example, Meyer, Semmelweiss, among others.

Finally, we believe that the use of humans as inadvertent laboratory animal as a consequence of residual risk of technological progress can be methodically avoided, provided an informed preventive policy is applied in Science and Technique. Some organizations such as Ethikschuetz-Initiative (ESI), INES/INESPE, which focus on global responsibility and ethical commitment, will be a highly valuable and essential contribution to achieve this aim.

VIII. Technopathogenology and the need of an ethical objector in Science and Technique

'Don't accept the habitual as a natural thing. In times of disorder, of organized confusion, of de-humanized humanity, nothing should seem natural. Nothing should seem impossible to change'
Bertolt Brecht

Introduction

There are several cases in which people find themselves facing risky situations at their workplace, either directly or indirectly. These situations involve unethical acts that may have an adverse effect on the whole society. When facing these acts, people must decide whether to remain silent, resist passively, or openly denounce them (Bultmann, 1996). If they choose the last option, they may be called altruists, since they put all their dedication and indulgence on the good of others, even at their own expense.

This mainly happens in occupations that are connected with high-risk technologies.

Moreover, and going deeper in the approach described in this book, we can add, due to its causal importance, those *occupations* related with the origin of the knowledge, creation and application of technologies.

In general, when these people reach a limit situation in which they discover a risk for the community, they find themselves in a dilemma between speaking out or not. In most cases, they must remain silent since they are afraid of reprisals. Several cases have been described about people who have suffered reprisals as they tried to uncover serious situations that harmed the community. In some cases, these people were even sent to prison (Bultmann, 1997).

The magnitude and importance that harassing acts may take due to ethical reasons have led to the creation of protection organizations in some countries. For instance, and inspired on Dr Günter Emde's initiative and work, which we will describe below, we can mention the creation of the Initiative of Ethical Protection in Germany by A. Bultmann. Our disciplinary proposal was considered of such relevance by the Director of this organization in relation to the scientist's ethical commitment that she allowed the inclusion of Technopathogenology in one of the articles submitted to the UNESCO, whose glossary includes this term (Bultmann).

Despite the possibility of reprisals, unethical acts represent a problem that forces people to decide between the responsible attitude of trying to solve it, or the irresponsible attitude of remaining static and not doing anything about it (Denevi, 2002).

The attitude of ethical responsibility is not only applied to those aspects that are directly connected to humans, but also with problems that may represent a risk for the ecosystem (Huisman Fuentes, 2001).

Facing a non-ethical act responsibly implies, as we have said, the possibility of reprisals. For that reason, INES created the Initiative of Ethical Protection (INESPE-International Network of Engineers and Scientists' Projects on Ethics), which is an international movement that helps concrete people with their ethical commitment without interfering with the normal legal channels (Tengstrom, 1985).

When we deal with the description of the acts that ethical objectors in Science and Technique may suffer, we will mention certain paradigmatic cases in order to illustrate some of them.

We will also describe a case mentioned by Dr. Hirigoyen, a psychiatrist of great relevance for the present reading: Paul's case (his surname is concealed to maintain the professional secret). Likewise, we will not give any names in the cases we describe; we even consider it irrelevant.

In order to illustrate the present reading, we have also turned to a few personalities such as philosophers and writers. We have taken their thoughts, because since they can say so much with so little, it encourages others to think of the way of acting, so as to have a harmonious relationship in human life.

History of the ethical protection initiative

The Ethical Protection Initiative was created by Dr. Günter Emde, in Germany, in 1992 (Schraeder, 1995). Dr. Emde had been a researcher in a cybernetics company where he found out that his inventions were used in intelligent missile heads that were sold without any restriction. As a pacifist he resisted such use of his inventions, but the company decided to solve the conflict by dismissing him. Later, Dr. Emde presented the

Ethical Protection Initiative at the International Network of Engineers and Scientist for Global Responsibility (INES), which included it as a project called International Network of Engineers and Scientists to Protect and Promote the Ethical Engagement (INESPE), becoming its first Director.

Some persons, who receive support form INES/INESPE, include: A. Nikitin, M. Vanunu, van Buitenen, M. Herbst and one of the writers of the present book, A. Motta, who was expelled from the University due to the whistleblower nature of our work. All these cases have in common people who in their regular occupation found situations that are incompatible with ethics, situations that presented a risk to the whole community. They refused to play along with these situations; they refused to benefit from them either by action (by actively participating in the unethical act) or by omission (by covering them and benefiting from the silence). The decision of not participating in *foul play*, forces the system to try to keep them silent. This brings to them difficulties of various kinds when facing power and authority, including economic and even more serious ones such as the loss of freedom (Deiserot, 1997). They are people who, in spite of all this, assume an ethical commitment. They are people who experience that deep feeling which was so clearly described by the British writer and politician, Edmund Burke (1729-1797): "All that is necessary for the triumph of evil is that good men do nothing" (Burke).

In other cases, since the system cannot expel or imprison the person, it makes him or her undergo a constant moral harassment, with the intention of making him or her resign voluntarily or collapse physically and psychologically.

The Ethical Protection Initiative has the purpose of helping these people in different ways. Nowadays, the aspects of the Ethical Protection Initiative that actually motivated its creation (helping people around the world who have proved that their tasks are deeply related with ethics (INESPE/Ethikschuetzinitiative, 2000) and are thus being persecuted) are managed by the ESI (Ethikschutz-Initiative) organization under the direction of Antje Bultmann. The INESPE Project is more oriented to the academic/scientific aspects of the problem, its current director being Professor Tom Boersen Hansen.

INES is an independent non-profit organization interested in the impact of science and technology on society and is mainly devoted to the prevention of nuclear war. INES was founded in 1991 in Berlin at the

Challenges – Science and Peace in a rapidly changing environment Congress.

The INES efforts focus on international peace and disarmament, science ethics, scientists' responsibilities and the responsible use of science and technology, justice and sustainable development.

The ethical protection in Science and Technique

Science and Technique are nowadays undergoing a process of self-criticism. From a dogmatic position, in which the positive Comtian doctrine had emphasized the importance of replacing the religious dogmas in order to be able to do a true and objective scientific work, a similar mistake to the one they were trying to avoid was committed. Thus, religious dogmas were, consciously or unconsciously, replaced by scientific dogmas. They were dogmas all the same, not less strict and even more questionable due to their imperfection, since they pretend to have the character of absolute and indisputable explanations of reality. Moreover, the religious dogma is based on blind faith and as such, if it does not have any explanation, it can at least be justified for being religious. But when science requests blind faith from those who follow a theory and give a dogmatic character, a tragedy strikes when no explanation or justification is found.

Therefore, the dogma of the innocuousness of the concrete technological object (based on a supposed infallibility of the scientific method used to generate it) was supported. If unexpected and harmful to health side effects appeared, they were considered an exception to the rule. The accumulations of cases that contradict the dogma have made it stagger. As we concluded when we referred to the innocuousness of the technological object *the lack of consideration of human values will lead Technology to an irreducible antithesis with the own essence of the human being.* The criterion of the *exception to the rule* is not enough to justify damage to human beings' health. Nowadays, more realistic solutions are being sought for the more and more burning issue of the unexpected side effects in Technique, which leads to evident conflicts among different schools or even better, different programs (Lakatos, 1982) and paradigms (Kuhn, 1995). Here is where there should be more room for those who have the systematic study of those side effects or persistent anomalies as their own object of study in an unconditional search of its causes (Eguiazu & Motta, 2001b).

The unexpected verification of the fallibility of the scientific knowledge has contributed to this search. As we have said above, it was mainly expressed by the environmental issue and the technopathogenic issue.

The technopathogenic issue is a very particular case involving ethical faults. People can find unethical situations during the entire process that goes from the genesis of knowledge and the development, testing and dissemination of technologies. As we have seen, there are bodies of knowledge (Technologies) that are used even though there is evidence or suspicion of voids in them. These voids can mean that in the Techniques developed from them, flaws that manifest themselves in the short or long term can exist, resulting in damage to human health. If they manifest themselves in the long term, we define them as Technopathogenies (Motta, 1994). This application of knowledge and techniques without enough evidence of innocuousness, obeys to giving priority, mainly, to economic benefit instead of the safety of the community (Eguiazu & Motta, 2001a).

Finally, we enter the international normative aspect, when evident side effects are verified in certain technologies and – as it happens in the case of pesticides – this does not prevent these from being sent to another part of the world. In this way, a big business is done by keeping silent its side effects (Eguiazu, 1996). In these cases, many times one counts on the complicity of the customs' departments employees.

We can see, then, that the ethical protection in Science and Technique must be present or may be necessary in all the stages of development up to the application of the knowledge, such as:

- Genesis of knowledge
- Development of technologies
- Pilot testing of these technologies
- Dissemination of these technologies
- Stop or permission to use or export after side effects of late manifestation have been detected

This chart briefly indicates the five critical points where ethical protection is necessary since, in each of them, not only strict quality controls must be applied but also strict ethical controls. If the people involved in each of these stages detect that some of these controls are not carried out or there is an attempt to avoid them, they may find it necessary to report it. If there is an attempt to silence such people, they become ethical objectors that require support and protection. The quality control during each stage is essential so as not to get to the next point without a previous control, and if possible, to avoid the genesis of a technological object with potential technopathogenies. In some cases, one runs out of chances to know more, despite the actors' good will. In other cases, little ethical faults that are deliberately tolerated carry their consequences to each of the stages, leading to a final object that carries unacceptable side effects.

The ethics in the academic-scientific world: Is it obvious or should it be made explicit?

It is widely accepted that scientists must not lie. So their best virtue must be veracity. Nobel Prize winner Dr. Leloir always responded to whoever asked him about the qualities researchers should have: "mainly not to lie." He gave more importance to this virtue over vocation, talent or diligence, and he was not wrong. However, in scientific research, fraud and deception are also present (Gomez Herrera, 1984) (Hansson, 1999).

Besides the rightness of Dr. Leloir's response, we consider that watching over the researcher's virtues there must be a system that respects Freedom of Thought, which, as we have already mentioned in the first reading, is a basic characteristic of an Authentic scientific system. We can ask ourselves: is it worthwhile for researchers to be truthful in their affirmations if they are not allowed to investigate critical topics they think they should, or those which their *instinct* leads them to? In our system, for instance, that claims to respect freedom of thought, the Science and Technique system will classify the research areas into commissions. A new researcher will have the *freedom* to choose the subject he or she wants to work on as far as it falls within the framework of a commission that can evaluate it, or else he or she will encounter all sort of problems. In other words, you can choose any color, as far as it is red, yellow or blue.

Now, this sounds ambiguous since there are also different degrees of truth or falseness. It is not the same to plagiarize a book or a whole project than to take a phrase or part from the book or project without making references to the source. One must wonder:

- In which situations does a researcher face the temptation to lie?
- When has a result been purposely modified so that it does not contradict the expected phenomenon or curve?
- How much is a little and how much is a lot?
- When has the power given by belonging to an examination board been used so that the director, the disciples or members of his or her own workgroup could obtain privileges?
- How much of this is allowed? In which situations should this not be allowed at all?
- When has an innovative work been excluded for its essential faults and when simply because of the examiner's envy or anger, who thinks: why gas this occurred to me?
- How can we detect, at an early stage, if the examiner shows emotional faults in the evaluation?
- Which efficient mechanisms can we have for real revisions of negative reports that go beyond the administrative?
- How can we notice when an examiner says no, *just because*, in an authoritarian way, without any explanation?
- Has such rejection happened due to laziness or fear of the new or because what has been presented was essentially of low quality?
- Which efficient mechanisms exist in order to control the quality of the evaluative act?
- Who examines whom and under which objective rules?
- How can we distinguish between relations of mutual enrichment for the work groups or work directions, and the inexcusable relations of parasitism?
- How can we avoid and recognize at an early stage the maneuvers of an authoritarian system that exhausts the youth's talents while exploiting them, maneuvers which are performed by the most advanced researchers of the system?
- How can we detect when a researcher is being discriminated by the critical nature of the research subject he or she chose?

In general, these questions were supposed to be implicit in all evaluative acts and were rarely stated explicitly. The evaluators' honesty was not questioned. The existence of Aloentic scientific systems was unthinkable.

Just as the application of knowledge and techniques without sufficient evidence of innocuousness happens due to giving more importance to economic benefit, it is easy to detect in all the noted non-ethical attitudes the economic interest or corporate favoritism that motivates them. Some of them tend to discriminate against researchers that could irritate established interests, others to benefit some and discriminate others in terms of incentives, research subsidies, etc. Apart from the reasons described, and as it is mentioned in one of the points, some personal reasons such as envy or professional jealousy can be the cause of non-ethical attitudes.

In the first reading, we have analyzed the characteristics of two Science and Technique systems, the Authentic and the Aloentic. We have seen the results produced by each of them. In relation to the subject we are dealing with in this reading, we can add that, since in an Authentic system the ethical faults can be denounced, the figure of the persecuted or *resister*, to the system may not exist. You will find an example of that below:

In an Aloentic system, if a young person who starts to research and has the ethical commitment to do so finds faults in the system – a system that will try to control, condition or *tame* him or her so that he or she does not *snoop around* - he or she may never get to carve out a career.

Recalling what we described in the first reading about the transgressive character that an Authentic scientific researcher has when working within an Aloentic system, we can surely state that the ethical objector in Science and Technique is par excellence a transgressor, since by breaking the obstacles that compromise his or her freedom to uncover problems that are crucial to society, he or she becomes a victim of the system, a system that will try to silence him or her. There are some humanists who are branded as transgressors because they worry about affairs that are kept hidden by society in order not to be shocked by them. Similarly, scientists can also be transgressors when they *shock* the ruling scientific group with their statements. A researcher of this kind will fight for an idea. He or she will resist for years, becoming a *Resister*; he or she will persevere in his or her ethical commitment, but will be left out of all kind of benefits. If the person is a researcher who has already been trained in the Aloentic system and because of an *explosion* of conscience pretends to denounce some ethical faults, he or she will become an ethical objector and will suffer the corresponding consequences. In most of the cases, though, the privileges received from the system and, perhaps, some previous misdemeanor made on behalf of the corporation that supported, favored or even empowered him or her, determine that this researcher ignores deliberately all ethical faults and continues profiting from the situation. In the best of cases, he or she will retire, leaving things as they were. Such researcher does not commit. By retiring, he or she does not become an ethical objector by omission, a concept that we will refer to later. This last position, i.e. the attitude of leaving all as it is, of not stepping in the defense of a colleague by keeping silence, damages the true ethical objector. This is not the ethical objector's silence before a situation in which a non-ethical act is proposed that sooner or later will damage him or her, but the silence of somebody who is not an ethical objector but, recognizing a colleague who is, leaves him or her to be persecuted and damaged by keeping silence. By being loyal to the corporation, he or she will neither denounce the ethical faults nor support those who commit to do so.

The Swedish Parliament

Paradoxically, in one of the countries with the fewest and less important faults in Science and Technique, the idea of evaluating and systematizing the most common faults was proposed. The ethical scientists' performance was criticized during complex debates in a commission created by the Swedish Parliament.

Therefore, well-known but relatively harmless cases such as the Piltdown fraud, common occurrences like innocent plagiarism in thesis presentations, and serious ethical faults have been evaluated in detail (Westerholm, 1999). These faults include mobbing and moral harassment to scientists (Hirigoyen, 2001).

The university ombudsman

At some universities, the *University Ombudsman* figure has been established, for instance in the University of Karlsruhe which is essentially technological.

This system has been established because people harmed by a non-ethical behavior prefer to use the Ombudsman instead of regular administrative channels.

In general, the administrative channels of certain universities which are not so respectful of people, do not consider the reason on which the administrative act was based, but only evaluate their formal correctness. This administrative attitude makes it possible for injustices and persecutions to be carried out in the name of a clumsy statutory logic. Student persecution, currently called *mobbing,* is hidden by subtle administrative reasons. The legal system hardly revises any report or administrative act since it does not question the good or bad faith of the ones who made them but only takes into account its formal perfection. This, in the academic scientific world, leaves the one who turns to the justice of the system totally defenseless. All reports that are well written without internal contradictions are sustained, no matter how many appeals are lodged. They are irrevocable. In a previous chapter, we quoted Albert Einstein in connection to the technological problem "Problems cannot be solved by those who have caused them." We can say the same about our situation regarding persecution. Evidently, an ethical objector cannot expect his or her problems to be solved by the ones who have caused them. The system that generates the moral harassment against ethical objectors will not recognize its existence, so it will hardly be forced to solve it.

The corporate character of the system is clearly expressed in the reports. Each main or ad-hoc commission will always endorse the report handed out by the first evaluative commission. It is obvious that the report is sent to different commissions just to comply with an administrative requirement. We can also think that in this way, the corporation group that harasses the researcher compromises the rest of the corporation. This is an internal control mechanism.

The true modifications to erroneous reports are only achieved by political action, and this is related to discretion, as we have said, to "the freedom or power to make one's own judgment" (Standard Encyclopedic Dictionary) and in some cases to the arbitrariness of the acts of authority (Universitaet Karlsruhe, 2000) (Volmar, 2002).

Thus, for instance, by the simple method of ignoring what has been done and focusing on what it has not, or in the simple subversion of giving values to certain rules, any report of an evaluative commission can be hatched either for or against the evaluated person. The legal or administrative channels are useful only to confirm the report, but not for its essential revision. It can only be considered invalid if there are formal mistakes in what is written. What is interesting about this is that what is written is only examined in its formal correctness, without investigating its basis. It is like a theorem coming from false premises: although all its development is correct, the result will be wrong. The administrative mechanism is not interested in all this, but only in the formal perfection of the intermediary steps.

Oddly enough, when administrative clumsiness joins a persecutory corporate intent, every researcher or university professor is defenseless.

On the other hand, a University Ombudsman can interpret the equity of a report beyond its formal perfection.

Our involvement as technopathogenologists within the INESPE project

Within the INESPE project, our proposal has the aim of:
1. Respecting the ethical commitment in a field so crucial and relevant to humans as Technology is.
2. Intending to comply with the values of an Authentic scientific system against the values of an Aloentic system, widely described in the reading corresponding to that topic.
3. Developing educative and preventive work for new researchers regarding a reality they may have to face in their scientific activity, so that from the very beginning they can adopt attitudes that may protect their intellectual property as well as their own heath.
4. Training professionals and future professionals of technological areas concerning non-evident technological risks and the ethical principles related to them.
5. Helping ethical objectors, mainly in Science and Technique.

These were the reasons why we were invited to be members of the INES organization and the INESPE project, which diagnosed our situation and described it as typical of ethical objectors. At the beginning, this diagnosis surprised us. In fact, we did not understand the attitudes we were facing were characteristic of ethical objectors until the INES report was handed out. All these attitudes have already been described in the first reading and will be expanded afterwards. Such attitudes have a common factor: the lack of respect, not only as researchers but also the lack of the minimal respect any human being has the right to receive.

The fact that the harassed person does not understand those attitudes can also be explained by the fact that an Authentic researcher always starts from *trust*, while in the Aloentic system, he or she starts from *distrust*. This trust is based on a certain amount of naivety that leads him or her to the unconditional search for knowledge, thus forgetting about him or herself. The system definitely knows it can take advantage whenever it finds a naive person who trusts it. The researcher who trusts ends up being a naive person who offers ideas freely, receiving some kind of reciprocity by the system. In some way, the naive person thinks: *If I give away ideas freely, I will receive their respect and the minimal means to continue working.* But this is not so.

The Authentic researcher does not know that within the Aloentic system, as well as in the wilderness, he or she should adopt a distrust attitude as a means of survival. A scientific person who values ethics and the given word finds it incomprehensible and unacceptable to distrust people who should be better than the common mortals. A person who is used to keeping his or her given word cannot accept that others act differently. This is why he or she is always at a disadvantage within an Aloentic system. Such ethical culture leads the Authentic researcher to be a predator's victim. After some time, he or she discovers bitterly that he or she was plundered and that the expected respect and means of work never arrived.

Consequently, the aim of training new researchers in the risks that may exist in the Science and Technique system where they will develop their work is oriented towards new researchers who have ideas, enthusiasm, will to work and idealism; i.e. researchers with true vocation. In the system there are also researchers that only enter it because after finishing their university studies they have not received any offer by a private company, so they accept a grant as a paid waiting time. In other cases, they may apply in search for the social position that being a scientific researcher gives them, or because the grant was offered by a friend or a friend of a friend who happens to be a director. We do not think it is necessary to train those people since they do not usually have ideas to be stolen. They are not people who wish to assume an ethical commitment either; they just want a position. For them, scientific work is simply another job and their director is just a boss who gives them orders they have to follow without thinking too much.

To continue with the case of the Authentic researcher, the situation gets complicated for the system when it does not destroy its victim quickly. As in the jungle, the prey already knows the existing dangers and will try to be safe; thus appears the figure of the *Resister*.

The concept of *Resister* is very important to us since it is the attitude we were forced to take throughout our work. The open or veiled opposition was so intense that we had to display an extraordinary resistance so as not to abandon the work completely. The support given by INES in the last years made us strong enough so as not to weaken when the action taken against us became clumsy and open.

It is important to emphasize, as we consider it a support our task would deserve to receive, that after having studied in depth mycotoxins in Germany, as we mentioned in Chapter II, we asked the Commission on International Migration (CIM) to support its continuity in Argentina.

During discussions with some of the members of this Committee, it was agreed that it was necessary to create a university program and a specific institute for the development of our line of work. The Committee arranged the chair in the Conicet and in the local University. After some rounds of negotiations, working conditions were agreed upon with the Committee.

But the promises made by our official organizations to the Committee were never fulfilled and we only got precarious working conditions that meant an enormous personal effort. This shows that research subjects in which the consumer's health is at risk are sidelined or poorly supported.

Although authorities of our country had promised this International Organization that we would have space and support to develop our chair and institute in order to be able to work on our research question, such promises were never kept. All the subsequent work we carried out for over two decades was due to effort and *resistance*.

We requested support to many organizations such as ministries, private companies, Conicet, Secyt, Foncyt; yet, we were rejected by all of them. Why? Then we asked ourselves the following question: why is not a direct defense of society and human health directly promoted without hesitation? Is it because this health risks are related to highly profitable technological processes? Is it because by showing the side effects of these highly profitable technological processes there could be substantial economic losses? Or maybe because non-ethical practices in science and technology would be made evident?

The *administrative process* that tried to destroy our work can be considered a *lapidary process*. Lapidary is a word that means stoning, a punishment by which a condemned person is stoned to death. Stoning assures in some way individual impunity since it is a group of people who collectively throw stones to the condemned person.

The concrete killer, the concrete stone that kills the condemned person, can never be identified. The person who may suffer pangs of conscience could say: *I didn't kill him, I just threw a stone*. But what kills is the whole group, the collectiveness. The same happens with the moral harassment we have suffered at work. Nobody could be blamed. As we will see later, it is common in cases like this to hear the people involved saying *I didn't do it*. Actually, in a certain way, there is not an individual culprit. Therefore, in the present reading, we will use the term *corporation*, in which each individual *throws a stone*. It could be small or big, but each of them hurts the person, who unless is rescued from the *stoning*, will eventually succumb.

Attacks against the ethical objector:
Psychopathic process – Four consequences

The system's reaction to our position of ethical objectors in Science and Technology for pretending to approach our investigations outside the described criteria of an Aloentic system has made us suffer different attitudes or situations that can be classified into three categories, as we will see in table 36.

No matter how serious the attitudes may be it is not wrong to consider them *aggressions*, since their aim is to hurt, a term that in its full meaning can be applied to what is done to ethical objectors: they are hurt, ill-treated or spoiled. The latter can be applied both to researchers, who are wasted or *spoiled* as such, and to their work. It is important to make clear that considering the attitudes as simply aggressions may not be enough. As we will see, the final aim of some of them is to eliminate the attacked person.

For these attitudes' characteristics, degree of violence and way of occurring, our own experience – either for personal suffering and/or just observation – we will describe a process to which an ethical objector is submitted.

Psychopathic process

Even though the different psychopathies related to harassment in the workplace are described by specialists, we are really interested in analyzing other aspects related to this problem in the scientific/academic field which allows us to define the above mentioned *stoning* as a *psychopathic process*. We would like to make it clear that we are making the following proposal with full respect of psychiatry specialists. What is described in this reading is the consequence of our experience; we would like to emphasize that we refer only to the scientific/academic environment where we developed our work. This experience has also led us to suffer the described attitudes, many of which, according to specialists, can match several of the 45 actions described by Dr Heinz Leymann within the moral harassment framework (Anonymous (c)).

Perhaps the attitudes we will describe have already been studied and have a more suitable nomenclature than the one we propose.

We find it interesting to explain an aspect we have observed: it is very common to mistakenly consider that all the negative acts a person suffers at work constitute moral harassment.

Unlike moral harassment – which is widely dealt with in the context of the workplace – we find it appropriate to consider all the difficult situations an ethical objector goes through in Science and Technique, including moral harassment, as a psychopathic process. Such phenomenon can be defined as a: *Degenerative, systematic/corporative, and diachronic process, which is progressive in intensity*.

According to the definition of each term, we can say:

1. *Process*: because it is a set of successive phases of a phenomenon.
2. *Degenerative*: because it tends to go from a condition or state to another one which is the opposite or worse. Its aim is the person's *decay*, i.e. turning gradually a person or thing from a perfection or prosperity state to that of imperfection, dissolution or adversity.

3. *Systematic/Corporative*: because it follows or adjusts to a doctrinaire system.
4. *Diachronic*: because it is a phenomenon that occurs throughout
time.
5. *Progressive*: because it continuously increases.

The 5 aspects clearly differentiate this process from regular moral harassment.

In order to support this, we can also argue the following:

A. The degenerative effect influences both the person and his or her
own project. We could even state that in the case of the ethical
objector in Science and Technique, the attack on his or her research program is the most important thing. That means that
whereas in moral harassment harassers make the individual abandon his or her workplace, in the psychopathic process, the
main interest of the corporation is to profit from the researcher's
professional skill, and/or avoid, if the case requires so, the introduction or advancement in areas which the corporation considers
dangerous or forbidden. The motives can go far beyond personal
or group trivial reasons such as envy, in fact, a whole system can
be implicated. This risk can be present in the case where the researcher's activity endangers the sustainment of the canons established by the system dogma or doctrine on which it rests. The
canons at risk are the values listed for an Aloentic system seen in
the first reading, and/or when they can bring to light knowledge
that may affect big interests. It is in these situations when the ethical objector is of crucial importance.

B. As we have seen before, the phenomenon we are analyzing, by
being Systematic/Corporative, depends on a system. Recalling its
definition, system is the set of things or parts coordinated under a
law, which are orderly related to each other and contribute to a
certain object or function. In the case of the psychopathic
process, the attitudes detailed in table 36 show a set of acts,
coordinated under a *law* – the corporation rule – a non-written
law that is followed blindly as if its non-fulfillment were a taboo.
Just as a secret society, it is run by implacable codes and with the
omerta or code of silence. These attitudes are orderly related to
each other and contribute to a certain object or aim. In the case of

moral harassment, to control or destroy a person. It is an environmental problem of the institution and not of a group of people that may play a secondary role. Consequently, we use the term Corporation, although we could also use the following terms, perhaps with more accuracy: *Fraternity*: since its members make up a union, company or group of people for a certain aim. *Clique*: since it is a group of people that influence surreptitiously the State business and other acts or decisions. *Sect*: we could even use this term, for being a group of believers in a particular doctrine. That is why we use the term *doctrinaire*. The psychopathic process is influenced by deeper interests than the ones that can simply trigger moral harassment in the workplace, as we saw in the previous item. In general, within the psychopathic process the responsible people cannot be identified. Even the ones who sign resolutions, regulations or make aggravating and discrediting judgments against the persecuted person must do so because they must follow the *group's* orders. The group can remain in total anonymity. Instead, moral harassment refers to a group of people as identified harassers.

C. Furthermore, when saying systematic/corporative, we are referring to the important doctrinaire and dogmatic component that lies in the motives of the psychopathic process. This shows that due to the person's activity, a whole system may be implicated, as we have already mentioned.

D. Moreover, since the phenomenon is progressive in intensity, at the beginning the acts are practically *innocent*. In moral harassment, the intention as defined by Leymann is an extreme psychological violence, it is destructive. It could be considered literally as stalking: term that defines an insistent attack that has the intention to bother somebody persistently and with certain intent. In the Science and Technique System, these pretensions make reference to vanity, the presumption of the members of the corporation to the arbitrary right that they claim to have over a person or his or her production. Moral harassment makes the harassed person abandon the workplace. The psychopathic process first tries to take advantage of his or her ideas. For all the above described, this kind of phenomenon can last more than two decades.

E. As a victim of moral harassment is considered every person who, among other peculiarities, has suffered the following one or more times a week, during at least a six month period...(the author then mentions some of the 45 acts observed by Leymann) (Gutiérrez, 2003). In the psychopathic process the listed acts in table 36 do not follow a regular frequency: once a week, twice a week, etc. The corporation does not need to follow a routine since it has a researcher *in its hands*, who depends on it and who it will try to control and take advantage of his or her ideas. Perhaps a more appropriate term would be *ruling*, in the sense of governing or dominating. That is why it is common to hear that the ones who cannot be *ruled* are branded as *anarchists*. If they cannot be ruled, the next intention of the corporation is to destroy them, knowing it has all the time to do so. It is the figure of the *military siege* where the enemy has a city besieged and has all the necessary time to attack. By knowing that sooner or later the besieged will have to surrender or commit suicide, the enemy does not need to act intensely or with certain regularity, but can attack sporadically, without worrying about the results, knowing that a more direct attack will only result in unneeded damages to the attacker. The enemy knows that the besieged cannot abandon the site and that he is victim of such uncertainty and fear that may affect him more than any direct attacks. If this uncertainty is not enough, starvation by hunger and thirst will finish the job. This is the best example of the corporative moral harassment in public institutions. An ethical objector in Science and Technique is a *besieged* researcher, victim at times, in a system that expects his or her surrender or elimination, pretending it to be the researcher's own decision so that the corporation does not seem to be directly responsible. Even the arguments the corporation uses to justify certain attitudes are infuriating. For this last reason, the moral damage caused can hardly be proved. Continuing with the military example, it is as if in the well-known siege of Masada, the Roman army would have said: *They committed suicide, we didn't do anything.* If while trying to eliminate the ethical objector the corporation turns to extreme measures such as the ones that characterize moral harassment, there could be members of the corporation at that level that may seem directly responsible.

F. Although the psychopathic process motive is dogmatic or doctrinaire, within the acting corporation there are people who can have other reasons for attacking the person. What's more, the corporation members that protect their dogmatic interests – who, as we have said in item b (and will repeat below) are unknown since they do not want to be put in evidence – take advantage of other members that have spurious interests against the person so as to see him or her decline. Take for instance the case of a researcher whom the corporation wanted to dominate, and in order to do so, tampered with a competition, which eventually declared him incompetent. The evaluating commission was composed of a professor who had personal hostility – due to envy for not having graduated as a doctor – against another person who benefited from an academic position, and against another one whose unfavorable report was the payment for a political favor.

Returning to the example of the siege, if in our case in particular one wonders which the *siege* was, the answer would be: not assigning subsidies, positions, leaving us outside the incentive system, not providing us with resources, etc. If the question is: which was the *harassment*? The answer would be: false accusations, compulsive eviction from the workplace, dismissal, forged trial, etc.

The last moments of this long process are the ones that increase in intensity and brutality, thus reaching – in the last stages – the levels described by Leymann though not with the indicated frequency of one or more times a week, until the harassed persons end up destroyed.

The classification of attitudes into the three categories grouped in table 36 is to show the different magnitude and aim in each of them. Besides, even though we refer to this phenomenon as progressive, we are not suggesting that the different attitudes follow the order indicated in table 36. Surely the acts are more violent as the psychopathic process advances. However, we consider it convenient to state that after the initial attitudes, more serious ones will enter the picture. Therefore, in an advanced stage of the process, there will be situations of *mobbing, moral harassment, pressing, mocking,* as well as others we will describe in this reading.

All these situations are caused by the members of a corporation. Among the actors of the corporation, no matter what the hierarchical level is, there is a *tacit complicity*. It seems to be inevitable that *target persons* have to be persecuted even with joyful impunity at times. We say *joyful* attitude because the corporation enjoys seeing who cleverly manages to stop or prevent target persons from doing their activity. Of course, this only takes place at the beginning. In later stages the attitude changes, it turns into cold indifference and finally, into brutal aggression.

It would seem that the set of situations to which ethical objectors in Science and Technique are subjected, responds to the insane curiosity of *let's see how much they can take*, i.e., how much they are able to resist, term that originates the figure of *resister* and which we will describe soon.

Although we refer to this process as Psychopathic because it mainly affects the individual's psyche, if we described it generally, it would be a Morbid Process. That is the reason why its intentionality is precisely, as its name indicates, to make people ill. As we have said, even though manifestations are mainly psychopathies, there can also be somatic diseases related to them – therefore the use of the word *Morbid* – as well as social consequences of such a process, especially on the harassed person's family.

Psychiatry has widely described the main psychopathies associated with moral harassment. Of course, it is definitely not the intention of this work to describe psychopathies associated with moral harassment. Dr Heinz Leymann, who popularized the term *mobbing* in the 1980's, and Dr Hirigoyen, to whom we will often refer, have done a great and extensive job regarding this subject. As we will see, moral harassment includes acts which are highly aggressive. As Dr Hirigoyen explains, they must have an aggressive tone since the harasser wants to destroy the harassed.

Moral harassment is known to cause serious health problems. Since the phenomenon we are dealing with is a process with particular features that comes as consequence of the acts performed within the frame of this phenomenon and that are listed in table 36, we have observed the possibility of occurrence of four consequences.

Mithridatism, irreversible cumulative effect,
reversible cumulative effect and anesthesia

We have said that it would seem that the aggressions ethical objectors suffer would respond to the insane curiosity: Let's see how much they can take, or how much they are able to resist.

There would be two kinds of resisters:

A. The ethical objector who resists non-ethical proposals and acts. This is a moral resister: one who has a deep sense of justice and equity, and who does not want to be involved in non-ethical acts. This negative act, according to what the corporation pretends to get from him or her, leads to psychic maltreatment, which either destroys the ethical objector's active life – or life, period – or else gives way to the following concept:

B. The ethical objector who resists. This is the consequence of the previous concept, the difference being that in this case he or she resists psychologically and/or resists the physical consequences caused by the psychic maltreatment.

Many times, due to the harassers' arrogance, contempt to the harassed or meanness, the moral harassment attitudes are light at the beginning thinking that by taking light attitudes they will manage to break the harassed. Yet, this could be counterproductive for the harasser, since every situation that is resisted by the harassed forces the harasser to use more violence the next time.

We now can refer to the first consequence of this title, *Mithridatism.*

There is a well-known phenomenon in medicine, a resistance to poison acquired by the progressive administration of it starting from a harmless dose. This phenomenon is called Mithridatism.

Even though the attitudes against an ethical objector can lead him or her to serious health problems, in the case of the resister the concept used by medicine should perhaps be applied, since as in Mithridatism, the acts are also progressive in intensity – the acts are also *harmless and innocent* at the beginning. For the case analyzed in this reading, we could talk about *mithridatism to moral harassment.* Or else, if we call the first kind somatic Mithridatism, for being the body the one that resists poison, in our case we could call it *Psychological Mithridatism,* which is related to point B; the ethical objector resists because his or her psyche becomes resistant. Therefore, regarding the ethical objector, the *resister* could be called *Mithridates* as well.

We cannot assure, however, that this psychological Mithridatism can be sustained indefinitely. Most surely the person will be unemployed before an irreversible damage occurred. In this respect and if we continue with the comparison of the resistance to poison, apparently, Mithridatism would only apply to poisonous substances whose toxic effect depends on the dose. We have already quoted Paracelso when we discussed error as a cause of Technopathogeny in Chapter I: "The dose makes the poison." We have also said that nowadays there are hypotheses that talk about a cumulative effect for even small doses of carcinogenic substances, which only after several years of exposure would have their effects on health made manifest. That is to say, Mithridatism does not apply to substances that may have the effect of inducing or promoting a carcinogenic process.

Although we think this could be a more extensive subject of study for other specialists, we consider that psychological Mithridatism will only apply to certain types of aggression or to some people, who, for special circumstances, are able to experience it.

On the other hand, and as we have said above, even with the existence of a psychological Mithridatism, the individual may suffer other organic disorders, and/or members of his or her family be the ones affected. Eventually, the individual will always be damaged.

However, even though we accept the possibility of a psychological Mithridatism, the fact that the person is a resister does not justify the harassment.

Mithridatism can evolve in two other consequences. The comparison to the substances that may lead to a neoplastic damage let us think of the second consequence: the *Irreversible Cumulative Effect*. We wondered if all or some of these aggression acts of higher or lower degree (such as the ones listed in the columns Discouragement and Discrimination in table 36) may have a cumulative effect. In this case, the acts would be *harmless only in appearance*, since eventually they will end up showing the unexpected damage, unexpected for the apparent little importance of each individual act. On the other hand, as in the case of a neoplastic process where different factors may intervene with different properties (physical, chemical, initiator, promoter, synergistic, etc., in the case of the psychopathic process we are analyzing, different attitudes also intervene. If the psychic attitudes had behaved as the factors that trigger neoplastic processes, the apparent psychic Mithridatism would not be such because finally and inevitably they damage the individual's psyche. In this case, we could call this cumulative effect the *Irreversible Cumulative Effect*, also to differentiate it from the one we will describe below.

548

The other consequence that may be related to Mithridatism and that we have also observed in this psychopathic process we are analyzing is an effect we could call *Reversible Cumulative Effect*.

To analyze this, we will continue with the similarity with chemical substances. For a poison that acts in an acute way to manifest its effect, it needs to reach certain levels of concentration in the organism, the level varying according to the substance. There are poisons – a pesticide for instance – that have the property of accumulating in the organism. If a poison needs to reach, for example, 100 units to show signs of acute poisoning in a person, and the person has received 90, he or she will not manifest any effect. But if later the person is exposed to the same poison again, even though it is a light exposition but enough to reach the 100 units when added up to the 90 the organism had collected, the person will show signs of poisoning. We have noticed this same effect within the framework of the phenomenon we are analyzing. Take the case of a researcher who was a victim of persecution at his work but did not show any critical psychological sign. It happened that while being in an official organization doing an errand which was unconnected to his scientific activity, he had to endure a situation that could be described as maltreatment. Although it was insignificant, he suffered a crisis episode when he arrived home that could only be overcome after some hours. Despite being able to get over the unpleasant situation caused by maltreatment, he knew he had to avoid similar situations, since because of the anguish *accumulated* by the persecution process, a new crisis could be triggered. When we described toxicology tests in Chapter II, we said that in order to predict or prevent potential risks due to exposure to xenobiotics one can turn to biomarkers. In the same manner, an emotional situation, unpleasant but trivial, could perhaps be a *psychomarker* of non-manifested psychological damages that then triggers a psychological crisis. We could call this an effect psychomarker since it is the result of a previous act. But as there are biomarkers of susceptibility, it would be highly valuable to be able to investigate the existence of susceptibility psychomarkers as well. The early identification of these psychomarkers in new researchers would make it possible to advise and warn them about the risks they face concerning their emotional and intellectual integrity and even their own physical health, unless they try to group around people with common interests, people who share the same sensitivity and commitment to the work they are doing, people who would not hurt them.

The damage an authentic researcher – i.e. a sensitive intellectual – can suffer from constant harassment and pressure from insensitive people or groups in order to force an impossible integration can be huge. The nervous breakdown, burnout or mental fatigue caused by having to politely refuse to that integration can wreak havoc on the person.

We must not confuse the psychic Mithridatism with the fourth consequence of this title, another effect that we have also observed and that we will afterwards refer to, and which we will describe as *Psychic Anesthesia*. Due to this effect, the researcher does not feel the health damage caused by aggression as a consequence of the passion put at work, which is typical of new researchers. They will continue working even when on the brink of exhaustion, thus reaching critical levels of fatigue that make it necessary to get medical treatment.

In the effect *Psychic Anesthesia* there is damage while in the *Psychic Mithridatism* there is not.

Psychopathic process evolution

If harassers do not want to show themselves openly as enemies, the harassed resistance forces them to do the harassment increasingly overtly. That is why the process must be diachronic and progressive in intensity. In that sense, we can mention the case of a researcher the authority tried to manipulate with a not so extreme measure of forcing him to do an activity which, due to a disability he had, he was not able to do. Although the public health system justified his disability, a person close to the researcher commented: *The authority was very upset with it.*

Moreover, not only the situations get more violent, but also the harasser weakens by the exasperation that the harassed resistance provokes, which means an advantage to the latter.

However, it is essential to be able to detect the underlying situations or original indicators of the process so as to stop it on time or else so that the person can develop defensive measures, i.e. to be even stronger against the attacks.

These situations, then, seem to be *innocent* acts of Discouragement at the beginning: we can include attitudes that attempt to curb the interest or enthusiasm of achieving the objective. They continue with sporadic or isolated acts of Discrimination, which generally show the obvious intention to try to stop the work. Finally, serious Persecutory acts enter the picture: more perverse, refined and open, with a clear intention of damaging.

For its purpose, the two first attitudes of Discouragement and Discrimination can be described as Persuasive, and that of Persecution as Destructive. The latter are manifested when the system proves that it cannot crush a person, spoil his or her integrity, manipulate his or her conscience, or does not manage to make him or her surrender. It is interesting to emphasize this last point, since apart from the list seen in the first reading about the harassers' characteristics that are worth repeating:

- They lack sense of guilt.
- They are inefficient at work.
- They are compulsive controllers and liars.
- They hide under the position of director.
- They are cowards if confronted.
- They use unfounded excuses to harassment (Treviño Ghioldi, 2005).
- They say the victim is a masochist (Le Nouvel Observateur, 2006).

and the characteristic included by us:

- They are great pretenders and liars

Now we can also include six more characteristics:

- They are person who have no ideals or ideas.
- Because in order to achieve power they lose their dignity, they are enormously infuriated by the harassed person's integrity, morale and dignity.
- They are enormously infuriated by the harassed resistance to the psychopathic process.
- They are notably intolerant to the researcher's diverging opinion and unexpected success.
- They suffer from the syndrome AIM (Active Ineffective Mediocrity) (Marian, 2003)
- They have a psychopathic disturbance with a disturbance of the sense of moral norms (Marian, 2003).

Psychopathic process: A new phenomenon?

Paradoxically, in this book we are referring to a phenomenon caused by non-evident aspects of technique that produce long term damage to human health and that we call Technopathogeny. The ethical objector's health is also damaged by attitudes in the scientific academic environment, *factors that are present in the workplace, a subtle hostility, non-evident at the beginning but that it ends up by undermining the person's health* We can then wonder: how can we call the non-evident health damage caused by the scientific system and which the researcher suffers without noticing at the beginning? We could ironically say: which is the word that defines the researcher's health damage that is not manifested immediately but after a period of activity as a consequence of non-evident attitudes of the Science and Technique system, generated by cultural, scientific and academic differences between the researcher and the system? This damage differs from Technopathogeny in that it is not generated by what the person produces – a certain technological object or product – but by people in the scientific and academic system. Whereas Technopathogeny is damage related to a Technological Factor, this psychopathic process is related to the Human Factor. Therefore, another way of formulating the question could be: which name would this psychopathic process have, defined as: *The damage to a person's health that is not manifested immediately but after a long period of activity as a consequence of being exposed to wicked attitudes, non-evident at the beginning, from people from the corporation who were set up as the victim's authority,* a process we have described as a: Degenerative, systematic/corporative and diachronic, progressive in intensity process?

Although we speak about the person's health damage, in the particular case we deal with in this reading – that of the ethical objector researcher – it is worth repeating that the harassment also has a negative effect on the researcher's family environment.

This damage is so subtle that it is only known by those who cause it and for the effect it has on the researcher's health, but not by the rest of the people around. When the scientific ethical objector's health collapses because he or she cannot resist any longer, everyone is astonished since most well-intended people did not expect it. Only the members of the scientific corporation responsible for the attitudes know that they achieved their objectives though externally they throw their hands up in horror.

As we say that the Technopathogeny is caused by factors created by Technique, we can also suggest that due to its characteristics, the attitudes against an ethical objector in Science and Technique are so *vague* regarding their origin that an expert who became interested in an ethical objector researcher's situation told him: *It is a problem of environmental hostility.*

As we will define when we refer to moral harassment, corporative harassment *has no face.* Unlike moral harassment situations in other working activities where it is possible to identify the perpetrator, in Science and Technique it is not so. Even regarding the most reliable people, from whom one would expect help, one does not know if they respond to the corporation interests, are negotiating or just think about their own interests. Even for people who are responsible of an adverse measure, it is common to hear expressions with which they want to justify themselves such as: *I have to follow orders, I'd do you the favor but I am not in the position to go against authority.* Even the maximum authority can always cite a person or group that is over him or her to which he or she *cannot go against* or whose pressure forces him or her to adopt an adverse measure. Therefore, nobody can ever identify whoever is responsible for the adverse action. When confronting the damage done to the ethical objector, some people will say *I didn't do it* and others; *I couldn't do anything; I can't be exposed*; etc.

In order to exemplify even more the environmental character of the persecution process to the ethical objectors in Science and Technique, we can mention the case of the destruction of an institute, where it is very interesting to observe that the last person who made its physical dissolution effective, i.e. the final executer of its destruction, was only the last link of a chronological chain. That person was just the one who culminated several decades of moral harassment with a destructive purpose suffered by the members of that institute. The person just followed the corporation's order.

Psychopathic process – Classification of attitudes

After this brief introduction about how the figure of the ethical objector in Science and Technique can emerge, in the following table we list some attitudes that can be included into each of the three categories above described. They are attitudes that we have observed as a consequence of our experience or that we had to suffer and therefore must be considered to have been observed in an academic and scientific environment. Many readers will surely be able to include other attitudes.

Table 36: Opposition Acts classified according to the three proposed categories.

Discouragement	Discrimination	Persecution
• Teasing, mocking nicknames. • Losing files. • Undermining the proposal: You won't be able to do it. Don't bother to try it. • False and mocking excuses: Oh! I didn't know, I didn't do it, I have to follow orders, I'll solve the problem for you in two months, Don't worry, nothing wrong will happen, Oh, we were wrong! • The harasser blames the victim of some unfulfilled errand. • Interviews permanently interrupted by telephone calls or staff requirement. • Distortion of merit-credit relation. The system may take credit from the one who has merit and on the contrary give credit to the one who doesn't have any merit. • The same but even worse: the one who has merit is dispossessed of the credit. For example, a researcher can be divested of a co – authorship of an article to incorporate another	• Not assigning research subsidies. • Robbing of rights. • Giving the victim an unfavorable position in the ranking for a grant. • Leaving the victim aside in the promotion system. • Not assigning staff to do service tasks forcing the victims to perform them by themselves. • Making the teaching task difficult: by not giving classrooms or equipment (projector, etc.). • Not informing about administrative aspects that would allow getting a subsidy, a better teaching category, etc. • Assigning dangerous and unworthy physical workplaces. • Not assigning suitable evaluators. • Giving false excuses so as not to comply with a request: Everything has been put in the refrigerator. • Arranging interviews that do not take place, many times after a long wait. • Denying recognition to the achievements and	• Dismissal. • Moral harassment. • Reducing the harassed person's work tasks. • Taking advantage of a health physical problem to describe the victim as intellectually incompetent. • Forcing early retirement. • Removal of incentives or other economic benefits. • Forge academic evaluations. • False accusations. • Defamation. • Removal of Social Security and Medical Assistance. • Abandonment. • Destruction of the performed task: removal of physical premises, destruction of lab trials. • Administrative mockery: creating false expectations in the presence of imminent serious facts such as a project cancellation, job loss or workplace destruction. • Encouraging the victim to have false expectations. For example, starting and managing negotiations personally, arguing that in that way the procedure will be faster in order to have a positive change in the situation, yet the ha-

Discouragement	Discrimination	Persecution
one.	prizes obtained. • Disregard and discredit for the performed tasks. • Reproaching the victim for looking for external support. • Raising doubts about the person's seriousness by saying: He's a loony, He's a little bit crazy, He lacks common sense. He's getting crazy ideas into his head. • Neither consulting nor calling the victim about questions related to him or her. Others make decisions for him or her that can even be damaging. • To diminish a local researcher who is the first author in a publication that was written together with a foreign researcher, by only mentioning the foreigner name. • Not communicating the interested party about the result of the report of an application for a position, subsidy, or doing it too late, when it is not possible to claim it. The system resorts to this attitude when the person can represent a competition for the evaluating corporation since it does not have to inform. • Discrediting the research subject on no	rasser knows beforehand that it is impossible. • Arranging an appointment that implies a long and tedious trip of hundreds of kilometers, promising a profitable dialogue, but when the victim arrives at his or her destination, he or she is told that the staff member is out of the office or, what is even worse, that the person you came to see is too busy to see you. • Forging selection processes with a clear intention of damaging. • Maliciously failing to recognize previous work and achievements. • Appropriation of assets the Victim obtained through personal negotiations. • Not helping to finish a procedure that could have avoided a serious negative consequence: for example, making the workplace safe. • Force the victim to do tasks which due to some disability cannot be performed. • Force the Victim to do academic tasks which are below his or her academic level. • Submitting the victim to the authority of a person of significantly less rank. • Publicly question his or her authority. This can be

Discouragement	Discrimination	Persecution
	grounds.	in front of students at evaluation boards.
	• Refusing any kind of application without any grounds. Saying NO without saying how or why. Saying NO just because.	• Personal or telephone threats, if the victim does not accept to participate in non-scientific activities such as political activities.
	• False expectations on the part of the adminis-trative staff promising a procedure will be speeded up or done in the right way.	

All the acts listed in the table, which we can also describe as *hostility* or, during the first stages, of *vague environmental aggression*, can also be described as Direct Hostility and Indirect Hostility. Direct Hostility refers to acts that are openly performed by clearly identified people, accompanied by writings, etc. Indirect Hostility refers to acts that are not clearly manifested, in which there is not a formal person who is evidently involved.

Some extreme actions of the persecution

> *'The spark of rage is the consciousness or threat of failure'*
> E. Mira y López

As we have already described, the psychopathic process to which an ethical objector in Science and Technique is subjected to starts with apparently minor actions, which could even be described as petty jokes, product of the person having *good humor*.

We have started this section with E. Mira y López's quote because in the last stages of the process, the actions are so perverse that can only be explained by plain rage on the part of the person. We could say that academic or corporate moral harassment in Science and Technique, due to the perversion level it can reach, could be defined as a true and subtle modern way of torture. Uncertainty is the main tool of this torture. The final act of the process is given by moral harassment, which we will deal with firstly.

We have said that the processes against ethical objectors in Science and Technique start with actions that could be the result of the *good humor* of the person that generates them. However, and taking the concepts used by the author whose phrase opens this section, rather than actions of *good humor* we should say *humorous* attitudes. The author (Mira y López, 1950) says that:

> One cannot confuse humorous attitudes with 'good humor.' The former is generally 'bad humor' trying to copy the latter. The proof is that when great 'humorists' are examined in detail, they turn out to be mostly hypochondriac, resentful, <u>consumed with envy</u>, incapable of accepting a serious criticism or being generous. If humorists are in any kind of humor, they are often in an ill humor a terribly ill humor.

It is this kind of people that ethical objectors in Science and Technique must face.

To describe some attitudes we will mention Paul's case, presented by Dr Hirigoyen as an example of a researcher who was subjected to moral harassment. We will also include several cases known by us without giving any names, since we consider it irrelevant to this reading.

Flattery or cynical praise

Before starting to analyze the subject of some extreme actions of the persecution, we would like to refer to a very interesting aspect that cannot be defined as Discouragement, Discrimination or Persecution: Flattery or Cynical Praise.

Unless, and as we will refer to later when we deal with Envy, the harasser is an envious individual whose only aim will be that of destroying the person. The harasser's interest is generally that of controlling the person, forcing him or her to negotiate so as to profit from his or her knowledge, initiatives and willingness to work. In other words, the harasser's only interest is to *take advantage of the harassed* for his or her own personal benefit.

For that reason, in order to achieve that objective, harassers use the trick to affect the researcher's *self-esteem* to take him or her to their *battlefield* and therefore be able to act against him or her. In this case, harassers also resort to a trick that is more than related to self-esteem, it is related to the researchers' ego.

Harassers can thus enhance the harassed person's ability, intelligence, *invite* him or her to join the team, etc.

Now, it is interesting to mention again the case of a researcher who was told by the director: *You have an inner engine*. The director's interest in emphasizing his ability and creativity was that the *engine* he had detected in the researcher was used to *tow* both the director the team. The enthusiasm created by an authentic vocation can lead to great achievements, but towing a group of people who follow a researcher without making the same effort (or any effort at all), produces a huge wear that can shorten his or her *lifespan*, as it happens with any engine that is subject to a great effort. The literal meaning of the term *tow* is such that what the director who uttered the expression *inner engine*, was telling this young researcher in reference to his colleagues was: *these people have to be pushed to work*.

The director even said to this same researcher: *You are my right hand*. At first, the expression would seem to be a flattery but in this case it had the opposite effect since the researcher, knowing that he had contributed with the subject of study, felt undermined – an attitude we will analyze later. The expression quoted can be flattery in an Authentic system, in which the Tutor is a prestigious researcher who wants to highlight the new researcher's vocation, dedication and ability.

Another case is that of a researcher who in his beginnings as a student went to see his professor, who was also a powerful researcher of the corporation, with questions about a work that had been requested by the professor in the class he taught. When the professor saw that the student had been able to solve the complex task requested, invited him to join his team, and even highlighted his ability and dedication in front of the other members of the team. Since the young student was devoted to another line of study, he rejected the invitation. The young student made a great career in the new field of knowledge and the powerful professor, by noticing such development in the scientific field, became his opponent and main force in the destructive persecution.

For a new researcher, the fact that a superior highlights his or her qualities and vocation for science is an incentive as long as it is from a tutor in an Authentic system. It becomes unnatural when the person who emphasizes the qualities is a researcher who by exhibiting his or her position of director only wickedly aims at showing the young student his or her interest in *incorporating* him or her into the team with a double intention. Once the incorporation has taken place, the young researcher is forced to suffer a parasitism which, if aware of it, can lead him or her to a serious decay of interest in his or her activity. It is worth remembering here what we said about the value of *collectivism* in an Aloentic system, concerning the difference in productivity among the members of a team in a working environment. Rejection of efficient people to integration is one of the reasons for moral harassment.

Moral harassment

In table 36, in the column of Persecution, we included moral harassment and other attitudes that are not only persuasive but also destructive. Although they are listed separately, they could actually and most surely be all grouped within moral harassment. However, we prefer to describe them separately, including within moral harassment those attitudes that clearly try to eliminate or destroy the harassed.

Moral harassment is also called *mobbing*. This term was coined by the German psychologist Dr Heinz Leymann, who studied this situation in the workplace for the first time in the 1980's (Leymann, 1996). Although in the bibliography moral harassment and mobbing can be used as synonyms, in this book we differentiate the terms. The term *mobbing* refers to being *attacked* by a group of persons: Group Harassment (Gutiérrez, 2003), and *Harassment* can be the attack of one person. Another term used in the bibliography is *emotional abuse*, but as well as Mobbing, we prefer the term *moral harassment*. It is mentioned that it may be appropriate to use the term *Abuse*, but Abuse implies actions that are beyond harassment. Harassment is usually a continual, annoying behavior, whereas Abuse can be a single intense incident where harm occurs.

Anyway, the term *Emotional* refers to the feeling, whereas *Moral* refers to: values, morality and principles of a person. They are the qualities that the harasser actually expects or tries to corrupt in the harassed person.

Therefore, in reference to our experience, we prefer to use the more general term *moral harassment*.

According to an author's report (Marian, 2003), Dr. Heinz Leymann:

...started to study in detail that phenomenon, arguing 'that mobbing in the working life involves hostile and unethical communication which is directed in a systematic manner by one or more individuals, mainly towards another individual, who, due to mobbing, is pushed into a helpless and defenseless position, and held there for a long time.'

Whole books have been devoted to this subject matter. It is not our intention to approach it from Psychology or Psychiatry. What we are interested in, as we have done in our first reading when we referred to the figure of harasser and harassed, is to highlight the aspects that as ethical objectors we have noticed in our activity of Science and Technique.

Although there is not an international definition of Harassment (Marian, 2003), we can mention the following:

Just as it is defined by Dr. Leymann (Leymann, 1996), moral harassment is:

That situation in which a person exercises extreme psychological violence in a systematic and recurrent manner, towards one or more individuals at the workplace over a long period of time in order to destroy the harassed person's communication channels, destroy their reputation, disturb their work, and finally manage to make that person or people leave their workplace.

The persecution is such that Dr. Leymann himself defines it as *psychoterror* (Leymann, 1996).

The European Commission (Marian, 2003), defines harassment as:

Negative behavior among workmates or among superiors and inferiors. As a consequence, the harassed is object of harassment and systematic attacks and for long time, directly or indirectly, one or more persons do this with the objective and/or effect of ostracizing the harassed.

Dr. Hirigoyen (Mujeres en Red), who has also thoroughly studied the problem, defines Harassment as:

An indirect violence which does not leave any marks or injuries but a psychological damage that may last forever. Harassment is a frequent, intentioned, destructive and invisible repetition. It is a phenomenon of indirect destruction of another person, frequently exercised and throughout time. It is performed by narcissistic perverse individuals.

In the first reading we have seen that one of the harasser's features is that of cowardice. In that respect, and as we have mentioned above, we can confirm this feature with the following statement: *corporate harassment has no face*. When asking the harasser about where that harassment comes from or why he or she applies that adverse measure on the harassed, he or she will answer: *If it were for me I wouldn't do it, but I have to follow orders*.

Moral harassment is described by Dr. Hirigoyen as a way to take power, to be superior (Bembibre).

She indicates that (Bruno):

> When we speak about phenomena of violence in the workplace, we refer to problems that imply violent, recurrent, non-episodic, and unique phenomena and behaviors. Abusing is restlessly subduing. The harassed person, at the beginning, and contrary to what harassers pretend others to believe, neither show any pathology or weakness. Harassment may start precisely when a harassed person reacts against a superior's authoritarianism and does not let others push him or her around. His or her ability to resist authority despite pressures makes him or her a target.

The figures of *harasser* and *harassed* have already been described in the first reading in the item Harasser-Harassed vs. Demand-Progress. For that reason, we will now only cover the aspects of moral harassment that are important to the ethical objector in the Science and Technique system where we had to develop our work.

Moral harassment can be exercised vertically (vertical moral harassment) and horizontally (horizontal moral harassment). Vertical moral harassment can be upwards (upward moral harassment) when the harassment is exercised by a subordinate or subordinates, and downwards (downward moral harassment) from an authority to a subordinate (Marian, 2003). Downward moral harassment is also called *subordinate's harassment*. Horizontal moral harassment occurs among workmates of the same rank (Marian, 2003) (for instance, when several colleagues see another one working too much thus jeopardizing their promotion or making it evident that they are not complying with their duty efficiently); or *upstream* (when the harassment is exercised by a subordinate).

Although moral harassment in the workplace can occur in three directions, our experience lets us observe that in the whole *Pychopathic Process* we have referred to, there are actions in the three described directions as well. To exemplify this, we can mention the situation of two researchers who had asked the authority for some furniture they needed for their institute. The authority agreed on their request, but the researchers themselves had to pick the furniture up from a filthy warehouse, with the personnel who should have helped them just mockingly observing them. The situation continued when they arrived to a site that was only a few blocks from their destination where the above mentioned personnel abruptly refused to continue working alleging that their workday was about to end (completing the delivery of the furniture would have taken them only half an hour more). The researchers asked the authority for a solution, but they supported the personnel by saying *they had worked too much,* thus refusing to pay the extra time needed to complete the task. The researchers requested then permission to leave the furniture in the vehicle in order to complete the job in the afternoon, which was also denied since that vehicle had to be used for another service. As a consequence, the researchers themselves had to remove the furniture from the vehicle, leave it temporarily in the site and load it again the following day. Here we do not see a serious situation of moral harassment but a simple mockery, an initial act of discouragement to the researchers *upstream,* but with the *vertical* complicity of the authority. In that moment, the researchers did not imagine that this act was part of the systematic opposition of the corporation.

When the supporting personnel can exert the power of standing in the way of a researcher's task, knowing that he or she will not be able to do anything, in many cases it could be said that: *They are inefficient out of sheer boredom.* Administrative employees create unexpected obstacles just to amuse themselves, though in some cases they do it so as to show their power or authority.

In the case of the phenomenon we are describing about the ethical objector, an interesting aspect to highlight concerning vertical harassment (authority-subordinate) is that we have observed that in our environment the harassment is worse since there is no clear, real, and permanent authority. The authority looks to the other side and lets persecutory corporate lobbies do as they please. The fact that the persons in authority change permanently actually protects them, since in case any measure taken mistakenly or intentionally causes damage, they will probably not be in their post to give an explanation. Due to the periodical renewal of authorities, the person responsible for the damage caused may not be there to give any explanations when the time comes. Another consequence is that this allows the new authority to say: *I didn't do it.* This can be seen in public institutions where authorities are renewed periodically in representation of certain corporate and political parties.

Going back to moral harassment, our experience in Science and Technique, allowed to verify that while this can occur in the three directions described above, the most common one is vertical harassment, since the other two also generally respond to the interests of the authority. For instance, among colleagues or peers, harassment can be motivated by the harassed exposing the lack of creativity or good ideas of his or her colleagues, but it can also happen that the colleagues respond to the authority's interests as well. In the case of a person of a lower rank, a support personnel or a researcher's subordinate that for instance destroys his or her work or just makes it more difficult, that attitude will always come as a request of the authority.

Our experience with the system also let us observe (or, why not, suffer) attitudes that allow to differentiate two aspects – one less extreme than the other – within moral harassment which we will describe below.

Likewise, we'd like to emphasize the relationship between dialogue and harassment. We have already mentioned in the first reading the difficulties of dialogue among scientists with different cultural criteria. Our experience allows us to state that moral harassment starts when the authority or harasser realizes that the person does not respond to the initial proposals of *integration* for ethical reasons, thus cutting all kind of communication. We should not forget that the person who has an intuitive and deep sense of integrity does not accept the integration if its ethical implications are not clear. The cultural clash or differences with the harassed make them stop any kind of communication and start with moral harassment, with subtle measures first and more serious ones later. All the attitudes included in table 36 were adopted with a complete lack of dialogue. Such dialogue clarifying and bringing to light the spurious reason for these attitudes, or what is worse, the lack of scientific academic grounds for denying work tools, a promotion, etc. must be avoided at all costs by the harasser. If the harassed happens to question the harasser for an adopted measure, the latter may just remain silent or give *tangential* answers which are not answers at all.

Pressing and Mobbing

We have explained now why we prefer to use the term moral harassment. Now we will refer to other differences in the attitudes enclosed as moral harassment. Our experience let us observe attitudes of Harassment, some of them more extreme than others. For that reason, we believe that it can be interesting to distinguish between two kinds of moral harassment: *pressing* and *mobbing*.

Pressing

In its least extreme aspects, moral harassment manifests itself through attitudes of *pressure* or *oppression*, which we dare call *Pressing*, attitudes by which a Director of a work group, by definition, subjects the person to coercion, compelling him or her to quickly complete a task; i.e. the director forces his or her subordinates to do things by making use of his or her authority. These actions are kept within a certain normality or causing light damage. As we have already seen in the first reading, arguments are used, depending on its seriousness, tend to bother, annoy, scare or intimidate the person.

Common ways to do it is by insinuating subordinates that a task was badly executed, or that they are not qualified for the position, or that they are not worthy of the responsibilities they have been given. When the harassed asks the harasser to clearly state the reasons why they have failed, the harasser finds ways not to do it, avoiding direct confrontation or turning to arguments as the ones we will quote below.

The research reports graded as negative or unacceptable without enough grounds, are an example of this. They try to destroy the harassed resistance, exposing him or her to an uncertainty of *half-truths* and reproaches, such as:

- *You know what you have to change.*
- *We have tolerated enough so far.*
- *There are many researchers that in their situation have made brilliant achievements.*
- *It is not necessary for me to explain the reason for your problem, you know it.*
- *There are many researchers like you, we don't need you.*
- *Your achievements are neither important nor original.*

- *Submit the report urgently because your position can be jeopardized.*
- *The report was incorrectly laid out.*
- *We have done a lot for you, you should be grateful.*
- *You have included me in this project, you cannot leave the team.*
- *If it weren't for me, you wouldn't have received anything.*
- *Do you know how hard it was for me to get what I have obtained?*
- *Do you know how much I've been criticized for what I've given you?*

These last reproaches are very commonly used by authority. In general, what the harassed receives (a position, a subsidy, a grant, etc.) does not mean any kind of effort for the authority since it only distributes what it has been assigned and it will not make any effort to offer what it does not have. In the public academic scientific systems, authorities are simple distributors of work tools that do not belong to them since they are provided by the State. It is their obligation to distribute them fairly and, if it is an Authentic system, make an effort to get them to new researchers that have shown, as we have said in the first reading, initiative, enthusiasm and devotion. In an Aloentic system, the authority abuses its power of distribution and does it arbitrarily in order to increase its power. The authority then turns to reproaches simply to have the harassed under its superiority and in a permanent condition of debt and gratitude. The authority makes the harassed notice in this way that what he or she has achieved is not due to the harassed merits but because he or she has been done a favor.

Pressing attitudes are a blatant human manipulation and tend to demoralize the person so as to subject his or her work to the team and the director. As there are attitudes whose intention is to damage the researcher's self-esteem or ego, pressing attitudes, specially the last four we have listed, resort to the researchers' sensitivity.

A typical case of hurting the researchers' sensitivity was the one of a researcher who by his own effort had obtained the chance of temporarily continuing his research abroad; the director reproached him by saying: *you leave after we gave you the possibility to begin your researching career?* The researcher had been working as a grant holder at the time. Since the researcher had already accepted the impossible-to-reject opportunity to work abroad, the pressing attitude continued with more drastic measures of punishing him by forcing him to unnecessarily resign his post.

If by adopting Pressing attitudes, the harasser has not achieved his or her objectives yet, he or she will turn to more aggressive attitudes.

Mobbing

We consider that in the most extreme aspects of moral harassment, the so-called Mobbing, the harassers wants to get rid of the harassed. As Dr. Hirigoyen suggested, the harasser wants to *eliminate* the harassed (Hirigoyen, 2001). That is the reason why after the first Pressing attitudes, the harasser moves to other forms of harassment. In order to understand such attitudes, we should consider what was indicated by Dr. Hirigoyen (Mujeres en Red):

- The harasser rejects and denies the harassed as a person. Without a fight, and without ever saying it clearly, the harasser gets rid of the victim because he or she bothers him or her. When the harassed finally realizes what is going on, the harasser blackmails him or her into keeping quiet.
- The harasser must hold on to his or her power. Deep down they are very insecure individuals.
- He or she harasses the victim more and more often until the latter reaches the limit of his or her strength, succumbing and getting ill.
- It is then when the harasser says clearly to the harassed that he or she is incapable of doing anything right, with the intention of finishing him or her off in order to be able to dismiss him or her on health grounds. The victim is a worthless object now, despised by the harasser.

We can add to those characteristics:

- The harasser's aim is to destroy the harassed person's hope.

It is interesting to refer to this last harasser's aim against a person who has devoted his or her life to an endeavor that implied a great effort and sacrifice. In Chapter II we described the disciplines or special fields of study that were excluded in our effort to frame the issue of mycotoxins in order to find a more precise framework to approach this subject from the point of view of its relevance for the consumer. We say so because for the development of an initiative, the researcher must abandon already consolidated disciplines. It is important to emphasize that each discipline or excluded science meant leaving aside a field of study where it could have been easily *hosted*. This would have been prestigious and profitable, and would have offered the possibility of receiving a better income. The development of an initiative demands an incredible amount of time and effort. A great effort made against not only the inertia of the matter but also, and more importantly, against the inertia and animosity of colleagues and authorities.

Possibility and concretion are not the same things. Achievement implies renouncing. Are we ready to renounce in order to achieve? Each discipline that, in our case in particular, was excluded because we resisted framing the study of mycotoxins under what the system defines as politically correct meant a resignation. Every renounce hurts. Most of the time, every idea that was not concreted was eliminated or substituted by a better one. But this only became clear at the end. In the meantime, one lives nostalgically thinking about what could have been. It is the nostalgia of the abandonment. We, as researchers always have the sense of nostalgia, that sorrow of having lost a possibility of working *comfortably*. The nostalgia of the abandonment of a possibility, of *establishing* ourselves in a field of knowledge we had already mastered. This mastery was not searched but came as a consequence of trying to answer a question. For example, in a moment when we were devoted to the subject of mycotoxins we thought of establishing ourselves in the field of Mycology, but this science was just a step towards a deeper question. However, the nostalgia becomes traumatic when it is strengthened by the feeling of guilt for not continuing in the discipline despite the colleagues' request because they needed us. In an Authentic system, it is the Tutors themselves who encourage their Disciples when they see they have achieved a degree of depth that goes beyond the Tutor's discipline, to leave, to *move* from the discipline in which they began in order to get into other fields of knowledge where Tutors know their Disciples will achieve a greater progress.

This nostalgia could appear as many times as disciplines the researcher could have established him or herself in. This is counteracted by the hope in the new initiative. When the Corporation notices this, it first tries to control and then, if it does not work, to destroy.

In these cases, even the authority can offer to the researcher support at the beginning. This promise is perverse and then in an unexpected way (so as to have the greatest effect on the harassed regarding his or her hopes) it destroys completely what has been done. Unlike an Authentic system where the researcher's effort is rewarded and means a merit for him or her, in an Aloentic system the effort can become against him or her. The harasser knows that the more effort the person has made, the bigger the negative impact of his or her attitude will be over the harassed. In an Aloentic system, as we have seen in the first reading, the harassed, because of what we can define as the *harassed logic*, tends not to or finds it hard to be aware of the harassment, since it is not within his or her respectability canons. For that reason, by seeing the system's opposition and so as to provide arguments to support or defend his or her work without knowing how counterproductive it can be, he or she describes his or her effort to the authority, without knowing that is giving harassers elements for them to discover *the place where it hurts the most, or where to hit.* This ironic destruction can have even a bigger effect against the harassed by showing them that, for example, goods acquired through their effort are shared out as *war booty.*

Then, as Dr. Hirigoyen showed in the last two points quoted above, the harasser wants to eliminate the harassed. This is really so. The harassed is first relegated by the system with discouragement and discrimination. He or she always remains in the same position without any promotions seeing his or her colleagues continue with their careers by having better positions and therefore better income. In fact, they have the regular and logical career expected from any researcher. If the harassed bears this situation and does not quit voluntarily, the system will try to eliminate him or her. This elimination may go from a simple symbolic elimination to a physical evident elimination. The last one takes place in four ways:

1. The harassed voluntarily resigns when seeing more aggressive attitudes than that of simply being relegated.
2. Harassing the harassed until, irritated with the moral harassment received for a long time, the harassed reacts violently against the authority or against the person close to it who generated the harassment. This may lead to, as it is included in the next point, a leave for psychiatric disability and/or even a criminal trial in case the aggression is against a person. A trial whose sentence, whatever that be, will be enough to cause the researcher's *scientific death.*

3. The harassed suffers illness or sick leave, retirement for psychiatric disability, or dismissal, according to what is allowed by the harassed administrative situation.
4. The harassed died, although it seems an incredible and unacceptable case, either for natural reasons or by suicide, or an irreversible damage to health. Leymann mentions that a great number, between 10% and 20% of the harassed get serious illnesses or commit suicide (Leymann, 1996). The irritation described in point 2 can also be caused by the Authority wanting to generate a sudden or imminent death by a violent emotion, or to provoke a health damage that leads to a permanent disability.

This harasser's aim is so real that according to Dr. Leymann (Gutiérrez, 2003):

> In the societies of the highly industrialized western world, the workplace is the only remaining battlefield where a person can kill another without running any risk of being taken to Court.

Regarding point 2, in one opportunity and after a succession of harassing acts, the Authority ordered a compulsive eviction of an institute upon no notice to its directors. In order to intensify the effects of the aggression and without the directors giving any reason that justified such decision, the authority threatened them with using the public force and with the destruction of the door, if they resisted. It was a threat with an exaggerated use of force towards peaceful people. The aim of this attitude is to immobilize and intimidate. To inform about the acts, resolutions or dispositions of the authority through certified notification is an obligatory administrative act. That is why the failure of justifying the lack of previous notification makes the authority's perverse attitude evident, which clearly was not only a continuity of the moral harassment but also intended to provoke a violent reaction on the part of the directors, either physical or verbal, due to such unexpected destructive act so as to apply the extreme measures mentioned in point 2. At the very least, the authority wanted the directors to be so demoralized that they resigned. This was made evident when the directors communicated the event to another authority, the authority said: *I would have resigned.* In this case, the authority wanted to continue pressing and demoralizing the researchers so that they abandoned their resistance.

Regarding point 4, as incredible as it may seem, moral harassment, organized by an anonymous group of people toward whoever is *different* or *distinct*, can be exacerbated to a self-feeding paroxysm until it causes the harassed person's death.

These attitudes, as indicated, are not stopped by any health problem or physical or mental disability the harassed may have. On the contrary, in some cases, the harasser maliciously may use a disability in order to further mock the harassed. The harasser can sometimes even deny such a disability, surreptitiously accusing the harassed of having forged his or her disability certificate. We can refer to a case of a harassed researcher who was being pressed by the authority to commute to a work site which was 40 km from his city of residence, which he could not do due to a disability. As it happened, the harasser openly doubted about the harassed disability by saying: *The authority has confirmed that you must present to work, but surprisingly you cannot travel.* This person knew about the harassed health problem since a disability certificate made by an official public health medical entity had been presented. The harassment did not finish there but continued with the researcher's dismissal without previous notice, therefore making him lose his salary and medical benefits, which because of his illness he needed and used. We do not think it is necessary to be more explicit about the intentions of somebody who takes away medical benefits from a sick person.

Further on, when we refer to how envy can lead to harassing attitudes, we will exemplify it with the case of a researcher, Paul, described by Dr. Hirigoyen. In order to describe the degree of perversion the harassment system can reach, we will now mention the case of two researchers, victims to several years of moral harassment – the situation of one of them is similar to that of Paul's. This researcher, after a series of psychiatric studies, receives the following diagnosis: *The patient presents a progressive psychosis, the early melancholic depression with the emerging variables of this case advancing in such a way that the patient perceives it and stresses it all throughout his process of psychological diagnosis showing the damage of his ego. This impedes him of finding coherent answers to his life.*

There is also an important neurological cognitive damage that encloses him more and more in a world of loneliness, he is overwhelmed by feelings of disability, insecurity and lack of reaction against the external world.

It is urgent for the patient to remain isolated from all that produces stress, anxiety and anguish. He needs to have access to a life where his connection with reading, his loved ones and with his own personality let him get a better quality life.

That is why it is so important and urgent for him to retire from work through a pension. The Burnout syndrome suffered when his research was ruined and when his dreamed laboratory – put together with effort with a colleague and in which he deposited all his vital expectations in terms of vocation and professional projects — was dismantled, negatively affected the researcher, being a relevant variable in his pathology of physical and mental damage. Like Paul's case, he is offered a compulsory early retirement. Although the authority was forced to comply with the medical report request, it deliberately made an administrative mistake so that the researcher received a pension worth 10% of what he was supposed to receive by law. This forced the researcher to begin anew with the proceedings, which took 18 months until the administrative *mistake* was corrected. We should take into account the fact that the researcher had a psychiatric condition which did not get any better with all those administrative proceedings, which were tedious even for a healthy person and which contributed to trouble him even more.

The other researcher, when consulting a doctor about some health problems that had no manifestation before the destruction of the laboratory, was diagnosed with a serious case of hypertension. Fortunately for the researcher, that did not lead to any crisis of more severe or irreversible damage.

These researchers had been enthusiastic people that had projects for the future and yet suffered from a slow deterioration by having to face the permanent administrative mockery for decades, this being light at the beginning but perverse at the end. What we have just described clearly shows how harmful this harassing procedure is, if there is no way to detect it prematurely and thus protect the harassed in time. It is common for the harasser to mockingly minimize the harassed health deterioration, encouraging him or her to continue resisting. Many times the harassed mistakenly resists moral harassment beyond its strength so as not to show signs of weakness. But their health deteriorates dramatically. There may be cases where the harassed resists the system perversion without reaching the serious consequences described by Leymann. Even so, a protection mechanism is essential so that there is no irreversible damage or even death. As we will mention later, we should not apply the inhuman Darwinism ideology: *survival of the fittest and elimination of the weakest.* Needless to say, it would be a mistake to select who will survive in the system for their resistance to harassment instead of for their creativity, intelligence, hard-work, etc.; then the system would be selecting for the capacity of submission. In addition, if the system confirms that the researcher resists harassment, it will get rid of the person by dismissing or retiring him or her.

Taking into account what we just have described, and considering the person's health and life so unimportant, the harasser can make absurd demands such as asking to make a physical effort to somebody with spinal damage, to work on heights to somebody who suffers vertigo, to let somebody who is epilepsy-prone, work alone, etc. Needless to say, after working under these conditions, the physical and/or mental health reach such a damaging degree that the person must resign or ask for a sick leave.

Authentic researchers with true vocation are very susceptible to moral harassment since by being completely devoted to and overwhelmed by a difficult scientific problem, they forget about themselves and their pains. Regarding this point, it is interesting to highlight what Dr. Hirigoyen (Mujeres en Red) says:

> The harassed falls into the harasser's trap, not out of masochism or being a sufferer, but because the perversion degree is such that it prevents him or her from understanding this kind of situations. The harassed person does not react before as the contradiction seduction-threat he or she is so continuously submitted to, submerges him or her into a sea of doubt.

Some psychologists have confused the symptoms described by people who suffer from moral harassment with this false preconception of masochism (Bembibre). In that respect, we can mention that the harasser, by accusing the harassed of being a masochist, is trying to make him or her responsible for his or her own situation so as to present him or herself to the system as a harassed person and the real harassed as the aggressor. This is another tool of moral harassment: making the harassed responsible for his or her own adversity, generating guilt feelings and continuing to undermine the victim's spirit and morale.

The harasser knows the harassed person's personality, morale and meticulousness, as well as the harassed logic – which makes them doubt about their innocence and believe that they are responsible for the adversity they are undergoing.

Let us return to the example of the General Practitioner and the specialist. One day a patient noticed that he did not respond to the treatment the specialized doctor had given him; even worse, it was causing him certain discomfort. The specialist, far from recognizing a possible mistake, told the patient that he himself was responsible for the failure of the treatment by *believing the treatment was not doing him any good*. He practically implied he was crazy. In our case in particular, the corporation, rather than admitting that the framing proposals they offered for our research did not respond to our needs for the efficient study of the technopathogeny phenomenon, tried to force us to accept those proposals. In response to our denial and rejecting our grounds, just like with the patient, the arguments were *you are crazy*.

The perversion is such that along with damaging attitudes, the harasser uses, as defined by Hirigoyen, seductive acts. It is a double game of *give and take*. The harasser pulls the rope and causes damage, then immediately loosens the rope and just to make a good impression says in a sickly-sweet tone of voice: *This is terrible! What happened to you?* In many cases, the harasser does not assume his or her character in any way and even accuses the harassed of being the aggressor and responsible of the difficulties and troubles generated on other people. The victimized harasser is thus seen as a victim of an apparent intransigence of the harassed *who does not want to negotiate*. The harasser's speech is: *Despite all my good will and having tried to help these people with many alternative proposals to improve their situation, their own intransigency condemned them. How hard it was for me and how much I've tried to help them.* What the harasser does not say is that the apparent intransigency is simply moral integrity so as not to fall into proposals of doubtful ethics. It is interesting to quote the case of a persecuted and harassed researcher to whom the authority said: *We forgive you for causing us problems. We forgive you for not having accepted our friendship, for not having accepted to join us.* The aggressor becoming the victim is the utmost perversion; a victim of the resister who did not succumb to his or her treacherous manipulation. The same authority did not doubt after some time about admitting without shame its perversion by having said to somebody close to the researcher: *I tried to help, the point is he or she won't negotiate.* By the term *negotiate* we must understand accepting *indecent proposals* using the public funds.

It is said that *burn out* appears in all professions whose aim is to help the other. An emotional tiredness is generated in such a way that the patient acquires an attitude of *throwing it all away.* The destruction of all hope is an important aim of harassers so as to make the victim feel hopeless. In order to do so, as we have seen, they cause this syndrome through pressing or mobbing attitudes. In the case of researchers who are strongly committed to a scientific question that would help others which make them ethical objectors, the burnout happens after a slow and permanent accumulation of disappointments. Such disappointments are caused by the constant rejections by the official evaluation and financing. The researchers ask themselves the following question: why are all our proposals ignored, when our training and background are similar to or the same as for other researchers that approach other research subjects that are unrelated to the immediate help of others? The constant accumulation of more or less veiled denials, indifference and harassment, take them gradually to the destruction of all hope – which is aimed by the harasser as we have mentioned above – and to burnout. Victims realize that all the help and effort offered, to which the authority could have even promised recognition, will not be reciprocal. All that effort means to them an irretrievable and irreparable loss. While other researchers of a similar age – who perhaps started their careers around the same time – have had so far bright careers, researchers who are committed to helping others and who have become ethical objectors, end up undergoing psychiatric treatment due to burnout.

If victims manage to recover, defend themselves, or not succumb to the harasser's pressing aggressions and, in order to look for a relief from the harassment situation ask for a transfer, an evaluation commission change, etc. the harasser will systematically refuse any kind of permission. On the one hand, he or she will refuse the permission so that the evil game played on the harassed does not finish. But on the other hand, and perhaps most importantly, when the harasser harasses other people of great capacity and academic and scientific level, he or she would not authorize the transfer because he or she knows that the harassed will surely be successful and would or could be rewarded in the new environment. This way, the harasser's vile deeds would be put on the spotlight. It is an absurd relationship in which, on the one hand, the harasser persecutes and prevents the harassed manifestation, but on the other, he or she believes to have the sole right to manipulate and examine them. This perversion quickly leads to the harassed person's health deterioration.

There are two interesting elements to highlight regarding the scientific-academic work. The first one refers to the groundless denial to value the harassed work; the second one, the dismissal of the harassed person on *disability* grounds after having caused the harassed physical and emotional downfall.

Envy as a motive for moral harassment

Above all, we would like to explain that although we are analyzing moral harassment, we consider that envy may motivate other attitudes included in table 36, besides moral harassment itself.

Perhaps in order to be able to understand some of the motives of these slander attitudes in the Science and Technique system, we can emphasize what has been stated by an author concerning envy (Montoya) since these are attitudes that we have also observed. The author mentions that:

> Envy is that psychological mechanism that does not let anybody have more or be better than oneself.
> Why him and not me? Wonders the envious person who does not accept the other person's success.
> There is nothing more enviable in life than the luck owned by the one who has the toy which oneself would like to own. So that in this open competition, where one wishes to be or have what the other is or has, it is almost natural for the envious person to wish by all means the opponent's downfall, forced by that innate belief that no one is more capable and perfect than oneself.
> Everything goes when it comes to envy: the law of the jungle and every man for himself.
> In order to achieve their opponent's downfall, envious people slander, insult, accuse, and what is worse, when they have no more arguments to speak against them, turn lies into truths and turn the truth into rubbish, in fact, envious people are like poisonous snakes and double-edged knives.

Envious people are characterized by the following features:
1. They usually slander and
2. They are fault-finders
3. With the aim of emphasizing the others' weaknesses and
4. Undervalue their virtues.

Although it is not our intention to study Envy thoroughly, since like harassment it is a subject for other professionals, we would like to draw our attention to the fact that the attitudes referred to by the author (Montoya) have been suffered by researchers. We have observed aspects in our activity such as: the authority not tolerating or accepting its subordinate higher ability; its wish to destroy researchers if it could not own or share their intellectual property; its accusations, slanders, etc.

Since Envy generates enemies, it is interesting to remember Seneca's thought: "If you have no enemies because you did not insult anyone, there will be others who become one out of envy." (Séneca)

Causes generating envy

Our experience allowed us to observe the following causes generate envy in scientific activity:
1. The intellectual capacity and the researcher's concrete achievements
2. The Researcher's Integrity and Morale
3. The Researcher's Resistance
4. Independence from the system arbitrary or non-arbitrary obligations
5. Allies who protect or help the researcher

It is common to think that Envy is grounded on what we can call the person's professional virtues: a good artist, composer, designer, researcher, etc. As Horace wisely said: "he who likes what belongs to others is unhappy with his own lot" (Horace). The same was said in a more lapidary way by St. Thomas Aquinas: "Envy is sadness for the other's property."

But not only professional virtues are motive for envy. The fact that harassers are incredibly exasperated by the harassed integrity and morale is absolutely relevant as a motive of envy and finally of moral harassment. In the same way, we can say that the harassed resistance to the psychopathic process also exasperates the harasser. We believe that the harasser envies the harassed for such strength. Regarding the fourth motive, we could say that the corporation takes the harassed as the *scapegoat* of situations with which he or she has nothing to do. It may happen, for instance, that corporation members must perform some arbitrary or non-arbitrary requirements asked by the system, obligations that because of the researcher's nature of his or her own job, or for health reasons, among others, even the system itself is obliged to waive for him or her. This is also a motive for envy and therefore moral harassment. Harassers say: Why aren't they forced to do what we are? and thus there is another motive for spite. In that respect, we can quote the case of two researchers who had developed an institute that had its own building and that was based in the same city where the head office it depended administratively on was. Since the head office had been transferred to a nearby town, the authority ruled against the academic and scientific arguments that determined the opposite, and also arranged the unnecessary transfer of the institute. This measure meant such a difficulty for the institute concerning its research and teaching activities that its continuity would be impossible. Finally, the measure was made effective showing that the real interest was the dissolution of the institute. In one of the meetings which the institute directors had with the organization authorities in order to avoid the damaging consequences of the transfer, one of them told them: *If you don't travel, other people won't be willing to.* The head office transfer was not necessary either and like any obligatory groundless provision, this generates annoyance on the part of the ones who have to comply with it. That is the reason why the corporation members pressed for the institute transfer.

In that respect, Dr. Hirigoyen says that neither manifested capacity nor quality work are enough to relieve researchers from arbitrary bureaucratic obligations (Hirigoyen, 2001). As Pierre Corneille clearly says: "An envious person never forgives a merit." (Corneille). If for some reason, the system is forced to give certain privileged work conditions to someone who deserves them due to proved work quality, a consequent spite is generated in those not earning such privilege.

An author defined the existence of the *incorruptible accountant* (conscience) within a person (Payot, 1947): as in an accounting book, people's bad and good deeds are registered in the Debit and Credit columns. Everybody is aware of that and so are harassers, and no matter how much they try, they cannot fool themselves or get rid of the evil and corruption within them, to which they had to turn in order to obtain all they have. As a play on words, we can say that harassers are conscious of their bad conscience. By being aware of their corruptness, they want to corrupt others. That is why, as we have seen, they are exasperated when they see that another person wants to and can achieve his or her goals by respecting moral values. Harassers can even wonder: *Who do they think they are to pretend to develop an institute or research program without being corrupted?* When we refer to researchers' need for help in critical situations, we will give an example about that.

When we analyzed Ethics in the scientific–academic world, we commented that for a researcher of the corporation it would be practically impossible to become an ethical objector. In the best case, he or she would retire and leave everything the way it was, i.e. without committing. Among other reasons, we argued that the privileges received from the system would *force* such a researcher to have a certain loyalty to the corporation that supported him or her, gave him or her favors or even more, power. The fact that the system gives the corporation members things for privilege and not for merit is a tool, a powerful weapon to control its members. As a result, researchers' intellectual capacity, concrete achievements, integrity and moral become motives for envy and exclusion when it is the time to grant subsidies, promotions, etc. Indeed, the corporation knows that all authentic researchers can receive will be for their own merit, i.e. as a right, and not for privilege. Thus, it will not have a pressure tool to obtain from them whatever it wants to, such as to support a negative measure against another researcher who perhaps they do not even know about. In the corporation, everything is assigned by privileges and not for merits, even awards. They are all benefits or favors given without the awarded particularly deserving them.

The privilege criterion even allows the corporation to establish justice rules, i.e. what is just and what is unjust. Therefore, a person with sufficient merits to obtain a position, for example, would be rejected by the corporation out of envy, adducing arbitrary regulatory reasons, and stating that if they agreed to such request it *would be an act of injustice* since other candidates are applying for the position. Although the argument can be true, what the corporation does not admit is that while there are other candidates that have applied for the position for perhaps a longer time than the researcher who is requesting so, his or her merits are far better than the other applicants.' That is a complete distortion of reality. For the system, choosing a candidate for professional merits, as it should be, would be unfair! So, let us return to what we have said about merit and privilege. As we will see below, harassers never admit the harassed professional superiority, which will be systematically discredited by trivial arguments.

Regarding justice, we can quote the Spanish playwright Jacinto Benavente (1866-1954): "Envy is so ugly that it goes around disguised, and is never more hateful than whenever it pretends to disguise itself as justice."

Envy, when associated to Wrath and Fear (two soul giants who are related as defined by an author: "Wrath, unfaithful woman whose favorite spouse is her incestuous progenitor, Fear" (Mira y López, 1950)), leads to perverse attitudes against the harassed. Harassers' wrath is generated by their being aware of being corrupt, by seeing their own vile deeds and weaknesses in a mirror, and not being able to accept their limitations; and Fear of all that being exposed and therefore losing all its possessions. Wrath is thus the result of a huge fear of their world, their fragile house of cards, being thrown down. As we have mentioned, the spark of wrath is the conscience or threat of failure (Mira y López, 1950). We have quoted before a case in which we showed that when the harassed manages to avoid or resist a harasser's attitude, it annoys the latter.

In the first reading, in points 20 (Grant Holder vs. Disciple) and, 21 (Director vs. Tutor), we included hatred of the old against the young within professional jealousy. In this reading, it is worth emphasizing another motive of hatred: from the incompetent person towards the competent one (Mira y López, 1950). Although the author also mentions that there can be hatred from the competent person towards the incompetent one, in fact, and in our view, in the case of the ethical objector and due to his or her moral values, more than hatred what the competent person feels towards the incompetent one is compassion. However, even accepting this, the author (Mira y López, 1950) draws attention to:

> The hatred from the incompetent towards the competent one is, of course, more intense and deeper, because it is less caused for differences in position, prestige, etc. than for the irremediable fact of the competent person's technical superiority, which is associated with essential conditions of his or her psyche and therefore inherent to his or her existence. The incompetent person can never aim at 'being' like the competent one; at the most, he or she can try to replace the other and pretend to be 'equal.' Facing that impotence, he or she has no other way than that of the intrigue and no other attitude than that of spite. It is not unusual then to see the psychic 'projection' process at work: the incompetent person rationalizes his or her hatred by saying that the competent one is 'conceited,' and that he (or she) despises and diminishes him (or her) without any reason or even that the competent person persecutes him or her due to his or her professional superiority (the only way of admitting this superiority is by affirming simultaneously that competent person abuses of it).

In such conditions, each adversary gathers motives of anger and starts to use less recommendable weapons for the fight, which is more and more spiteful and hypocritical. At the same time, he or she needs to find allies who support his or her position and soon enters in some professional or technical (scientific, artistic, industrial, etc,) group or society, from where – as a captain or soldier, according to his or her conditions — will continue acting against the workmates of the opposite camp. This is how they set up a sort of small professional army in each place...

We can include here one thought by Napoleon (1769-1821): "Envy is a declaration of inferiority."

From what has been expressed by the psychologist, and from what we were able to observe in the case of the ethical objector in Science and Technique, since the corporation members have authority over the harassed, they will not need to admit the harassed *professional superiority,* which as an act of conceit the harassed would manifest against the authority. No doubt the harassed professional superiority generates jealousy on the part of authorities, but they will never admit it; if they did, they would be putting their incompetence for their position in the spotlight. They never admit the harassed professional, intellectual or technical superiority, but they certainly try to profit from it.

Moreover, an attitude in which harassers have become evident is that of looking for *supporters of their position,* who can be directly benefited from the ethical objector's destruction or else from what they can *negotiate* with the ones who want to destroy the victim (usually, what they want to obtain is the victim's work position). This is really so, indeed, according to the British expert Guy Dehn, on the subject of the Whistleblower: When the whistleblower persecution is exacerbated, this is generated by 5% of the people around but there is another 5% who honestly try to defend them and a 90% of opportunists, who can be easily bought or convinced by the 5% of the whistleblower's enemies (Dehn, 2000). What this British jurist has observed in his country can be applied to our situation. An interesting aspect worth emphasizing about the opportunists is that once the harassers' aim has been achieved, and, in the best of cases, the harassed has resigned or been dismissed, their attitude basically changes: while at the beginning they avoided contact with the victims since they felt they were accomplices of their persecution (or even guilty by omission), then they look for affectionate contact as a way of limiting their responsibility for such a hideous act.

In the scientific world, it is possible for the harassing scientific group to find the necessary allies for destroying another researcher(s) within the authorities. Due to our experience, we can say that the intellectual authors of our harassment or persecution – that 5% Guy Dehn refers to – do not show themselves; instead, the authorities are the ones who make the final decision sometimes even ignoring the victims' work. Harassers prefer to remain unknown and look for allies who support and follow their position, and then an executioner so as to achieve their goal: the ethical objector's elimination.

A previous attitude to the incompetent person's jealousy is that of discrediting the competent person's virtues. First, the incompetent person undervalues the competent one's achievements; and when the other realizes that the competent person's achievements, postulates, and ideas are real, mockery turns into envy. As the psychologist has said, when bullies finally understand that they are incompetent or less competent, creative, etc. – qualities which are irremediably unreachable for them — they start to attack the competent person by first trying to negotiate with him or her. If they do not get what they want, as we have seen, they will try to destroy him or her.

We have also seen that whenever harassers cannot subjugate the harassed, they aim at destroying him or her. When the harassment has Envy as a motive, and having said that the technical superiority is an irremediable fact for the harasser, destruction is the final goal. It is worth mentioning here Quevedo's thought: "Envy is thin and yellow because it bites but it does not eat."

We would like to underline what has been expressed in Item 5 as a motive for envy: the possibility that the victim finds allies who protect him or her. Our situation was paradigmatic, with the recognition and support obtained from INES/INESPE, which ruined the project of total destruction on the part of the corporation. This recognition generated envy and wrath in members of the corporation since we had been able to find in INES *allies* for our fight and resistance in this true psychological war between harassers and harassed. War in which there is a powerful person, the harasser, and a weak person, the harassed, who has to continuously survive this permanent injustice and inequality. Wrath and Envy appeared mainly among the members who created the destructive project and who acted destructively, going as far as they were administratively allowed to.

Undervaluing the harassed

Let us continue with Envy, and refer to what has been indicated in point 4 about the envious person's features: undervaluing the harassed person's virtues.

This is a very common attitude: the authority adopts it in order to discourage, demoralize and undervalue researchers so that they do not think that they can count on some merit of their own to make use of their rights.

The authority always has false, untimely, irrelevant and even laughable arguments, i.e. all groundless, to argue against researchers and therefore try to refute, reject or counteract their arguments or else make them go against themselves.

Although it can have envy as a motive, this can also be used so as not to recognize an effort applied to some work, some task done beyond any obligation, for pure enthusiasm and out of love to the task being performed, etc.

So as to undermine or despise researchers, the authority can turn to undervalue, among other virtues, the following:
1. Vocation
2. Devotion
3. Will
4. Inventiveness and creativity
5. Production: books, projects, inventions, scientific proposals, etc.
6. Achievements: awards, degrees, positions, promotions, rewards, etc.
7. Training and competence

Among some cases of undervaluing we can mention the following:

A junior employee says to the authority that he has worked a number of extra hours without having the obligation to do it, to which the authority answered with an argument which was completely out of place: *I have also changed the car's flat tire* (he was referring to the Institute official car).

A researcher who told the authority that he was entitled to some kind of recognition because he had worked hard for many years to develop an institute, to whom the authority responded: *We have all worked hard, we have all made the same sacrifice.*

Another case is the one of a persecuted researcher who, in spite of this, had succeeded in developing an institute together with his colleague. When this researcher made a comment on the sacrifice involved in creating it to another junior researcher who belonged to the same institute but who had joined it several years after its creation, the subordinate answered: *Other people have also founded universities.* Out of this remark, we can observe the obvious undervaluing of the director of the institute by comparing its development (made through the two researchers own vocational effort) to the creation of a university, knowing that they are created by political provisions. Such undervaluing of vocational effort in the creation of institutes or programs is typical of official institutions. This case could, for what we have already described, be considered as *upstream* harassment, which happens when authorities both allow it and encourage it. The authority remains unhurt maintaining a friendly relationship with the harassed while it sends its *agent* to do what it does not want to do personally in order not to shake the confidence of the harassed.

Another case is the one of a researcher who as a victim of a persecution had been left outside a system of promotions. Although his merits entitled him to be promoted to Category I (the maximum in a ranking from I to V), one of the members of the harassing corporation said: *If you work with us, perhaps you are promoted to category III.* Not only did he offer him a lower level category, but also he put it as if he was offered that because he was doing him a favor. The harasser perfectly knew that the researcher deserved the maximum category, which he did not assign in order to keep the harassed in a lower rank than his own as to be able to control him (the harasser himself had been promoted to category II for belonging to the corporation and not due to personal merits).

Regarding the undervaluing of the researcher's inventiveness and creativity, we can quote the case of a researcher who after a previous vocational independent and thorough investigation process managed to think up an original question. On administrative demand, to be able to enter the Science and Technique system he had to turn to a formal *director*. This director was really interested in the young person's question and after gathering some more information about the subject, he tried to teach the young researcher. In an Authentic system, the tutor may share with his or her disciple any new knowledge that come up during an investigation, but in the Aloentic system, the director adopts an attitude of intellectual superiority even in a subject he or she primarily knew about through the junior researcher. In the mentioned case, the director undervalued the researcher's competence. He turned a formal direction where the truth was that the grant holder had ideas of his own and intellectual high-quality work into an aloentically *real* direction where all those merits and talents belonged to the director. That *suction* of ideas on the part of research directors in an Aloentic system only contributes to the mental damage of new researchers.

Regarding point 6, undervaluing the achievements (awards, degrees, positions, promotions, rewards, etc.) we can quote here the case of a researcher who, for not having a PhD, the corporation undervalued all his achievements (such as an award, an important position in the researchers' seniority listing, etc.), murmuring around that he had obtained all those achievements through a colleague who did have a PhD. Another example of undervaluing the achievements is the case of a researcher who, after an arduous investigation process and several attempts, developed a very practical design. When he presented the finished device to his Director, he said to the researcher: *Well, from the dinosaurs to present, animals have also evolved in several attempts.'*

Another case of undervaluing achievements is that one of a persecuted researcher who after having obtained his PhD, the corporation adopted the attitude of ignoring, both verbally and in paper, the postgraduate degree that he had obtained, always addressing him with his lesser degree.

In the case of point 7, undervaluing training and competence, we can be more specific and say *undervaluing the knowledge's authority.* For instance, we can mention the case of a professor with high-academic qualifications who gave a good mark to a student in an exam. By having to be approved by the managing chair professor, who had a lower academic level than the examining professor, arbitrarily and without having been present in the exam, considered the mark was excessively high and lowered it in front of the professor and the student examined. The examining professor did not consider that act important, although he was part of the phenomenon we are analyzing.

Another case is that of a researcher who in his own home country had gained a great experience in an original and relevant subject but was undervalued regarding his ideas and projects. When he went abroad to continue his research, his new supervising professor, in an attitude that astonished the researcher, also undervalued all the previous training and knowledge he had obtained in the subject that he now wanted to continue studying thoroughly. As the researcher showed his competence, going beyond what the supervising professor wanted, he started to be persecuted; then the professor told him: *you are asking too many questions*. After finishing the thesis, he was promptly dismissed. On the tutor's supervising professor defense, we can at least say that he did not steal any idea or project from the researcher, as it had happened in his home country.

Undervaluing virtues is an attitude the harassed is generally aware of. However, in the last mentioned case, the harasser tried to make the victim doubt about his own merits.

Attacking the weakest

Undervaluing virtues or discrediting attitudes are very commonly used by people who are part of a work team, where although everybody works with the same devotion and everybody makes the same intellectual contribution, the academic degrees held by its members are different. Take for example the case of a team where only one member has a postgraduate degree while the others have university degrees.

In this situation, the system aims at discrediting the person holding a lower degree against the one (or ones) holding a higher degree. This is another way of affecting the researcher's self-esteem by observing the unfair attitude of the system towards him or her, of being considered a *subordinate* or *junior*. Naturally, by affecting a member of the team, the whole team activity is also affected. It is a fundamental strategy in all battles: attacking the enemy on its weakest side.

The observed actions regarding this attitude of undervaluing the member holding the lowest academic degree in a team can be as follows:

- Referring to him or her simply as an assistant.
- Referring to the researcher as the main researcher's right hand.
- Relating the researcher's achievements, such as publications and awards, to an undeserved consequence of the work of the researcher with the highest degree.
- Not speaking to him or her by his or her name, but through his or her relationship with the person of higher academic degree: a person who works with, or the assistant of.
- If he or she has not graduated, and completely ignoring his or her competence and capacity, they will refer to him or her as *the apprentice of.*

- If the highest degree member requests a subordinate researcher that after finishing a report he or she hands it to a lower degree member for its revision, this subordinate researcher may even adopt the harassing attitude of telling the higher rank member concerning the lower rank one: *I don't need intermediaries.*

It is worth mentioning the case of a researcher who for his merits obtained a very good category in the seniority listing, but his opponents argued that it had been due to the work of the highest academic degree member in the team, who was absent abroad when the commission ad hoc submitted the evaluation, ignoring the higher degree member who composed such commission.

This situation of undervaluing the person of lower degree is easy to understand; at the heart of it lies the fact that the person doing the undervaluing (and who always holds a higher academic level than the person being undervalued, although less intellectual capacity) would like to be in the position of the person being undervalued, which – as the psychologist quoted above would say – is irremediably impossible for the envious person.

Regarding undervaluing, further on we will turn to the example of a circus in order to analyze moral harassment attitudes. Yet, we can also use this example now to analyze what was previously said and turn to the analogy of the man on stilts. The harassing system acts as if a man 1,50 meters tall uses stilts in order to go higher than two meters and thus pretends to show another man 1,80 meters tall that he is shorter. In the quoted case, the member of the harassing corporation with a higher category than his real merits, pretended to make the researcher of a higher academic and scientific level to feel inferior. In the case of a harassed person who has been tolerating harassing attitudes for a long time, he or she can be in such a psychological situation to fall into this trap.

Other characteristics of envy

We can also say that due to its ubiquity, Envy can be responsible for many negative groundless reports about researchers of recognized capacity, and naturally, for many attitudes from persons in authority tending to destroy former colleagues' laborious work.

An author (Montoya) suggests that:

Art, culture, politics, and, of course, journalism, abound in those who plot against others of the same profession behind their backs; not in vain the saying goes: 'Your colleague is your worst enemy,' because your colleague's rivalry manifests itself not only as jealousy and hatred, but also as treason and crime.

Nevertheless, our experience allowed us to verify that this also perfectly applies to Science and Technique. Leymann, in a study on patients performed in the so-called Swedish Mobbing Clinic, found an over-representation of patients coming from universities (Leymann, 1996). Another author discovered that moral harassment is most frequently found in Public Administration, and within this area, in Health, Education, and Social Work (Gutiérrez, 2003).

The first mentioned author also states that "envy is a psychological mechanism that does not allow anybody to be better than oneself." There is a paradigmatic harassment case referred to by Dr Hirigoyen in her book (Hirigoyen, 2001) that was motivated by the authorities' fear of a researcher's progress, about which she wrote:

If researchers are too bright, then their superiors can fear they progress too fast and overshadow them. In this case, they can prevent them from working in the established competitive areas and stop providing them with the material means to continue with their investigations.

It is the case of Paul, the researcher who, as we have said, is a perfect example due to its paradigmatic character.

Paul underwent the following process of harassment:

- He was a recognized, award-winning, prestigious researcher. He published articles in several international magazines.
- He was denied a vested moral right for his previous performance so as to continue his work through a thesis.
- In spite of that, he went on and finished his work without the support of the authority.
- When he returned, he was denied the new acquired merit.
- The entity of his new work was denied and he was asked to do tasks that did not correspond to his newly obtained and verified training.
- Work tools were denied.
- Financial means were denied.
- Disciplinary action was taken against him when he did not comply with the authority's arbitrary requests.
- He was forced to retire.

Envy is a passion to which authentic researchers will not give any value at all; on the contrary, they may feel that by showing their achievements they will be well regarded by their colleagues or by the authorities. This criterion may work in an Authentic system, but in an Aloentic system it could be catastrophic, since it will only create resentment among their colleagues and the authorities. For example, a researcher in an Aloentic system who wanted to exhibit his publications so that the people who were interested could request them received the following director's advice: *Remove your work from the display cabinet; it can be taken the wrong way.*

Another common envious reaction in these systems, generated by the researcher's creativity and good ideas, is that of *why it didn't occur to me!* which we already quoted when we referred to the relevant aspects of Ethics in the scientific-academic world. This reaction, when on the part of an authority, will inevitably lead to the researcher's harassment. Obviously, the authority will try to appropriate that idea. At first, it will try to sweet talk the researcher into *sharing the idea*, or *integrating with the group.* If the researcher, in order to defend his or her intellectual property, does not abide, the authority will turn increasingly extreme attitudes that could include getting rid of the researcher and appropriating ideas, projects, or more advanced achievements like an Institute or a Program. If it cannot manage to do any of that, it will abandon the researcher to his or her own luck, as we will exemplify later when we analyze the Extortive attitude.

Another place where the *why it didn't occur to me!* reaction can manifest itself and therefore lead to an unfavorable act for the person, are scientific magazines. We know a case where an article was accepted by the Refereeing Commission of a scientific magazine, which even sent the authors a written approval that stated *Your excellent work will be published.* But after that, the article publication started to be delayed. Although the authors were able to contact one of the members of the Refereeing Commission of the magazine, they were not given a reasonable explanation for the delay. The article was never published. When the authors telephoned the magazine asking them for the reasons for not publishing it, they gave evasive answers, even rudely demanding not to communicate with the evaluator anymore. Evidently, some prestigious scientist connected with the Refereeing Commission of the magazine, after learning that it would be published, pressed the committee not to do it. The reason for the rejection may have perfectly been envious passion.

Another similar situation happened when a new and very original idea which was philosophically grounded was sent upon request to a prestigious researcher in order to be published. Although the person who made the request assured it would be published, that never happened. When the researchers who had developed the idea asked about the reasons, they were also given evasive answers. In the meantime, the authors sent the researcher publications that expanded and further supported the proposal. No matter how many times they tried, they never received an answer or even a return notice for the letters or e-mails sent. Every new idea generates expectation, but this prestigious researcher must have evidently observed that the idea went beyond the expectations he had of the subject. Perhaps, his prestige was not enough; the recognition for such an original idea could mean discredit. He was exceeded by the idea.

The malicious pride as a motive for moral harassment

As it was the case with envy, the feeling of Malicious Pride can be a motive for other attitudes besides moral harassment.

It is interesting to underline that Pride has two contrasting meanings that can be both found in the scientific world.

On the one hand, it refers to the legitimate feeling of self-esteem arising from noble and virtuous causes, as in *feeling* proud. As an example to this meaning we could go back to what we said when we referred to the persistent anomaly as a key for innovation; we said then that stern commitment to their own ideas is typical of scientists. It is the *scientific pride* Umberto Eco speaks about. Pride, which in case it resists an authoritarian measure, we must say it is not out of superiority but out of the strength to resist injustice and defend truth, as we will see further on.

On the other hand, pride refers to the excessive self-appraisal, by which one believes to be superior to others, as in *being* proud, which results in an arrogant person.

Naturally, the Pride we refer to in this title is the one that corresponds to the second definition. Now, why – though apparently unnecessary – do we make a specific distinction between malicious Pride and this kind of Pride? The answer is simple: nothing happens while an authority *is proud* for considering itself superior but does not interfere in the researcher's life, who *feels proud* of his or her noble and virtuous causes. The problem arises when an authority who believes to be superior, also believes he or she can interfere and decide over the researcher's activities, not backing down even though this attitude (which the authority has even verbally admitted to be wrong) destroys an institute, a project or a researcher's career. In table 36, we indicated that the authority can say *we made a mistake* as a mocking excuse. However, there are opportunities in which this expression does not have that mocking connotation. We can quote here the case of a researcher who, when discussing with an authority about a provision that had been adopted that meant an institute's destruction, was told: We made a mistake. In a different meeting, the same authority, when asked why they had stubbornly made the decision stand though it was an admitted mistake, said: *People have their pride*. It seems that the authority is not very wise and quite stupid since gross stupidity and blind pride go hand in hand.

As we will see later, the harassing system supports its attitude with an unwritten law: The authority will not back down on any of its decisions. It is worth remembering a phrase uttered after the compulsive transfer of an institute: *We decided to move the workplace and we don't accept excuses for not complying with this decision.* They do not put forward any academic or scientific reasons for the transfer, just the superiority pride of having complied with what was established on no grounds. This pride wanted to force a disabled person to perform a task that was impossible for him to do. The pride led to a blindness that even denied medical evidence.

Infallibility is a quality that cannot be demanded from any person. Authorities can make mistakes. Yet, we consider that in an authentic scientific-academic system, they will be modest enough to accept and correct their mistakes. In an Aloentic scientific-academic system, though, the countermarch on any provision – or its revision – does not exist. They are strictly complied without thinking about the consequences. Its aloenticity makes sure the authority's decisions are never questioned while the authority is in charge. Also, the cyclical recurrence of authorities and corporations of power within the public system allows for a misuse of the impunity bestowed upon the authority. It is common that big and little mistakes are tolerated and even deliberately caused in a frivolous and humorous rejoicing environment just for the sake of making ostentation of power. The public money assures that nobody will question the inefficient use of human resources and materials. The administrative jumble that justifies the expenses can also justify the cost generated by the proud and inefficient authorities' mistakes.

It is interesting to highlight that malicious pride does not surprise anybody in the academic and scientific world, even when this pride is present in occupations where modesty should be a virtue.

Authentic scientist's altruist work goes beyond them, transcending them. The simple and proud authority, since its *work* is the discretionary exercise of power, is only transcended by its failures and iniquities.

Psychopathic process and harassment

We have defined the adverse situations an ethical objector in Science and Technique undergoes as a *degenerative, systematic/corporative, and diachronic process, which is progressive in intensity*. We have said that this last aspect is the one that most clearly differentiates this process from plain moral harassment since the intention of the later is to destroy.

After this superficial analysis of envy as a motive for moral harassment, and continuing with this topic, we see that the attitudes described – that begin with discouragement until they become persecution – are also suffered by other researchers such as Paul. The procedure follows quite regular steps; by applying the characteristics of scientific knowledge, we can say that this is a universal phenomenon.

If the authority takes advantage of the passivity of a researcher who does not understand those situations, if it takes advantage of his or her vulnerability creating obstacles, it becomes very difficult to avoid the collapse of the researcher's health.

Since the harasser accuses the harassed, among other things, of not participating or integrating, it is interesting to underline a concept from Dr. Hirigoyen (Le Nouvel Observateur, 2006):

> The staff is asked to discuss, express itself, participate. It is requested to speak, but everyone knows that the most convenient thing is to always follow the interests of the unanimous culture of the company: the defense and promotion of the collectiveness.

While the harasser wants to protect his or her own interests and those of the *collective* and corporate group, the harassed runs out of the typical vital energy of the researcher due to the demand to analyze and contribute to trivial initiatives.

The accusation to the persecuted researcher of not wanting to integrate, or being selfish and conceited, i.e. individualistic, is a blatant maneuver of the system to achieve its aim: manipulating the researcher so as to affect his or her self-esteem. As we have said in the first reading when we referred to point 10 (Individualism), by this we do not mean that the researcher must be selfish. In the same reading, in point 22, we have also said that in order to protect themselves from moral harassment, harassed persons want to isolate themselves from the harassing environment – an attitude which is interpreted by the system as *they do not want to integrate*. That is the reason why the researcher must be individualistic and the system must respect this individualism which should not be understood as selfishness. Individualism is defined as the ethical doctrine that puts the human individuals as the object in which the purpose of the moral acts must be applied. Depending on what the purpose of this moral act is, individualism may be selfishness or altruism. Therefore, when we refer to Individualism, we are making reference to Altruism or *Ethical Individualism* – opposite to selfishness – which puts other people as the object of the moral act, people who are not the subject of that act.

The system accuses the researcher of being individualistic and selfish, but what it really wants is to manipulate the researcher so that the purpose of the moral act works for the selfish interests of the corporate group and not for the community.

One must not confuse Individualism with *non obvious acting* or, as it is commonly known, with *do it your own way*. Many times, researchers isolate themselves out of the need to be alone so as not to be absorbed by the obvious acting of the corporate group. Thus they are accused of being individualistic (selfish) when in fact they should be *accused* of being resistant against abdicating from their deep sense of justice. It is not superiority pride, but the courage to resist against injustice and defend the truth.

An authentic researcher focused on his or her tasks is usually bad at preventing risky situations, since he or she is generally a little naïve. Furthermore, we must highlight that extreme situations of moral harassment are also placed in an extreme level of persecution. Before facing such an attitude, as we have seen, the researcher was a victim of less aggressive discouragement and discrimination attitudes, which in some way acted like the frog in the frying pan. To illustrate with examples the difference between the psychopathic process and moral harassment, it is interesting to turn to this example: it is said that if we put a frog in a frying pan with boiling water, it would jump to safety. If, instead, we put the frog when the water is cold and we slowly turn the temperature up, it will not try to escape from danger and will die. Similarly, people who suffer the slow damaging process end up by generally succumbing without escaping the risk, as it would occur if the aggression were evident.

Another characteristic of this psychopathic process – which we mentioned in the first reading when we described values 13 (Tirany vs Openness) – is the harassed persons' lack of understanding their situation. In that respect, Dr Hirigoyen (Bembibre) speaks about some patients who went to see her:

> They complained about their depression but could not understand what was wrong with them. It was a pattern that appeared in very different situations, and that could be defined as a series of harassing procedures – gestures, words, looks — that attack the person's dignity, and physical and mental integrity. There are little things that seem to be unimportant but which through repetition and systematization become serious.

Strategies for moral harassment

In the academic-scientific environment, different strategies can be used for moral harassment, some of which we referred to in the text. However, we can also mention:
1. Intimidating measures.
2. Acts of derision.
3. Humiliating workplace.
4. Manipulation of the researcher's staff.
5. Extreme arbitrary regulations.
6. Forged trials.
7. Impeding Communication or making it difficult.

Regarding intimidating measures, we have already mentioned them when we spoke about Pressing. Now we will give examples for the other strategies used in moral harassment.
2. Acts of derision will be described under a separate title.
3. Concerning humiliating workplace, this is very common. We have already commented on the researchers who had requested furniture for their institute and were ordered to pick it up from a filthy warehouse, which is also humiliating. But regarding the

workplace, it is interesting to mention that the authority assigned these researchers an abandoned house in poor conditions in a totally unsafe location of the city as a physical place – in a so-called *villa miseria* which is the equivalent to a *favela* in Brazil. Another case is that of a researcher who was removed from the office he had been assigned to at the institute, in order to work in a small place near the restrooms. In another case, a group of researchers were removed from their workplace and if they wished to continue working, they would have to do it in a newly assigned place, which was precarious and filthy.

4. Regarding the fourth strategy, manipulation of the researcher's staff, it is common for the corporation to use this in order to deteriorate the researcher. We have observed two possibilities in that regard. One is when the researcher does not have any staff and is not assigned any – an issue we will deal with later. The other possibility – the most perverse one – is when the corporation starts to meddle with the researcher's already consolidated work group, such as the support staff, group of researchers, etc. so as to damage that group and leave the researcher alone. It is the case of a researcher to whose work group the corporation offered better positions at other university chairs or institutes. The group members feared that since their director *had problems* they could have problems too, putting their positions at risk. The researcher was finally left alone and had to retire.

5. The extreme arbitrary regulations are authoritarian, compulsive, discretionary measures that the authority demands the researcher to comply with without previous notice. By *extreme* we do not mean those situations which, though bothersome, can be solved by the researcher, such as denying at the last minute a device that he or she needed to deliver a speech. It is easy to imagine how destructive it can be to a person's mental health to find himself or herself in a surprising and serious situation against which he or she can do nothing. Among such regulations we can mention cases of: eviction from the workplace, impeding entry to the workplace, destruction of essays, property seizure, dismissal, etc. Concerning impeding entry to the workplace, we can mention a case in which the directors of an institute arrived there and found that none of their door keys opened. Thinking that the lock did

not work and was damaged, they asked for the locksmith's service. When opening the lock, for which he had to destroy and put a new one, he communicated to the directors that the lock had been changed. This led the researchers to the conclusion that the authority, as another act of persecution, had got the lock changed without previous notice. It is interesting to observe that when adopting such measure they did not care about the institute staff having to remove their personal items or the existence of tests that needed to be controlled, etc.

6. Regarding the sixth element of harassment, a strategy for moral harassment very much used in the Academic and Scientific environment is the so-called *Academic Trial*. This strategy is used as a last resort, when all the dispossessions the harassed has suffered have not affected him or her enough as to voluntarily resign. It is then when the system tries to dispossess him or her of the last thing ever possible: his or her honor. A trial is conceived for trivial or absurd motives that are simply forged by the system. It does not need any evidence. Perhaps, even more, the evidence in favor of the victim is destroyed in order to have the elements needed to start a trial. Through an impeccable lawyer-like logic, the trial becomes detached from the cause. In a certain moment, the cause is not important anymore and the trial is what only matters. Thus the harassed is subjected to this mechanism of endless police-like questioning, derision and countless accusations of lies or incompetence. Very few people resist this harassment, which by being authoritarian cannot be stopped by any legal protection. This reminds us of the guilt confessions in totalitarian regimes that are obtained under pressure. The harassing system supports its attitude with the unwritten law that states that the authority will not back down on any of its decisions. The harassed have no protection. Following Quevedo's advice: "Where there is no justice, it is dangerous to be right." (Quevedo) We can consider the Academic Trial as an evil display that puts the system *delight* on the spotlight, since despite being able to simply retire the person, as with the quoted case of Dr Emde, it wants to play cat and mouse with him or her. Besides aiming at the person's dishonor, academic trials aim to disgracefully expel the accused. In order to do so, a trial is set in aspects where the person must prove the

highest honesty. Also, once a trial started and the accusations maliciously advance, it is simple for the lawyer-like inner group of the corporation to start *finding* or *inventing* unexpected consequences. It becomes a real *snowball*, whose size will be in the corporation hands, which will create more accusations until the harassed is subdued and resigns.

7. Regarding impeding communication or making it difficult, when we tackle the subject of the courtesy Interviews as acts of derision, we will mention the case of interviews permanently interrupted by telephone calls. But in order to illustrate this point, we can mention two researchers who were summoned by the authority of an institute to attend an academic meeting about changes in the academic program. One of them was not allowed to express his ideas and the other one, though he was able to do it, received a despising attitude from the group. It seemed that everybody was thinking *when is this guy going to finish speaking?* Their proposals, which were completely logical and reasonable, were not considered. Another case is that of a researcher who, when attending a meeting where they would decide on the future of an institute, when asking an authority permission to speak to put forward arguments in defense of the institute's continuity, that right was completely denied. Regarding the intention of preventing communication, we can state that the harasser wants to isolate the harassed. Take the case of the researcher who, by being dispossessed from his workplace, had to work in borrowed places such as the library.

One of the harasser's strategies: The lack of solidarity

Among the virtues of the harassed person referred to in the first reading we can mention: strong sense of comradeship, good team worker, independent and with initiative, valued by his or her workmates, having a great aversion to using people for his or her own aims. Notwithstanding, in the typical situations of an ethical objector, it may happen that the person does not count on any support, especially from his or her workmates. We should remember here the case quoted in the fourth point. In that respect, Dr Hirigoyen (Le Nouvel Observateur, 2006) comments the following:

The colleagues' fear of losing their jobs is very strong, but this also happens because the work organization divides more and more each individual's work into sections. In this context of 'each man for himself,' it is easier to isolate the person who they want to get rid of.

This is known by the harasser, who takes advantage of it.

Although the harassed person is valued by his or her workmates, some of them telling him or her about it privately, when he or she needs help is generally left alone. The workmates group as such will never support him or her since they are afraid of being exposed. In fact, they are in that institution to receive a salary rather than for intellectual or idealistic reasons. Thus, they can be in a research group today and in another one tomorrow. In the first reading, we commented that in an Aloentic system the scientific arguments used by a researcher to defend his or her ideas are responded by the system with administrative arguments. It is for this same reason that even scientists that occupy a position of authority in the evaluation system and who could help a researcher who by his or her ideas has become a dissident or persecuted scientist, do not do so. They do not do it not because their scientific prestige would be at risk but because their administrative career would. The lack of scientific competence is replaced by fulfilling the rules to the very detail and not doing anything that could compromise them. This assuming the actors' good faith; they may act moved by orders that come from dark interests so that evident but unpleasant-for-the-corporation truths would not come to light.

When the person is creative and for that reason is valued by his or her workmates, and does not reach the harassed person's level, i.e. when he or she is lucky, we can say that he or she will never know who really values him or her sincerely. As the Italian poet Ludovico Arioso (1474-1533) expresses it: "…we cannot know who really loves us when luck is on our side" (Arioso). But when the valued person starts to be harassed, i.e. when *luck is not in our side anymore*, the harassed person will be able to prove who really loves him or her. Perhaps he or she does not find anyone and has to suffer the loneliness of abandonment. In that respect, we can also quote a Polish proverb that goes: "When adversity knocks on your door, all your friends are sleeping" (Anonymous (b)).

Every work group has its union, and so we can think that a persecuted or dissident researcher professor should be protected by it. However, at least in our situation, this has not happened. We think that this is so because the union protects the common workers' interests: better income, longer breaks, sick leave, etc. Yet, the reasons that make a researcher dissident or ethical objector are not shared by his or her workmates. The ethical commitment, for example, is not a common objective. That is why during good times, he or she is valued by his or her workmates, but in bad times, he or she will be left alone. The dissident or ethical objector has no union. Ironically, when we tried to found an INESPE Argentine branch, after submitting the first document to the corresponding official organization, the main argument against it to deny our request was: *unions and professional associations already exist for that purpose.* (We will later expand on this.)

Other characteristics of harassment

An author refers to harassment as the *hidden damage* (Pérez Soliva), stating that:

> In a campaign of personal discredit, as in cases of moral harassment at work, and despite the victim having distanced him or herself from the focus of harassment, we find that some of the accusations made still cause damage over time.
> I have seen it in harassed workmates, where though the actual harassment had long stopped, some of the accusations made are still there, eroding. I call it the hidden damage.
> Out of all the accusations the victim has had to endure there is one that hurts the most. It is not the same one for each victim and he or she rarely names it.
> From what I was able to verify, that accusation 'in singular' contains a high stigmatization level in the ethical aspect and is centered on paracriminal features.
> They also want to affect the victim's mental integrity.
> It is based on accusing the victim of derangement through attacks to the victim's mental integrity, with accusations of insanity, drug addiction etc.
> The victim is hurt by being accused, even though he or she knows it is not true, this kind of accusation continues to hurt throughout the years.

From this, our experience let us underline the concepts of hidden damage, personal discredit, damage throughout time, fraudulent and false accusations – some more painful than others –, ethical stigmatization and paracriminal features.

As a last aspect included in table 36 for the persecutory attitudes, we can add personal or telephone threats if one does not accept to participate in non-scientific activities, such as being forced to take part in political activities.

Regarding this, it is interesting to again quote Dr. Hirigoyen (Bruno):

> In fact, in order to psychologically tie up an individual, it is enough to induce him or her to lie or to take certain compromises so as to turn him or her into an accomplice of the perverse process.

The induction to certain compromises may have an intimidating and coercive result. However, it can have a *seductive* connotation at the beginning. This term is perfect since the intention is to persuade slowly into evil – in this case, seducing the person one wants to persecute. We can mention the case of a researcher whose colleague was offered a high hierarchical post and who was said by a member of the corporation: *You're going up*. That is to say, not only would the colleague have a better position but the researcher would also be benefited from working together with him. It was a real *seductive* proposal. The offering deceit and the clear intention of control and manipulation by the authority were revealed by the fact that when the offer was not accepted, the persecutory attitudes intensified.

In table 36, under the Persecution column, we underlined attitudes, for some of which we have referred to concrete cases. It is worth mentioning some of them again, along with others whose intention is to generate moral harassment.

- Taking advantage of a physical health problem to classify the harassed as intellectually incompetent.
- Removal of incentives or other economic benefit or bonus.
- Removal of social security and medical care.
- Libel.
- Destruction of work: removing of the physical place, destruction of tests.
- Obligation to do tasks that due to disability problems cannot be performed.
- Obligation to perform auxiliary tasks which are not appropriate to the academic level.
- Submitting the harassed to the authority of a person who has a lower or much lower academic hierarchy.
- Publicly questioning the victim's authority in front of his or her students – in examining boards, for example.
- Personal or telephone threats if he or she does not accept to participate in non-scientific activities such as political activities.

- Changing the workplace lock without previous notice so that when the researchers arrive they cannot enter. This is a measure taken without any consideration of the possible deterioration of experiments.
- As we have described, compulsive eviction and without previous notice from the workplace with an unusual violence and threat of using the public force. This could cause the victim to be charged of resisting authority, if he or she does not comply in due time.
- Dismissing the victim without previous notice so that he or she is informed when getting paid.
- Groundless academic trials.
- Threatening mail (of dismissal, for instance).

We draw attention to these acts since there is a law in Argentina (13.168) dealing with Workplace Violence in Argentina. This is defined as the violence provoked by civil servants and/or government employees who, by taking advantage of their hierarchical position or circumstances related to their duties, behave in such a way that affect the worker's physical, sexual, psychological and/or social dignity and integrity, and which manifests itself as power harassment through threats, intimidation, frightening, salary inequality, harassment and physical, psychological and/or social maltreatment.

Among other aspects, psychological and social maltreatment is remarked and it is defined by an author (Bruno) as follows:

> The continuous and repetitive hostility in the form of insult, psychological harassment, despise and criticism. For instance: to force somebody to do denigrating tasks, unnecessary or senseless duties just to humiliate him or her; to give offensive opinions about work performance; to move offices or the usual workplace to separate the person from his or her workmates; to block initiatives; to impede communication; to request impossible-to-perform tasks; to promote harassment through plotting; to threaten repeatedly with groundless dismissals; etc..

The similarity between the acts we suffered and the ones provided by the Law is not just coincidental.

Then a question arises: if there is a law, why isn't there a protection? Probably, because the system has the necessary means to find a justification to block any law that may affect it. The scientific/technical corporation, in a public institution like the one in which we have worked, has automatic skillful mechanisms of self-defense. They make such Law sound as if its provisions were things that happen to somebody else, as if it would be impossible to think it necessary to apply it in a public institution of a democratic government. The concrete individual can paradoxically be completely unprotected in a public organization where seminars about Law 13.168 are given. Much is known about the Law but it would never be applied in concrete cases within the institution itself. It is worth repeating here what we have said before: all attitudes follow the *Unwritten Law*. The authority will not back down on any of its decisions, even if this goes against the law. The harassed has no protection. Regarding mobbing or corporate harassment, we dare say that it will never be legally recognized by the Science and Technique system since every corporate system (even the corporate/legal) reserves the right to harass and expel its dissidents without suffering any legal sanction. The law can only be applied when the crime is committed by a Private Company and judged by the state; within public organizations, the law is not effective.

From what has been exposed and because of the consequences the harassed may suffer from moral harassment, Dr. Hirigoyen (Le Nouvel Observateur, 2006) advises that:

> Victims should not ignore the situation. Victims must escape the situation in some way or another. Above all, victims must speak. Yielding, ignoring and waiting for the harassment to go away are the worst solutions. If a victim remains motionless, his or her family life will soon be destroyed; his is or her life as a whole will soon be destroyed.

With regard to Dr. Hirigoyen's advice, at least in our personal case in which we realized after several years that we were in a moral harassment situation, we can say that since the psychopathic process is degenerative, it has the *frog effect* and conclude that even when not ignoring the harassment you cannot escape from the pain. This is really so. Not ignoring the harassment meant not yielding to the harasser demands as if the harassment did not exist. Examples of this would be accepting a workplace transfer as if the harasser's false arguments were valid, changing the subject of study in order to please the harasser, incorporating or eliminating people of the work group to please the harasser, etc. By accepting such things, one would ignore the real problem: Harassment. Accepting the harasser's arbitrary demands does not diminish harassment but exacerbates it. Negotiating with the harassing bloc would be, as indicated by the author, *ignoring the situation*. The individual or collective narcissistic perversion is not appeased by concessions; on the contrary, it becomes more and more demanding.

Nevertheless, the slow progressive damage makes the person unaware of his or her *final destiny* and despite having faced all acts, from the most incipient to the most serious ones, his or her health can be seriously damaged, especially psychologically speaking. But again, ignoring the harassment would probably lead to even more serious damage.

In order to illustrate this last point (that ignoring the harassment can lead to the victim's life destruction), we can imagine the case of a circus where an excellent magician is maliciously forced – as a clear underlying act of moral harassment – to perform as a trapeze artist if he wants to continue working in the circus. If the magician agrees to the harassment his prestige may be damaged due to his lack of training or skills; he would even risk his life as he can have a serious accident. If the magician agrees to the harassment and gets on stage as a trapeze artist, it would be like ignoring the harassment by believing that he will later be able to work as a magician. He does not see that his lost prestige and his impaired health due to the possible accident are both damages that would finally prevent him from working as a magician, which is his real specialty and for which he has talent. The only solution for the magician to face the harassment is to refuse working as a trapeze artist. Then the harasser may cunningly say to him: *You are such an excellent magician that the trapeze work will be completely simple for you, you will not find it hard at all.* Appealing thus to the magician's ego, if he falls into the trap, the harasser will have achieved his or her goal.

What we have just exemplified is very common at some universities, where to distract committed researchers from their subject of study they are offered better paid or superior posts but to do activities that are not of their interest. If, for instance, a researcher is working on a subject related to biology as a teaching assistant, he or she will be offered to work as full professor in Social Sciences. If a researcher has obtained a high training abroad, he or she will be fallaciously told that such training allows him or her to teach any subject. At the same time, all his or her requests of recognition for the subject he or she and his or her collaborators would have created will be maliciously ignored.

We should not forget that the corporation tolerates resistant or dissident people as long as they totally or partially agree on its demands with a smile on their face. When the conflict between integrity and demands becomes as big as to make resistant people resort to some legal resistance, the harassers will show all their brutality. The huge asymmetry between organized power and the resistant or dissident person is displayed in all its harshness.

For that reason, apart from not ignoring harassment, we dare call for the development of a mechanism that protects dissidents from being buried in a defenseless system, as we will see later.

Administrative mockery

Among the persecutory attitudes, we also underlined attitudes that are characterized by *mockery* and *injurious mockery*. When such mockery takes place within the frame of the administrative paperwork necessary to obtain means of work, subsidies, etc. we can define it as Administrative mockery. Such attitudes also constitute a kind of moral harassment. These are attitudes used indirectly by the establishment in order to dissuade, discourage, and finally make the victim resign. These aims are different from Pressing, which is lighter. Pressing, as we have seen, tends to bother, pester and frighten the person, while Mockery has the intention of hurting the person.

The common factor of all the Mockery attitudes as a strategy of moral harassment is the fact that the generator knows perfectly well beforehand that the harassed request will never be granted, using this knowledge in order to mock. The mockery would be more offensive if it is connected to something the harassed truly needs.

The system turns to different procedures in order to Mock, among which we can mention:

The courtesy interviews

Interviews as a mockery strategy are very common and simple to apply by the authority. Although in table 36 they are presented as discouragement and discrimination strategies, we also want to include them as a form of Mockery. Courtesy interviews usually end with false promises that can be defined as *pompous courtesy promises*.

The following case is paradigmatic: Two persecuted researchers requested to have an interview with an authority, which they trusted, to explain the need of support for their work so this authority could furnish the necessary measures. The authority agreed to meet them, the date and time set, the researchers presented themselves for the meeting. They waited for more than one hour but the authority never arrived. Instead they received an excuse from his secretary – that for all they know could be totally false – and also a new date for the meeting.

The researchers presented themselves again for the meeting, receiving from the secretary the communication that the authority had not arrived yet but would do it soon. After less than an hour, the authority arrived and welcomed the researchers. A few minutes into their presentation, they were interrupted by the authority's cell phone. After the authority's apology, the researchers resumed their presentation, only to be interrupted again by the authority's cell phone. After a new apology, the dialogue is interrupted again when the authority receives a telephone call from his desk telephone. After that, the dialogue continued for a while, until the authority's secretary entered the room saying that another authority was waiting for him in another office for a meeting that cannot wait. In the short time the meeting lasted, the researchers could barely outline a comment on their situation for which they received the answer *I will deal with this matter.* This was no more than a false promise that was never fulfilled. The truth is the authority only conceded the interview out of courtesy in order not to reveal that he would not do anything because of interests of the harassing group.

The Mockery effect was more intense since the researchers had to make a more than 300 kilometers trip to attend the meetings.

An attitude we classified in table 36 as discriminatory is that of leaving the person outside the system of promotions. To justify why we include it as Mockery we give the example of the case of a researcher who had worked full time for 20 years but received an income equivalent to that of an assistant professor who only works 5 hours a week. The researcher requested a higher hierarchical position that not only considered the academic and scientific level achieved but that also would provide him with an income coherent to his ability and dedication. For this, certain paperwork was requested, after which, the authority finally answered: *We don't give you the position so as not to set a precedent.* The answer is a mockery since other people with much lower achievements than the researcher's had obtained hierarchical positions in the institution. If they had known that the position would not be given, the authority should have not requested the formal paperwork. But this was asked as an act of mockery.

Another Mockery attitude is possible through the answers given by the authority to the researcher after a brief meeting. It is interesting to mention the case of a researcher who inquired about an unfavorable measure: the loss of the workplace where he was working on his research program. When asking if such measure was going to be adopted, he received as an answer: *Have no doubts about such a thing happening.* The phrase – and above all the way the authority expressed – gave the researcher the impression that nothing would go wrong. But it was actually a play on words. The adverse measure was adopted, and the authority was able to argue that he had been misinterpreted.

Another example of mockery is the case of a researcher who turned to an authority whom he trusted in order to solve a situation regarding the loss of a paid position. It was an urgent situation since the researcher was working without being paid. During the courtesy interview the authority granted him, he received the following answer: *Endure this situation for six months, even if you don't get paid. I'm going to solve this problem. What's more, I'm going to improve your situation.* The promise was never fulfilled. In fact, the authority who had made the promise always knew the position would not be assigned.

Another case of courtesy interview was that of the researchers who had been conceded an interview to deal with the imminent closure of an institute. They submitted a note to the institution's legal advisor requesting the measure to be revised – which was not a formal appeal and, as such, had not been accepted. The legal advisor told them that *submitting a new note with the same tone would be a simple complaint. You should lodge a formal appeal.* The researchers, innocently and even at their own expense since they had to resort to a private lawyer, lodged the appeal. Ironically, the same person who had suggested the appeal was the one who had to evaluate it and pass the final judgment, which he already knew – for being a member of the corporation – would be adverse to the researchers. When recommending the appeal he already knew it would not be favorable. Yet, the researchers were not told so. In this way, he contributed to feed the administrative bureaucratic machinery, pretending to be nice with the researchers and providing them with the illusion of the possibility of a favorable outcome. In this same case, one of the advisor's legal assistants asked the researchers for further documentation to raise their expectations. What's more, she also promised to include aspects that would support the continuity of the institute. These aspects were never included. It is interesting to underline the fact that the administrative legal bureaucratic machinery of the corporation pretended to make a supposedly fair evaluation when in fact the negative result had been previously decided. The institute was finally closed. After this happened, the legal advisor encouraged the researchers to take the case to the ordinary justice outside the university legal system. The researchers did not accept the advisor's suggestion and stopped the process mainly because, as we will see later, by being a closed system, no ordinary court interferes. That is, if a public organization takes a decision, it will not be contradicted by a higher authority. The proceedings may be initiated, but nothing will happen at the end except for the psychical damage caused to the person being subjected to a new mockery. The legal Advisor, who knew that a filing to a higher court would not be successful, recommended it anyway as another way of mockery. The corporate cynicism seems to use these attitudes to vent its fury on the ones who resist, on the different ones.

This kind of attitudes on the part of the corporation authority could be defined as a true *administration of lies*. These people possess so much power and cynicism that tell subtle and bare-faced lies just to temporarily appease the harassed who request their help. The authorities' ability is such that the harassed always believes them. It seems almost impossible for victims to doubt the authority. They never deny help nor tell the victims the truth about the fact that they already agreed with their harassers on not giving it to them. We can mention the case of researchers who turned to the highest authority of an organization to support the idea of maintaining a research institute. After a very pleasant meeting, where the authority even recognized the value of their research program, he promised them to talk about the problem with the authorities where the researchers' harassment came from. The researchers were very pleased after the meeting. However, the institute was closed a few months later and their goods were distributed among other members of the corporation who were loyal to the harassing authority. The less valuable items were distributed as remains in a ritual act.

After some time, they learned that a few days before the meeting with the highest authority, the resolution of the institute closure had already been signed. The highest authority had already agreed upon closure with the researchers' harassers. These hypocritical attitudes are usually the rule more than the exception and contribute to a lower scientific and academic level. That is to say, as we have said in the first reading, to keeping the system within aloenticity.

The fact that the resolution had been already signed reveals the interest in closing the institute as soon as possible. In order to support this authoritarian attitude, the authority used the uncertainty produced by libel. Reliable information was never requested, and the reports presented annually for more than two decades were not consulted either. In order to adopt a measure against dissident researchers in an authoritarian system that always go unpunished, it is obvious to say that academic and/or scientific arguments are unnecessary. If the authority wants to adopt the measure, it is enough. The long research years were completely ignored to serve the haste and uncertainty that ended with the destructive measure requested by the defamatory corporation. On this matter, we can quote Tacitus: "Truth is confirmed by inspection and delay; falsehood by haste and uncertainty" (Tacitus). If the measure against the dissident or ethical objector researchers was *delayed*, the corporation would face the risk of the truth about such measure becoming public. All the authority's unfair decisions were always generated by lobbies or corporations based on defamatory envy stimulated by corporate interests.

We can quote here the phrase by the Russian novelist, Leon Tolstoi (1829-1910): "Writing laws is easy, but governing is difficult" (Tolstoi). *Governing* in a state organization means taking decisions, which are weighted regardless of regulations, always respecting the academic and scientific values at stake. Yet, so as to hurt, the easiest thing to do is to turn to the regulations that are completely out of reality, regulations that are conceived *over a cup of coffee* and are applied without caring about the damage caused by them. Instead of thinking about how to improve knowledge, they think about the simplest thing which is to regulate the activity. The authority cannot afford to make decisions superficially and even less by only listening to one defamatory group, disregarding what the soon-to-be victims have to say.

We can see that what they are in fact administrators of lies. This is a very easy trick to perform which appeases the inquiring party. If at some point, they are questioned by the harassed about the fact that his or her request was not solved, the authority will turn to a new lie. In spite of the obvious differences, this is similar to the mechanism used in science to repair theories, which was already discussed in former chapters. In this case, the *theory* is the authority's pretended good will and desire to help. So as not to reveal its falsehood, the authority repairs it with another *theory* which is also false, in this case, a new lie over the former lie. All this takes place trying to keep an apparent affability and good will.

The malicious challenge

For this item, as well as for the previous one, we can mention the case of a researcher who, on the verge of being dismissed from the organization, was repeatedly summoned to attend a meeting to analyze his situation.

When one authority (who three years before had been given a complete summary of the program objectives and of what had been done over many years) was consulted about the researcher's situation, the authority firstly resorted to the famous *not knowing anything* about the case. That gives him the impression of being a very busy person. The argument of *not knowing* was false since this authority even had personally discussed the researcher's situation with another member of the corporation. The authority requested that the report be sent to him again. After studying it, he *encouraged* the researcher to attend a meeting during which a certain consideration would be taken. The meeting was defined by the authority as of *good will* on the part of the organization. But the meeting was in fact just a courtesy interview in order to comply with the bureaucratic paperwork, since his situation had been already decided by the organization. The attitude of *good will* on the part of the organization was simply to comply with what had been administratively stipulated by its own regulations. The scientific background and the value of the subject of study did not matter at all. The researcher had been examined negatively and according to the regulations he had to attend to interview so that his negative evaluation would stand firm. The corporation became furious when the researcher did not attend the interview for health reasons since according to the regulations such formality was required to dismiss him. The corporation had to fulfill only one more administrative stage to be able to dismiss the scientist. In any case, the researcher could not expect a favorable resolution if he did not attend the meeting. That is why we call his situation *Malicious Challenge*, since the researcher was between the devil and the deep blue sea. If he attended the meeting, the authority would formally dismiss him; if he did not attend it, the authority would also have the excuse to dismiss him by accusing him of being a *rebel*.

The authority that falsely promised a certain consideration even appealed to the above described malicious trick of affecting the researcher's self-esteem by telling him that if he did not attend the meeting, it was because he *was not willing to*. This is a trick we can define as *ploy*, so as to set him a trap, or by using a military term, to lay an ambush to eliminate him. It is well-known that the ambush results in the enemy's surrender or destruction. The true objective of the meeting was brought to light when the authority refused to pass judgment about the values of the researcher's work. This refusal revealed that the supposed *good will* put forward by the organization was false.

This malicious trick of appealing to the victim's self-esteem, which is improper and unworthy of an authority, can be compared to the case of a young school boy who is labeled as a coward for not facing the schoolmate who dares him to fight but is physically beyond his size. If the boy succumbs to his self-esteem, he will be battered. If the researcher succumbs to his or her self-esteem when labeled as selfish or not willing, he or she will also be battered.

Useless paperwork

The method consists basically of creating trust and hope by doing more paperwork. Such paperwork does not only imply the simple preparation of a note, but also filling in several forms, drawing up a project, etc. This is mainly achieved by gaining the harassed trust, *by promising that now a new era will start, in which harassment will stop, and requesting the victim for 'the last time' to make a tedious administrative formal presentation*. The system can turn to trivial arguments to justify the lack of approval or acceptance of a previous presentation. Any person who showed doubts about making a new presentation was told by the authority: *Do not believe in black lists*. In view of this answer, we believe that all readers come up with the same comparison to the famous saying: *I do not believe in witches, but they do exist,* so we could also say: *I do not believe in black lists, but they do exist*.

Sometimes, the corporation official does not necessarily act in premeditated bad faith. In fact, more than once the person recognizes the importance of the victim's presentation out of common sense, for the interested parties' merits and humanitarianism. Therefore, such person can encourage it in good faith, ignoring the dark background of persecution surrounding those making the presentation. In addition, he or she can act in that way since, as we will refer to later under the title of the ethical objector in Science and Technique, the corporation moves in a closed system where nobody interferes in its decisions. Consequently, it can emphatically say yes today but say no tomorrow without the necessity to give any explanation. Today, I can accept a proposal saying that it is very good only to reject it tomorrow. This attitude is also useful for the authority who says yes today and no tomorrow, to blame the denial on a superior, thus appeasing the researchers. Just like the case of the Legal Advisor we commented on the last point, we can compare these authorities' attitudes to the *good cop – bad cop* cliché. The ones that play the role of the *good cop* get to know about the details, intentions and tools that will be used by the researchers to defend themselves.

We can mention the case of the director of an institute who was presented a researchers' proposal for a project to do academic activities. After several opportunities in which they tried to arrange a meeting to discuss the topic (which was permanently postponed for reasons such as the director being busy), this person agreed to see them, was nice to them and recognized the proposal's value and entity so much so that he said that: *I don't doubt about how valuable the topic is, if it weren't, we wouldn't be having this meeting.* He requested the researchers to submit a note and a summary of the activities to be developed. Having submitted the material, the director promised to discuss the matter with a higher authority. All indicated that the project would be accepted. When the director was requested for a new meeting a few months after the first one in order to continue discussing the topic, he used a trivial argument to dismiss the request, giving the researchers the false promise to deal with it in the future. He claimed that his refusal was due to the fact that the work program of his institute was complete for that year. That was an obvious lie since he could have said so in the first interview. The obvious thing to believe is that he received the order to act in this way from a *boss* of the corporation, whom he had not consulted before the first interview. This boss is the one who has access to the black lists of the system.

Another interesting aspect to comment about this case is regarding what we referred to above about the fact that only a few new researchers are vocational and the rest only enter the scientific world for economic reasons. When discussing the proposal, the researchers said to the director that they did not oppose to charge for its registration. The director obviously agreed on this aspect and also about the importance for the course to be officially recognized since he commented to them: *In general, the ones who sign up for courses like this one are only interested in obtaining a certificate to add to their CVs.* That is, for most of the attendants what only matters is the value it has in their CV; that is what justifies the cost of the tuition fees, while the training it may offer is a secondary matter.

Harassers act as great *pretenders,* pretending to accept the work done. This way, they always please the person they have in front. In some cases, the simulation and hypocrisy is such that the people who pretend to offer more support and recognition are the ones who are hiddenly persecuting the person. We can define this suffering as *tantalic pain.* For example, a researcher is about to get a subsidy, but in the last minute it is denied. Professor Schadel first applies the analogy of the tantalic pain in a paper on Kant (Schadel, 2005), though in this case, referring to Kant's personal sufferings while developing his philosophy.

In the case of Mockery, this takes place when the harassed person receives the same usual adverse result – final consequence that many times is recognized by the harassed since the harasser never says no. Fundamentally, the Mockery consists of creating a false expectation of help in a tired, hurt and hit harassed, pretending sincerity and will to support him or her. He or she is asked to make a new effort, assuring that if such formality is complied with, the needed support will be obtained. If the harassed does not accept this, he or she will be held responsible for the lack of will. As we have said about the malicious Challenge, the harassed is between the devil and the deep blue sea. He or she is presented with a dilemma in which the harassed knows beforehand that the result will be unfavorable anyway, but accepts to go through a new paperwork so as not to seem unwilling. We always have to underline that harassment does not have an evident face or person, and nobody openly speaks about it but its effects are felt.

These are attitudes that submit the person to what we can call *to be held captive of uncertainty*, with false promises and expectations that the people who make them already know that will never be fulfilled; they enslave the person to the system. Then the harassed realizes too late about the reality, either because of the faith he or she had placed on the project or his or her trust on the ones who have the power of making decisions.

We must remember that useless paperwork can be considered a useless job or task, an aspect that Leymann encloses as item 34, among the 45 actions that he described within the moral harassment framework (Anonymous (c)).

Malicious ignorance

This is a way of mockery that is based on the supposed lack of coordination among the different administrative areas.

Let us suppose that a dissident researcher is harassed in the following way: he or she receives some lab equipment which he or she then duly returns. After a few months, he or she is asked to return it since the equipment had apparently not been returned. The researcher will reply with a letter indicating he or she had already returned the requested set of instruments. However, a year later, for instance, the researcher may receive a new more aggressive letter in legal terms summoning him or her to return the equipment. If, after that, he or she does not receive either a new summoning letter or a letter indicating that the situation has been clarified, the researcher will always be waiting for such letter, without knowing the status of this situation and in a painful waiting for an unexpected and new summoning letter.

Another case is when the institution presents through its media the dissident or ethical objector researcher's background in a wrong or incomplete manner. This discredits such researcher since whoever looks for his or her records obtains them inefficiently. If the researcher manages to clarify the situation, he or she will be answered the classic: *Oh, I didn't know!* This expression was used by an authority after passing a negative judgment on some administrative procedure. In order to justify his decision to the researchers affected by this, he said he *had no idea* of the points that would have led him to the act differently.

Another case of malicious ignorance was that of some researchers who were called by the authority to evaluate the situation of their work project. When attending the meeting, the authority had only one report summarizing their work in only one area of their activity. He had not taken the time to investigate their background, which covered over two decades of work. The authority even said: *We think you haven't done an-*

ything. With that argument, the authority was trying to relocate the researchers to another academic/scientific activity, with the veiled objective of *controlling* the researchers and deflecting them from the critical question that made them dissident or ethical objector.

Concerning this case, there is another aspect that could be entitled *the foolish examiner*. The authority, having learned that the researchers had published a book which he had not even taken the time to have a look at, denied them the possibility of continuing publishing their articles and books without being previously revised – i.e. *censored* by him. The authority was completely incompetent in the researchers' scientific area of expertise, which leads to consider him a *foolish examiner*.

Another similar situation concerns a dissident or ethical objector researcher's health problem. This is a common practice when the researcher develops his or her work in a different city from where the head office of the organization is. This was the case of a researcher who had stopped attending the workplace due to a disability. This situation was known by the authorities since the researcher had informed them about it, by submitting the corresponding medical certificates and letters requesting that different tasks be assigned to him. In spite of that, he received a letter in which he was summoned to attend a meeting in order to discuss his situation in the head office of the organization, for which he had to travel hundreds of kilometers. This letter apparently indicated the administrative staff did not know of the researcher's situation. The researcher, of course, indicated his impossibility to attend the meeting due to his health problem, being on a sick leave and under medical treatment. Nevertheless, after a few months, he received a new aggressive letter summoning him to a new meeting. The researcher again expressed his impossibility to attend the meeting. He was deeply worried since the letters were clearly threatening to dismiss him. He was ignored again and after some time, instead of the usual letter summoning to a new meeting, he received a new letter that indicated his many *absences* since there was no register of him attending the workplace. Finally, after 3 years of being under sick leave, he received the following letter: I'm summoning you to justify your absences within the next 48 hours, on pain of establishing the abandonment of services under the terms of the current Law. The reader can surely see the system aggressiveness against the dissident or ethical objector researcher.

Since in a case like this the justification letters are received by an employee, the authority that insidiously summons the researcher can claim that he or she ignored that the medical certificates had been presented. This worsens the harassed person's health condition.

The authority fakes ignorance of what had been done by the persecuted researcher, blaming the administrative staff for the mistake.

This kind of harassment produces the victim's physical and psychological decline by keeping him or her in a constant uncertainty. The researcher suffers a kind of psychosis by every note sent by the authorities because fear of dismissal.

False promises

In this case, we include strategies to which the authority turns without pretending to receive anything in exchange, and sometimes even without requesting letters to be submitted, etc. An example of this can be a promise to solve a problem – the restitution of a post, for instance – even promising to improve the situation, asking the harassed to wait for some time, though the problem is never solved. In this case, the harassed person remains in a *Passive Expectant* attitude.

We can also include here what has been described in the point about Useless Paperwork, but the difference is that in Useless Paperwork the harassed must have an *Active Expectant* attitude, because she or he will have to fill in forms, applications, to submit letters, etc. For instance, we can quote a case in which promises for a subsidy assignation were made, requesting the harassed to apply and reapply many times. This subsidy was never given on groundless excuses. In cases like this, sometimes the application forms are even disposed of directly while the interested party waits expectantly for the decision.

The False Promise is a very useful strategy for the discriminatory system to *get rid of* a person whose work it wants to stop, discourage, etc. Although, as we have said, many times the authority does not demand a note to be presented, in general, and to give the person more expectations, it requests the harassed to comply with a simple paperwork. Just as we have previously referred to courtesy interviews, these would also be *courtesy letters* since the person who requested them knows beforehand the letter will never be replied. Therefore, there are many paradigmatic cases in which when facing a request, the authority will say:

Very well, very interesting... submit a letter, please. The researcher waits for months for a reply that never arrives. If after that time, the researcher inquires the authority about it, the answer is always *we're working on it* or *we're still dealing with your request.* We can define these answers as *courtesy answers*, like the ones used to finish any courtesy interview.

Harassment with false promises

Unlike the previous strategy, which can be defined as *free choice* regarding the decision of the harassed person, this strategy is *coercive*, since the system turns to False Promises in order to obtain some kind of benefit, and thus the harassed is put under a much greater pressure.

An example of this is the offering of false promises that a situation of harassment will stop if the harassed accepts to make a *gesture*, such as supporting the group led by the Organization administration management.

This is common in systems where the administration is renewed every four or eight years. Towards the end of the period, the administrators need to *gather* signatures or *references*, so as to remain for another period. In order to do so, they take advantage of the scientists they might have even harassed – or not defended if the harassment came from the harassed colleagues – practically forcing them to negotiate with them under the promise that in the new period they will support their work if they in turn sign their support. The mockery manifests itself since although the harassed makes the required *gesture*, if finally the group requesting the backing loses its bid, it abandons the harassed in spite of still having the political power to help him or her. It does not stop the harassment as promised. Rather than falling out with the new authorities, the political group negotiates with them positions or privileges for itself. In this respect, we know of a researcher who had been dismissed from an institution by a new administration. When he turned to a former authority he had supported to be re-elected – support that included continuity of the program and its staff – for help, he was ignored; he was told: *I'd help you but I cannot fall out with the new authority.* This is also an example of not keeping the word in an Aloentic system.

It has been said about wars: *At war there are neither friends nor enemies. There are only interests.* Therefore, each political group only gives priority to its interests which can be closer to the rival political group than to the harassed scientist who put his or her trust in the group.

To steal an idea and then invite the harassed to be part of it

Stealing ideas has already been dealt with when we discussed ethical faults in Science and Technique. A researcher can steal an idea or research subject, but when the thief is a powerful person – like the director of an institute or a program – he or she or one of his or her subordinates may propose the dispossessed person to join the work group. We can quote the case of a researcher whose results had been copied very original results obtained in four years of research in a first-rate international center. A subordinate researcher of the authority who had copied the idea, dared to tell him when they met by chance at a scientific Congress: *We have to work together because we're working on the same thing*, a mocking excuse we have already mentioned in Chapter III, in the example of the diver.

In this case, since the one who steals the idea is powerful, he or she can become a member of the evaluation committee which will decide against the researcher whose idea had been stolen so as to block him or her to ever develop it. If we return to the old and new paradigm concepts, slowing down the development of the idea is slowing down the possibility for the new paradigm to become established.

We can turn once more to the example of the architect, which we already used to illustrate our hypothesis of how potential faults which are responsible for damage can be detected in an architect's plan. In the old days, in order to make a technical drawing they had to use a drawing pen. This drawing tool was charged with ink in small quantities between two blades which let it flow down into the paper in a constant thickness. The drawer needed to be very skillful to use it. Pencils were not allowed to draw plans. With the popularization of the photocopier, it was discovered that although a plan was made in pencil, the photocopier could make a copy that seemed to be drawn in ink. The first photocopy was better than the original. Therefore, if an architect laboriously developed a good idea on a plan using pencil (not having the means to do it otherwise), he or she would be rejected by the director, simply because a plan drawn in pencil was not worthy of consideration. Yet, the director would take the young architect's drawing and make a good photocopy of the pencil drawing. When presented to an evaluation board, the copy was accepted since it actually seemed to be an ink original. In the case we are analyzing, the Director who steals the idea would be the unscrupulous architect who steals the plan in pencil, the original idea, makes and ink-like copy, destroys the original, signs the copy as a new original and appropriates it. It is essential to destroy the original. If the author does not accept the director's rules, he or she can also be attacked – both subtly and grossly – until a health collapse occurs. The photocopy represents the administrative procedures: an author presents an idea to the authority, for instance, the creation of a program or institute. The authority appropriates the paperwork and shapes it in the right administrative way; it draws up the resolution and thus creates the program or institute that of course will be managed by a member of the corporation. This is a dispossession, or better still, usurpation. The creator could be suggested first and forced later to *contribute* with ideas since the usurpers do not know how to develop the copied idea. The corporation's indirect acceptance of the need of the original author in order to develop the idea is recognition of its own deficiency. But it may happen that, if the author of the idea does not accept to negotiate and is therefore finally dismissed, the corporation would still believe that by appropriating the idea, they will be able to develop it. But they will eventually discover how useless it is. To the belief of appropriating someone else's idea and trying to make it work we can apply a well-known text of Pirandello: The glasses. An ignorant man believed that by wearing glasses he would be able to read when in fact he should learn how to read first. Likewise, if the corporation wants to develop an idea, it should have first gone through the whole creative process that generated it. We can thus define the corporation (which, taking the psychologist's concept already quoted, is composed by the *allies* against the harassed (Mira y López, 1950)) as *corporate fools*. That is why, in order to achieve their goals, they can really act with indescribable clumsiness.

Hierarchical ostentation

This strategy is applied when a researcher manages to grow scientifically with all the effort implied, in spite of enduring discouraging, discriminatory and persecutory attitudes. This researcher, as another sign of despise of the system, can see that colleagues who started their careers at the same time he or she did in different areas of science succeed in having much higher positions or categories in the system than his or hers. The mockery manifests itself when the researchers of the corporation make ostentation of their position to the dissident or ethical objector research-er, while even pretending to pity him or her. This position does not only give them more prestige but also a higher economic level. It is the case of a dissident or ethical objector researcher who was relegated in the promotion ladder; a researcher of the same age who had started his scientific work at the same time told him during a meeting: *Are you still an assistant researcher? I'm a senior researcher already!* The dissident or ethical objector researcher observes how with little scientific merits others can obtain positions or promotions in the system just by doing what is politically, or administratively correct.

Another case is when people with lower academic level than the ha-rassed obtain a hierarchical position by which they attempt to put him or her under their authority.

Maliciousness can reach such a level that these people who are hie-rarchically placed in higher positions may try to obtain from the harassed useful ideas for their own projects. They consult the person who at the same time they are trying to maintain in an inferiority situation. The con-sultation must seem casual, as if it wasn't happening at all. Harassers wish to learn from the harassed but trying to make him or her believe that they are doing him or her a great favor without receiving anything in exchange.

To steal a development to gain from it

In the first reading, in the items Grant Holder vs. Disciple / Director vs. Tutor, we mentioned the case of a professor who told his student – who was very creative and enthusiastic, and who had created technological concrete objects that were even patentable an had written excellent ar-ticles – that he would take the article personally to present it at a con-gress because the student would not be allowed to do so due to the high level of the congress.

In this extreme case, those who steal a development are the mem-bers of the corporation. They would steal an invention and present it as if it was theirs at a congress or seminar, to which the true owner has not been invited. Apart from being an act of mockery, the members of the corporation use it to do *scientific tourism*. We are talking about people who want to obtain scientific subsidies to travel and, in their despair to obtain them, present others' results as if they were their own in order to comply with the bureaucratic formality. Since the evaluative system is generally away from the concrete situation, and is only interested in the compliance of the form, these attitudes are usually successful. Besides, this is done by members of the corporation and for that reason they will never be questioned.

Devaluation of initiatives

We have mentioned that destroying and maliciously ignoring the work done are typical attitudes of moral harassment.

We consider that devaluation of initiatives is also an element of mockery, for instance, when not giving a work done the due value it is worth. With the following case, the reader will perfectly understand what we mean. It is the case of a researcher who, having no support on the part of the authority to have the minimal means of work, and acting – as we have already said in the first reading, as a *cartonero*, could obtain modest substitutes to replace those means. In a meeting with the authority, where they were discussing the continuity of the project, this researcher supported the importance of the studies by saying that results of entity were obtained using these minimal substitute means of work he had personally obtained, but with official support, the results would be even better. The authority, far from recognizing the effort by deciding to support his work, pretended to be shocked, reproaching him: *Why do you beg for things?* thus deliberately ignoring the vocational effort of the researcher who was committed to an idea, and also pretending not to realize that the researcher was begging for means of work as the only possible way to do his work in the face of the fierce and systematic refusal of the corporation to give him the minimal means.

Since you can't continue with your work, give us your support so that we can continue with it ourselves

In the first reading, we said that the indignity of the Aloentic system reaches such level that one can hear: *Your idea is not working, but if I co-author it or even conduct it, it will.* In spite of being a disgraceful attitude, at least in this case the researcher is offered to continue working.

In this section, we would like to discuss an even more disgraceful strategy, which is to take advantage of a researcher who has been persecuted and dismissed by the system by trying to steal the subject and the path the researcher had opened with his work. To make matters worse, the usurper would ask the researcher to support him or her *for the importance of the work's sake*. It is similar to tell a person who has been wrongfully sentenced to death *leave me all your belongings*, instead of trying to find ways to stop the execution. This is the case of two researchers who had created an academic field, which they could not continue teaching because one of them had been dismissed and the other was given a disability retirement (a disability caused by the suffered persecution). Shortly after, a person who had familiarized with the subject some years before, for belonging to a political faction was associated with the system, came to them. This person told one of the researchers to *support him and his associates on their bid to teach the subject*. This group did not care to help the researchers to continue their work, although they had the political power to do so. They were only interested in taking advantage of their work. We also have to clarify that they had no intention to spend the knowledge developed by the two researchers, they just wanted to distort or politically misappropriate an intellectual capital that had been cumulated with effort, thus distorting the very objectives of the discipline they wanted to teach. In other words: the discipline has been already developed through its creators' effort and sacrifice; it can be used now as a platform for other objectives. It may be expected that if the group does not obtain the creators' support, it can even plagiarize the signature and use it for other purposes. As we have seen before, due to the authoritarian and discretionary character of the system, the deed will go unpunished. This strategy clearly shows the opportunistic nature of most of the people who surround whistleblowers.

Other persecutory strategies

Malicious arbitrary obligations

The use of Malicious Arbitrary Obligations is another strategy of the system to persecute a person.

We define them as *malicious* to differentiate them from the Arbitrary Obligations already mentioned when we referred to Envy, which include regulations of a general nature that the corporation members must perform. As we have said before, due to the nature of the researcher's work, health reasons, etc. the system is forced to waive such obligations and therefore comes the envy.

The Malicious Arbitrary Obligations, instead, are regulations that the system deliberately applies to the persecuted person with the purpose of damaging him or her. That is what gives them a particular nature.

As we have said, they can also be framed within moral harassment and could also have been discussed under Malicious Ignorance because since the system should not show its game, it will always have an excuse to justify itself.

Among these regulations we can quote the following:

1. To oblige persons to do tasks that due to disability problems they cannot perform.
2. To oblige persons to do academic tasks that are not appropriate to their academic specialty.
3. To oblige persons to participate in tasks that are inappropriate or insignificant for their project, such as political meetings.
4. To arrange mandatory meetings when the person required is busy with another task.
5. To oblige persons to commute daily to workplaces where they cannot attend.

We can illustrate point four with the case of a person who worked part time in an institution and was summoned by the Director for a meeting precisely the day that the person was in his other part time job. This person received a sanction for his absence.

Even when the persecuted person may manage to explain and justify why he or she did not comply with the obligation, he or she has already suffered psychological strain. In a real case regarding point four, the person resigned. As another element of mockery, his director tried to convince him not to do it. While the aim of the harassment is mocking so as to wear down the harassed, some harassers get frightened when facing the harassed resignation and do not want to show their perversion. They wish to continue playing cat and mouse, mocking the mouse but without killing it. If the person resigns, it is like killing the mouse.

For point five, we can mention the case of the relocation of some researchers' work, which had neither academic nor scientific grounds, to a place the harassed could not attend due to health reasons.

Destruction of work

We have already discussed this strategy under Extreme Arbitrary Regulations and as one of the tools used by moral harassment.

Among other persecutory attitudes, we have also mentioned that of having to do tasks that first seem to be useful, but which the system knows useless. Unlike the tasks described under Administrative Mockery that include administrative tasks, such as files or proceedings, the ones considered in this point are tasks that the system gives permission to perform but that will end up destroying. For instance, to allow researchers to make a great effort and spend a lot of time to build a project that then is dismantled. Or authorizing the use of a field to be sown as part of a scientific test only to shamelessly destroy it later (without anybody ever being held responsible) and then having to start the experiment all over again. Going back to Greek mythology, doesn't this remind us of the myth of Sisyphus? Sisyphus was punished for his cruelty, but the dissident or ethical objector researchers for trying to maintain the unconditional search of knowledge. Take the case of a researcher who, in order to provide the poor workplace the authority had given him with equipment and in view of the authority's lack of help, he himself furnished two offices and a lab with its electrical installation using materials he had bought himself. Shortly afterwards, the authority ordered to abandon the office and in front of the researcher dismantled all his work.

Extortion

It is common for a researcher who starts his or her work, to be given some subsidies by the Corporation, typical of every researcher who gives the first steps in the investigation. A researcher can pretend to develop his or her own project, which was developed after hard research theoretical work that had a bearing by saying of an author (Abrahamson, 2007): "…in the encounter of an unexplored niche," If the project has a potential of considerable growth and the researcher want not accept the false figure of the director, in spite of that, it is possible that the system with a total unworthy attitude gives him or her some minimal subsidies. In that way, the help the researcher will receive will not be from vocational people but from others who will charge one hundred per cent for their help. As History shows us in these cases, at the beginning, these people are considered *crazy* just like many other innovators of the most diverse areas are tried to be seen ridiculous.

Nevertheless, if the researcher shows that his or her proposal was not wrong and the corporation is interested in it – either to participate in the project or to prevent it from progressing – the corporation will try to control this innovator. That is why, if those researchers who are wanted to be controlled do not accept the figure of the *interested party assistant* but work with other people who have joined the project vocationally and succeed, extortion begins. Once the researcher is inside the system and working with other people and managed to progress on the project, the system starts to harass him or her with the attitude that can be defined as *extortion* and say subtly*: Now, if you want to continue your work and receive more subsidies, you must strictly comply with our conditions.* These conditions are usually very promising. It is the attitude that Dr Hirigoyen described before as *seduction-threats*. If the harassed person does not comply with these conditions, he or she can start to fear for his or her position and income. Paradoxically, these conditions will imply changing the object of study, allowing the participation of people who the system wants to incorporate, or other interests. Somebody said once that *changing the subject to be accepted is treason.* It would refer to that person who, in order to be accepted by a group, resigns to defend his or her ideals, most precious principles, moral values, etc.

He or she would not only betray himself or herself but those who trust and have hope on him or her.

For system we understand here the corporation of examiners who were given the *privilege* of setting themselves as examiners of this work. With this, it is expected a quick submission from the researchers to the corporation conditions. It is a malicious attitude. Through threats, the system aims at *stealing* the idea or what it is trying to obtain from the harassed. We could compare this humorously with assuring a sports person crossing the desert in a sports competition with water supply and then denying him or her new supply when he or she has run out of water unless the person shares the prize with a corporation sports person. If he or she does not accept the conditions, the sports person will have to count on nature to get water (through rain or an unexpected water spring), or perhaps a charitable group of Bedouins.

One aspect of the *Corporation* is that its loyal members believe they belong to an elite. They think they are intellectually superior to the harassed. Consequently, they reserve the right to copy or steal the harassed ideas and rewrite them under their own name appropriating them with the excuse of being more suitable to develop them. That is, they are given carte blanche to copy and increase their own status.

A paradigmatic case is that already quoted of a student whose professor requests him or her to hand in the paper he or she has written in order to present it at a congress, since as a student he or she will not be able to. The article will only be signed by the professor's name. The argument, as we have seen, is that the professor has a higher academic level and, because he is well-known, he considers he will be able to explain or defend the article in a better way. The professor's higher *prestige* – or perhaps we should call it better position in the corporation – will make him or her think he or she will be more suitable, even to deal with an idea that is not his or her own. What is not said is that the article can be defended by the student who developed it and that it is not necessary to remove his or her name and put the *prestigious* professor's instead. What's more, if the professor is honest he or she must defend his or her student and not plagiarize him or her.

A professor with a great sense of integrity would never remove his or her student's name in an invention or article just to include his or her own. What the professor would lose in a supposed illegitimate authorship, he or she would gain it in dignity and integrity. In addition, we consider that in an Authentic system, the last thing we mentioned is impossible to occur since the professor will have enough prestige, dignity and integrity so as not have to turn to any unworthy act for his or her own benefit.

If a middle-aged professor has so little prestige gained by his or her own merits, or perhaps so few original publications that he or she needs to steal a new student's original idea he or she completely trusts, we could doubt that his or her former merits were obtained legally. These cases are some of so many situations of those who are placed in higher and higher positions in an Aloentic system.

Another way of Extortion is to give a position to the person and after some time, when the person could have structured his or her life to that position, he or she is told to comply with some kind of political claim, for example, if he or she wants to continue keeping the position. The aim of the extortion can be that the other person or anyone related complies with the authority's request. Take the case of a dissident or ethical objector harassed researcher who had been removed from his position, and whose colleagues support the authority tried to take advantage of – though he should not, ethically speaking – and ordered this researcher's colleague: *Tell your colleague to do what I say, if not, I'll kick him out.* The dissident or ethical objector researcher did not accept the extortion and finally, since his colleague did not come up, he lost his job. The situation of the damaged party situation was much more painful and humiliating since before passing the final *judgment* the authority forced the person for half an hour to offer him or her arguments in order to keep his position while the authority was distracted doing other tasks and was not paying attention to what the person was saying. This attitude could be defined as ridicule or treating somebody like dirt.

An interesting aspect to highlight in this kind of extortion is the fact that when the authority gives the position, can even tell the person that he or she *deserves it.* The given position or promotion is thus not only an economic benefit but also a recognition for the receiver, which creates a positive expectation. Therefore, if the authority does not manage to obtain what it wanted through extortion, by removing the person's position or promotion, damages the person both economically and morally. What is even more, although the position or promotion is not essential for the receiver, its removal will cause a moral damage to the harassed by making him or her feel diminished personally and in front of his or her family.

We have said that the purpose of the corporation is at first to incorporate the person they want to control. If the person resists due to his or her ethical commitment, because he or she sees that the incorporation would distort his or her purpose of study and ethical integrity, he or she will start to suffer more bloody acts. However, and as a justification for the adversities the harassed undergoes, the corporation will reproach him or her using the argument of having adopted a sober resistance faced with the scholar's request of joining the group in order to *discern together.* It is worth remembering the case of the harassed researcher to whom the authority said: *We forgive you for causing us problems. We forgive you for not having accepted our friendship, for not having agreed to join us.*

The corporation uses the expression *discern together*, which could indicate an exchange and discussion of ideas, when in fact the intention is that of taking advantage one hundred per cent of the harassed ideas and work.

If the harassed does not accept Extortion, the next step is abandonment.

Libel

Another strategy of the system to damage the pursued person is Libel. This can be manifested in different ways as you can see in the following cases:

1. One case is when the ethical objector is dismissed but he or she manages to continue with the work thanks to a small support from some institution or simply with the help of his or her family. A libeler once said about a harassed researcher who was dismissed but continued working due to his modest lifestyle and the help he received: *He can work without getting paid because he must have money or a personal fortune of his own.* This aims to make the sacrifice done unworthy. If the researcher is single, they might also say that *he can accept being taken his salary away because he has no responsibilities or family to support.*

2. In that same sense, it may happen that some people achieve an original development with great effort and personal sacrifice, which can be presented to the public highlighting the effort and sacrifice involved. Now, if the authorities to which these people report are consulted on the people's achievement and the effort applied, they may answer: *We have all made similar sacrifices*, even knowing that was a lie and undermining those people's effort and therefore generating doubts on the real effort implied. The vocational effort is thus made unworthy and the ones who made it are seen as exaggerated and whiners. The authority will only recognize the corporation members' effort.

3. Another variant is underrating health problems. If the harassed has health problems caused by persecution, the harasser may say about this: *It is just a stress problem; he (or she) will be able to continue working after a little rest.* Here the harassed real cause and suffering is underrated. It is as if a former concentration camp prisoner goes public to tell his story showing himself extremely underweight and with psychiatric disorders, but people, without an understanding what this person has gone through say that with the right diet and rest the person will recover. They can even say that the story told was exaggerated. Or as if some international commission of human rights inquired the camp director about the prisoner's health and he ironically told them that he

was just tired but with a few days of rest in Marbella he will be able to return to work.

4. Another possibility is accusing the harassed of lying about the situation he or she describes. This is very common for those who expose ethical faults in the scientific community. In some cases, this persecution becomes so furious and violent that some scientific corporation members are forced to declare lies or fallacies regarding certain ethical objectors in order to discredit them internationally.

5. If the person is performing his or her tasks in another location or has been assigned different duties for certificated medical reasons, they will say that he or she does not fulfill his or her duties, never goes to work, attend meetings, etc. The systematic reports containing true scientific production will be deliberately ignored and shelved. The aim of the authority is to show people he or she is avoiding responsibilities.

6. If a person has an original idea and challenges the scientific community to have an open and critical debate about it, this will never take place since the most important members of the scientific corporation would say: *He (or she) is a loony, we won't take his (or her) ideas seriously.* This concept is supported even by those who must give subsidies, promotions, etc. And in this way, any development of this person and his or her group is blocked.

7. Another case is also related with the already mentioned academic trial and it is to make the harassed look like a thief or at least a negligent and irresponsible person. The most important thing is that although the system cannot dismiss the person for not having enough evidence, it aims at generating doubts in order to discredit the person and to collect formal legal elements to threaten or exonerate him or her. This is also related with extortion.

So as to indicate the reason for these attitudes, we can quote the famous phrase erroneously attributed to Goebbels: "If you tell a lie big enough and keep repeating it, people will eventually come to believe it."

A common factor in all the described persecutory attitudes is that the authority, real originator of the persecution, in most cases does not show itself and spread the gossip through its subordinates. We think this is so since the authority is aware of the lack of arguments or grounds that justify any of the adopted measures.

The authority's coward shame is very well illustrated in the answer they usually ask their secretaries to give harassed researchers who demand to see them: *Tell them I'm out of the office.*

If a researcher is working in a critical and compromised area, the authority will never either ask to see such researcher nor tell him or her that such subject should not be investigated anymore. The Authority will say through a secretary: *If you continue with this subject, you'll be destroyed and you will resign in a few years' time.* In that way, he or she can deny everything, saying it was just a secretary's opinion.

Another example is the case of some researchers who wanted their papers to be publicized through the official media structure of the institution they worked at. The administrative staff requested to hand out all the data and to fill the corresponding report, which they did. In view of the final result of this paperwork, we could say it was a waste of the researchers' time: when ready to submit it, at the last minute, they were told that their work would not be publicized. When the researchers asked for an explanation for this last-minute exclusion, the subordinate staff was unwilling to give any answers. The researchers continued insisting on finding out the reasons but the administrative staff informed them that they could not give the authorities' names who had adopted the measure and that they had made them assume full responsibility for it. This was a clear example of the corporate *Omertá*. Anyway, the fact that the subordinate staff assumes responsibility means nothing to the researchers. The true motive of the act always remains hidden. That is their way of being protected. This is similar to what was discussed in the first reading in connection to an anonymous evaluator when we referred to Authoritarianism vs. Freedom values. Both anonymous evaluation and malicious ignorance are two coward ways of exercising authoritarianism. Cowardice is one of the characteristics of harassers already mentioned in the first reading on point 22: Harasser-Harassed.

Ultimate motive of the persecution

All these systematic persecutory attitudes are a common phenomenon to many researchers worldwide. In the past, this situation was suffered without attributing it to an organic and systematic cause. The persecution is not always based on an immediate ethical denunciation. Sometimes, the persecution is caused by professional jealousy or envy, or simply by the examiners' perseverance in an old paradigm. The disciplinary commissions' evaluators can fall into authoritarianism; they just become controllers of the researchers' ideas. This could be defined as follows: *Either you return to the fold or we will indefinitely persecute you.*

That is, in Science and Technique, a researcher can be forced to become an ethical objector simply because of resisting to the old researchers' whims. Even so, we believe ethical objectors only emerge within subjects that have humanitarian implications. We personally believe that Darwin was not an ethical objector, though Semmelweiss was.

Paradigms must not change: if somebody discerns a new paradigm and pretends to abandon the old one, he or she will be punished, mocked and harassed to make him or her return. If the harassed requests, begs, implores to be let go, it will be denied. The authentic researcher searches for the truth; if in an Authentic system, the authority must serve to such truth, while in the harassing Aloentic system, the authority will serve its own interests. The people in power in the old paradigm will continue with the innovator's harassment, going to the extreme of damaging his or her health. This will cause the innovator to retire due to disability. If after this process the innovator has some strength, will or enthusiasm left, then, he or she can continue working in the new paradigm, but outside the institutional and collegiate conditionings; outside the Science and Technique system.

Paradigms and their representatives are implacable not only in the rejection to the new but also in not releasing people from the corset with which they were oppressed. The eternal return to the old paradigm on the part of the harassed happens over and over again.

There is no pity for the one who says: *This is new, please, take it seriously and evaluate it well.* This lack of mercy is stressed when the corporation researchers fear the harassed has identified a critical and fundamental subject which they never thought of studying or never dared to.

This is so in the coarsest aspects. Yet, in the highest and most intellectual aspects what they fear is that their paradigm may crack.

Considering some described strategies of harassment, we can define the system's attitude as of *marches and countermarches*. This means that the system never says no at the beginning, on the contrary, it encourages all kinds of presentations, even if they are critical. Sometimes, if the researcher must hand in a presentation again to a new employee, he or she blames it on the previous employee's lack of understanding of the subject. Once the presentation is in, the corporation is consulted, which indicates that the researchers are on a black list, interdict, dangerous, etc. From that moment onwards, the presentation enters a stage of manipulation during which the corporation tries to control the researcher's work. If it does not succeed, it destroys it. As we have seen, the researcher does have some support at the beginning. Then, if the researcher does not agree to negotiate, it is not that he or she will lose the possibility of receiving substantial amounts of funds as other corporation members do; it is that he or she will lose the possibility of receiving the minimum work tools any researcher should be entitled to. One of the signs that show that a researcher is an ethical objector is the fact he or she is persistently denied those minimal means of work. If a researcher can continue working after some time with fewer means than the minimum, he or she is not just an ethical objector but also a *resister*.

In the light of the current research, persecution could be defined as moral harassment and mobbing. Moral harassment results in the harassed person's fast health deterioration. If moral harassment is very subtle it may go completely unnoticed. The harassers smile when observing the harassed collapse and they always treat him or her with a smile on their lips and honeyed courtesy.

As Dr. Hirigoyen (Hirogoyen, 2001) states, harassment is longer and more subtle in the public sector than in the private one. The case of the public sector we are dealing with is special since it is composed by the intelligent *elite*: universities, research councils, etc. Therefore, the duration of the harassment is more evident as well as its subtlety.

Our situation as ethical objectors – as regarded by INESPE – became more and more critical as our acts became more explicit in resisting the corporation's insinuations. We mentioned above the example of the Emperor's New Clothes. We believe this can also be applied to the case of the ethical objector since all the attitudes adopted against him or her also aim at avoiding the fact that situations generated by the science and technique system *are exposed* or brought to light. Such situations are typical of an Aloentic system which does not respect academic capacity.

The Aloentic system gets furious when an authentic researcher does his or her job demolishing the canons that rule and give support to the system he or she is in.

That is, when succeeding in his or her work and thus having succeeded in getting out of the false system.

For example – as we have mentioned as another sign of the need of an ethical objector in Science and Technique – since 2004, the authorities have forbidden us to continue teaching the subject Environmental Technogeny. As we said in the first reading about the Structured vs. Non-structured values, our academic proposal was never formalized since it was not a political establishment creation but it originated from the research itself. Our subject was too much for them: bringing to light and at the same time disseminating information about so many critical and non-ethical attitudes of technological risk that for a corporate *omertà* nobody dared to.

Besides teaching this subject, our explicit activity as ethical objectors also manifested itself through conferences, publications and by our intent to give legal status to an association we tried to create in our city.

We have said that our goals as ethical objectors are:

- Respecting the ethical commitment in such a crucial field with such an implication for human beings as Technology is.
- Being prone to the compliance with the values of an Authentic system against the values of an Aloentic system.
- Helping ethical objectors, mainly in Science and Technique.

For that reason, we tried to create the Argentine branch of the INESPE Network, which we called RIPCE and which had similar goals, mainly to be applied in the Science and Technique system in our country. The organization was created with a corporate charter on May 12th, 2000.

On June 4th, 2002, the application for legal status was formally incorporated (File number 37633/02). On June 25th of the same year, we were communicated by court ruling number 311, the need to correct the articles of association to comply with the Legal Status requirements of the State Prosecutor's department. One of the strongest objections, as we have said, was: *we already have organizations (unions and professional associations) that can protect ethical objectors.* This is a legal/administrative example of what has already been indicated for *automatic reduction* in Science. Anyway, the argument is fallacious. According to a report, in Argentina there are many Non Governmental Organizations, the report cites three – apart from one national agency – that deal with safety in traffic. Therefore, even if there are other NGOs for protecting ethical objectors, why can't other NGOs be created to deal with this issue? Then the question could be, what is the real reason for the denial? They tried to convince us that unions could assume the function of protecting ethical objectors, without considering the fact that they did not solve the dilemma of who would protect ethical objectors who denounce irregularities within the unions or professional associations themselves.

What greatly caught our attention was that after our attempt of creating this organization, corporate aggressiveness from colleagues and authorities clearly increased. We were told that it had caused an unfavorable reaction within the corporate circles, which worked in such a way that we were not given the legal status. Finally, on August 15th, 2002, less than two months after the association had been proposed, our institute was closed with unusual violence.

Some evidence of the false argument referred by the authority that justified the lack of need of an association to protect ethical objectors is the fact that in our personal case, the union we belonged to did not protect us from the persecution received from the Academic/Scientific system. One of us was dismissed and left without medical benefits despite being ill and the other one was subjected to a continuous moral harassment by being falsely accused, his salary reduced to the minimum and having to endure an uncommon prolongation in his retirement procedure. The union did not do anything about it, always alleging puerile excuses.

According to what we discussed in the reading about culture in Science and Technique (Squandering vs. Economizing), one of the reasons that made us become harassed by the described attitudes was the rejection of the *director, or administrator, or guarantor-of-subsidies* figures. In our beginnings, our first experience had already been unfavorable: The requested funds for a project arrived in the director's hands, who used them to acquire equipment for a different project. If we give the director the benefit of the doubt, we could say that the problem was that the funds took too long to arrive in the author's hands.

To sum up, the utmost aim of persecution is, at first, to control the researcher. Then, if that is not achieved, to destroy him or her.

Society's lack of understanding

We have seen that one of the persecution strategies is Libel and we mentioned that one of its goals is to discredit the person in front of society, either society in general or, most commonly, in front of the scientific and academic society: researchers, professors, support staff, students and people related with them.

Therefore, the authorities try to make the community echo of the libel so that it thinks badly of the objector and doubts about him or her. By this, the entity of the harassed person's work or denunciation is doubted as well. There is perhaps a tendency *of justifying the harasser and doubting the harassed.*

This means that in addition to those attitudes the ethical objector must face from the system he or she is confronting, he or she must bear another attitude: Society's *Lack of Understanding*.

For instance, society may dare to say about ethical objectors that:

- There must be a reason for them not getting research subsidies.
- Their work may not have a good level or value since they work in conditions of little infrastructure.
- They are misfits. They do not know their place.
- There must be a reason for them to be in this situation.
- They do not respect authority.
- They do not want to work their set hours.
- They do not want to be controlled.
- Why don't they want to travel?
- Why don't they request the necessary subsidies before starting to work?
- Why didn't they leave when they didn't receive any answers?
- They want to work alone. Why don't they integrate?
- Why don't they want to change their subject of study?
- Why don't they accept to fit into another discipline?
- Why didn't they realize before about their situation?
- Why don't they agree to the authority's request?
- Why haven't they employed new staff?
- Why don't they attend meetings?
- They are anarchists.
- They are troublemakers. They are schemers.
- Who do they think they are? Einstein?

Society's lack of understanding of the ethical objector is increased even more by another attitude that corporation members adopt in front of society: showing their own merits – in some cases exaggeratedly and falsely. Consequently, it is common to observe an attitude of admiration in society – almost of reverence – towards certain researchers who are corporation or establishment members. This attitude is supported by different reasons: the huge amounts of money they receive in subsidies, very expensive research devices that were bought for the researcher or group of researchers, attitudes of false modesty or humbleness they adopt with society, veiled display of erudition, a continuous state of frenzy and concentration and extreme nervousness, a permanent state of occupation even to answer a question, obviously the huge effort invested in achieving what they got, etc. In view of these attitudes, it is easy for society to doubt about those researchers who do not enjoy the same benefits. The doubt is obvious: How can anybody be a persecuted researcher in a *system of wonders*? Looking for an answer to this question in the previous list has a logical consequence: the belief in a system where science works as a promotion mechanism for the best, the evaluators are infallible; they do not run out of resources which are definitely given to the best, etc. Society is then deceived. This mechanism gives authority to the people who have risen to that position. As we saw in the first reading, society in this case confuses:

- Erudition with intelligence
- Equipment accumulation with efficient laboratories
- Obvious questions that have high-cost answers with deep questions
- Frenzy, concentration, extreme nervousness and permanent occupation with the concentration of the wise, etc.

It is easy to give authority to a person who shows erudition, economic power, etc.

Without reaching libel, the lack of understanding of the ethical objectors' sacrifice and effort leave them alone in front of society.

Even the media can deny them some space. In that regard, it is interesting to mention the case of some researchers who by recommendation of a person who valued their work tried to contact some media social communicator. This person had defined the social communicator as an *honest person*. The researchers told this person about their skepticism since corporations (media, universities, research organizations, etc.) never interfered in areas that may affect another one. As this person insisted so much, one of the researchers tried to communicate with the social communicator and was told by the secretary to call back in a few days. The researcher called again after some days and as soon as the secretary recognized his voice she hanged up. The researcher commented what had happened to the person who recommended the interview, and who therefore tried to find out about it personally. Unfortunately, he confirmed that the researchers were right in their skepticism.

Questions like the ones listed above are left unanswered, thus helping those who libel in bad faith.

Another attitude that contributes to society's lack of understanding is the *political speech*. A harassing system will never expose itself. On the contrary, it will use a political speech by which it will show virtues typical of first-rate international systems. Thus society hears that for high positions *extremely high* background is required, when in fact the person who will occupy the position may have the required academic degrees but which were illegitimately obtained. Another example is the common saying that students must be *educated as thinking people*, and be encouraged to develop independent thinking: nothing like that really happens. If somebody in the system, deceived by the saying, considers that by having an independent way of thinking he or she will be recognized, he or she couldn't be more mistaken. Such person will be persecuted and will likely collapse physically and psychologically after some years. The independent way of thinking cannot be allowed in an implacably controlling system, especially if that independence leads them to discover unsustainable ethical situations that must be brought to light. The corporation forgives a lot of things except for the ethical objector. The political speech does not only deceive society but also those who will try to be trained as authentic researchers in an Aloentic system.

Although society's lack of understanding is not a bad faith attitude as Libel, it also contributes to the ethical objector's psychological damage. For that reason, organizations that protect ethical objectors must educate and inform society as a whole so that they can also support these people morally.

The constructive value of pain in the will of sense

Perhaps we can start by referring to a saying from the Spanish writer Miguel de Cervantes (1547-1616) (Cervantes) "The evils that are not strong enough to end life will not end patience either."

We can also mention a similar saying attributed to the German philosopher Friedrich Nietzsche (1844-1900) (Nietzsche): "That which does not kill me makes me stronger."

We do not want to place ethical objectors at the same level of the greatest martyrs of humanity, whose sufferings and death left a lasting mark in history, and who were a life example for different societies and/or cultures.

But we do want here to refer to the case of resistant people for whom circumstances let them overcome, bear and endure their opponents' destructive attempts. They overcome an unwanted pain that has been provoked by others – unlike what some psychologists want to make us believe when they call them masochists. A resistant person, according to Burke, is "He who wrestles with us, strengthens our nerves and sharpens our skill. Our antagonist is a helper" (Burke).

Despite their heroic efforts, some of them cannot recover and therefore succumb.

In Chapter III, by dealing with the subject of the Innocuousness of the technological object and briefly including concepts some thinkers put forward regarding hypotheses, new ideas, programs and paradigms, we mentioned that *it seems that innovators must have a personality that endures pressure, inconvenience, indifference, discrimination and persecution in order to allow for innovation in the scientific world.* We also added that Kuhn postulated that: "The psychological nature of innovators should be more important than brilliant demonstrations" (Kuhn, 1995). In the case of ethical objectors, we dare say that it would be wrong to think that those who despite their efforts cannot overcome the harassment are not psychologically gifted, unlike others who are *stronger* and survive the harassment. In fact, we think that ethical objectors, the so-called *Resisters* – we call them *Mithridates* – who can resist the poison of harassment can do it because of the circumstances of their activity and not because they are stronger and the ones who succumb, weaker. Apart from that, the fact that they are stronger does not mean that they must bear harassment.

Our experience, and surely that of many others, shows that when a person manages to overcome the evilness and/or protect him or herself from the opponents' evil the saying above may come true. This may be so because *necessity is the mother of invention.* Just like pain, it may originate a creativity that allows for the birth of ideas of such entity and meaning that would not have been conceived in calm and natural work circumstances.

That is how the disciplinary proposal described in this book developed. The opposition from the Science and Technology system to our activity, the countless tolerated attitudes of different degrees of seriousness including moral harassment, and above all, the enormous lack of resources that isolated us in a space of reflection and analysis, led to the proposal of this new science.

We do not justify the opponents' acts, which many times do not even come from peers but from intellectually and scientifically inferior people that set themselves up as peers and gave themselves the right to have an opinion and make a decision about something they did not know. These acts are different from what we discussed in the first reading when we described how demanding a tutor should be with a disciple in order to get the best out of him or her.

We also used Dr. Frankl's concepts on Dimensional Ontology applied to psychiatry so as to explain the basics of Technopathogenology. We can turn to Frankl again to confirm what we are analyzing now. Frankl helped to acquire sense in a sad and inhuman situation making the concentration camp prisoners understand about the *value of the attitude in front of pain* as a sense provider. Frankl gives a great value to Pain as an element that increases the quality of the biographical product of a person. He is the creator of the last Viennese School of Psychiatry (based on the will of sense). Frankl speaks about the historicity of the human person, who *writes the novel of his or her life* (Frankl, 1978). In Science, the dullest and most boring novels are those where everything happens as it is expected and there is no pain for the protagonist. However, the deepest novels are those where the protagonists or heroes give sense to their own pain or destiny.

We can also say that pain lets us test and shape the person's vocation though we definitely do not wish these situations to happen. Although History shows us that these facts although unacceptable, are unavoidable and they simply will occur.

The nature of the ethical objector in Science and Technique

*The expeditious or acute ethical objector and the patient
or chronic ethical objector*

By seeing the need of also considering the figure of the ethical objector in Science and Technique, we have seen the possibility of distinguishing between two kinds of ethical objectors: the *acute* ones who could also be called *active* or *expeditious*, and the *chronic* ones who could also be called *passive* or *patient* ones.

Acute ethical objectors are the ethical objectors mentioned at the beginning of this reading, who by being integrated into the system, surprisingly discover an obvious lack of ethics, which is therefore of great importance and that represents a risk to the community. Despite the authority's suggestion of being indifferent to or hiding it, they publicly denounce what they have seen.

- They are researchers who have carved out a career in the corporation.
- They have never run out of tools for their research.
- Perhaps they do not become resisters: by swiftly wanting to solve the situation on their own they may not have to bear the ongoing punishment.
- Their manifestation comes as a surprise. In a moment, they face the decision on whether publish, spread or make public or not results that have not been expected by the corporation. They become Whistleblowers.
- They express and reveal their denunciations, which have been simplified by the obvious nature of them such as ecological denunciations, nuclear material leaks in nuclear stations, chemical industry emissions, and ecosystem damages, among others.
- They are easy to identify.

Dr Günter Emde and Dr Arpad Puztai are typical cases of Acute Objectors.

The chronic ethical objector is defined as the one who resists being part of or supporting the little non-evident ethical faults, which together contribute to the general inefficiency and corruption of the Science and Technique system. This corruption may lead to the production and dissemination of knowledge with voids that is wrongly considered as true and which finally – when applied to a technique of human relevance – can cause either short or long-term damage to people.

About the chronic ethical objector, we can give as qualities that:

- They do carve a career in the corporation. We can say that they vegetate in the system being completely left aside from promotions, which can be clearly seen by the asymmetry between objective merits and credit given by the system.
- They may not receive the work tools they request to investigate their critical question.
- Their manifestation does not come as a surprise. In general, the passive or chronic ethical objectors are people whom we can define as *resisters*, i.e. those who refuse to play the game. We have referred to Dr. Hirigoyen's concept of moral harassment, which starts precisely when the person resists to being overwhelmed by authority. Perhaps there is no evident reason, as in the case of the active ethical objector, that encourages them to take a fighting attitude. Their fight comes down to the fact that for many years or decades they have had to resist non-ethical proposals from the corporation. As we said when describing the psychopathic process, non-ethical acts are light at the beginning but become more serious after some time like the ones that must be faced by the active ethical objector. Finally, the sufferings they must undergo by the system make their own life a denunciation.
- They are persevering. They tend to ignore punishment and to not take measures to protect themselves until it becomes unavoidable due to the risk to their health.
- They discover the bad will of the system when it is too late. That is why they try to adapt as much as they can to the precarious and subhuman conditions they are subject to.
- At the beginning, the denunciation reasons are generally not evident. They have a rather persevering and resistant attitude of non-acceptance of the corporation non-ethical proposals.
- They are not easy to identify, mainly by society. This objector is much more difficult to detect than the expeditious or acute ethical objector. The authorities easily distract the attention from their proposals or attitudes in order to make them object of discrediting.
- Basically, they do not accept being diverted from the unconditional search for knowledge to investigate certain subjects.

Now we will refer to a patient or chronic ethical objector: the ethical objector in Science and Technique.

The ethical objector in Science and Technique

An ethical objector in Science and Technique can be interpreted in different ways in all stages of a product research, application, development process and commercialization. It can be both acute and chronic.

In the scientific stage, an ethical objector can be the person who does not accept to negotiate the unconditional search for knowledge in critical subjects or subjects that may compromise human health or the environment, or the way the inventors or creators' ideas and moral intellectual property are respected. We can mention, for instance, resistance to forced co-authorships, non-ethical funds distribution, resistance to being manipulated by a spurious director, resistance to being part of courtesy work groups, among the already mentioned ethical faults.

In the technological stage, an ethical objector can be the person who does not accept to keep side effects of the product in question to him or herself. This case is very common when it comes to chemical substances which show a great efficiency with economic implications such as the control of a pest. If an independent researcher finds side effects in a product, he or she can be put under pressure so as not to publish them since they oppose a massive business (Pusztai, 2000).

In the sale and marketing stage, an ethical objector can be a person who observes frauds and adulterations, even the most common ones, that generate risky situations to the community, and resists being part of it.

The denunciation, in whatever stage, bothers the system members. Nowadays, people speak about a *Technocracy* that pretends to dominate or rule the progress of mankind. It is defined as the technicians' intervention in or influence over the political direction of a country or the technicians' group who exercises this power.

In order to understand how much the figure of the ethical objector's in Science and Technique upsets the *Ruling Technologists*, we can draw an analogy between them and aristocracy. Although this is defined as the government by society's upper class, we should turn to the purely etymological meaning, by which Aristocracy would mean the ruling of the best. Let us consider which attitude will the members of an aristocratic government adopt if somebody denounces that in the government there are people who are not precisely the best? Not only that but also that these people *are quite worse than what was expected from them.* The possible reaction will be that of imprisoning or killing the person who reports the crime so as not become exposed. The same can be said of an objector in Science and Technique who denounces the system's weaknesses, faults or immoralities.

These are well-known cases of whistleblowers or ethical objectors in companies such as nuclear stations in the USA. There is also the important case of Dr. Margrit Herbst, who denounced the existence of bovine spongiform encephalopathy in Germany (Deiserot, 2001), being this another case of an acute ethical objector.

The ethical objector is defenseless against the pressures put by the medium he or she is in, which benefits from the non-ethical acts, and despite the promises of help or good will it is usually very difficult for him or her to receive any help from the environment that produces the non-ethical behavior.

It is also interesting to repeat what we commented on when referring to moral harassment about the researcher having been *submerged in a defenselessness system.* Both the person and – also important to include – his or her work do not have any protection from the corporation attitudes. This can act openly and in an authoritarian way since nobody will interfere with its decisions. In that respect, it is interesting to comment on our experience when we tried to avoid the destruction of our institute. When we asked for help to the highest authority regarding citizens' protection (the Nation's Ombudsman), we received the following answer: "Once the decision taken by the High Council regarding the institute is firm, the Ombudsman has no competence to modify the administrative decisions. The present procedure is closed" (Defensor del Pueblo de la Nación, 2000). That is to say, neither the researchers nor their institute or the importance it had for society were important to the Ombudsman. Justice remains absent and expectant in the eyes of the injustice that has taken place within a corporate organization. Here we can observe that the State itself, which should protect its own patrimony, simply leaves it to be unjustly wasted and destroyed. In this way, a State's organization is discretionally and arbitrarily destroyed, leaving aside several decades of work. Paradoxically, the state itself represented by the Dean and the Higher Council of a University had authorized the researchers to develop the organization (Universidad Nacional de Rosario, 1985). An excuse to avoid the *interfering* among the different departments is to turn to the *separation of powers* principle, by which an organization that does not want to interfere with another one's affairs can easily claim that *it is forbidden* to do so or refer the interested party to another department. Some matters are thus avoided though they are of great importance for citizens such as violation of human rights. It is interesting to emphasize how easy it is, even in a democratic system, for a citizen to be completely defenseless against the administrative, bureaucratic and political mishandling. The final result is of total arbitrariness and authoritarianism. The organizations that should defend become only responsible for what happened several decades ago or at some other politically correct critical points. The human rights of the persecuted and discriminated researchers of today are not considered.

The consequence of this attitude is a huge waste of resources both material and human. If those researchers who managed to be trained for years on a relevant subject for society do not take responsibility for becoming ethical objectors with a huge personal *resistance,* they may have to face the dilemma of changing subjects or retiring, which is an intellectual waste. This waste includes both the researchers of the cancelled Program as well as the other researchers who were, are or wish to be trained. This of course infringes the right and freedom of teaching and learning stated by our National Constitution.

If – as we mentioned above – a wrong ruling, made in good faith, is not easily changed, even less it will be changed if it involves the hiding of non-ethical attitudes.

Concerning what has been described under this title, it is worth considering Professor Beck's concepts (Beck, 1970) on Technique:

> Through the technical act, human beings destroy the given structures of reality and dissolve them in their elemental and basic functions, and with them they build new structures, which respond more to human beings' goals. Thus, the aim of the 'technical ideology' seems to be the creation of a new world according to human beings' ideas and wishes – which then tempts them to think that they can resign to an Almighty God and take his place.

We can thus see that the ethical objector in Science and Technique is an unavoidable figure since we can conclude by saying that if the *technical act* or the *technical ideology* aim to make human beings' wishes come true, this can – and in fact does – lead to the human beings' own destruction. The presence of the ethical objector, as we have said, is then necessary in those contexts of Science and Technique that may affect human beings or – using Beck's term — threaten them with their own destruction. Perhaps that scientific religion at which Positivism (Sanguinetti, 1977) aims has to give in when faced with the facts that science itself generated. The apparent solid God of the *scientific religion* was just a hero with feet of clay. Technopathogeny with all its consequences is the clearest example of this.

The ethical objector by action and the ethical objector by omission

Besides the acute and chronic figures, ethical objectors in Science and Technique can be differentiated between two types in terms of the attitudes they can adopt when faced with the system: the ethical objector by action and the ethical objector by omission.

The ethical objector by action will cover the following cases:

A. When the researcher pretends to make public scientific truths that contradict a powerful corporation that sustains opposite results. For instance, the case of Arpad Pusztai.

B. When the person, without being a researcher but working for a big non-scientific corporation, denounces that he or she is tolerating practices which are damaging health. In spite of not being a researcher, the person is nevertheless considered an ethical objector in science and technique since his or her denunciation is framed within science and technology. It is the case of M. Herbst.

C. When the researcher denounces non-ethical acts he or she has deeply known and experienced in the scientific community that are wished to be kept hidden. These non-ethical acts have become so deeply rooted that are taken as common habits and customs.

This ethical objector is the one who suffers the hardest attacks from the corporation in the form of persecution. It can be considered the ethical objector par excellence.

The ethical objector by omission will cover the following cases: when, for instance, the researcher is requested:

A. To join a team, supporting or covering non-ethical behaviors taken as common habits and customs by the corporation.
B. To support a work project so that the organization where he or she works can benefit from the allocation of subsidies when in fact the corporation members are the ones who want to profit from the funds in order to obtain personal advantages.

The researcher can reject it in two ways:
A. By openly rejecting the veiled proposals to join or incorporate into it.
B. By passively ignoring such veiled proposals although not rejecting them openly.

By adopting a less critical or committed attitude, this ethical objector may suffer less harsh attitudes like discouragement and/or discrimination.

The need to help researchers in critical situations

We know that *advancing knowledge* is a very broad phrase that covers countless elements.

Here we focus on researchers who decide to advance in the knowledge of issues which are highly relevant to community. This is done without accepting any compromise or non-ethical proposals from the Aloentic Scientific community – which makes these researchers extremely vulnerable. Even though these people can endure this and are actually called *resisters*, how long can they resist? The aim of helping these people is to be able to hold them afloat so that they can resist staunchly.

A person who decides unconditionally and without making concessions to advance in a specific field that involves bringing to light compromising situations will be usually stopped by the administrative and evaluative machinery (Westerholm, 1999).

The freedom to research and teach is considered to be basic in the academic scientific world. In some countries, it is assured by the Constitution itself. For this reason, the collegiate pressure to block some issues from being investigated or to restrict the researcher freedom cannot be openly done. Consequently, the discrimination against researchers who must lean on the necessary academic and scientific freedom takes place in the form of indirect obstruction. They are denied a minimum of work tools and the minimal institutionalization of their object of study. They are forced to work in borrowed places, both literally and in terms of the disciplinary framing of their subject.

In those countries where there is no protection – or if there is, it is just formal – the persecution takes place openly, degenerating into a crude moral harassment or harassment, *tolerated or even supported* by the authorities, who will obviously deny knowing anything about such persecution.

The obstruction to the *target* researchers almost never aims directly at deeply questioning their object of study – scientific discussion is totally avoided. The best way of avoiding the scientific discussion is by ignoring the object of study.

In order to illustrate how harassment is carried out in these cases, let us take three examples:

A. When deciding to investigate a pesticide waste in the fine dust thrown by a device of dust separation of a silo or terminal elevator.
B. When deciding to investigate coal dust impregnated with benzopyrene that can be thrown into the air as combustion product.
C. When deciding to investigate the practice of wetting the grain so that it weighs more, which has the undesired possible consequence of generating aflatoxins due to the increase in humidity.

Actually, these investigations – which may have critical consequences by showing that flawed or non-ethical technological practices must be replaced – would not be directly prohibited. Yet, the questioning will come indirectly: in the first example, by saying that *determining pesticides is not a step forward in knowledge since the technique has already been described*. In the second case, that *the coal dust and the benzopyrene have also been widely described*. In the third example, *that investigating excess water is simply determined with a technique which has already been widely described*. That is, they are trying to divert the attention towards what is obvious and well-known such as the analytical techniques employed in order to ignore or deny the entity of the problem. It is as if we discredited an electrician who wants to find out why some installation does not work with the following report: *The work he wants to do has no originality at all since the screwdriver he will use has already been invented.*

In this way, the core of the problem is left aside and the deep question is discredited by tangential evaluations. The exclusion mechanism consists of leaving aside the core of the question and evaluating a number of tangential aspects. Thus, the object of study is ignored as if it were non-existent and the number of tangential aspects are not enough to assign the subsidy, or to promote the work or the persons involved in it (Westerholm, 1999).

It is clear that the exclusion mechanism begins with evaluating committees composed by colleagues that are the only ones who know the deep consequences of the proposed research. At the same time, it is possible that a minimum shame generated by blocking research of relevance to the community leads to permanent indirect arguments and to avoid any open discussion over the proposal. It is common to argue about the non-fulfillment of unimportant formalities or use tangential arguments to deny the proposal's entity. The in-depth question presented by the problem is always denied.

However, if the person who does some work of this kind resists to be part of a courtesy team with powerful researchers, who despite not understanding the question or taking it as of secondary interest are ready to co-authorize any project, he or she will be simply left aside. This abandonment will not be attributed to a logical reaction of rejection to the researcher's resistance who reasonably wants to protect his or her intellectual property. This would be too honest and obvious. In order to justify the researcher's rejection and abandonment, they search secondary and incidental elements that are made fundamental by evaluators. These elements will be, for example, not having a numerous group of people in the group, or nor having enough analytical equipment or not wanting to integrate, etc. This happens despite having made progresses of entity (Westerholm, 1999). What they do not say is that both the lack of people, tools and sophisticated analytical means are nothing more than the consequence of the continuous obstruction made by the evaluators themselves. They neither explain about their systematic obstruction and denial to all the presentations made by the ones interested when requesting more paid people in the work group. They do not say either that they have systematically prevented examiners other than themselves or their corporate groups from evaluating the presentations. Perhaps they do so because they fear that the researcher can be examined positively if he or she gets out of the examining circle he or she is trapped in.

Furthermore, the possibility of incorporating personnel through fellowships is blocked by denying the existence of the object of study, thus closing a vicious circle: the training of human resources is only allowed within the discipline which the powerful researchers of the courtesy team belong to. This denial of the existence of the object of study seems to be incompatible with what is usually said about science and scientists' freedom. This is also known by the evaluators who damage the researcher. It may be for this reason that they do it hiddenly and silently, since they feel ashamed. The researcher is thus faced with the dilemma of finding a *Director* of an old and consolidated discipline to obtain means of work. If one falls into the trap, he or she will shortly abandon the original question.

For the development of the scientific activity, subsidies to obtain means of work are necessary in a greater or lesser extent according to the research subject. With the analyzed subjects, we can see how the system has a considerable amount of tools so as not to assign these subsidies to any researcher who is ethically committed so as to abandon such researcher to his or her own luck. The system does not even need scientific arguments to leave the researcher it wants to persecute without support. Generally, the abandonment has as a motive the fact that for ethical reasons the researcher does not want to distort his or her subject of study by sharing his or her idea with others who are not committed in the same way. However, there are much more crude situations of abandonment that have the same origin: the authority's reaction to the researchers' refusal to take part of *shady deals* with state money. We have mentioned that the harasser *is aware of his or her bad conscience* and is exasperated at observing that a person tries and succeeds in achieving his or her goals while respecting moral values. We have also stated that the harasser can dare to say: *Who does he think he is to pretend to develop an Institute or research program without becoming corrupted?* It is the case of a researcher to whom, when summoned to attend a meeting to deal with his situation, the authority insinuated that he had to allow the misuse of funds. Faced with the researcher's passive resistance to be involved in this manipulation, the authority – pretending to be blinded by rage – said: *You don't want to share anything.* This is a clear example of an attempt to corrupt the researcher, as we have seen when discussing Envy. The authority stood up, opened the door so that the researcher left, thus finishing the interview. From that moment on, the abandonment became bigger and bigger.

We have already mentioned that the corporation searches for arguments to justify the researcher's rejection and abandonment, and that, in general, secondary and incidental elements are considered fundamental by evaluators. Examples of such arguments are: *The institute does not have enough infrastructure,* or *does not have enough publications,* or *does not have enough staff.* Next, we will refer to these three arguments.

Infrastructure, number of publications and critical mass:
Three fallacious arguments to support obstruction and exclusion

Infrastructure

The argument of *lack of infrastructure* is many times used in order not to assign subsidies. Although below we will refer to an argument that we could at least say that has a certain scientific connotation (number of publications), in this item we want to go back to the fact that the system does not need any scientific arguments to block a researcher. Here the system does not claim lack of infrastructure but openly denies every possibility for the researcher to count on it to develop his or her work. Take the case of the researchers who were denied financial aid for their research on the grounds that *what the researchers really want is to support an institute.* They ignored the fact that the institute, despite not having a great infrastructure, was already working and having all the administrative formalities complied with. For the study of a phenomenon, some equipment can be requested which once the study is finished will be available for another study, that is, it will stay in the Institute. The argument for the denial clearly shows how the corporation tries to prevent an Institute from receiving equipment that would be part of its equipping in order to later be able to say that it lacks infrastructure. The question is: if the phenomenon under study is worthy, why cannot a researcher create an institute? The lack of infrastructure is also invoked in case the institute production is big enough so that they cannot use this (lack of production) to justify the denial. We can thus see how the Corporation prevents any attempt to develop some work without its participation. In that case the goal is: *Stop the researcher!*

Small number of publications

As we commented when we discussed the method of Yunus, the Corporation only gives subsidies to consolidated groups. In greater or lesser extent, subsidies are necessary in order to be able to develop any research and thus be able to have papers to publish.

If the researcher who is ethically committed to develop an idea does not accept to adapt to the system or its conditions so as not to distort the object of study, he or she will not obtain either means or staff. Therefore, by lacking them, he or she will not be given subsidies. This is a circular argument which the evaluative system uses to justify pushing researchers to the background.

The argument of the number of publications is mentioned as a *sine qua non* to be able to carve out a scientific career. It is so much so that when a corporation member was consulted about a researcher who did not receive the corresponding promotions, far from searching for a solid argument about his scientific project he said: *He will never publish enough.*

If the researcher develops his or her work in a consolidated area, it is natural that he or she is asked to have some papers published. But if he or she is working on a new subject, it may happen that his or her question is so advanced that does it not fit in the existing publishing media yet. Besides, the publication frequency will depend on the subject. The researcher should not be pressured to remain studying a familiar subject so that in this way he or she can publish as frequently as the system demands so.

However, if one does not have any subsidies, staff and equipment, papers will not be able to be published, and if they are not published, funds will not be given, and without funds, how can one have any staff and equipment to be able to publish? Thus the system creates a *vicious circle of ineffectiveness*. In fact, as we have said, it is a circular argument, *the vicious circle of the deliberate exclusion* of *target researchers*. The Corporation offers a simple choice to break the vicious circle: to fit into a consolidated group and *share* his or her ideas with it, that is, the researcher must resign him or herself to sharing his or her intellectual property. This integration proposal hides a pressure to obtain a change in the direction of the investigations and thus, under a different perspective from the one the researcher wanted to direct his or her original idea: to be able to publish. As we mentioned in Items 20 – Grant Holder vs Disciple – and 21 – Director vs Tutor – from the first reading, there are researchers who think of cheating the examining system by presenting a work subject and then pretending to develop another one, the one that really interests them. In this case, it is the researcher himself or herself who wants to hide the subject he or she wants to investigate. If the researcher thinks that after having a number of publications he or she will be able to be independent from the group and develop his or her own project, he or she will be making a terrible mistake.

If, despite being pushed into the background, the researcher manages to obtain help outside the system and publish his or her papers, the authoritarian corporation will always have arguments to discredit him or her. For instance, the journal does not have enough refereeing (this regardless the fact that the referee is an expert in the subject) or the article does not strictly tackle the project's subject matter. Finally, the researcher will only be recognized for a few publications and will therefore receive a disapproving report: *The number of publications is small.*

The critical mass

This is another argument that is also quoted as a *sine qua non* for being able to develop the scientific work. It is very common to hear the corporation scientists saying that it is not until a *critical mass* is achieved that they have enough researchers so that *the necessary ideas come out in order to carry out a project.* Not only do they minimize the individual ability in this way, but they also take for granted that by accumulating people, ideas will necessarily arise. The more people there are, the more ideas there will be. If we put together ten lamps of 40 watts each, the light would equal one of 400 watts. Conversely, if we gather 100 persons without any ideas, it would be the same as having one person with ideas. If people do not have any ideas, no matter how many of them get together, an idea will hardly emerge. What is really positive is gathering up many people with ideas: by sharing them the results will be better.

With the explanation of the *Critical Mass*, every researcher who does not have access by ethical commitment to join aloentic workgroups will be doomed to be exiled from the system of Science and Technique. This regardless of his or her valuable ideas. That is, if the Science and Technique system wants to control an Authentic researcher when he or she requests human resources, scholars, technical staff, among others, instead of assigning that to him or her, the system will offer a group already made up, even with a director. The researcher will of course have to obey such director as well as allow him or her to co-author all his or her work – even if the director and the other researchers' participation is minimal. If an Authentic researcher completely driven by his or her question carries it out almost without means, with a great effort and exhaustion, and desperately asks the system for minimal resources such as a small subsidy or grants for the researchers, instead of giving the researcher what he or she has required, the system will try to integrate him or her into a group formed for something else. Within scientific work we can apply the paradigmatic example of numerous sports where it is necessary to have *mutual understanding*, i.e. people identifying with each other's ideas and feelings apart from how the team members complement each other in order to be successful. That is the reason why if there is no mutual understanding within the workgroup, they will not be able to achieve significant knowledge. Paradoxically, the system does not allow the integration of researchers or persons who understand and are committed to an idea. The price of this ideal is that team members will have to work in low posts or ad honorem while the system distributes posts to other people who are working on projects that are politically correct.

The argument of the critical mass can be valid for certain phenomena but it is fallacious to apply it extensively to all the scientific activity. We will illustrate this with different sports. In marathon, the necessary critical mass is that of one athlete. In table tennis, the critical mass could be of one or two people per team. In football, the critical mass is of eleven players per team. It could have fewer players, but not many, for if there were only two players per team, that sport would lose its essence.

The same concept can be applied to Science. A phenomenon that needs a multidisciplinary frame, such as a Bioethics or Technological Evaluation, for example, will require a critical mass of several specialists. Yet, and taking the case of the Theory of Relativity, the critical mass for its deduction and postulate was of only one person: Albert Einstein. This example helps to illustrate the fact that our work would have been completely disregarded by the system since, as a researcher who recognized the system's faults said: *Einstein would not have made a career in our system since he did not promote human resources.*

If just like the argument of the number of publications, the researcher wrongly thought of accepting the idea of participating in a critical mass of researchers to then be able to continue with their project, the only critical mass they will obtain will be that of a psychological oppression. This burden, as in the case of the thermonuclear bomb, will explode in some moment causing serious psychological damages for this researcher.

We can illustrate how irrelevant the criterion of the *critical mass* can be with how armies were conformed in the Antiquity. Ancient armies were conformed by companies of professional soldiers and by companies of recruits coming from the most diverse occupations. Although the latter greatly outnumbered the former, the victory in general accompanied the professional companies. Modern armies aim at a greater professionalization and modernization, so that fewer soldiers can be used: a small group of professional and highly modernized soldiers can be as powerful as a large number of less professional and less modernized ones.

Similarly, a small group of Authentic researchers can produce more than a large group of aloentic ones. In a harassing system, – i.e. Aloentic – society will see all the researchers as *professional soldiers*. Everyone believes that all the researchers are equally motivated by their question, ready to devote their lives to it. Yet, this is pure fiction.

A vocation based on the initiative, dedication, enthusiasm and perseverance, together with the necessary tools, greatly outnumbers the simple amount achieved by the association of people who were barely motivated by the salary or economic incentives.

For an Aloentic system that lacks ideas, the critical mass is in fact that researcher who can provide that idea which the group cannot. By no means, everybody will have ideas and together with others will investigate the phenomenon. In the Aloentic system, the only phenomenon which practically interests the Director is his or her continuity in the system and his or her access to funds distribution. With the argument of the critical mass in an Aloentic system, the lack of deep or significant ideas is tried to be justified.

We can then sum up these three points – the Infrastructure, the Small Number of Publications and the Critical Mass – by saying that just like in art, one cannot do science when the researcher is denied the right of freedom to be the architect of his or her own work and the minimal work tools. Or else, when each work tool is only given to the researcher after a hard political negotiation, which in any case will condition his or her work.

Summarizing what has been analyzed under this title about the need for help to researchers in critical situations, this is a common story for researchers who culminate without noticing within a subject which is more and more compromising and critical for its nature. The system excludes them indirectly since it does not mention the study purpose as an argument to justify the lack of support for the project. If they did so, the discriminatory attitude would become very evident.

The need for a protection mechanism for the ethical objector in Science and Technique is to break the structure of *neglect* in which he or she works. Neglect that occurs despite the existing laws, but which – as we have said – are subordinated to a non-written law that always agrees with the authority. In that respect, it is interesting to underline what has been said by some authors (Bruno):

> The population that composes the Administration performs its tasks having been affected by a learned neglect. This defenselessness is the one that according to Inés Izaguirre 'covers and perpetuates the existence and functioning of the most frequent and everyday violent relations of our society, where one does not see the material strength exercise and that is why they have become naturalized.' This violence requires a context in which some members of the system have the power of deciding what will be validated as legitimate for all the members of the public administrative system.

The researcher of the system that we defined above as aloentic instead of being treated as *subject* is treated as *object*.

Nevertheless, and due to our experience, we would like to emphasize the fact that before the harassment is motivated by the researcher's attitude of not letting themselves be overwhelmed by the authorities, there are a number of respectful but firm attitudes that show the person is not easy to manipulate. These being acts we described above in table 36 such as discouragement and discrimination.

Now, how and who can help them?

It is obvious that if they give in to the two pressures: a) change of study purpose and b) that of integrating into the courtesy team, in both ways, sooner or later, their program will be *restructured* or *normalized* and will not perform their original purposes. Although there will be possible economic benefits for the participants, the improvement of the knowledge in a scientific subject of community transcendence will finally be the only one affected.

Here is where the ethical protection organizations can help (INESPE/Ethikschuetzinitiative, 2000).

Technopathogenology has revealed the existence of a phenomenon typical of Technique which is risky to the human being.

The search led to the discovery of this phenomenon and the science foundation has also made it obvious that in the system of Science and Technique, by making incursions into certain fields of knowledge, may motivate the appearance and need of a protection mechanism for the ethical objectors.

We can then say that in the scientific context they are people who:

- Can be described as "brave people who can create amid oppressions," quoting poetry.
- Scandalize modern science by showing that the ruling canons and paradigms on which the knowledge generation is based are apocryphal: making voids within that knowledge, which could lead to a risk that exceeds the limit of the unreasonable.
- By seeing the consequences of phenomena that are being or were studied and that can give rise to a real damage to the human being with an unwavering vocation, feel the inevitable need to denounce them and bring that truth to light. We could say, by using a familiar phrase: *bringing that pressing truth to light.*
- Disturb at the beginning and then scandalize or infuriate the Corporation when, and taking the words of a poem, "They want to silence him but could not."
- By quoting Kuhn, the corporation detects the ethical objector as a *persistent anomaly.* For progress in Science, for all general process of innovation or discovery, it has already been written that by altering the expected theory, it ends up by being recognized as a phenomenon itself. But also, and unexpectedly, it is the key to Aloentic systems, old paradigms, degenerated programs, all being crucial aspects when the Human Being himself can be affected by the application of a Technique that was ill conceived. Yet, the difference is obvious: while in the case of the innovator scientist the anomaly leads to novelty, in the case of the ethical objector the corporation detects it as an anomaly and, just like it acts with anomalies that could demolish its theories – such as eliminating that curve data that does not coincide with the regression already obtained – also tries to eliminate it, remov-

ing it from the system for considering it *dangerous*. The reason for this being so is that as an anomaly the ethical objector can demolish not only a theory but also the system itself. His or her resistance makes harassers more evident. Finally, the innovation occurs when the ethical objector himself or herself, i.e. the *human anomaly*, manages to stand up on his or her own.

From what we have observed, in the case of the ethical objector in Science and Technique, more than with an initial and evident moral harassment, when the corporation tries to take advantage of the ethical objector and/or control him or her, he or she is subjected to a degenerative, systematic/corporate and diachronic process, which is progressive in intensity. A process in which, just like in *The Castle* by Kafka (Kafka, 2011), the corporation will try to prevent the researcher from doing his or her work.

If we compare the psychopathic process that we described in this reading with the process of the novel *The Trial* of the cited author, we could define our process as a *Kafkaesque Process*, because as well as in the novel of Kafka (Kafka, 2002), once that the corporation *pronounce a sentence*, although absurd, this is irrevocable. Nobody can revert it. All arguments will be in vain. *Roma locuta, causa finita.*

In words of Kafka at the end of his novel *The Trial* we also could say: *On a morning two lawyers arrived at the institute. They arrived with a removal van. After expelling us from the institute, they proceeded to dismantle it. Our expectations, projects and plans were ruined.*

We have also observed that unlike the workplace moral harassment, the ethical objector harassment in an academic scientific environment is focused on the question. The question seems to be more important than the person. For this reason, as in all civilized countries, freedom to investigate and teach is assured, and it becomes embarrassing for the establishment or state corporation to accept that some questions are on *black lists* but others are not. Consequently, the critics aim at the people without referring to the questions. Thus, the corporation hopes the hit or badly hurt people sooner or later will resign to eliminating the challenged question.

In addition, we have observed that it is important for the adoption of protection measures for the ethical objector in the scientific environment to establish the difference from the researcher who, by performing the

655

corporation's requirements and investigating questions that are not on black lists, obtains unexpected results that are highly critical to the economic interests of the corporation. This is a precise phenomenon. But the researcher's great merit is to make results public despite the corporation pressures. This is a case of precise and acute moral harassment of the ethical objector we call expeditious or acute. However, in our case we are always referring to researchers who from the beginning choose an ethical position related to a behavior that finally selects a question of human and critical interest. They are unconditionally loyal to this question persevering throughout the time despite its unpleasant derivations. Here we are witnessing an ethical objector we call patient or chronic. In this case, if these researchers work for a state corporation, the moral harassment will be subtle and in some cases it will be done in a shy and embarrassing way since the formal objective of a state corporation is precisely to give an ethical service to society.

In our particular case, perhaps for what we saw in the first reading about the productive differential of the people of the same group, after the first attempt to take advantage of our enthusiasm, where they failed, they opposed fiercely to our work. All the effort we made in the creation of new ideas, publications, etc. highly efficiently since the expenses were minimal and with a great hope of success, i.e. formal recognition by the distributors of subsidies, had no answer, or else this answer was not more than the usufruct of our ideas and the increasing pressure for integrating. How was this going to be successful if our effort was evaluated and surrounded by people who did not understand our efficiency? How can anybody recognize something that lacks and at the same time does not have the dignity to recognize it? After seeing the high efficiency at work, one person requested official funds, in order to be able to continue the work; yet, all answers we obtained were integration proposals deliberately ignoring what had been done.

Efficiency by itself is mercilessly punished unless it is integrated into the already established groups in order to enrich them. We can state then that the forced integration will always be inefficient since although the director researcher of the group can be efficient in his or her discipline, it will be inefficient for the new idea proposed by the researcher whom this director wants to integrate. Obviously, it will be totally inefficient if the group that wants to integrate the researcher is a group with neither skills nor scientific vocation. Generally, these groups are more interested in adding another item to the curriculum than to what has been produced.

In the first reading, we commented on a case where a director proposed a researcher to remove his or her collaborator researcher from the authorship of an article and incorporate another person who had not participated. That incorrect proposal, as we called it, which occurred in the beginnings of the researcher's scientific activity, in the light of what we have described in this reading, was already indicating aloenticity and evil of the system they were in. This kind of attitudes experienced by young researchers at the beginning of their careers already gave a hint of the dilemma between joining the system or becoming ethical objectors. Since it happens at the beginning, and is due to the *logic of the harassed,* he or she finds it hard to recognize the harassment because it is not within his or her canons of decency.

That is why one of the purposes of this reading is to show the new researchers the reality of a world where they may have the fortune, or rather misfortune, to develop their work.

This corporation attitude of wanting to silence the ethical objector, to destroy his or her hopes or goals, which in the case of these people go beyond the individual, in some cases is so close. An attitude secret and indirect with the inexistence of true black lists only known by its members and initiated ones, that it greatly resembles a familiar secret society whose members fit into the so-called *family.*

In order to understand all the corporation attitudes we have described, we should also consider that, as we saw in the first reading, a harassing system is an Aloentic system, which is not interested in searching for the truth and opposes to it or its search.

As what has been developed in this reading is a phenomenon framed in human relations, if we examine this phenomenon in detail we can reach the essence of its reality and say in philosophical and metaphysical terms that it is about a fight between Good and Evil. A philosopher said about a research subject: *He or she must be searching for a very deep and irritating truth for the intensity with which they are trying to destroy him or her.* Therefore, every ethical objector who searches for the truth must be ready – just like a battlefield soldier – to protect himself or herself against the enemy army. This militia is even organized in different ranks in the scientific world and can even be represented by a perverse opponent who aims at his or her destruction.

One has already heard the cases in which the manifestation and denunciation of situations that can be included in the frame of this phenomenon, such as Pusztai's potatoes, motivate the need for an Ethical Protection system. We have proved that this is very difficult since the system ignores, hinders and rejects every attempt to generate organizations that propose those goals. As we described above, our proposal of creating RIPCE is paradigmatic.

We described the ethical objector's difficulties in Science and Technique. These difficulties are similar to those that must be faced by ethical objectors in other fields and that are assumed by them for being motivated by *something* that only an ethical objector knows. It is said that when one prophet was asked why he insisted on his sermon if he did not convince anyone, he answered: *I do not preach to convince them, but not to be convinced by them.* That is how the ethical objector acts: he or she does not want to accept being convinced of taking irregularities of the system in which he or she is immersed as something normal and respectable, mainly the lack of freedom in the activity, but to be able to finally teach those who do want to listen to him or her. We can remember at this point Bertolt Brecht's quotation we used as an epigraph to this reading: "Don't accept the habitual as a natural thing." Ethical objectors do not want the system to convince them of the convenience of joining it. The system will never be convinced by the ethical objector, it will only change its stance if obliged by big pressure. He or she resists to succumb to the indignity to obtain easy benefits in the system. That resistance of being dragged by indignity is the ethical objector's essence.

In the case of Technopathogenology, we believe we have soundly proved that a mechanism of ethical protection in Science and Technique, apart from protecting those who denounce risky Techniques to people, is necessary already in the initial stages of the technological process.

Therefore, it is necessary to have a mechanism that allows:

- Freedom is guaranteed in the knowledge generation, in issues which are considered irritating by some people, but of a significant community impact.
- Release these researchers – quoting Descartes – from the *Methodical Mock*, *Methodical Discrimination* and *Methodical Persecution*. That is to say, from a *Methodical Process* on the part of the system that we have defined as Aloentic, that first searches to incorporate the person into it by the seductive proposal of bene-

fiting and encouraging his or her work, but whose hidden background was the interest of the system in benefiting itself and, as it is already known, controlling the person.

It is well known in that respect that the person who belongs to a group must renounce to certain liberties. If the group has been freely chosen and is grouped around a common goal, it is natural that these liberties are spontaneously renounced in the name of the proposed work. We are referring to the system's attempt to impose a group under pressure with different goals from the ones that could have been freely chosen by the interested parties. When researchers advance too much in knowledge areas which are compromised, critical or simply areas which the corporate group does not want to be investigated, it tries to impose being a group or part of a group in the corporation oriented to other goals in order to stop their spontaneous task. Although the project keeps the title or subject the researcher proposed, the insertion in the corporation and the obliged presence of the *Director* will completely distort it.

If the system does not achieve that goal, it then tries to stop or destroy the person's work.

- Protection to these researchers from Discouragement, Discrimination and Persecution acts that can both limit or prevent their work and damage their health.
- Protection and help to those defined by some authors as *Resisters* (Tenner, 2004), *those who do not take part in the game,* Those who resist pressures to be absorbed by a non-ethical environment and which can tell on his or her own health.
- Protection to the ethical objector, both acute and chronic, by developing – mainly for the second one – a mechanism of early detection of this kind of people and offering them help or a help mechanism these people can turn to.
- Protection of the ethical objector because besides affecting society regarding health problems and early retirement, as it is mentioned (Leymann, 1996), society is also affected, or rather damaged by the loss of a person who is fighting to defend it.

The development process of Technopathogenology and the lack of understanding from society also prove the need of ethical protection organizations to include training and information of society among their goals.

This training implies or may have as a consequence the fact that common citizens know ethical objectors' activity and value, thus seeing in them persons who, though risking their career and even their health, are fighting to protect them. Just like we saw in the reading of consumers' protection that an informed consumer could be protected from the hidden risks, for the ethical objector's activity, a trained society can be of great help and support in its acting.

Many times, the ethical objector ends up by being a martyr. It would be right to early recognize what he or she would have to denounce, either to neutralize it before it is too late or spread it among enough people who get to know the problem and support him or her so that the corporate power withdraws from its destructive intention.

To the question: *Why do harassed people resist for such a long time defending their ideal, enduring moral and physical damages until then they become aware of reality?* we have said that they do so due to the trust and faith they have in their project. The *innocent* trust in those who have the power of deciding is easily understood if we take and apply the authentic researcher as it is synthetically and brilliantly defined by Ortega y Gasset: "Because there is something inside the authentic researcher that struggles to be performed."

Terms we have taken from the following quotation of this philosopher:

> A human being is never a series of events, things that happen, but a path with a dynamic tension, like that of a drama. Every life has a plot. And this plot consists of something inside us that struggles to be performed and crashes into the environment so that this lets it out. The vicissitudes involved constitute a human life. That 'something' is what each person names when he or she always says: I.

Summarizing, the authentic scientist's passion – which struggles inside himself or herself to be performed – for the unconditional search for knowledge is so strong that leads him or her to *be anesthetized* against every opposition and pain caused by the system's harassment and rejection.

We then ought to obtain a protection mechanism in the scientific activity that first may avoid the need of an ethical objector in Science and Technique or of helping him or her if he or she was attacked by the system members. We should not forget that the ethical objector is under anesthesia by his or her own work, and as it occurs with anything under anesthesia, he or she does not feel the pain of the damage, which can lead him or her to death.

Final Conclusion

Technological development has made undeniable contributions to humankind. The work and effort of scientists is worthy of recognition, as well as the enormous investment by the Industry and State. This is why the risk they take is so significant.

The diversity and complexity of Technology is enormous. Within such complexity, based on a *particular situation that brought to light a general problem*, we detected a problem which, given its characteristics, magnitude and entity, we defined as a new phenomenon or a phenomenon still to be described, of high relevance to human health: The Technopathogeny Phenomenon.

We proved such phenomenon as well as the fact that technique, as a cultural object – notwithstanding its degree of sophistication – is a fallible object that can manifest at any moment unexpected side effects. We want to stress once more the fact that we arrived to this conclusion motivated by the concepts on Technique and Culture that had been postulated by Prof. Heinrich Beck in his work *Kulturphilosophie der Technik*.

This thinker states that: "Technique, nowadays and in the future, determines and will determine our being in a more radical and universal manner."

He asks himself:

> What is technique in essence and as a global historical fact? Does Technique lead us to new dimensions of meaning or being? Or does it lead us to our end? What does the cultural obligation consist of? Is it of improvement or of the spiritual integration of technique? Also, how will the social structure of the future look in relation to Technique?

These questions have also led us, as technologists, to review our own particular situations. For example, they made us ask ourselves about agronomical production techniques and finding its limitations. After asking question upon question we ended up running out of answers within our disciplines. These questions eventually led to support the need to create Technopathogenology.

Prof. Beck's work provided us with an excellent intellectual impulse, since we further make questions on what seemed already answered but, it actually still remained in the dark. Borrowing a term from Chemistry, we could say his work *catalyzed* the cognitive process. We can thus speak of two stages in our concept of technique: Before Beck and after Beck.

By proving the phenomenon and observing its dimension we also realized the lack of a disciplinary *home* to it.

We arrived to this conclusion, as we have said, after starting with a problem in particular – a natural contaminant – and then incorporating Technique in general. Then we found that the Technopathogeny phenomenon could not be framed within the disciplinary system.

We have also seen the logical connection of hypotheses and theories that enabled us to arrive to this conclusion, a connection that arose in an unforced and natural way. We were not obsessed with the idea of creating a new science. The need arose as a consequence *a posteriori* since the knowledge came or depended on experience or, in other words, it was a reasoning that arose from the effect to the cause or from the properties of the thing to its essence.

The benefits of technological development are undeniable and, knowing the efforts involved in its search, it is our wish to also contribute to such development by:

A. Unveiling a problem which, due to the already mentioned complexity, has only recently become evident, and framing it due to its unique entity, as a phenomenon in its own we call Technopathogeny.

B. Having defined it as a phenomenon, just like any other phenomenon, Technopathogeny needed to be framed within a specific disciplinary field. Our initial attempt of framing it within the existent always led us to a dead-end alley. As we have mentioned, we proved the disciplinary orphanage of the phenomenon. None of the proposed disciplines allowed to tackle its study as efficiently as the phenomenon required.

C. Supporting and proposing Technopathogenology as a discipline to study this phenomenon. This new discipline proposes its own criteria as well as a methodology and tools for its prevention.

In point "B" we mentioned our attempt to frame the study of this phenomenon in different disciplinary or multidisciplinary fields, some of which were abstract and some concrete. With diverse levels of detail, we considered:

- Philosophy
- Ethics
- Science, Technology and Society
- Health Sciences: Epidemiology, Toxicology, Bioethics
- Ecology
- Environmental Sciences
- Anthropology
- Social Sciences
- Risk Assessment and Risk Management
- Technological Assessment
- Environmental Impact Assessment
- Life Cycle Assessment
- Technical Consequences Assessment
- Technological Genesis
- Analytical Chemistry

The fact that Technopathogenology did not emerge from any of these existing disciplines that had already dealt with technique – not even from the techniques in particular – meant that this discipline had to emerge from Technique itself as a general discipline. This required a thorough training in the sciences that allow the creation of techniques, as well as having had a vast experience in solving problems of a technical nature. The constant verification of the imperfection of the new discipline and of Technique was also needed, as well as continuously finding how hard it is to achieve perfection in a technical object. Most times perfection is not achieved and the product is launched into the market even if it is not quite ready yet. In many cases, as we have jokingly said, not even *fully invented*. This leads to an important self-revision and search for those voids that allow dangerous imperfections. On the other hand, only someone with biological training understands the delicate balance of a living organism, the delicate balance of thousands of years of evolution in nature and realizes how easy it is to alter this balance negatively in the long term by wanting to obtain a questionable good in the short term.

We can see then that Technopathogenology did neither emerge from the purely abstract neither from the purely concrete. The abstract without the concrete or vice versa do not give real solutions to the problem. This science did not emerge from thinkers alone or from technicians alone. It emerged from technicians that were thinking about technique. Technopathogenology is a science that emerged from observation. It emerged as the science of Technology that reflects upon itself and upon its own fallibility.

The principles that say that *problems cannot be solved by those who have caused them* could be expanded as: Problems cannot be solved by those who have caused them *unless there are consistent strategies that enable the causers to detect such problems early enough, even before they can be called problems.*

We have been suggested that the prefix *pathos* sounds negative to name a science because it refers to an illness and that it could even be the reason why the concept was resisted. This was Prof. Jacobsson's perception, whose letter we include in the Annex. As we will see in such analysis, the prefix *pathos* was included to further specify the field of action of Technopathogenology – this prefix is used in health to refer to illnesses including their preventive study (prophylaxis). In our case, we study a subject that also deals with illnesses, whether caused by Technique in humans or also, in a more metaphorical way, by the illnesses of the technique itself – i.e. the alterations in its *health (*which we defined as flaws) or state that allows it to carry out all the functions for which it was conceived. This is why there is no other way to refer to these concepts.

Technopathogenology does not study an illness. It studies the possibility that a technological flaw can cause an illness or the technological causes that might eventually lead to an illness. In other words: it studies the non-evident etiological technological causes that might engender a morbid state, in order to achieve their prevention.

Technopathogenology does not study the patient, it studies the Technique.

The specific study of an illness caused by Technique could be a part of Medicine called Technopathology.

We know that in certain human diseases preventive medicine aims to identify the patient – whether he or she has symptoms or is a healthy carrier that can spread the disease – isolate him or her or create adequate conditions to avoid other people catching the disease. If it is a new disease, it is studied to avoid it is spread. In this sense, Technopathogenology is similar to medicine: it aims to identify techniques that can make humans sick and, if such is the case, isolate the technique or create conditions for it not to be harmful – as well as studying ways of developing safer techniques that are not harmful to humans. Just like preventive medicine does it with the healthy carrier, Technopathogenology also aims to identify which of those apparently safe techniques or *apparently healthy techniques* are potential health hazards.

In this sense, the prefix *pathos* used to name the new science is accurate and we believe that with time it will eventually be accepted.

The difference with preventive medicine lies within the fact that Medicine does not study how pathogens are generated (they are generated by Nature and a new virus can appear through mutation) but how they affect humans and Technopathogenology not only studies the presence of technopathogens in Technique but also their genesis and prevention. This is the apparently inevitable condition: Technopathogens are generated by concrete techniques which were ill conceived from the very beginning.

We believe that Technopathogenology is the consistent tool of Technology. It is a science that tries to solve and prevent a problem that another science which, in spite of its good will, *has not noticed*, and, due to its imperfect method or tools the problem cannot be avoided. If our proposal was included in Technology, it would enable technologists to slowly begin to prevent non-evident risks on human health. This is a science for technology, an auxiliary science which is part of the technological process.

As we have mentioned when we referred to Bioethics, we can say that in technological progress there are, on the one hand, "the enthusiasts who want to progress fast" and, on the other, "the critics that put obstacles on the way" (Pompidou, 1997).

Technopathogenology does not try to put obstacles on the way. In Chapter I we conclude *that the voids in knowledge that are responsible for Technopathogenies are a consequence of the hasty generation or of the eager attitude for obtaining such knowledge.* This thesis supports the technopathogenological criteria of *patience* and *prudence* we referred to in Chapter III, but this does not imply putting obstacles. For example, in reference to toxicological methods, it is mentioned that the *hasty generation of new toxicological methods may result in faulty assays. Despite pressure to rapidly develop new assays for toxicological assessment, careful attention to assay design is imperative for producing assays that provide interpretable and relevant data.* We know how relevant the toxicological methods to predict technopathogenic risks are. Therefore, we can generalize and say that the eager and hasty generation of new technologies may result in faulty Techniques. Despite the pressure to develop new Techniques rapidly, careful attention to technological design is imperative for producing Techniques that satisfy the necessities but without risks for human beings.

Therefore, Technopathogenology does not want to put obstacles on the way, it tries to contribute to a well gestated technology.

Technopathogenology aims to lie at an intermediate position. Not to escape commitments but to contribute with preventive measures that cannot be found in any of the *affiliates* to either extreme position. Enthusiasts disregard the risks while critics exaggerate them. An article defined these two positions as technophilia and technophobia (Eguiazu, 1999b).

We have also analyzed the attempt of framing Technopathogeny within the Social Sciences framework. We have commented that a few researches coming from this field had proposed studying the impact of Technology. We have resorted and we will resort to use different sciences to support the creation of Technopathogenology. Therefore, in order to further support our proposal, we will mention some comments used for Sociology.

"Max Weber conceives Sociology as the science in charge of understanding and interpreting social reality as it is". (Anonymous (a)) Similarly, we can say that Technopathogenology aims at understanding and interpreting the reality of Technology as it is. That is to say, to get to know Technology in an authentic manner, by focusing on non-described aspects or on aspects that are deliberately disregarded for being *not nice*, as are the non-evident negative side effects inherent to it.

Technopathogenology does not pretend to be completely thorough or to give a full answer to a technological problem – even less to substitute a discipline or multidiscipline already focused on the problem. Some problems of economic, ecological, social, labor risk, etc. interest are not considered by it. We do believe that it can cover the voids left by other disciplines that focus on other aspects of Technology.

In connection to what is new in Technopathogenology, we could say that *the small imperfections prove the rule.* Only Technopathogenology can deal completely with the problem. It gathers everything that has been said and done about the phenomenon and puts them in the same bowl. The question is thus valued as a scientific object.

If, after all the arguments we have used to support the need of Technopathogenology it is still argued that there are not enough elements yet to consider it a science, we can at least say, maybe leaving aside any epistemological principle, that we believe that this science proposes applicable principles and that it is, in addition, useful.

Going back to Sociology, "Max Weber considers sociology as a science that aims at understanding and interpreting social action in order to explain its development and effects from its causes" (Anonymous (a)). The same could be said of Technopathogenology, which aims at understanding and interpreting technological side effects in order to explain its development and effects from its causes. We could add to this the aim of achieving an effective prophylaxis of these side effects.

It is interesting to observe that these two concepts can be applied both to Sociology and to Technopathogenology – and perhaps too to other sciences. This does not mean that Technopathogenology wants to *meddle* in fields which are specific to Sociology or to any other science. We mention this relationship in order to show that Technopathogenology has the same aims that Sociology has for other phenomena it studies, and that such aims are used to support their existence as sciences.

Today Technique can get into fields which seemed unthought-of in the past. As we have already said, technological development has contributed and keeps on contributing enormously to humankind. However, the enthusiasm it has generated has caused certain achievements to produce adverse effects – effects qualified as *aggression* by some medical practices.

Maybe we could go back here to ancient wisdom remembering a piece of advice on morality that could also be applied for technological development: "All things are lawful unto me, but all things are not expedient: all things are lawful for me, but I will not be brought under the power of any" (San Pablo (b)).

The exegetist who analyzed this advice comments that "it is not about knowing what lawful is and what is not, but it is about determining what favors or jeopardizes the growth of Man..." (San Pablo (b)).

The technical man has achieved such a degree of development that today we can talk of a *Technocracy*: Technique as a *ruler* of life and human progress. Technologists, enthusiastic about their power, should meditate about such power and arrive to the conclusion that they must not be dominated by it. Several multidisciplines have been created in order to analyze these consequences (for example, Bioethics).

We believe that the Technopathogeny phenomenon is one of the consequences of this Technocracy.

Technopathogenology can then be summoned and participate in an interdisciplinary or multidisciplinary environment in order to evaluate, within a global framework, any problem associated to technology *to protect present and future Humans* so that risks associated to the undeniable benefits of Technology are not justified as *the price of progress* and that such benefits can be defined as *a priceless progress*.

As we have said in the Introduction, Technopathogenology contributes to the control or prevention *a posteriori* of technological risks, but this aim is also pursued by other disciplines such as Risk Assessment, Technological Assessment, etc. The most important and substantial goal of Technopathogenology is to achieve a control *a priori* of such risk. An *a priori* control means the early recognition of indicators or signs that a certain Technique is being generated with potential errors or flaws which are hazardous to human health. In Chapter III we included proposals or criteria that Technopathogenology can contribute with.

Technologists, whose knowledge will be applied to humans themselves, will have to behave without going against their own nature. We can also apply to all technicians the principle that must rule the physician's work: *primun non nocere.*

In Chapter II we mentioned some philosophers who analyzed the question of Technology. They established technological postulates from a philosophical perspective. Similarly, we established philosophical postulates from a technological perspective. If applied to train people either directly or indirectly connected to Technology, such postulates would prevent or reduce the risk of technopathogenic harm.

We have received several criticism and objections to our proposal. Even if we considered such criticism right, the consequences of this problem are objectively more important than the theoretical objectivity the criticism may have. That is to say, just warning about the problem and finding its roots in Science and Technique was worth the effort.

Apart from presenting our disciplinary proposal, we have described the enormous amount of difficulties we have encountered in the Science and Technique System. This is why, even though we have devoted a specific reading to deal with this, we would like to conclude our work with this issue. If Technopathogenology is finally considered an innovation or a useful contribution to Science, maybe the difficulties we encountered are typical difficulties any scientist who dares to explore unexplored fields must encounter. The work of these scientists is not like the story of Elzeard Bouffier, Jean Giono's character from *The Man who Planted Trees*[1]. In the story, Bouffier, "armed only with his physical and moral resources", started a hard and persistent work that took him half a century. Day after day, one by one, he planted seeds in the French Alps and he eventually managed to turn a wasteland into an 8100 acre paradise, full of life. He worked completely alone.

> That is why no one meddled with Elzeard Bouffier's work. If he had been detected, he would have had opposition. He was undetectable. Who in the villages or in the administration could have dreamed of such perseverance in a magnificent generosity?

Unlike Bouffier, the work of scientists engaged with ethics brings to light issues which cannot remain in anonymity. Their inevitable accusation makes them public and the system starts *meddling* with them. Sometimes, there is a short period of bonanza until they are discovered and the persecutory process begins.

However, their ethical commitment strengthens their physical and moral strength, which enables them to endure. It is our wish that every researcher committed with ethics and human life has the ability to overcome all these obstacles and manage to see, like Bouffier, the results of his or her work.

An author says that humankind is driven by gold and technique, which show a progressive materialization of intelligence and the world. The author continues saying that "it is not necessary to relinquish Technique" and he adds that "reason must impose its human regulation" (Maritain, 1978). According to this postulate, Technopathogenology – with its aims to contribute to the establishment of *cannons* which Technology should respect – wishes to establish scientific *reasons* as *regulations* for the technological development.

The Greeks considered that every single good could be reached by using the truth as a starting point.

---

1   Copy from Jean Giono's "Der Mann der Bäume pflanzte" (The Man who Planted Trees), given by Dr. Otmar Wassermann in a meeting in 1990.

We have supported the fact that both the lack of truth and the existence of a void in the bodies of knowledge used for the development of a Technique can result in immanent and hidden flaws in Technique. This can produce the generation of factors (Technopathogens) which can be harmful to humans in the long term. If we cannot search for the truth in the scientific technological knowledge, we may suffer adverse consequences.

So, we can finish this Final Conclusion with a quote from Saint Augustine: "Those who do not want to be beaten by the truth will be beaten by the error."

Annex

In this book we have commented that the Technopathogeny phenomenon was discussed with several scientists. Naturally, we must first mention our mentor, Prof. Heinrich Beck, PhD. Among other people who have expressed their opinion about our book and comments about our phenomenon and Program we can mention: Prof. Dr. Otmar Wassermann (Germany), Prof. Per Jacobsson (Royal Institute of Technology, Stockholm), Dr. Christian Hedinger (SAGUF, Swisse), Dr. Hector José Huyke, Prof. Dr. Carl Mitcham, (Penn State, U.S.A.), Prof. U. Beck, and Prof. H. Gadamer, (Bamberg, Germany). They have all contributed with valuable opinion and advice.

In this Annex we include:

I. Prof. Beck's statement on our work. Professor Beck is Emeritus Professor of the Philosophy I Chair, University of Bamberg.

II. Opinions, comments and general criticism received.

III. An important evaluation by Prof. Dr. Otmar Wassermann, on our Program from 1996. Prof. Wassermann is the highest authority in toxicological-environmental research in Germany. This was an evaluation of the report that was revised and corrected by Dr. Günter Emde. There has been great progress since that year – which must be considered in order to adequately appreciate this evaluation.

IV. A note we addressed to Prof. Per Jacobsson, from the Royal Institute of Technology, Stockholm, with whom we exchanged valuable correspondence and who evaluated our technopathogenological concept.

V. Comments in the letter sent by Dr. Christian Hedinger, secretary of the Swiss Academic Society for Environmental Research and Ecology (Schweizerische Arbeitsgemeinschaft für Umweltforschung – SAGUF) to the President of CONICET, Argentina (February 28, 1992), a copy of which was sent to the Rector of Universidad Nacional de Rosario(UNR).

VI.   Opinions by Dr. Hector José Huyke in a letter sent to the President of CONICET (July, 1994) and by Dr. Carl Mitcham in a letter to the Rector of UNR (July, 1994).

VII. Letter by International Network of Engineers and Scientist for Global Responsibility (INES) to the Rector of Universidad Nacional de Rosario (January 27, 2000). Chairman: Prof. Dr. Armin Tenner.

VIII. Letter by Greenpeace Argentina to the Rector of Universidad Nacional de Rosario (August, 2002).

I.   Prof. Heinrich Beck's statement

(Translated from the Spanish version of Prof. Beck's statement approving the publication of this book)

Intention of the work

In the past, it was thought that technical inventions could be applied provided no negative effect was found. Today this has changed. The "ethics of responsibility" state that new technologies must not be applied until possible negative effects are excluded from the very beginning. The work of Nobel Prize Hans Jonas was an essential contribution to this change of paradigm and Guillermo Eguiazu and Alberto Motta wish to materialize this principle.

For the evaluation of Technical innovations through certain processes of natural and technological sciences, it must be admitted that certain harmful effects on health are not expected using the laws of causality. In this manner, the evaluation of factual effects and philosophical principles that search for the vision of totality are fundamental.

It is about answering the following questions: Are there actual damages on health (frequently connected with medicines and agricultural techniques)? How are such damages accepted according to ethical norms? The principle of the lesser evil could also be used to defend its use. This is done by comparing the disadvantages and harm that can be caused if such new technique is not applied. A fundamental logic problem for the scientific prediction of side effects – whether expected or not – lies within the limitation of the current methods of knowledge, i.e., of our capacity of knowing. The fact that a negative effect cannot be known does not mean knowing that it could not *factually materialize.*

This is why it is crucial to find in the structures to be investigated the capacities or aspects through which the negative effects are impossible. This is why in many cases a *complete impossibility* will be impossible to recognize. This is an evaluation of *degrees of impossibility*, that is, probability or improbability.

Within this lies a problem – either of theory of knowledge or of theory of science – which, just like the ethical problem above mentioned, requires a philosophical treatment.

It is obvious that for the concrete realization of an ethics of responsibility in that which is crucial for life, such as technical progress in our society, it *is essential to establish a specific science: Technopathogenology.* This science must accompany the process of production of new technologies in every possible field. The book thoroughly supports this relationship and specifically defines its conditions.

Contents and organization of the Book

The book will be divided in four chapters which come after a short introduction and finishes with the bibliography.

Chapter I introduces the phenomenon of Technopathogeny. The most accurate way of indicating it would be the scientific considerations of the apparition (or generation) of damages through technique. In this sense, the questions about a harmonious relationship between humans and the environment are essential, as are, regarding this, the following questions: a) What causes the alterations? b) How can they be recognized? The aim is to develop methods to recognize such characteristics of Technology that can be harmful to health and, in the deepest sense, the development of methods and technologies that do not have such characteristics.

The second chapter shows that given the fact that the existent sciences study other issues, they do not consider this phenomenon. Biochemical correlations are also mentioned in this chapter.

In addition, Chapter 2 describes in which circle of related sciences and auxiliary disciplines this new science could not be included: Chemistry, Biology, Medicine, Agricultural Sciences, Foodstuff Sciences, Environmental Sciences, Sociology and Cultural Sciences as well as Philosophy of Natural Sciences and Ethics.

A large amount of sciences that do not have the same object of study as Technopathogenology are mentioned

This is used in Chapter 3 to present the structure of the internal methodology of this new science. Different relevant empirical and philosophical methods related to the ethical object are discussed in this chapter.

A fundamental value is given to the a posteriori nature of the technopathogenological studies. This first stage states that instead of arriving to conclusions of given facts and expected effects, Technopathogenology studies certain negative effects from which it goes back to the causes that might be harmful to health (the substance is systematically proved in various situations).

In Chapter 4, various complementary issues are discussed, which stress and further describe the need of this new science. This is why, for example, the social and cultural relevance of biological quality and scientific innovations tests are studied, as well as the "promotion of trust among consumers and producers" (both in international commerce and in the positive effect of human and political relationships). The authors propose to further develop this point and discuss the different aspects. The aim and criterion here is human life as both its individual and social wholeness.

Finally, equally important is the inclusion of opinions of scientists and public life representatives about Technopathogenology as object of study – both to be interpreted or to be corrected. These opinions can promote new discussions on the field and further stress its importance.

Final conclusion

As we have clearly seen, this book deals with a current issue which is soundly scientifically supported and presented in a very rich and multifaceted manner. The authors show they are committed to pursue their aims but are also open to dialogue. They are oriented towards totality.

Readers can feel the commitment towards humanity of these authors, which can attract readers too.

The publication of this book will help the authors improve their precarious situation, as well as to the "thing itself" and to human society, which is subjected to serious stress regarding its health.

The *clear and dynamic nature* of this book makes it readable to both experts and the general public interested in this issue.

I recommend its publication.

II.   Opinions, comments and general criticism received

We have seen that in order to prevent a concrete problem for human health such as Technopathogeny, Technopathogenology has the following elements:

A. A methodological process on its own to apply before the technological development stage and a classic methodology coming from empirical sciences: Hypothetic-deductive, Experimental, Observational.

B. It also resorts to auxiliary disciplines to accomplish its aims.

C. It has a series of criteria to follow in order to avoid the risk or to reduce it as much as possible.

We believe that by considering the methodological process a Centrifugal and Centripetal evolution and with the cases taken from other disciplines, as well as with the analogy with Criminology, we have further clarified our proposal.

Below we will list the objections or criticism we have received and we will reply to each point.

Of course we will only refer to constructive criticism, although because of the tone of some of the remarks we could say that they constitute a veiled attempt to ridicule our work. Such critiques contribute to the attempt of falsifying the Theory which, if it can be sustained, will have more entity. Such constructive criticism forces the author of the Theory to find further supporting grounds to sustain it. We will not refer to ill-conceived criticism from colleagues, led by human passions wanting to undermine or destroy. This is ungrounded criticism which does not attempt to contribute with scientific grounds to refute or improve an idea. We believe that this kind of criticism is part of the history of science. Such destructive criticism must be endured by scientists who dare to approach an idea from a different perspective and refuse to let pre-existent structures distort such idea. This leads to the following reasoning: Maybe such criticism only proves the entity of a new Theory.

Perhaps such criticism leads to a new project which some readers of this book might find interesting.

Below we will list each criticism followed by our counterargument.

- Why is a specific discipline necessary?
- Are Ecotoxicology and Environmental Sciences not enough?
- Why is preventive medicine not enough?
- Is Toxicology not enough?
- Is what you are saying new or has this been known for a long time?
- Why is Environmental Medicine not enough?
- Why is Workplace Medicine not enough?
- Isn't Technopathogenology an esoteric or metaphysical approach?
- Isn't it a pedestrian proposal that came as the result of a play on words?
- This looks like a clever synthesis of philosophical and scientific thinking. Is this really of any value?
- We have never known of a technopathogeny.
- The methodology seems imperfect.
- The proposal does not represent anything new. The science does not describe any new concept.
- Can this phenomenon be really prevented?
- Is Epidemiology not enough?
- Isn't Technopathogeny a rather narrow concept?
- What is the difference between this science and Technological Assessment?
- Isn't the prefix patho too strong? It seems as if it attacked Technique. Shouldn't it be better if this prefix were removed? It wouldn't sound so striking. The prefix patho sounds scary.
- They are inventors who want to make their idea known through the Internet.

- Are they not exaggerating? Maybe Technopathogeny is only found in third world countries due to bad practices which are common there, or due to the higher level of corruption in those countries.
- Technopathogeny is an obvious flaw that is impossible to fore-see. It is part of technique and we are doomed to suffer it.
- The Technopathogenic problem is so complex that a scientific approach is impossible.
- Isn't it too pretentious to develop such a vast concept as Techno-pathogenology based solely on a few experimental works?
- Their concept is obvious. The Science and Technique System has been dealing with the Technopathogenic problem for a long time and we are positive it will be solved without the need of a specif-ic science.
- The work is too focused on medicine.
- The term Technopathogenology is too long and heavy. It seems baroque. Isn't there a shorter term to express the same idea?
- Why Technopathogenology and not Technopathology?
- Are there no qualified evaluators coming from other sciences that could prevent this problem?

Below we will analyze each question individually.

Why is a specific discipline necessary?

Bearing in mind that there are sciences which already contemplate the relationship Technique/Human Health, the question sounds reasonable.

We have already dealt with this point in articles quoted in this book. The need of Technopathogenology is based on the fact that we believe that the existing disciplines such as Medicine, Toxicology, Philosophy, Ecology, Ecotoxicology, Environmental Sciences, etc. cannot approach the problem in a holistic manner (Eguiazu & Motta, 2005b, 2005c) (Mot-ta & Eguiazu, 2003).

It is worth remembering here the remark of a specialist in Ecotox-icology who, when asked on the Chernobyl incident, he declared *I am not a specialist in Chernobyl.*

Everyone wants to avoid Technopathogenies from happening, but they do happen. Why is this? The answer is very simple: because there is no specific science. Everyone wants to avoid it, but nobody knows how. Technopathogenology studies what happens *before* the exposure and *why* it takes place. Physiology studies what happens *after* the exposure. This question is connected to the next:

Are Ecotoxicology and Environmental Sciences not enough?

The need of Technopathogenology is based on the fact that we believe that the existing disciplines such as Medicine, Toxicology, Philosophy, Ecology, Ecotoxicology and Environmental Sciences, etc. cannot approach the problem in a holistic manner (Eguiazu & Motta, 2005b, 2005c) (Motta & Eguiazu, 2003).

Environmental Sciences, for example, study the negative effects that a specific Technology can have on the environment. The analysis can include the processes that may lead to such negative aspects. The difference between this discipline and Ecology is that the latter analyzes the damage on the environment outside the company, whilst Environmental Sciences does it within the company. In this sense, Technopathogenology can further explore this since it gets into the field of knowledge, or of theories which gave origin to the technique/s that are used by a company, for example.

As for the differences between Technopathogenology and Environmental Sciences, the latter would investigate non-evident damages caused by Technique in the Environment in order to correct its defect and help the company avoid getting fined. What is important to Environmental Sciences is the compliance with existing regulations on environmental control. For instance, it helps determining if, due to the level of environmental damage, the company must have insurance or not. Optimizing productive processes in order to avoid environmental damage – even though they might imply a higher cost for the company – can represent a higher profit in the future. Environmental Sciences does not study Technique in relation to the potential environmental damage it can cause before any concrete damage is observed. Moreover, Environmental Sciences only concentrates on the Environment – which is more closely related to Ecology – whilst Technopathogenology studies the Human Environment.

To generalize this concept, we could say that all the existing disciplines have the effects of technique as a starting point, but not technique itself.

Why is preventive medicine not enough?

Because Technopathogeny as a phenomenon is substantially different from any disease or common pathology. When dealing with a disease, a pathogen is to be detected and then controlled. But a technopathogeny can even be caused by the actual medicine used to control the pathogen.

Is Toxicology not enough?

Toxicology is in itself a very useful tool for risk control and of course for Technopathogenology. However, it is not enough because this science refers to toxic substances and does not bear in mind its technical application, which is what would determine its potential technopathogenic risk. There are also a wide range of Technopathogenies caused by, for example, radiation or electromagnetic waves, which are not borne in mind by classic Toxicology.

In addition, this discipline requires a concrete element already developed to investigate its potential risk.

In the case of risk caused by chemical substances, an interesting preventive approximation, and a very useful one for Technopathogenology, is to consider the relationship between structure and activity – i.e., the relationship between the chemical structure of a molecule and its potential toxicological activity.

Is what you are saying new or has this been known for a long time?

The fact that some techniques can have a negative effect on health is not new. What is new is supporting the fact that due to its complexity and unique nature, Technopathogeny could be framed as a phenomenon – also because we said it was immanent to technique. The immanent nature of technique constitutes a substantially new program (compared to the traditional programs of technological studies).

Why is Environmental Medicine not enough?

Because this science studies a human being inside a pathogenic environment without considering the causalities that made such environment technopathogenic. It does focus, however, on how to treat and cure the patient. All the medical sciences study the human being, not the technique.

Why is Workplace Medicine not enough?

Because there are many technopathogenies that do not originate in the workplace. Many of them can appear in technologies which are not related to the workplace, for example, medicines or foodstuffs to which humans or consumers are exposed regardless of the place in which they work.

Isn't Technopathogenology an esoteric or metaphysical approach?

It is not esoteric, since it does not look for magical solutions. It investigates what causes the problem, which is complex but real. It is not metaphysical either: technopathogeny as a phenomenon is a concrete problem. It would be esoteric or metaphysical to observe the technopathogenic disease and deny its cause or divert its explanation towards non-existent causes, i.e. to defend the *non-causality of the phenomenon*. This is commonly found in the explanations of scientists that deny the existence of the phenomenon.

Isn't it a pedestrian proposal that came as the result of a play on words?

It is not pedestrian since it aims to contribute to the study and solution of a problem of great entity in terms of the global survival of humankind. This aspect was highlighted by the scientific committee of a specific magazine (Eguiazu & Motta, 2005b, 2005c). The authors are not experts in literature or rhetoric so as to play with words.

This looks like a clever synthesis of philosophical and scientific thinking. Is this really of any value?

What is new is not to have made a synthesis; it would not look clever or original since in the works of philosophers such as Aristotle there was not a great separation between philosophical and scientific thought. More recently, thinkers coming from biology and medicine like Nobel Prize Alexis Carrel have made brilliant synthesis between philosophical and scientific thought (Carrel, 1949). Therefore, we do not believe we have made any new contribution on this aspect.

What we do consider original is the identification of the phenomenon in all its identity and complexity. This will be falsified – or not – by the confrontation with criticism, reality and history.

We have never known of a technopathogeny.

Whoever says this has probably not observed with an open spirit the myriad of cases that prove otherwise.

Furthermore, if it never occurred to whoever said this to consider the immanent and hidden effects of technique that have adverse consequences on human health, it is not possible for him or her to declare the contrary. Nobody can know what it doesn't even consider as new, nor know something new that does not call up on his or her attention. Fleming could have been told: *We don't know of any substance generated by the Penicillum mold that inhibits the development of bacteria.* Instead, the bacterial culture that was contaminated by mold caught Fleming's attention, which enabled him to find or know something new and unknown.

The methodology seems imperfect.

We have already long discussed this subject. Nevertheless, it is reasonable to reiterate that as in any new science, there are methodological aspects that need to be developed or perfected. As we explained when we described Criminology and Criminalistics, we see that every new science has rudimentary methodology and tools in the beginning.

We can also repeat the example of seismology, which even though it has a well developed methodology, it does not have yet the tools to accurately predict all the earthquakes.

The proposal does not represent anything new.
The science does not describe any new concept.

The adverse effects of Technique on human health are not new, but technopathogeny as a phenomenon is. Even when it is a problem of technique that involves health, it is not a medical or toxicological problem. Otherwise, medicine or toxicology could have predicted, for instance, the effect asbestos has on human health, which was discovered after many years of use.

Medicine and/or toxicology cannot solve the technopathogenic problem because they run behind it. If we keep thinking they will solve the problem, we will have to accept *thalidomide children* and discover that a substance is carcinogenic or teratogenic in humans after many years of use. In short, it would mean accepting that humans are technique's ultimate laboratory animal.

Today Toxicology aims to prevent, though imperfectly, the non-evident and unexpected effects substances have on human health. Short term trials, structural alerts and the development of Toxicogenomics are examples of this intention. Nevertheless, it still works on techniques that are being applied or in development. Also, ecotoxicology only deals with *boomerang* substances: substances that although introduced into the environment with a positive intention, come back with negative effects on humans (Petrosyan, 2005). This concept only focuses on a partial prophylaxis of the problem, since it detects the negative effects on the ecosystem after the application of the technique.

Boomerang substances are those that are released into the environment with a certain interest, but that return to human beings with a negative, unwanted effect. It is like a boomerang that, instead of returning to the hand that sent it, hits somebody standing nearby. In this case, the study of the deviations in the return path of the boomerang would be the object of study of Technology Assessment (Technikfolgenabschaetzung). Technopathogenology, on the other hand, would study the effects of a boomerang that against what is expected would not turn at all.

We need a discipline that is at the forefront of the technopathogenic problem; we believe such discipline is Technopathogenology.

The technopathogenic problem is very complex. It is not just a Medical or toxicological problem. It begins, as we have already said, in the stage during which the knowledge that will originate the technique is generated.

Regarding whether Technopathogenology is something new, we can go back to the example of the soil. The soil in itself is not new at all, but when all its complexity was discovered, it became a phenomenon worth to be studied for which a new science was necessary: Edafology.

We can also mention volcanoes. They are not new. They have existed since the earth crust began to solidify. But to study them as a new phenomenon due to its complexity, Volcanology was developed.

The same happened with rivers. They are not new either. We could ask ourselves, what is rare in a river, in a simple stream of water? But when its complexity was observed, a new discipline was developed with its own methodology: Hydrology.

Edafology, Volcanology and Hydrology are new sciences that describe new ideas. Technopathogenology also describes new ideas.

Can this phenomenon be really prevented?

In Chapter III we have proved that some technopathogenies can be prevented.

When we discussed the fourth approach to the technopathogenic phenomenon, we proved that the voids in the knowledge used during the development of a technique are the cause of the defects it may carry within it. We have also said that among the attitudes a scientist can adopt regarding the truth, only two are ethical: Ignorance and Error.

Others, like Doubt, Uncertainty, Opinion and Mendacity are not ethical. We can say that if we advance in the knowledge that will give birth to a new technique up to the point where the non-ethical causes of voids in such knowledge are eliminated, many technopathogenies will be prevented.

Epidemiology is an auxiliary science to Technopathogenology. It is a tool to establish which technique in use proves to cause damage on health in the long term. A typical example of this is the establishment of the cause-effect relationship between neoplastic diseases in humans and carcinogenic substances.

We have already made reference to it when we tried to disciplinary frame the technopathogenic phenomenon. Even when the usefulness of this discipline is out of discussion, we can reiterate its limitations.

1. The damage has to have already been manifested.
2. Many times it is difficult to establish a relationship with the causing agent.
3. It needs a minimum number of affected people for the results to be statistically significant.
4. The carcinogenic agent may not be concentrated enough so as to generate a statistically significant response.

We can therefore outline two objections:

a. The technique has been or it is currently being applied. Although the verification of a cause-effect relationship can help to recall the technique from the market, the damage has already been done. The risk may have been minimized at the beginning due to economic or political interests but it will surface through the appearance of victims. The manifestation of the risk as a concrete damage can be seen at first with skepticism by the scientific community; only when its manifestation is overwhelming it will consider adopting control measures.

b. It requires the existence of a significant number of persons that had shown the adverse effect in order to relate it to a substance as etiological factor. The number of affected persons may be small in relation to the exposed ones thus making the relation difficult, but this does not mean that the technopathogenic damage has not occurred. Nobody with a minimal ethical commitment can say: *Since the number of affected people is small, let us continue using the technique; the number of people benefiting from it is bigger.* To endorse this criterion would be accepting Nietzsche's concept according to which everything that helped the weak to survive is despicable. Any scientist defending this criterion would be going back to the sadly well-known ideas that proposed the elimination of the weak. This goes against the principles of the mayor religions and especially against the Christian principles of charity and love for your neighbor.

Isn't Technopathogeny a rather narrow concept?

This question was formulated by Dr. Werner Rammert a Social Sciences researcher specialized in Genesis of Technique' (Technikgenese) (Rammert, 1991). Even when he considered Technopathogenology to be a very interesting proposal, recognizing that the troublesome consequences of technique were immanent to it, he did put forward some objections. He considered that Technological Genesis, a discipline that originated in social sciences, was enough to prevent the problem. He believed that it was not enough to extrapolate the concept of iatrogenesis to Technopathogeny only in relation with the damages to health caused by technique. He thought the concept was rather narrow.

Genesis of Technique is also a new discipline, but one that, coming from Social Sciences, is applied to problems related to them. It tries to find the social and cultural factors that lead to the genesis of a technique, both in its positive and negative aspects. We can see how Technopathogeny appears to be a narrow concept when analyzed from the general concept of Genesis of Technique. We could reiterate here the arguments used to explain why Technopathogeny cannot be framed within Cultural Anthropology, or what we said in relation to social sciences. We consider it is enough to say that the Genesis of Technique approach misses the *hard* section of the biological-toxicological-technological knowledge, which is the specific aspect of the damage to health caused by the particular techniques.

At the same time, we consider that focusing on a phenomenon that has its own singularity allows for a greater depth by only concentrating in the non-evident and non-acceptable damages to health. The social and cultural aspects, even when relevant from the Social Sciences point of view, are purposely left aside of our field of study. These ideas were discussed with Prof. Ivan Illich from Penn State University in 1994.

What is the difference between this science and Technological Assessment?

Since this question has already been put forward by Prof. Jacobsson, and so as to not repeat ourselves, to answer this question we can refer the reader to Chapter II.

Isn't the prefix patho too strong? It seems as if it attacked Technique. Shouldn't it be better if this prefix were removed? It wouldn't sound so striking. The prefix patho sounds scary.

This observation was made by Prof. Per Jacobsson, from Kungliga Tekniska Högskolan (Stockholm). We will comment on it when we discuss his letter below.

They are inventors who want to make their idea known through the Internet.

Even when we said we would only include criticism made on good faith, we decided to include this for considering it interesting. When we tried to include Technopathogenology in a well-known internet based free encyclopedia, one of the reasons given for its exclusion was that it had not been requested by many sources at the same time. The person submitting the exclusion proposal indicated that there were not enough quotes in English, emphasizing the lack of volume of presence on web sites. This is again a circular argument: a new concept is excluded only because it is new, without even discussing its value. If something new cannot be disseminated, how is it going to reach the volume of dissemination required to be discussed and maybe be accepted? In the same encyclopedia one can find many completely insignificant novelties that are there due to their wide dissemination.

It is interesting to highlight that our proposal, which implies a strong criticism to an established scientific paradigm, is also fiercely excluded from the web site were anybody can supposedly propose anything without being excluded.

Another interesting aspect is that none of the criticisms was signed by a specialized Scientist or even by anybody with knowledge in Technological risks.

If we hypothetically consider Technopathogenology to be an *invention* then Edison could have never disseminated the incandescent lamp, since he was the only one to know about it. The administrator of the encyclopedia would have rejected the dissemination of his invention claiming that *there are not enough web sites talking about the lamp.* They could also say that *the inventor only wants to disseminate his own invention.*

It is deplorable that such authoritarian system of selection and exclusion calls itself free.

Are they not exaggerating? Maybe Technopathogeny is only found in third world countries due to bad practices which are common there, or due to the higher level of corruption in those countries.

Actually, it is the opposite: Technopathogenies are created in the first world from where they are *spilled out* to the third world. The hiding of side effects begins in the first world where the technologies are created. Regarding corruption, we can ask ourselves: Though more subtle, wouldn't the biggest corruption be where the technique is created, which is generally in the first world? In the third world there are only mere executors at the service of the directives of dissemination and use of technologies coming from the first world.

Technopathogeny is an obvious flaw that is impossible to foresee. It is part of technique and we are doomed to suffer it.

This is a non-scientific argument. As Scientists we must believe in the human ability to know, and therefore to prevent.

The Technopathogenic problem is so complex that a scientific approach is impossible.

The fact that it is a complex scientific problem does not make it less scientific, nor prevents the possibility of working through it with the help of auxiliary sciences.

Isn't it too pretentious to develop such a vast concept as Technopathogenology based solely on a few experimental works?

It is not pretentious, it is simple scientific. By reading Popper we see that the number of cases does not determine in itself the scientific quality of a hypothesis which is determined by being falsifiable. That is to say, the truth or cohesion with the truth of an idea is not defined by the number of cases but by its internal coherence. Technopathogeny is true.

Their concept is obvious. The Science and Technique System has been dealing with the Technopathogenic problem for a long time and we are positive it will be solved without the need of a specific science.

The science and technique system does not appear to be such an efficient system, since the cases of side effects of late manifestation that cause astonishing damages to health are innumerable. It is so in such a way that there are economic interests involved. In order not to obstruct the use of products, enormous efforts are made to hide these unexpected side effects; such efforts include corruption and bribery in the official institutions that must certify the innocuousness of a product. There is a mechanism called *Revolving door* where scientists who must evaluate products to protect consumers or the general population are or were part of the same companies that created such products. That way, many officials in public institutions are directly selected by the companies; instead of defending the interests of the population they defend those of the companies they answer to. In other words, they circulate between the private companies and the public institutions. Furthermore, as we have discussed in the previous chapter, to trust that future science will solve the problems caused by present science is a fallacious argument that only tries to justify the flaws in technology.

The work is too focused on medicine.

It is not so when evaluated globally. The medical aspects are necessary to understand that Technopathogenology is grounded in positive sciences; otherwise it will appear as a mere theoretical lucubration. Even when the approach seems sometimes too medical, medicine is only an auxiliary science to it.

The term Technopathogenology is too long and heavy. It seems baroque. Isn't there a shorter term to express the same idea?

It is a very interesting criticism. Actually, if there was a shorter term to express the idea, we would have used it. The problem is that any attempt to reduce the word only leads to conceptual ambiguities or inaccuracies. For instance, if we had kept our original choice (technogenology) we would be missing the reference to the damages to health that lay at the core of our proposal. The term technogenology exactly means *what is generated by Technique*, which includes all the good things generated by technique as well as a few bad things, some of which can cause damages to health. By adding *patho* to the word, we circumscribe its meaning to the damages to health. We couldn't devise a shorter word that expressed this idea.

We must clarify that the sole extension of the term is not a motive of objection. Otorhinolaryngology is a discipline with a more reduced object of study than Technopathogenology and uses a longer word to define itself.

Why Technopathogenology and not Technopathology?

We were asked why, among the existing disciplines, the technopathogenic phenomenon couldn't be studied by Technopathology. This discipline studies diseases generated by a technological factor that have already manifested themselves. The term is used to describe, for instance, the addictions or health problems associated with the use of computers. It aims to study the disease as well as to cure it. Technopathogenology, on the other hand, aims to study the causes of those diseases that are immanent or inherent to technique in order to limit them and, if possible, to deactivate them. It is more important to study the technopathogen as the cause of the disease as a constitutive defect of the technique that the disease that will come as the result of the technique interacting with humans.

Technopathology is the realm of the physician; Technopathogenology is the realm of the technologist.

Are there no qualified evaluators coming from other sciences that could prevent this problem?

In this regard, it is interesting to point out what happened when transgenic seeds were approved in the USA. Some independent scientists were of the opinion that genetically modified organisms represented such a complex and new subject that there were not too many experts to evaluate it, not to talk about the field of its possible side effects, which was even more unknown. The officials that in all good faith were to approve the use of these organisms had no knowledge of the complex problem of their side effects, despite being many of them recognized scientists. So as not to admit their ignorance, they took as valid the information provided by the interested companies. We see here how there are many other examples of total absence of qualified evaluators, as well as the incapacity of experts from other disciplines to prevent the complex problem of the side effects.

III.   Professor Otmar Wassermann's evaluation

In 1996 we submitted Prof. Wassermann, the highest authority in Germany in Toxicological-Environmental research, a summary describing the aims and projects of the PROCABIE program, which was then under development, for its evaluation. Prof. Wassermann's prestige in this field of knowledge gave us an invaluable authorized opinion for such a new program as PROCABIE was.

We would like to state that even though we have referred to our program as Program of Biological and Biopathological quality of the Human Environment (PROCABIE) we had originally submitted it as Biological and Ecotoxicological Quality of Human Environment Research Program (INCABIE).

The research – both the experiments and the logical-formal process – was developed in the INCABIE Institute, for which we had presented a founding project in 1984 – and which was formalized by Universidad de Rosario in 1985. However, in 2002 INCABIE was dismantled. We then continued our activities focusing on the logical-formal aspect of Techno-pathogenology.

INCABIE was an honest attempt to find a physical space to develop this kind of research in a region that was craving for it. Some experimental research was developed in prophylaxis for the apparition of mycotoxins as well as theoretical/experimental research on the identification of mutagens in the environment and a great amount of paradigmatic theoretical research. We created two series of publications: Colección Tecnogenia (Technogeny Collection) and Cuadernos del INCABIE (INCABIE Journals), published by Universidad Nacional de Rosario.

Below we will list the projects that were being under development within the Biological and Biopathological Quality of Human Environment Research Program (PROCABIE). It must be taken into account that for practical reasons, the dates indicated in the description – just like other references (personal, aims, etc.) refer to the project status in 1996. This is why the original name of the institute is used (INCABIE), and the terms Technogeny and Technogenology are used (instead of the current Technopathogeny and Technopathogenology). Some explanatory footnotes are also included. After that, we include Prof. Wassermann's evaluation.

Project submitted to Prof. Otmar Wassermann

Contents

   I. The problem of Environmental Research in Argentina and our Program.
   II. Area of Concern
   III. Different Areas of Concern:
      A. The problem of Aflatoxins and Mycotoxins in General
      B. The problem of the transference of agrochemicals from countries with strict regulations to countries with lenient or insufficient regulations.
      C. The problem of industrial emission of mutagens and the presence of mutagens in chlorine water,
      D. The problem of the lack of training programs of technological risks both in university and in technical schools
   IV. First Results

I.   The problem of Environmental Research in Argentina and our Program

It is proven fact that the application of techniques bring about not only advantages but also unwanted side effects with negative consequences to human health. We call this phenomenon Technopathogeny. Until this day, these consequences which are studied by epidemiologists and toxicologists are very difficult to foresee. One could say that, because of the way in which it is done, science nowadays has inherent technological risks.

This is why a sense of responsibility must be developed in all the people who must carry out these activities.

Today, those researchers who study such risks can be eliminated or discriminated against by the scientific community.

Such researchers are generally denied of a fair evaluation of their projects. As a consequence, they are denied of resources to carry out their work.

That is to say, the scientific projects that must contribute to knowledge on the relation between human health and the harmful effects of technologies are disregarded by the traditional unions or scientific commissions.

Examples of this are the environmental toxicology programs. This situation is particularly negative in third world countries, where the interests of contaminating industries and the scientific groups are not balanced by alternative evaluators like in Europe or the USA.

The Nordic Council of Ministers proposes as a fundamental human right the right to have environmental information. That is to say, the right of every free citizen to have all the information available in connection to the risk generated by environmental influences.

Most of those risks are associated to techniques (Technopathogenies). In third world countries there are certain projects, such as PRO-CABIE, which attempt to receive or produce information in connection to biological and biopathological quality independently from scientific and commercial interests. This program, however, is not adequately evaluated by groups of experts since there is no proper framework to deal with these matters in Argentina.

692

For many years, this program was negatively evaluated because the people working on it refused to give in to the pressure of the groups of interest.

Therefore, the common citizen has no way of receiving scientific environmental information. The aim of our program is to make this information available to citizens and disseminate it. This is why it is important that specialized, independent scientists evaluate and support our work. Such specialists must aim at working in the interest of human beings, not of industrial or commercial interests or scientific lobbies.

Summary

In our region, the common citizen is subjected to receive distorted environmental information due to commercial or scientific interests. Our program attempts to make environmental information available for all citizens.

This is the reason why this program not only did not obtain a minimum financial support, but also its members were persecuted.

II. Area of concern

The following questions were based on the aims of the United Nations Conference on Human Environment, held in Stockholm in 1972.

Which role does technique play for the general question on the environment?

Are the negative side effects of Technique predictable?

Is the technical scientific system really a low risk system? Are the experts' statements as infallible as it has always been said?

Based on three long years of reflections on the interaction between Technique, Environment and Human Health, we arrived to the conclusion that we had to focus our research on the unwanted side effects of technical processes. Having a basic training in Agriculture and research, we began our work on environmental problems in that field. We observed that the quality of grains used for human consumption was decreasing fast as a consequence of the apparition of molds that generated carcinogenic substances. Evidently, the grain post-harvest handling system was not using a method to avoid the problem. The crucial question was: Do aflatoxins appear spontaneously as a natural consequence or are they caused by technical processes whose defects or flaws were not recognized in time?

In order to answer to this question, we started to apply analytical techniques. In 1976, we found the contaminant in Argentine corn. We therefore started a campaign to inform consumers. We also informed the relevant authorities on the measures that should be taken. However, in spite of receiving support from the State, in 1979 G.M. Eguiazu was asked to renounce his position at CONICET. His work continued in Germany, where he developed an analytical Technique and he studied the conditions in which contaminant substances are developed. From Germany, he kept insisting Argentine officials to take the necessary control measures. He never received satisfactory answers.

The research on the apparition of contaminating substances in different types of seeds allowed the development of an anthropo-ecological hypothesis about the causes that led to the deterioration of seed storage conditions.[1]

From 1983 onwards, once the Program was already created, different studies were made which seemed appropriate to improve the knowledge on negative consequences caused by technique in the region. A critical work on agrochemicals[2] proved how inadequate the control mechanism was for the international transfer of agrochemicals from regions with a strict control to regions with lenient legislation (North to South).

The Prior Informed Consent principle (PIC) from the FAO Code was analyzed and criticized and there was an attempt to incorporate two new principles: The Principle of Automatic Exclusion and the Principle of Responsibility. This was carried out in a FAO Seminar in 1994.

Later, a doctorate student was incorporated in the program. She worked on the quality of drinking water and on the control of industrial emissions. The topic she worked on was: detection of mutagenic substances using the Ames test.[3]

---

1   Refers to the work *Las Micotoxinas desde una perspectiva antropoecológica* (Mycotoxins from an anthropo-ecological perspective), presented in the San Luis Congress, Argentina, 1985.

2   Refers to the work *Plaguicidas y Error Tecnogénico* (Pesticides and the Technogenic Error), presented in 1987.

3   In 1999, the doctorate candidate left her post for personal reasons.

Using this test (with and without metabolic activity) we tried to investigate if there were mutagens in the Paraná River (the river from which the waterworks plants take the water).

Our aim with these works – both with the mutagens test and with the study on agrochemicals – was to call the attention of the people exposed, to raise awareness on the quality of the air in the application of these products. We wanted to raise awareness on consumers about the possible residues in foodstuffs as well as on the quality of water. This takes us back to the right of environmental information advocated by the Nordic Council of Ministers. We wanted to support citizens in asking for their right to obtain real environmental information.

Summary

All the research works were oriented towards the detection and prophylaxis of environmental noxas. Until 1996, the following research areas where studied:
    A. Detection and prophylaxis of aflatoxins and mycotoxins in general.
    B. Critical research on the transfer of agrochemicals from North to South. Proposal of new principles for the PIC of the FAO Code.
    C. Detection and prophylaxis in waters through the application of the Ames test.
    D. Development of a basic methodology to evaluate the negative consequences of Technique.

Comments on each topic:

Topic A. This is the most thoroughly developed topic, since the research has been carried out for over two decades.

Topic B. Only critical works on the legal legislation applicable at the time were carried out. We have still been unable to develop a method of analysis of agrochemical residues. We were forbidden – without scientific grounds – to use a gas chromatographer that had been available for ten years.

Topic C. Was an incipient doctorate project.

Topic D. Development of concepts that aimed towards the construction of a specific discipline (Technopathogenology: a science to study technological consequences).

III. Concrete points in each of the research areas

We can say that we have obtained concrete results for the problem of aflatoxins and mycotoxins (Topic A). Most of the experiments were conducted in relation to this topic. In reference to the agrochemicals (Topic B), we suggested solutions to the transfer of agrochemical products from North to South (with teratogenic, mutagenic, carcinogenic and late fetal damage). This was done not only for the flaws in administrative control, but also for the flaws in the analysis of residues. The solution of such flaws was planned as a future research.[4]

We will be able to discuss solutions for the mutagens in water (Topic C) when we obtain results through the application of the Ames test.[5]

We have developed several concepts regarding the systematic study of the unwanted consequences of Technique (Topic D).

Below we will describe in detail the topics we were planning to develop for each item (A to D). This would be divided in two groups: 1) Short term – which was partly already at work – and 2) Long term.

All the topics mentioned were part of the work in our Institute. They can be summarized as *Detection and Prophylaxis of Contaminants or Environment Noxas.*

Topic A. The problem of Aflatoxins and Mycotoxins in General

1) Short Term:

A1) Development of a simple and safe method for the first selection of contaminated grain batches. Proposals for legal regulations and control.
A2) Distribution of information of the potential damage to groups of risk (such as organizations of protection to consumers) so that they can require public organizations to apply control policies.

2) Long Term:

A3) Critical research (with the aid of a methodology developed for this purpose) of the natural resistance of the most important seed species humans use for consumption (including hybrid seeds) in their capacity to

---

4   This topic was only developed in theory. Due to the reasons already explained, we were unable to carry out the experimental stage.
5   Due to the same reasons, we were unable to carry out the experimental stage. It led to the publication of a pre-doctorate book that initiated the series "Cuadernos del INCABIE".

resist long term storage in poor conditions (high relative humidity, high temperature, fungal attack, etc.). Publication of the most resistant seeds available in the market. Ancient cultivars (used by natives, Incas, coyas, etc.) would also be born in mind.

Difficulties:

The ones who produce and sell highly genetically modified seeds are against proper investigations on the natural resistance against fungal attack and appearance of mycotoxins. They fear that modern hybrids have little resistance to this type of contamination and that using ancient or traditional cultivars, although being more resistant, might lead to economic loss. Those who sell seeds for internal consumption know that the seeds highly contaminated with *verdin* – the commercial name given to grains attacked by *Aspergillus flavus* or *Aspergillus parasiticus*, the causing factors of aflatoxins – generally surpass the tolerance for B1aflatoxins. They are also against the development of regular controls.

The exporters, however, have their own methods of control, but they are applied to exportation. There is no interest whatsoever in domestic consumption.

The industry for internal consumption is also against controls since the instrumentation of systematic controls would raise the cost of its products.

Topic B. The problem of transferring agrochemicals from countries with strict regulations to countries with lenient or insufficient regulations (North-South transfer of risky agrochemicals)

1) Short Term:

B1) Comparative study of the agrochemicals which are imported in our region with the agrochemicals in strict regions (for example, those that are banned in California or in Scandinavia). Study the reason why highly risky agrochemicals were allowed in our region when they were banned in other regions.

This study can lead to find out that in our market highly risky substances are used. This research must be accompanied by an analysis of banned substances residues – or other highly risky substances. This will enable a realistic analysis of the situation in the region.

B2) Distribution of information about the actual potential risk. Development of political will in groups of risk (Organizations of Protection to Consumers) and in students so as to exercise pressure on the relevant instances. This could help recalling products from the market and stopping the importation of new products.

2) Long Term:

B3) Studying the process that allows public institutions to permit the consumption of highly risky substances in developing countries. The aim of this study would be, on the one hand, to cast some light on the weak points and, on the other, to support organizations to protect consumers or the press.

Initiation of trials when there is enough information available.

Difficulties:

The commercialization of products with agrochemicals that are banned in developed countries – that is to say, products that cannot be sold any longer in developed countries but are exported to developing countries – is of the utmost relevance. It is suspected that local officials, bribed by foreigner exporters, are tempted to produce favorable statements on these products. This also interrupts any attempt to solve this problem.

This is proved, for example, by the enormous quantity of lab instruments in public institutions that are used in insignificant projects and, at the same time, not allowed to use to analyze residues in pesticides.

Topic C. The problem of industrial emission of mutagens and the presence of mutagens in chlorine water

1) Short Term:

C1) Development of a simple and safe method of analysis to give a first approximation or alarm signal on the presence of mutagens in the emissions and effluents discharge points as well as in the intake of water to be used as drinking water in Rosario (1,000,000 inhabitants). Determination of possible residues of chlorocarbon after the chlorination process.

C2) Distribution of information about the potential damage as well as development of political will in groups of risk (Organizations of Protection to Consumers) to exercise pressure on the relevant instances so that, in case the detection proves positive, a control of the emission is developed.

2) Long Term:

C3) Critical investigation on the causes that lead to the presence of residual mutagens in water. Use of the test of Ames as a methodological tool. Apart from *Salmonella*, use of the micro or macroorganisms of water as indicators of quality. Training of highly qualified personnel. Tutoring of doctorate candidates.

Topic D. The lack of training to evaluate the negative consequences of technique in universities, higher education institutes and secondary schools

1) Short Term:

D1) Development of a methodology to evaluate the negative consequences of Technique. Systematization of known technological damage.

Systematic training at university, within the framework of the new discipline called Environmental Technogeny (Technological consequences found in humans, mediated by the environment) in a technological orientation at University.

D2) Motivation to future engineers in this phenomenon. Training in higher education institutes and universities as well as teaching in secondary schools the various technological damages so that this can be handled more reasonably by population. Also, systematic training of secondary school teachers.

2) Long Term:

D3) Send the information to different associations of scientists as well as to political institutions to encourage them to create an institution with the obligation of bringing to light the opportunities and risks of technological developments and its applications. Also, bring to light information about important harmful consequences and publish them. Develop a specific scientific discipline: Technogenology[6] (a science to study the negative consequences of Technique and its methodology).

---

6   The name was later changed to Technopathogenology to further specify its area of study.

This science would allow to detect negative consequences in a new technology prior to its existence. Work in collaboration with anthropologists who could support the early recognition of the phenomenon, and psychologists who could bring to light the unconscious forces that allow to plan, develop, distribute and even favor technologies with immanent risks.

Difficulties:

The scientific/academic communities are tied to carry on developing Science and Technique projects through the traditional model (science is neutral, the scientific knowledge and its technical application are always used for human progress). The concept of a specific science to address the hidden and unwanted collateral effects of technologies and prevent their risks is unacceptable to them.

There are also powerful interests in scientific/academic institutions that resist to any kind of change because either them or their lobbies would lose scientific prestige or privileges.

IV. First Results

As we can see, in 1996 the INCABIE program [7] was in its first stages. This is why there were not big results obtained back then. However, there were some concrete results for regional interest that could be proven.

Regional interest results:

- In 1975, aflatoxin B1 was detected for the first time in *Zea maize var indurata* (Argentine corn) for exportation. It was determined that 4,9% of the corn for exportation was contaminated over 5 ppb of Aflatoxin B1.
- Several groups were formed and promoted in the region to work on aflatoxins and mycotoxins in general as well as specifically on the improvement of the protection of harvest of different grains.
- Foundation of the Institute of Biological and Ecotoxicological Quality for consumer protection.
- Presentation of information and administrative request, just like sending bills to both parliamentary chambers asking for a law to regulate prophylaxis and control of mycotoxins in agricultural products.

---

7   After the Institute was dismantled in 2002, the program was called PROCABIE.

- Creation of the first Environmental Technogeny chair for the trans-disciplinary training of students in different careers at university.

Results of Experimental and Scientific Interest

- Development of an analyzing technique for Aflatoxin B1 with application of Blankophor P as a standard substitute for the first time.
- Development of a patented method in Argentina to carry out this analyzing technique.
- Development of a methodology to study the conditions of the formation of aflatoxins in sunflower and then on other seeds – especially corn.
- Development of a methodology for the prophylaxis of fungal growth based on the intergranular relative humidity of atmosphere in stored grain.
- Falsification of the hypothesis that blamed the loss of quality in stored grain to inevitable deeds of nature. Supporting of an anthropo-ecological hypothesis that blames the destruction of stored grain on technological processes that have influenced on their natural resistance.
- Support and application of the test of Ames to detect non-specific mutagens in the drinking water of the region.

Results of theoretical-scientific interest:

- Development of a methodology to evaluate the technological consequences and conception of a specific scientific discipline (Technopathogenology: Science of Technical Consequences.
- Development of an anthropo-ecological hypothesis that blames the loss of quality in grains, as well as its storage conditions and resowing capability to immanent defects in technique related to genetic selection and post-harvest handling. A few points to bear in mind: The resowing capacity is connected to the natural resistance of grains against molding and premature sprouting. The seeds which, as part of the natural evolution wait for the following spring to sprout, have higher chances of reproduction. The seeds of many highly developed hybrids (genetically modified), like corn and wheat, already sprout in the cob or ear. This

process means that if these plants were left to their natural reproduction, they would not exist any longer because they would have disappeared. The hypothesis above mentioned and its related works try to reconstruct the natural resistance of plants by reconstructing a primeval species that can be reproduced through natural resowing.

- Counsel to the professional agronomist in connection to actual risks of common pesticides.

V. Conclusions and final summary

The INCABIE Program is an example of the fight against a scientific-technological establishment that is not open to fundamental changes connected to the risks of modern techniques. If this program can be developed, it will not be only a model of organization for other institutions and projects that deal with the evaluation and limit of environmental damages caused by technique. It will also be an example of an ethical crusade against scientific-technological and political-administrative interests that act against the citizens' basic right to have environmental information.

INCABIE Institute had the following goals:

- Determination of environmental problems as a consequence of technological application.
- Development of concepts for the detection and prophylaxis of environmental noxas based on concrete examples (mycotoxins, pesticides, non-specific mutagens).
- Development of extremely simple and inexpensive devices to detect environmental noxas adapted to developing countries contexts (for example, a technique to detect aflatoxins in fields).
- Training human resources (in higher education, universities, graduate students, doctorate candidates) in environmental technogeny.
- Motivate, by means of example, the commitment of scholars, professors and students to fight against scientific-technological groups through a conceptual model appealing to moral values. In spite of the fierce opposition we had to endure, the Institute survived until 2002.[8]

---

8   After 1996, the harassment increased quantitatively and qualitatively to such an extent that, in order to stop our activities completely, the authorities resorted to evict

- Work along with other protection institutions (Consumer Protection, Greenpeace) especially on providing information about environmental data to Consumer Protection entities.
- Information to the general public about environmental technogenies and the possible harming factors. Preparation of environmental information for interested citizens.

In the long term, basic environmental information and the right of citizens to obtain such information should not be the consequence of the effort of a few individuals and the pressure of organizations of consumer protection. It should be guaranteed and legally protected. This information must be grounded by scientific-technological work. Especially within this framework, a specific technological-scientific discipline must be promoted.

Finally, this will eventually reach its maximum efficacy with total recognition and support from the scientific community that will recognize this as a scientific discipline. Its obligation will be fulfilled only when information on side effects and consequences of technologies are given and warn people before the consequences manifest themselves on humans used as laboratory animals without knowing so.

VI. Clarification of some concepts

Human Environment: In this context, it only refers to a means to transport negative effects introduced by technique on human health. These effects enter the body through various surfaces: Skin, respiratory system, digestive system.

Our concept of *human environment* here is simply an aid. The difference between our concept *human environment* and the ecologists' environment is that *environment* refers to nature in need of protection.

Environmental Technogeny (technogenies transmitted by the Human Environment) uses the term *environmental* to refer to the means that transports an effect. The central point is that Technogeny has immanent and hidden effects or defects of technique with negative effects on human health. This is why our concept of Technique is based on Prof. Henrich Beck's (Bamberg) cultural anthropology of technique. This is a dif-

---

us from the Institute on August 15, 2002, illegally distributing among themselves the equipment in the Institute.

ferent approach from the one generally used for the consequences of technique, for example, the one used by Günter Ropohl (Frankfurt).

Technological Assessment aims more specifically to political decisions. They are not necessarily interested in a systematic science we call Technogenology. Technogenology would study the phenomena caused by technogenies developing theories on its causes and/or methodologies that would enable the gestation of technologies balanced with health. This can happen if technogenies are avoided.

Prof. Otmar Wassermann's statement

Evaluation of the Report and Work of the Biological and Ecotoxicological Quality of Human Environment Institute (INCABIE) Rosario, Argentina. January 8, 1996. Dr. Otmar Wassermann, evaluator.

Introduction

For a better understanding of what I am about to say to the people responsible in policies, administration and universities in Argentina, I would like to say that here in Germany we are suffering the consequences of industrial development. For the last seven to eight generations there has been great progress and success as well as the greatest damage on human health and on nature. As a consequence, nowadays we are paying a very high price for the so-called progress.

This way of acting until approximately 1970 was determined by a general ignorance and indifference on the consequences of this irresponsible exploitation. All the voices that claimed against it were ignored and many accused of being "madmen". Looking back, the damage produced – which, on human scale is irreversible – forces to recognize that the "madmen" were right. The damage could have been avoided as well as so much human pain and the shortening of lives through diseases connected to contaminants. Furthermore, a clever environmental protection 100 years ago would have avoided the destruction of vegetation (death of forests) and of the animal world, as well as the destruction of the quality of underground waters, surface waters and seaside areas through a completely irresponsible contamination with complex and enormous quantities of harmful substances which implied huge economic loss in the long term.

In 1990, in former West Germany alone, the damages caused by the contamination of air in buildings, bridges, art masterpieces and vegetation, as well as the damages on human health, were estimated between 300 to 500 billion marks.

It is not surprising that this fatal development was possible thanks to the ambition of profit, corruption, minimization and silence of the possible harmful effects, as well as by pressuring and defaming opponents. All this, based on a squandering policy ruled by industrial interest. It was not until 1970 that the population started resisting against these actions: Thousands of initiatives were put forward by citizens who (locally, regionally or federally) started chasing out the corrupt and ignorant politicians as well as slowly developing an environmental awareness, at least managing that the phrase "environmental protection" entered the vocabulary of politics.

The governments of countries which have not gone through this in the past would be very well advised if they could learn from these mistakes, before the interests of a complete industrialization, without protecting the environment and promoting chemo-intensive systems in agriculture (including the widespread application of highly risky pesticides), act without respect; before the negative effects of genetic manipulation are perceived, before the catastrophic consequences of atomic energy, before the development of an industrial policy of burning garbage and other important risk technologies take place.

Since there are better alternatives for all this, the human beings from such countries must be protected against this new form of colonialism that industrialized nations impose making them use these technologies. Human beings must be aware that they constitute the State themselves since the State is only possible because they pay their taxes. Even the humblest agriculturist knows that he cannot send the cow he milks to the slaughterhouse. The myopic way in which we have treated nature has led to this destructive attitude – just like the little protection we have given to the ozone layer and to the oceans.

In this context, all the States in which there are constitutions that protect the people must allow the general public to have free access to the information on the emissions that damage the environment or health (an example of which is the Freedom Information Act in the United States). This must be a fundamental right.

Statement on the Report

1) In connection to the information received, it can be stated that the researchers evaluate the situation in Argentina in a very realistic manner since they have been receiving negative attitudes for the past 25 years. In addition, from my experience in Germany I can say that I myself have verified what they state in point I) and I fully support their needs.

As for point II) in the Report regarding the urgency and importance of the aims of INCABIE, I can state the following: Considering the great environmental problems in Argentina – which are caused by different factors – and the small number of scientists focusing on this field which is considered very annoying by politics, economy and administration, and who receive systematic discouragement, what I have observed as to what commitment is concerned in these two researchers is extraordinary.

It is outstanding that under the poor conditions they had to work, they managed to produce and publish a vast amount of works.

The core of their research work and the aims of INCABIE that are connected with environmental problems and which are fundamental for the population in general are:

1. Contamination of crops with highly toxic fungi (Aspergillus) and eventual increase of such damage through genetic modification.
2. Transference of agrochemicals from industrialized countries to developing countries.
3. Mutagens in drinking water.
4. Evaluation of negative consequences of Technology.

1. Contamination of crops with highly toxic fungi (Aspergillus) and eventual increase of such damage through genetic modification

It is widely known that in warm countries the contamination of food and crops with extremely dangerous fungi plays a major role. Some contaminants, like aflatoxins produced by the Aspergillus flavus fungi have been for a very long time of epidemiological interest due to the production of carcinogenic substances. Liver cancer is quite common in such countries. This is known in northern hemisphere industrialized countries, but it has never produced any interest whatsoever. However, northern hemisphere countries have suffered some economic loss, like for example, the massive death of turkeys in 1960 in the UK due to the consumption of aflatoxins contaminated peanuts.

After a series of studies and great economic loss on this issue, a high rate of liver cancer was found in African tribes with a high content of peanuts in their diet. Retrospectively, it was attributed to the same cause that caused the turkeys deaths in the UK. This is of no interest to industrialized countries, scientists, health departments, industries or politicians.

An effective solution to fungal attack in foodstuffs and crops is essential in Argentina. The government must feel ethically and morally compelled to apply the following measures:

- Establish a reliable register of cancer patients (register of incidence) and mortality (cancer as a cause of death and register of mortality). This must be done with a high statistic accuracy (population units must not be higher than 5000 persons because the regional causing factors will otherwise not be detected).
- Apply extensive and effective controls of foodstuff and crops. Methods to achieve this are known in INCABIE. This Institute can train on the usage of these methods, which are quite inexpensive.
- Inform the population about the high risk of cancer in molded foodstuffs and crops. Make this comprehensible for everyone.
- The cost of these preventive measures is much lower than the health treatment once the person has contracted the disease.

2. Transference of agrochemicals from industrialized countries to developing countries

It is widely known that chemical products multinationals are unscrupulous when it comes to expanding their market. For them, any means is acceptable. This includes deceit, corruption and the massive use of their products for military purposes. For example, Western chemical companies manage to sell almost half of the products they sell in Malaysia, by falsifying the toxicology data. They cheat the offices that authorize usage. Independent organizations have documented this kind of behavior, which is harmful for the community. This implies a series of risks for developing countries:

- The illegal sale or application of pesticides which are banned in other countries (including the producing countries).
- Unscrupulous use of lenient control systems (through inefficient offices) as well as abuse of illiterate or misinformed populations (illiteracy, poor work conditions, no protection to workers, sig-

nificant increase of toxicity when outdoor temperature rises or in greenhouses with mixtures of different pesticides).

- Serious damages on health and uncountable number of deaths connected to the use of pesticides as well as the consumption of products and water contaminated with pesticides.
- The widespread use of pesticides also leads ecologically sensitive tropical an sub-tropical countries to irreversible damage to the ecosystem and to the poisoning of drinking water, river water and underground water. This could be avoided if the adequate agricultural methods were used (adequate prevention).

Governments must protect the health of their population as well as nature (also as a basis for human life).

This obliges governments to:

- Avoid the indiscriminate import of pesticides.
- Promote ecological agriculture.
- Control the contamination of foodstuffs with pesticides. Punish severely those who surpass the tolerated maximum.

The measures proposed by the researchers Eguiazu and Motta would be of great help to governments that want to adopt them.

3. Mutagens in drinking water

Contamination of drinking water through pathogenic microorganisms and harmful substances plays an important role in industrialized countries. However, this situation is even worse in developing countries. Due to the increasing diminution of drinking water, this situation will worsen in the future.

Therefore, preventive measures for drinking water must be a priority. Waterworks plants must be improved and more should be built.

This should be an official obligation (protection of health population).

The research proposals to study drinking water (production and control) must be hailed and thanked by the officials who should support them financially.

4. Evaluation of negative consequences of Technology

Over the last decade, many institutes and work groups were established to study the consequences of technology. This was based on the increasing disappointment of the population for the frivolous way in which highly risky technologies (atomic energy, genetic engineering, pesticides, etc.) are used. An increasing prevention of risks is yet not observable, since short term economic and political interests stop this from happening.

It is not until great catastrophes take place (nuclear reactors, chemicals factories, contamination of large surfaces, wasting of aquifer through industry and subsequent loss of agriculture due to the lack of aquifer, etc.) that discussions on how to study and deal with the harmful consequences of technology arise. However, this is done in a temporary manner, although with a high temporary agitation.

INCABIE, the Institute for research, study and prevention of negative consequences of technique in different fields, must be hailed favorably by those in charge of the politics, administration and economy. This institute can contribute substantially to early recognition and prevention in order to put a stop not only to economic loss but also to harming the population health (in the workplace, for example, in the case of emissions due to technical flaws, or to population under risk). Developed countries have a vast amount of material to teach this.

A critical and transparent society represented by ethical and responsible persons in charge of politics and administration, must be manifested through the choice of technologies balanced with health and nature. This must have a substantial influence on the producers of these technologies, compelling them to use the best technologies under development or already in use.

5. First Results

The large amount of scientific publications by this group shows, on the one hand, their successful activity even under completely unfavorable conditions. On the other hand, it shows the need for Argentina to have institutions like INCABIE.

I strongly recommend this group is given the appropriate place to carry out their scientific work. I also recommend this Institute, which is so important for Argentine population, is given regular financial support. This minimal support will enable the group to obtain further financial support from other interested parties in order to improve their working conditions as well as allowing the group to travel to foreign institutions and to scientific congresses.

Kiel, May 6, 1996
Professor Dr. Otmar Wassermann

Note: Neither the authority and prestige of Prof. Wassermann nor his laudatory concepts to our Program and recommendation of support to our Program were considered by our authorities. We have never received financial support. What's more, our Institute was dismantled.

IV.   Comment on Prof. Per Jacobsson's letters

A very interesting exchange of correspondence began between us and Prof. Per Jacobsson, from Kungliga Tekniska Högskolan (Stockholm) after he learned about our disciplinary proposal.

We now include the comments we made in reference to Prof. Jacobsson's letters from January 7th, 2004, and to his reply to those comments on a letter dated June 30th, 2004.

Comment on Prof. Jacobsson's letter from January 7th, 2004

On your letter you express some concepts we endorse, which we have held for a long time. When you make reference to the ambiguity of the word *ethics* in Science and its possible usurpation to be used in a vain rhetoric we can't but agree with you. We believe the same, extending the concept to many other activities that easily lose objectivity and sense in order to be made political or ideological.

An example of this is the use (or we should say *bad use*) of the expression *Human Rights*. Where it says *human* it should actually say *some of the victims, but not all of them*. We have never heard of the *human right* of the researcher to not be morally harassed or persecuted for being an innovator, especially in fields nobody wants to objectify and bring to light. Nor we have heard of a human right to not being subject to political pressures to accept indecorous proposals regarding public money or hiding the truth. We attach a very interesting article on Dr. Favaloro's suicide in Argentina, which has similarities with Dr. Kelly's suicide in England. Both had to resist pressures after rejecting non-ethical proposals.

Persecution and harassment in the workplace in the scientific world are taboos within the scientific community itself.

Another case of usurpation of a term is *Ecology*. Contamination, technological risks etc., all have become *ecological* problems.

You make reference to the problem of *neutrality,* and here we also agree with you. That was our question ever since we learned about the 1972 Stockholm Conference on Environment: What is the most neutral way to express what is happening? What is the most exact and synthetic way to define, using the least possible words, the environmental problem? That is how we arrived to the narrow definition of a phenomenon: Error or defect immanent to technique with consequences on human health, for which we created the term Technopathogeny. This we consider the most neutral definition of our approach on environment and technique. Following your reasoning, the *neutral description good reasons* is what we have expressed and researched through Technopathogenology (as we expressed during the 2000 Stockholm INES conference).

After we isolated the technopathogenic phenomenon, we began to search for a discipline to explain it and provide prophylaxis to it. Soon we moved away from our technical-biological background to try to find such discipline. Our hypothesis was that a new specific discipline was needed, so we subjected this to a Popperian falsification by contrasting it with other disciplines. If we were able to totally frame the phenomenon within an existing discipline, we would have falsified our hypothesis, forcing us to forget about the problem. The hypothesis was not falsified, since we could not find an existing discipline to frame the phenomenon.

When we talk about the concept of *ethics* in relation to the technopathogenic phenomenon, we do it after having investigated several general human attitudes as well as several others that are specific to the scientist in the generation of knowledge. We can therefore talk about ethics in a non-vain way but specifically providing grounds for each attitude described. We attach two works that discuss such attitudes. We also attach a work in German on the necessity of the neutrality you talk about in order not to fall into a technophilia or a technophobia while contributing to a Techno-patho-geno-logy; a specific science we consider the only neutral way to study this phenomenon, which is a science in its own right that cannot be framed within the existing ones.

It is common in science to try to blame *another discipline* for an unexpected negative phenomenon. It is common to hear famous physicians talk about the risks of pesticides and about how bad and without ethics the agronomists work in the field. Those very physicians are silent about the calamities produced by the pharmaceutical industry (of which Thalidomide is a clear example).

Therefore – if we have grasped your concept – neutrality is lost and the term *ethics* is usurped in a banal way. An explanation for this is that every discipline defends itself, and that there is not a specific science for the phenomenon (which is the thesis we defend). In the cases that science admits the phenomenon as an effect, it tries to explain it with fallacious concepts. In other words, it only tries to repair the technopathogenic effects that have already clearly manifested themselves but making sure it does not call them techno-patho-genies. Instead it calls them *environmental diseases*, diluting the responsibility the technologist's should have of *doing things well*, of gestating from the beginning a technology that does not carry the *germ* of a flawed genesis which remains hidden until its manifestation.

For example, in the past, most of the genetic diseases were only recognized by their phenotypical manifestation in the already born organism – hemophilia, for example, was recognized in children for their tendency to bleed. Nowadays the gene responsible for hemophilia can be recognized way before birth. Nevertheless, we cannot say that hemophilia was not latent in the fetus, or even in the fecundated ovum, before the mother new she was pregnant, or better yet, before the egg got implanted. In the same way, technopathogenies are latent in the *fertilized egg* of the newly gestated technology, but we do not have the tools and methodology for its early detection. Thus the need for a Technopathogenology: to develop tools and methodology that grows in consistency for the detection of those errors in the conception of a technique.

Due to our attempt to study the problem of technique from a neutral perspective called Technopathogenology, our career as scientists had to endure a true evaluative exclusion that in some cases turned into a clear case of moral harassment. We had to resist enormous pressures to abandon the chosen road to establish ourselves in an existing discipline, with the consequent risk of being forced to abandon our object of study for others to *usurp it.* After more than 30 years of resistance in the search of a science which was inspired by the 1972 Stockholm Conference, we lost all our basic rights as researchers:

- To a decent workplace.
- To the basic research tools.
- To a fair evaluation, etc.
- To a salary and position that are adequate to our performance.

Even though our theoretical development might have benefited from the lack of material resources and the open persecution, this is not an ideal situation.

Today we consider ourselves Technopathogenologists. We have trained, against all sorts of odds, students and professionals that showed interest in this subject; yet we were paid with salary and research subsidies cuts. Changes in research programs, paradigms or simply in methodologies are usually attacked by colleagues. It is the price to be paid for innovation, especially if such innovations expose non-ethical practices.

Dear Professor Jacobsson, using your own terminology we take those non-ethical practices and *objectify* them by subjecting them to the scientific method. We bring to light non-ethical practices and declare: *This is an object of research as worthy as cell membranes or ATP molecules.* Nevertheless, when we talk about Technopathogenology we are fundamentally referring to that *gray area* we have already mentioned: What is the cause of the flawed gestation (in the technopathogenic sense) of a technology? That is the basic question. Everything else – the so-called *environmental problem* – is a consequence of this unanswered question.

Many of these ideas are included in the work in Spanish that we have submitted for your evaluation.

Prof. Jacobsson's comments: Our analysis

We have selected some opinions and observations made by Prof. Jacobsson on a letter dated June 30th, 2004 in response to our letter above. We have numbered the selections to facilitate the subsequent analysis.

1. "I understand the difficult situation of dissident scientists like you in Argentina. Here, in the relative tranquility of a Swedish University, it is easy to say that all the moral harassment that you have suffered is unacceptable and non-ethical."
2. "I have great hope that the combative spirit you have always shown will help you resist the moral and concrete oppression."
3. "Even when the Technopathogenology concept is relevant, it is still problematic. Analyzing the linguistic roots of the word "patho," which, as you know, comes from the Greek "pathos," we find that it means suffering. Nowadays it is associated with disease, hence its use in the word "pathology". Because of this, technopathogeny may be associated to the purely negative effects of technology. It is probable that for some people the term Technopathogenology minimizes technology's positive effects, which can be one of the reasons why there is resistance to the introduction of the concept."
4. "I propose you try to frame your subject within "Technological Assessment," which tries to study the balance between the positive and negative effects of the introduction of a new technology. An alternative could be "Environmental Impact Assessment," which is mandatory in the building of big infrastructures such as roads, bridges, etc., and which tries to predict the possible effects. It could also be included in "Life Cycle Assessment," which is internationally recognized as a good forecaster and assessor of the impact of technology, including its products, systems, etc. It may be easier for you to refer to these internationally recognized methods which would be essentially dealing with the same basic problem that Technopathogenology does."

Analysis of Professor Jacobsson's proposals

Regarding Point 1:

We see that our difficult situation is described by Professor Jacobsson as being truly persecutory, in the same way INES had done before.

Regarding Point 2:

Professor Jacobsson's recognition of our work filled us with satisfaction.

714

Regarding Point 3:

In reference to the use of the word *patho*, we consider that it is not negative; it is just precise. Its use in medicine is just so. In this case we refer to an unusual phenomenon, but one that does exist. It might be negative, even hurtful, for some persons that due to an excessive technophilia do not even want to recognize its existence. Professor Jacobsson's advice is based on fear of technologists. It would not be appropriate for an ethical conscience to modify the term out of fear. The word *patho* is shocking, but as a counter argument for its use we can say that what it is cannot be embellished. We are not criticizing every technique, just those that generate pathologies. The term is very precise and defines a pathogen that in this case is generated by a specific technique as part of Pathogenology, which is a recognized science. In other words, Technopathogenology is, if you may, a part of the science that studies pathogens, which is called Pathology.

In reference to the fact that Technopathogenology only considers negative aspects, we admit it is so; we think those negative aspects of technology must be focused conceptually in a precise manner. If, out of excessive technophilia, those negative aspects are not precisely and conceptually focused, it does not mean that they will cease to exist.

Regarding Point 4:

Something similar to what happens with Iatrogenesis happens in the so-called *hard* technologies. They also have their *iatrogenic diseases*. Unlike proper Iatrogenesis, they begin with an alteration of the environment that after a series of causalities will have a negative incidence in the human being exposed to such alteration.

The development of Technological Assessment in developed countries is proof of their importance (Bohret & Franz, 1982) (Daschen, 1983) (PNUMA, 1982).

Regardless of the possibility to frame our proposal within either *Technology Assessment, Environmental Impact Assessment*, or *Life Cycle Assessment*, after the wide description and justification presented in this work, we consider that is not possible. None of them proposes the criteria included in Technopathogenology, which we believe will achieve effective protection.

The above mentioned disciplines deal with the problem of the *introduction* of new technologies, and not with their creation process.

Another important aspect is that, as Risk Assessment and Risk Management do, they propose to deal with the problem in a Multidisciplinary manner, with the subsequent lack of framing for some problems. *Environmental Impact Assessment* for instance, assess the effect constructions have in the environment, but things that are related with the construction itself, as is the case of the *Sick building Syndrome, Tight Building Syndrome,* and/or *Closed Building Syndrome* are apparently not included.

Having discussed it when we analyzed Technological Assessment, we can apply what have we said about Risk Assessment and Risk Management to *Environmental Impact Assessment* and *Life Cycle Assessment*. These disciplines also focus on what we could call *Risks by Action*, or rather, *Risks by evident Action*. What they do not bear in mind are the aspects considered by Technopathogenology: unexpected risks, risks which, within this framework we could define as *Non-evident risks by Action*. They do not consider either the risks entailed by the absence of factors – which we have referred to when we dealt with new quality criteria, among them, Biological Quality – such as the diminishing or loss of vitamins, which we could call *Risks by Omission*.

The disciplines proposed by Prof. Jacobsson, like many others, only allow for an *a posteriori* control of the effects.

V. Comments by Dr. Christian Hedinger, secretary of SAGUF

A few explanatory points:
- SAGUF had known of our activities for ten years prior to this letter.
- G.M. Eguiazu became a member of the Association shortly after its creation.
- The fragments quoted from the letter are written in quotation marks.
- Some explanatory notes are included at the end.

"It is not customary of our organization to address the government of another State in this manner, but, given this is a case of special concern to us, we beg you to intervene in person."

"In fact, due to reasons we find unexplainable, the Institute INCA-BIE from Rosario is hindered from its possibility to carry out its research work. We beg you then to request an independent investigation to clarify the actual circumstances that have led to this situation."[9]

"The ideas that conduct their work in the field of Technogenology are extremely interesting and highly stimulating to collaborate in our European efforts to improve the research on Ecology. Moreover, we believe that their research and educational activity in Argentina constitute a strong impulse to protect the environment in your country."

"We have learnt through a series of letters and documents that for some time their work has been facing fierce opposition. We do not understand, for example, why was it not possible to provide to their basic needs in connection to the setting up of their laboratory. A member of the Directive Board of SAGUF [10], a professional chemist, could see for himself that it is impossible to carry out an efficient work with such lack of resources. This is particularly striking given the fact that apparently there is a gas chromatographer in good conditions stored in the basement of the University which the researchers are not allowed to use."

"This endangers a highly important research that is internationally recognized!" [11]

"SAGUF is an association affiliated to the Swiss Academy of Natural Sciences and an academic society whose aim is to promote and coordinate the research on Ecology in Switzerland and abroad. SAGUF organizes symposiums and fosters multidisciplinary research. It represents Swiss research on environment before international organizations. SAGUF supports new scientific approaches abroad which give new impulse to the international community of researchers."

---

9   In August 2002, INCABIE was dismantled.
10 Dr. Merian visited INCABIE in person.
11 Comment of Dr. Hedinger in reference to the lack of financial support and human resources for the Institute.

"Being a Swiss national organization of research it is not our aim to meddle arrogantly on Argentine internal affairs. Nevertheless, we wish to call your attention to the fact that INCABIE does not receive any financial support and beg you that you request an investigation to clarify and remediate this situation."

"We thank you in advance and we trust you will give this matter your urgent attention. Sincerely yours," [12]

VI. Opinions by Dr. Hector José Huyke and Prof. Karl Mitcham [13]

Prof. Carl Mitcham was the chairman and Dr. Hector J. Huyke participant in the seminar *Science, Technology and Society*, Penn State University. USA – 1994.

Dr. Héctor José Huyke's opinion

"... A special discipline is proposed to detect and prevent the harmful consequences inherent and hidden in technologies. Founded in the spirit of true social progress through responsible science and technology, Technopathogenology is an innovating proposal which is highly valuable

---

12 This letter and its laudatory remarks towards our work were never considered. We even consider they were counter-productive and further simulated the harassing acts against us. As we have mentioned in one of the footnotes, ten years after this letter, a period during which we did not receive any support whatsoever, the INCABIE as an institute of experimental research was dismantled.

13 None of the two notes, just like the letter from SAGUF, had a positive repercussion. They were suspiciously followed by unacceptable reports by CONICET and the violent looting and eviction from the first location assigned to the Institute, as well as by a suspiciously negative result in a selection process at the University. As we have said, the Institute was violently closed, its goods distributed among members of the institution that requested the eviction on August 15, 2002.

for humankind. We would like to show with this letter that the ideas given in a seminar in which more than thirty researchers from around the world participated were received with great interest. I support their work as an outstanding germinal work of highly importance to the world..."

Dr. Carl Mitcham's opinion

"... The article presented in the seminar Science, Technology and Society – Penn State University: Technopathogenology, an answer to the need of preventing hidden negative effects in Technology was very well received by thirty participants from the United States and six other countries. The general consensus was that a critical problem was identified, especially the proposal of an interdisciplinary research of specific social problems associated to contemporary technology, oriented towards highly desirable new developments in the field of science, technology and society. The importance of this work and its high quality in the seminar, contributed to a valuable perspective representing not only the University of Rosario but also Argentine culture. The fact that this was the only Latin American presentation, made it more important still. We hope that in the future this article can be published in English fully or in part. In the name of all the representatives of the seminar I would like to thank you for presenting this article in the seminar."

VII. Letter by International Network of Engineers and Scientist for Global Responsibility (INES) to the Rector of Universidad Nacional de Rosario

Amsterdam, 27 January 2000

Dear President,

As the Chairman of the Internacional Network of Engineers and Scientists for Global Responsibility (INES), I am writing you on behalf of Dr. G,M. Eguiazu and Mr. A. Motta and their research activities at the Instituto for Biological Quality and Ecotoxicology (INCABIE). INES is a non-profit internacional non-government organization (NGO), recognized by the United Nations and the European Community. The Ethics Protection Initiative INESPE, protecting and encouraging ethical engagement, is a project of INES.

INES stimulates and protects persons or groups of persons who try to bring ethics principles into practice in their professional work. We consider the principles and objectives of INCABIE highly praiseworthy and of implicit ethical content. Therefore, Dr. Eguiazu and Mr. Motta have been invited as participants of INESPE and Dr. Eguiazu is appointed as INESPE representative in Argentina. Moreover, Dr. Eguiazu has been invited as a speaker at the international INES conference "Challenges for Science and Engineering in the 21st Century" in June of this year in Stockholm, Sweden. Specifically, he should act at this conference in the workshop "Towards a culture of individual and institutional responsibility."

INCABIE should be supported and should enjoy the necessary academic and scientific freedom to carry out its objectives. With this letter we expect to contribute to the continúity of INCABIE's valuable investigations.

Yours sincerely,
Prof. Dr. Armin Tenner

Note: This letter and its laudatory remarks towards our work were never considered. On March, 2000 the University Superior Board provided the dismantling of the institute INCABIE.

VIII. Letter by Greenpeace Argentina to the Rector of Universidad Nacional de Rosario (August 3, 2002) [14]

Buenos Aires, August 3, 2002

Dear Sir,

I wish to draw your attention to the work carried out by the Institute of Biological and Ecotoxicological Quality (INCABIE), dependent on the Universidad Nacional de Rosario.

We have observed that this institute – which is a local representative of INESPE (International Network of Engineers and Scientists' Projects on Ethics) – makes an immense contribution to academic research and education.

The reason of this letter is to promote the work carried out in IN-CABIE by Dr. G.M. Eguiazu and Mr. Alberto Motta.

It is our wish that this letter contributes to the work of INCABIE.

With Best Wishes,

Emiliano Ezcurra Estrada
Biodiversity Campaign Coordinator
Greenpeace Argentina

---

14   The effect of this note sent on August 3, probably received two or three days later, was completely the opposite to what we expected. The INCABIE was violently closed on August 15th, its goods distributed among friends of the University heads. Its members were abandoned and ostracised by the University. The harassing attitudes continued systematically after that.

Detailed Table of Contents

CHAPTER II – Technopathogeny –
Its disciplinary orphanage and a framing proposal

729

CHAPTER IV – Technopathogenology and its impact on society

734

735

Bibliography

Abrahamson, E. (2007) "A perfect mess. The hidden benefits of disorder" (Interview to the author, Professor University of Columbia), *Diario La Nación* (Buenos Aires, 11 de febrero).

ADUIC (Asociación de Directivos de Unidades de Investigación del CONICET) *Observaciones Críticas a la Propuesta de Pautas Evaluativas para el CONICET* (Manuscript).

Aguayo, A.M. & H. Martínez Amores (1958) *Pedagogía* (7th edition, La Habana).

Albertini, R.J. & R.B. Hayes (1997) "Somatic Cell Mutations in Cancer Epidemiology", in: Toniolo, P., et al., eds., *Application of Biomarkers in Cancer Epidemiology, IARC Scientific Publication*, 142 (Lyon), 159-184.

Alfred (2011) *Que es la Nomofobia* (Document in internet) <http://www.yaestaellisto.com/que-es-la-nomofobia/>.

Amin, R.P., et al. (2002) "Genomic Interrogation of Mechanism(s) Underlying Cellular Responses to Toxicants", *Toxicology*, 181/182, 555-563.

Andersen, H.C. "El traje nuevo del emperador". Biblioteca Digital Ciudad Seva <http://www. ciudadseva.com /textos/cuentos/euro /andersen /trajenue.htm>.

Anger, W.K. (1993) "Behavioral Biomarkers to Identify Neurotoxic Effects", in: Travis, C.C., ed., *Use of Biomarkers in Assessing Health and Environmental Impacts of Chemical Pollutants* (New York), 159-168.

Anonymous (1993) Comment appeared in the newspaper: *Braunschweiger Zeitung* (Brunswig, 31 Juli).

Anonymous (1996) "*Cultivos modificados por ingeniería genética en los campos argentinos y sus impactos sobre el medio ambiente, la salud y la economía*" (Manuscript, Greenpeace).

Anonymous (1999) "*Centros de diversidad. La riqueza biológica de los cultivos tradicionales: una herencia mundial amenazada por la contaminación genética*" (Manuscript, Greenpeace).

Anonymous (2000a) "*Alimentos transgénicos en boca de todos: Debate y Acción desde los consumidores. Para Día mundial de los derechos del Consumidor*" (Greenpeace).

Anonymous (2000b) "Academic Freedom: is it dying out (the case of Arpad Pusztai)", *The Ecologist*, 30 (2).

Anonymous (a) Polish thought <www.rinconcastellano.com>.

Anonymous (b) *Risikomanagement* (Document in Internet) <http://www.elektro.de/lexikon.php?article=Kategorie:Risikomanagement>.

Anonymous (c) *Acoso Moral – Las 45 Acciones por Heinz Leymann* <http://www.acosomoral.org/leyman45.htm>.

Ariosto, L. (1474-1533) Thought <www.rinconcastellano.com>.

Asscher, W. (1999) *The impact of genetic Modification on Agriculture, Food and Health*, An Interim Statement Printed by the British Medical Association.

Bardoux, C. (1997) "Research on Biomedical Ethics in the European Community", in: Gindro, et al., eds., *Research on Bioethics – Bioethics Research: Policy, Methods and Strategies – Proceedings of a European Conference – Roma, 23-25 November 1995*, European Comission. Report EUR 17465 EN, 17-18.

Bateson, P.P.G. (1999) "Genetically modified potatoes", *The Lancet*, 354, 1382.

Baumgartner, A. (1988) „Postmoderne als babylonisches Sprachverwirrung", *Universitas*, 8, 885-894.

Beck, H. (1969) „Die philosophische Frage nach der Zukunft und das Ereignis der Technik", in: *Wissenschaft und Weltbild. Zeitschrift für Grundfragen der Forschung* (Wien), 122-132.

Beck, H. (1970) „Revokation des Todes? Zur ethischen und anthropologischen Problematik der modernen medizinischen Technik", *Philosophia naturalis. Archiv für Naturphilosophie und die philosophischen. Grenzgebiete der exakten Wissenschaften und Wissenschaftsgeschichte*, 12, 116-122.

Beck, H. (1972) „Der Mensch als freier Automat? Zur kybernetischen Struktur von Materie und Geist", in: Szydzik, St. E., Hsg., *Kritik – Autorität, Dienst* (Bonn), 127-144.

Beck, H. (1974) „Geist und Technik", in: Heitmann, C. & H. Mühlen, Hsg., *Erfahrung und Theologie des Heiligen Geistes* (Hamburg, München).

Beck, H. (1977) „Neufassung des Begriffs der ‚Solidarität' als Lösung fundamentaler Probleme der technisierten Gesellschaft", in: Braun, E., Hsg., *Gesellschaft als politischer Auftrag* (Graz, Wien, Köln), 171-192.

Beck, H. (1979a) *Kulturphilosophie der Technik*. Spee Verlag, Trier.

Beck, H. (1979b) „Thesen zur Kulturphilosophie der Technik", *Philos, Jahrb. der Görres-Gesellschaft*, 86, 262-272.

Beck, H. (1981) „Philosophische Probleme zu kybernetischen Prozessen in der Gesellschaft", in: Schauer, H. & M. Tauber, Hsg., *Informatik und Philosophie* (Wien, München).

Beck, H. (1982) "Tesis fundamentales sobre la ́Filosofía de la Cultura ́ en la época de la técnica", in: Gonzalez López, J., ed., *Crisis de valores* (Quito), 283-301.

Beck, H. (1984) "Técnica entre sentido y contrasentido. El desafio histórico de la cultura contemporánea" – *Confrontación de la Teología y la Cultura. Actas del III Simposio de la Teología Histórica* (Valencia), 211-223.

Beck, H. (1986) "Bio-social determination or responsible freedom?", in: Mitcham, C. & A. Huhnuing, eds., *Philosophy and technology* (Dordrecht, Boston, Lancaster, Tokyo), 85-95.

Beck, H. (1987) „Aufgabe der Geisteswissenschaften in der Technikkultur – Neue Technologien und die Herausforderung an die Geisteswissenschaften", in: Graf von Westphalien, von R., Hsg., *Studien zu Bildung und Wissenschaft 54* (Bonn), 44-64.

Beck, H. (1999a) "América Latina como Encuentro Cultural Creativo", Conferencia, U. N. R. (Rosario).

Beck, H. (1999b) "La Contrariedad Complementaria entre los Hemisferios Culturales de Europa, de Africa y de Asia en Punto de Partida de América". Lecture, summary of article "Europa – Africa – Asien. Komplementarietät der Weltkulturen", in: Schadel, E., ed., *Ganzheitliches Denken*. Festschrift für Arnulf Rieber zum 60. Geburtstag. Prologue: Heinrich Beck (*Schriften zur Triadik und Ontodinamik*) (Frankfurt, Berlin, Bern, New York, Wien), 10, 51-82.

Beck, H. (2000) "Letters" (personal communication).

Belitz, H.D. & W. Grosch (1992) *Lehrbuch der Lebensmittel – Chemie* (4. Auflage, Springer-Lehrbuch), (Berlin).

Bembibre, C. *Siempre ha existido el acoso moral*, Interview with Marie-France Hirigoyen <http://librosyrecuerdos.blogspot.com/2009_07_01_archive.html>.

Berger, A. (1999) "Hot Potato", *BMJ*, 318, 611.

Beringer, J. (1999) "Keeping watch over genetically modified crops and foods", *The Lancet*, 353, 605.

Bierce, A. (1842-1914) Thought. Viaje Literario <http://www.frasesycitas.com/verfrase-la-politica-conduccion-asuntos-publicos-provecho-p/cita-sin-clasificar-2566.html>.

Bingman, I. (1993) *Environmental Information als Basic Human Right.* Nordic Council of Ministers.

Bohme, G. (1986) „Hat der Fortschritt eine Zukunft?", *Universitas*, 41, 929-938.

Böhret, K. & P. Franz (1982) *Technologiefolgen – Abschätzung* (Speyer).

Bompiani, A. (2000) "Riflessioni etiche sulla produzione e commercializzazione di organismi vegetali ed animali geneticamente modificati", *Medicina e Morale*, 3, 449-504.

Borges, J.L. Humorous and ironic thought. Public communication.

Bracalentti, R & E. Mordini (1997) "Foreword", in: Gindro, et al., eds., *Research on Bioethics – Bioethics Research: Policy, Methods and Strategies – Proceedings of a European Conference* – Roma, 23-25 November 1995, European Comission. Report EUR 17465 EN, 15-16.

Bressan, R.A., et al. (1995) "Understanding the Structure/Function of PR-5 Anti-Fungal Proteins" – *Aflatoxin Elimination Workshop* – October 23-24, Atlanta, Georgia, USA, 13.

Brown, P. (1999) "Lancet editor defends decision to publish GM research paper", *BMJ*, 319, 1089.

Brown, P. (2000) *The promise of Plant Biotechnology – The Threat of Genetically Modified Organisms.* College of Agriculture and Environm Sci./University of California.

Brown, R., et al. (2001) "The Identification of Maize Kernel Resistance Traits through Comparative Evaluation of Aflatoxin-Resistant with Susceptible Germplasm" – *Proceedings of the 1st Fungal Genomics, 2nd Fumonisin Elimination and 14th Aflatoxin Elimination Workshops* – October 23-26, Arizona, U.S.A.

Brundtland, G.H. (1988) *Nuestro futuro común*, Alianza Editorial.

Bruno, M., et al. *De que estamos hablando.* <http://www.cta.org.ar/base/IMG/pdf/ate_violencia_laboral.pdf>.

Bultmann, A. (1996) *Gewissenlose Geschäfte* (München).

Bultmann, A. (1997) *Auf der Abschussliste – Wie kritische Wissenschafter mundtot gemach werden sollen* (München).

Bultmann, A. "World Transition, Whistleblowing und Civil Courage to Protect Social Peace", EOLSS – UNESCO Lexicon (forthcoming).

Bundesministerium für Jugend, Familie und Gesundheits (1976) „Verordnung über Höchstmengen an Aflatoxinen in Lebensmitteln" (Aflatoxin Verordnung), Bundesgesetzblatt, 1, 3313.

Bunge, M. (1988) *La ciencia su método y su filosofía* (Buenos Aires).

Buntzel, R. (2006) „Braucht man die Agro-Gentechnik, um die Welt zu ernähren?", *Umwelt Medizin Gesellschaft*, 19/2, 146-148.

Burke, E. (1729-1797) Thought < www.mundocitas.com>.

Burkhart, J.G., et al. (2000) "Strategies for Assessing the Implications of Malformed Frogs for Environmental Health", *Environmental Health Perspectives*, 108, 83-90.

Cantú, C. (1804-1895) Thought <http:/ /recursostic.educacion.es/observa torio/web/ca/cajon-de-sastre/38-cajon-de-sastre/622-monografico-radio-escolar-ii?start=2>.

Carrel, A. (1949) La Incógnita *del Hombre* (Buenos Aires).

Carrington, C.D., et al. (1988) "In Vivo 31P Nuclear Magnetic Resonance Studies on the Absorption of Triphenyl Phosphite and Tri-O-Cresyl Phosphate Following Subcutaneous Administration in Hens", *Drug Metabolism and Disposition*, 16/1, 104-109.

Cervantes, M. (1547-1616) Thoughts <www.rinconcastellano.com>.

Chadwick, R. & M. Levitt (1997) "Complementary: Multidisciplinary Research in Bioethics", in: Gindro, et al., eds., *Research on Bioethics – Bioethics Research: Policy, Methods and Strategies – Proceedings of a European Conference* – Roma, 23-25 November 1995, European Comission. Report EUR 17465 EN, 73-82.

Channarayappa, N.J. & T. Ong (1992) "Cytogenetic Effects of Vincristine Sulfate and Ethylene Dibromide in Human Peripheral Lymphocitoes: Micronucleus Análisis", *Env. And Mol. Mutagenesis*, 20, 117-126.

Chapin, R.E. & J. Phelps (1990) "Recent Advances in Testicular Cell Culture: Implications for Toxicology", *Toxic. In Vitro*, 4/4,5, 543-559.

Chargaff, E. (1989) „Erforschung der Natur und Denaturierung des Menschen", *Universitas*, 3, 205-214.

Chen, Z.Y., et al. (1997) "A Maize Kernel Trypsin Inhibitor is Associated with Resistence to Aspergillus flavus Infection" – *Aflatoxin Elimination Workshop* – October 26-28, Memphis, TN, USA.

Christie, B. (1999) "Scientists call for moratorium on genetically modified foods", *The Lancet*, 318, 483.

Clarín (2000) "Protesta ecologista en un supermercado por alimentos con cambios genéticos", Clarín Webpage, <http://www.clarin.com/>.

Colacilli de Muro, M. A. & J. C. (1978) *Elementos de Lógica Moderna y Filosofía* (Buenos Aires).

Comte, A. (1982) *Discurso sobre el espíritu positivo* (Buenos Aires).

Concejo Municipal de la Ciudad de Rosario (1991) Decreto 8270 Concejo Municipal "Programa de Investigación de la Calidad Biológica y Ecotoxicológica del Entorno Humano".

Congress of the United States – Office of Technology Assessment (1981) *Assessment of Technologies for Determining Cancer Risks from the Environment* – OTA.

Constitución de la Nación Argentina Art. 41. Constitución de la Nación Argentina – Artículo 41 de la Costitución Nacional, Jefatura de Gabinete de Ministros – Secretaría de Ambiente y Desarrollo Sustentable <http://www2.medioambiente.gov.ar /mlegal/consti/art41.htm>.

Corneille, P. (1606-1684) Thought <www.rinconcastellano.com>.

Cottam, C. (1946) "DDT and Its Effect on Fish and Wildlife". *Journal of Economic Enthomology,* 39/1, 44-52.

Crawford, M.A. (1999) "Genetically modified foods", *The Lancet*, 353, 1531.

Daschen, H. (1983) *Summary and Evaluation of the Internationales Symposium: Uber die Roller der Technologiefolgenabschätzung im Entscheidungsprozess*, Umwelbundesamt. BRD.

De Boer, W. (1984a) „Der Ursprung der Wissenschaft", *Universitas*, 39, 149-157.

De Boer, W. (1984b) „Der Ursprung der modernen Wissenschaft", *Universitas*, 39, 357-368.

De Boer, W. (1987) „Das Versagen der Aufklärung", *Universitas*, 42, 116-125.

De Gondi, P. (1613-1679) Reference of the author to Cardenal de Retz. France.

De Jouvenal, B. (1971) *La administraciòn de la Tierra* (Buenos Aires).

DeBord, D.G., et al. (1995) "Alterations of Histone Phosphorilation in Rat Spleen Cells After Treatment with Aromatic Amine, 4,4´-Methylene-bis(2-Chloroaniline)", *J. Biochem. Toxicology*, 10/1, 19-23.

Defensor del Pueblo de la Nación (2000) NOTA D.P. N° 07274 – 13/04/2000.

Dehn, G. (2000) Personal communication.

Deiserot, D. (1997) *Berufsethische Verantwortung in der Forschung* <http://www.friedenskooperative.de/ff/ff97/5-12.htm>.

Deiserot, D. (2001) *Whistleblowing in Zeiten von BSE – Der Fall der Tierärztin Dr. Margrit Herbst* (Berlin).

Denevi, M. (2002) Commentary in newspaper. Cited by Reichamn, *Diario La Nación* (Buenos Aires) .

Descartes, R. (1945) *Obras Filosóficas* (Buenos Aires).

DGUHT (2007) Personal communication. Letter January 10, 2007.

Diccionario "El Pequeño Larousse Ilustrado". Editorial Larousse, Barcelona, México, París, Buenos Aires, 1997.

Diccionario Enciclopédico Ilustrado de la Lengua Española. Editorial Ramonón Sopena, España, 1962.

Doucet, F. (1978) *Intuitions-Training* (München).

Druker, B. & B. Roth (1999) Press releaseAlianza por la BIO-integridad – 24 Junio.

Dubois, F. (2009) "¿Debemos tener miedo al. teléfono movil?", *Research eu, Revista del Espacio Eurpoeo de la Invesatigación,* 61, 38,39.

Dumur, L. Thought <www.citalandia.com.>.

Dutt, C. (1993) „Hans-Georg Gadamer im Gespräch", *Hermeneutik/Praktische Philosophie* (Heidelberg).

Eco, U. (2000) *¿Cómo se hace una tésis?* (Barcelona).

Eguiazu, G.D. Pbro. (2007) Personal communication.

Eguiazu, G.M. (1976) *Micotoxinas: Su Contaminación en Productos Agropecuarios. Segundo Premio Graduados – Ciencia y Tecnología al. Servicio de la Explotación Agropecuaria*, Bolsa de Comercio de Rosario (Rosario).

Eguiazu, G.M. (1977) "Investigaciones sobre aflatoxinas en maíz", *Segundas Jornadas de Comercialización Cerealista*, Bolsa de Comercio de Rosario, 30-31.

Eguiazu, G.M. (1978a) "Investigación sobre aflatoxinas en maíz. II parte", *Terceras Jornadas Nacionales de Comercialización Cerealista,* Bolsa de Comercio de Rosario, 59-66.

Eguiazu, G.M. (1978b) *Micotoxinas en Maíz. Resultados Analíticos del Aislamiento de Aflatoxina y su Agente Causal en Maíz de la Zona de Influencia de Rosario*, Bolsa de Comercio de Rosario (Rosario).

Eguiazu, G.M. (1979) "Exigencias del mercado internacional. Análisis de contaminantes: Aflatoxinas – (Estudio crítico del método Velazco)", *Cuartas Jornadas Nacionales de Comercialización Cerealista*, Bolsa de Comercio de Rosario, 33-36.

Eguiazu, G.M. (1983) „*Bildungsbedingungen von Aflatoxinen in Sonnenblumen*", Tesis Doctoral (Dr scienciarum agrarium) Universität von Stuttgart-Hohenheim (Stuttgart).

Eguiazu, G.M. (1984a) "Comportamiento de almacenaje del Girasol. I. Comportamiento de absorción de humedad atmosférica del aquenio, pericarpio y semilla del grano de girasol", *Grasas y Aceites*, 35, 246-250.

Eguiazu, G.M. (1984b) "Comportamiento de almacenaje del Girasol. III. Aparición del primer micelio visible como primer síntoma de deterioro, en función de la humedad crítica de la muestra, la humedad relativa ambiente y el tiempo de almacenaje", *Grasas y Aceites,* 35, 325-329.

Eguiazu, G.M. (1984c) "Comportamiento de almacenaje del girasol. IV. Efecto del alto porcentaje de anhídrido carbónico en la atmósfera del almacenaje sobre la conservabilidad del girasol", *Grasas y Aceites*, 35, 378-383.

Eguiazu, G.M. (1984d) "La contaminación ambiental en la legislación europea (Prevención de cancerígenos). I. Ley de Aflatoxina de la República Federal de Alemania", *Ambiente y Recursos Naturales*, 1/3, 103-106.

Eguiazu, G.M. (1985) "Las Micotoxinas desde una perspectiva antropoecológica" – *Actas XII Jornadas Argentinas de Micología* – San Luis – 9 al. 12 de Octubre, San Luís/Argentina, 95-109.

Eguiazu, G.M. (1986) "Comportamiento de almacenaje del girasol.V. Aparición espontánea de Aflatoxina y Esterigmatocistina en girasol almacenado bajo aire y 90 % CO2", *Grasas y Aceites*, 37, 25-28.

Eguiazu, G.M. (1987a) "Pesticidas y Profilaxis del Error Tecnológico", *Ambiente y Recursos Naturales*, 4/4, 81-91.

Eguiazu, G.M. (1987b) *Las Micotoxinas desde una perspectiva antropoecológica* (Rosario).

Eguiazu, G.M. (1988) *Plaguicidas y Error Tecnogénico – Primer Congreso Internacional de Ecotoxicología* (Rosario).

Eguiazu, G.M. (1990) "Fundamentación de una Ley de Profilaxis, Detección y Control de Micotoxinas en productos agropecuarios", *Ambiente y Recursos Naturales*, 7/1, 14-37.

744

Eguiazu, G.M. (1991) "Tecnogenología – Una respuesta a la necesidad de prevenir los efectos nocivos ocultos en la Técnica". Colección Tecnogenia 3, (Rosario).

Eguiazu, G.M. (1992) „Technogenologie: eine neue Präventivwissenschaft zur Früherkennung von Technikschäden", *Prima Philosophia*, 5, 161-165.

Eguiazu, G.M. (1993) *Profilaxis, Detección y Control de Micotoxinas.* Colección Tecnogenia 4, (Rosario).

Eguiazu, G.M. (1994) "El manejo de riesgos como nuevo modelo de la consulta agronómica", *Agrovisión Profesional*, 1/4, 6-10.

Eguiazu, G.M. (1996) "El Principio de Información y Consentimiento Previo (PICP) del Código de Conducta de la FAO: necesidad de una estricta norma universal", *UNR Ambiental*, 2, 46-58.

Eguiazu, G.M. (1998) *Manejo Postcosecha y calidad final para el consumidor.* Colección Tecnogenia 7, (Rosario).

Eguiazu, G.M. (1999a) "Aspectos tecnopatogenológicos de la aparición de micotoxinas: hipótesis antropoecológica", *UNR Ambiental*, 3, 95-124.

Eguiazu, G.M. (1999b) „Technopathogenologie: Aktive Gelassenheit in Hinblick auf extreme Technik-Auffassungen", *Schriften zur Triadik und Ontodynamik – Band 17 – Aktive Gelassenheit – Festschrift für H. Beck zum 70. Geburtstag* (Frankfurt am Main), 651-666.

Eguiazu, G.M. (2003) "Técnica Rápida, Simple y Económica para la Detección y Estimación Semicuantitativa de Aflatoxinas en Condiciones de Campo – Cámara Placa Autoactivada de Cromatografía", *Aposgrán*, 82/2, 49-62.

Eguiazu, G.M. & H.K. Frank (1982) "Rapid Method for the Detection of Aflatoxin B1 in Sunflower Seeds and Sunflower Seeds Products", *Handbook on Rapid Detection of Mycotoxins*, 32-36.

Eguiazu, G.M. & H.K. Frank (1983) "Demostration of Aflatoxins in Agricultural Products: A Simple Method suitable for Developing Countries", *European Journal of Appl. Microbiol and Biotechnology*, 18, 123-130.

Eguiazu, G.M. & H.K. Frank (1984) "Counts of Fungal Propagules and Acid number in Sunflower Seeds", *Fette Seifen Anstrichmittel*, 86/1, 16-18.

Eguiazu, G.M. & T. Grünewald (1984) "Comportamiento de almacenaje del Girasol. II. Cinética de la absorción para muestras de variado origen", *Grasas y Aceites*, 35, 320-324.

Eguiazu, G.M. & A. Motta (1985) "La Humedad Relativa Ambiente del Aire Intergranular como Parámetro del Deterioro Biológico del Girasol Almacenado" – *Actas XI Conferencia Internacional de Girasol*, Mar del Plata/Argentina, 821-826.

Eguiazu, G.M. & A. Motta (1986) "Relación entre contenido de agua y materia grasa en muestras comerciales de girasol para una humedad relativa ambiente del aire intergranular del 75%", *Grasas y Aceites*, 37, 307-312.

Eguiazu, G.M. & A. Motta (1991) *Programa de Investigación de la Calidad Biológica y Ecotoxicológica del Entorno Humano* (Rosario).

Eguiazu, G.M. & A. Motta (1992) "La calidad biológica y ecotoxicológica de Productos Agropecuarios. Un nuevo concepto en comercialización de granos", *Revista Bolsa de Comercio*, 1458, 26-28.

Eguiazu, G.M. & A. Motta (1996) "Calidad Total de Productos Agropecuarios: Fundamentos para un Proyecto Global", *Revista Bolsa de Comercio de Rosario,* 1470, 42-50.

Eguiazu, G.M. & A. Motta (1997) *Tecnogenia – Tecnología, Riesgos y Vías de Prevención*, UNR Editora (Rosario/Argentina).

Eguiazu, G.M. & A. Motta (2000) "Tecnopatogenología: una respuesta a la orfandad disciplinar de un fenómeno tecnológico", *Diosa Episteme*, VII, 6, 34-39.

Eguiazu, G.M. & A. Motta (2001a) "Tecnopatogenología: Sus Implicancias en Salud Humana y Económicas. Tecnogenia Ambiental: Necesidad de su Estudio Sistemático a fin de Evitar Pérdidas Económicas", *Realidad Económica*, 182, 94-114.

Eguiazu, G.M. & A. Motta (2001b) "Tecnopatogenología: Una Contribución Disciplinar para un Fenómeno Transdisciplinar", *UNR Ambiental,* 4, 48-64.

Eguiazu, G.M. & A. Motta (2001c) "Aspectos Tecnopatogenológicos de la Ingeniería Genética", *UNR Ambiental*, 4, 106-116.

Eguiazu, G.M. & A. Motta (2003) "Dificultades en el Diálogo Intercultural en Ciencia y Técnica y sus Consecuencias en el Avance Científico" – *1er Congreso Internacional de la AEI. ¿Cómo Conseguir el Diálogo Intercultural?* – Rosario, 26 al. 28 de Junio. Asociación de Estudios Interculturales (AEI), Centro de Producción Hipermedial, Instituto Rosario de Investigación en Ciencias de la Educación (IRICE) [Windows CD-ROM].

Eguiazu, G.M. & A. Motta (2004a) "Contribución a la Prevención del Deterioro por Ataque Fúngico Durante el Almacenaje, Análisis Tecnopatogenológico", *Aposgrán*, 87/3, 61-71.

Eguiazu, G.M. & A. Motta (2004b) „Nährungsqualität un Aflatoxine – Ergebnisse des Verbraucherschutz – Programms in Argentinien – Von Aflatoxinen zur Technopathogenologie" <http://www.schweisfurth.de/uploads/media/Vortrag_Schweissfurt_Internet_korr.pdf>.

Eguiazu, G.M. & A. Motta (2005a) "Evitar la Guerra y los Riesgos Tecnopatogénicos como Responsabilidad Global. Dos Iniciativas con una misma meta: la protección del ser humano". Presentation – *INES Council Meeting 2005* – Vaquerias, Córdoba, Argentina.

Eguiazu, G.M. & A. Motta (2005b) „Technopathogenologie – ein fachspezifischer Beitrag zu einem fachübergreifenden Phänomen – Teil 1: Transdisziplinäre Grundlagen", *Umwelt Medizin Gesellschaft*, 18/1, 41-48.

Eguiazu, G.M. & A. Motta (2005c) „Technopathogenologie – ein fachspezifischer Beitrag zu einem fachübergreifenden Phänomen – Teil 2: Entwicklung eines Forschungs- und Lehrprogramms", *Umwelt Medizin Gesellschaft*, 18/2, 137-141.

Eguiazu, G.M. & A. Motta (2006) "La evaluación tecnopatogenológica para la protección del consumidor. El caso de las aflatoxinas para su fundamentación", *UNR Ambiental*, 7, 267-297.

Eguiazu, G.M., et al. (2001) "Aparición de Mohos Potenciales Micotoxinógenos y Deterioro Controlado en Semillas de Zea mays de Uso Regular en la Argentina. Falsación de la Hipótesis Antropo-Ecológica", *Aposgrán*, 75/4, 36-42.

Eguiazu, G.M., et al. (2004) "Etica en Ciencia y Técnica – Fundamentos para un Mecanismo de Protección a los Objetores Eticos", *Humanitas 2004, Anuario del Centro de Estudios Humanísticos*, Universidad Autónoma de Nuevo León, 201-211.

Elmore, R. (2000) Communication, Nebraska University Institute of Agriculture and Natural Resources.

EMCA (2003) "Aceite Supresor de Polvo", *Aposgrán*, 81/1.

Emde, Günter / Ethikschutzinitiative (INESPE). (1995) *Wenn das Gewissen nein sagt – Ethisch handeln in der abhängigen Arbeit. Ein Ratgeber in Konfliktfällen.* (Pittenhart).

Ese, A. (1985) „Humangenetik in rechtlicher und sozialpolitischer Sicht", *Universitas*, 4, 735-748.

Esquivel, M.C. & M.L. Masteloni. *Tecnología 9° Año*, Escuela Superior de Comercio, Rosario.

European Commission (1997) *EURO-OP NEWS*. 3 – 1997.

Ewen, S.W. & A. Pusztai (1999) "Effects of diets containing genetically modified potatoes expressing Galanthus nivalis lectin on rat small intestine", *The Lancet*, 354, 1353-1354.

Ewen, S.W. & A. Pusztai (1999) "Health risks of genetically modified foods", *The Lancet,* 354, 684.

FAO (1982) Organización de las Naciones Unidas para la Agricultura y la Alimentación. *Perspectiva sobre Micotoxinas. Estudio FAO Alimentación y Nutrición*, 13, (Roma).

FAO (1985) Food and Agriculture Organization of the United Nations. "Residues of Veterinary Drugs in foods". FAO, *Food and Nutrition Paper*, 32, (Rome).

FAO (1986) Food and agriculture Organization of the United Nations. *International Code of Conduct on the Distribution an Use of Pesticides,* (Rome).

FAO (1990) Food and agriculture Organization of the United Nations. *Código Internacional de Conducta para la Distribución y Utilización de Plaguicidas – Versión enmendada,* (Roma).

FAO (1994) Food and Agriculture Organization of the United Nations. *Proceedings, Seminario Taller para Aplicación del Código de Conducta Para la Distribución y Utilización de Plaguicidas – 5 al. 8 de Diciembre,* Rosario.

Fatone, V. (1969) *Lógica e Introducción a la Filosofía*. (Buenos Aires).

Fedan, S.F. (2001) "Hard Metal-Induced Disease: Effects of Metal Cations in Vitro on Guinea Pig Isolated Airways", *Toxicology and Applied Pharmacology,* 174, 199-206.

Feijoo, B.J. (1676-1764) Thought <http://www.citasyrefranes.com /famosas/autor/399>.

Feldbaum, C.B. (1999) "Health Risks of genetically modified foods", *The Lancet*, 354, 70.

Ferioli, A., et al. (1986) "Drug-Induced Uroporphyria in Chicken Hepatocyte Cultures", in: Morris, C.R. & J.R.P. Cabral, eds., *Hexachlorobenzene: Proceedings of an International Symposium, IARC Scientific Publication*, 77 (Lyon), 465-466.

Fetscher, I. (1988) "Überlebensbedingungen der Menschheit – Zur Dialektik des Fortschritts", *Universitas Marksteine* 500, 266-275.

Feyerabend, P. (1986) *Tratado contra el Método* (Madrid).

Fisken, R A. (1999) "GM food debate", *The Lancet*, 354, 1729.

Fornallaz, P. (1986) *Die ökologische Wirtschaft* (Aarau, Stuttgart).

Fornallaz, P. (1988) „Früherkennung:Risiken und Risikomanagement", *Risiko und Risikomanagement Helbing und Lichtenhann*, 73-83.

FIBL (2006) *Qualität und Sicherheit von Bioprodukten,* Forschungs Institut für Biologische Landbau, Dossier Feb 2006 n 4 1 Auflage.

Frank, H.K. (1980-1983) Personal communications during the doctoral work.

Frankl, V. (1982) *Der Wille zum Sinn. Ausgewählte Vorträge über Logotherapie* (Bern).

Frankl, V. (1988) *The will to meaning – Foundations and Applications of logotherapy* (New York).

Fritsch, H. (1984) „Vom quantitativen zum qualitativen Wirtschaftswachstum", *Universitas*, 39, 639-650.

Fritsche, B. (1987) „Die zwei Gesichter des Fortschritts", *Universitas* 8, 747-752.

Fuch, Ch. (1972) <http://igw.tuwien.ac.at/christian/technsoz/technikfolgenabschaetzung.html>.

García de Ceretto, J. J. (2001) "El Desafío del Conocimiento en la Perspectiva del Pensamiento Complejo", *Forum 14*, 3/5, 6-15.

Gardner, M.J. (1991) "Father's Occupational Exposure to radiation and the raised levelof childhood leukemia near the Sellafield Nuclear Plant", *Environmental Health Perspectives*, 94, 5-7.

Gassen, H.G. (1988) „Abschätzung der Risiken in der Gentechnik, Bioinformatik und Biotechnologie", in: Gassen, H.G. and Knöpfel, P., *Risiko und Risikomanagement* (Basel), 11-29.

Gebhardm F. & K. Smalla (1998) "Transformation of Acinetobacter sp Strain BD413 by transgenic Sugar Beet DNA", *Applied and Environmental Microbiology*, 64, 1550-1554.

George, J.D., et al. (2002) "Evaluation of the Developmental toxicity of Formamide in New Zealand White Rabbits", *Toxicological Sciences*, 69/1, 165-174.

Germolec, D.R, et al. (1996) "Arsenic Induces Overexpression of Growth Factors in Human Keratinocytes", *Toxicology and Applied Pharmacology*, 141, 308-318.

Ghanem, M.M., et al. (2004) "Respirable Coal Dust Particles Modify Cytochrome P4501A1 (CYP1A1) Expression in Rat Alveolar Cells", *Am. J. Respir. Cell. Mol. Biol.*, 31, 171-183.

Goblot, E. (1943) *El Sistema de la Ciencias. Lo Verdadero, lo inteligible y lo real* (Buenos Aires).

Gomez Herrera, C. (1984) "El fraude y el engaño en la investigación científica", *Grasas y Aceites*, 35/1.

Gomez Perez, R. (1986) "Ciencia y Dignidad Humana – Cincuentenario de la Academia Pontificia de las Ciencias", *Aceprensa*, 39, sr153/86, 557-559.

Gomez, W. (2004) Personal communication.

Grafström, R.C., et al. (1987) "Pathobiological Effects of Aldehydes in Cultured Human Bronchial Cells", in: Bartsch, H., et al., eds., *Relevance of N-Nitroso Compounds to Human Cancer: Exposures and Mechanisms, IARC Scientific Publication,* 84 (Lyon), 443-445.

Greenpeace (1996) *Por que los productores agropecuarios deben evitar comprar la soja RR* (Manuscript).

Greenpeace (1998) *El costado peligroso de la ingeniería genetica* (Manuscript).

Greenpeace (2000) *Maíz transgénico. Una amenaza para la diversidad del maíz en México* (Manuscript).

Gu, Z.W., et al. (1992) "Micronucleus Induction and Phagocytosis in Mammalian Cells Treated with Diesel Emission Particles", *Mutation Research*, 279, 55-60.

Guggenberger, B. (1987) „Das Menschenrecht auf Irrtum", *Universitas,* 4, 307-317.

Guilford, J.P (1977) *La naturaleza de la inteligencia humana* (Buenos Aires).

Gutiérrez, A.A. (2003) *El acoso moral laboral: instrumentos jurídicos de defensa.* Dirección General de Trabajo y Seguridad Social de la Junta de Andalucía <http://www.acamlu.org/documents/ELACO-SOMORALLABORAL.pdf>.

Hansen, D.K. & T.F. Grafton (1994) "Comparison of Dexamethasone-Induced Embryotoxicity In Vitro in Mouse and Rat Embryos", *Teratogenesis, Carcinogenesis, and Mutagenesis*, 14, 281-289.

Hansen, M K. (1999) *Genetic engineering is not an extension of conventional Plant Breeding-How genetic engineering differs from conventional breeding, hybridization, wide crosses and horizontal gene transfer*. Research Association/Consumer Policy Institute/Consumers Union.

Hansson, M.G. (1999) *God sed i forskningen (Good conduct in research)* (Stockholm).

Heidegger, M. *Conceptos Fundamentales* (Barcelona).

Heisenberg, W. (1988) „Atomforschung und Kausalgesetz", *Universitas,* 500, 137-146.

Helgason, T., et al. (1984) "N-Nitrosamines in Smoked Meats and their Relation to Diabetes", in: O'Neil, I.K., et al., eds., *N-Nitroso Compounds: Occurrence, Biological Effects and Relevance to Human Cencer, IARC Scientific Publication,* 57 (Lyon), 911-920.

Herranz, G. (1982) "Límites Eticos de la Investigación Científica", *Sidec,* 419, 1-9.

Herskovits (1964) *El Hombre y sus Obras,* Fondo de Cultura Económica (México).

Hirigoyen, M.F. (2001) *El acoso moral en el trabajo* (Buenos Aires).

Hoffmann, M. (1997) *Vom Lebendigen in Lebensmitteln* (Holm).

Hoffner, J.K. (1980) *Mensch und Natur im technischen Zeitalter* (Bonn).

Hoffner, J.K. (1982) *Dimensionen der Zukunft,* SDB Verlag (Bonn).

Holden, P. (1999) "Safety of genetically engineered foods is still dubious", *BMJ,* 318, 332.

Horacio (65a.c-8a.c.) Thought <www.rinconcastellano.com>.

Horton, R. (1999a) "GM food debate – Comment of the editor", *The Lancet,* 354, 1729.

Horton, R. (1999b) "Health Risks of genetically modified foods", *The Lancet,* 353, 1811.

Huang, J.W., et al. (2003) "Using a combined assay of cell transformation and gene mutation in human fibroblasts to detect genotoxicity of chemicals", *Toxicology,* 191/1, Abstracts.

Huisman Fuentes, R.M. (2001) "Comentarios sobre las bases éticas de una conducta ecológicamente sostenible", *UNR Ambiental,* 4, 117-127.

IARC (1974) *IARC Monographs on the Evaluation of the Carcinogenic Risk of Chemical to Man – Some aromatic amines, hydrazine and related substances, N-Nitroso compounds and miscellaneous alkylating agents,* 4 (Lyon).

IARC (1975a) *IARC Monographs on the Evaluation of the Carcinogenic Risk of Chemical to Man – Some aromatic azo compounds,* 7 (Lyon).

IARC (1975b) *IARC Monographs on the Evaluation of the Carcinogenic Risk of Chemical to Man – Some aziridines, N-, S- & O-mustard and Selenium,* 9 (Lyon).

IARC (1976a) *IARC Monographs on the Evaluation of the Carcinogenic Risk of Chemical to Man – Some naturally occuring substances,* 10 (Lyon).

IARC (1976b) *IARC Monographs on the Evaluation of the Carcinogenic Risk of Chemical to Man – Cadmium, nickel, some epoxides, miscellaneous industrial chemicals and general considerations on volatile anaesthetics,* 11 (Lyon).

IARC (1976c) *IARC Monographs on the Evaluation of the Carcinogenic Risk of Chemical to Man – Some Carbamates, Thiocarbamates and Carbazides,* 12 (Lyon).

IARC (1977a) *IARC Monographs on the Evaluation of the Carcinogenic Risk of Chemical to Man – Some Miscellaneous Pharmaceutical Substances,* 13 (Lyon).

IARC (1977b) *IARC Monographs on the Evaluation of the Carcinogenic Risk of Chemical to Man – Asbestos,* 14 (Lyon).

IARC (1977c) *IARC Monographs on the Evaluation of the Carcinogenic Risk of Chemical to Humans – Some Fumigants, the Herbicides 2,4-D and 2,4,5-T, Chlorinated Dibenzodioxins and Miscellaneous Industrial Chemicals,* 15 (Lyon).

IARC (1978a) *IARC Monographs on the Evaluation of the Carcinogenic Risk of Chemical to Man – Some Aromatic Amines and Related Nitro Compounds – Hair Dyes, Colouring Agents and Miscellaneous Industrial Chemicals,* 16 (Lyon).

IARC (1978b) *IARC Monographs on the Evaluation of the Carcinogenic Risk of Chemical to Humans – Some N-Nitroso Compounds,* 17 (Lyon).

IARC (1978c) *IARC Monographs on the Evaluation of the Carcinogenic Risk of Chemical to Humans – Polychlorinated biphenyls and Polybrominated biphenyls,* 18 (Lyon).

IARC (1979a) *IARC Monographs on the Evaluation of the Carcinogenic Risk of Chemical to Humans – Some Monomers, Plastics and Synthetic Elastomers, and Acrolein,* 19 (Lyon).

IARC (1979b) *IARC Monographs on the Evaluation of the Carcinogenic Risk of Chemical to Humans – Some Halogenated Hydrocarbons,* 20 (Lyon).

IARC (1979c) *IARC Monographs on the Evaluation of the Carcinogenic Risk of Chemical to Humans – Sex Hormones (II)*, 21 (Lyon).

IARC (1980) *IARC Monographs on the Evaluation of the Carcinogenic Risk of Chemical to Humans – Some Pharmaceutical Drugs*, 24 (Lyon).

IARC (1981) *IARC Monographs on the Evaluation of the Carcinogenic Risk of Chemical to Humans – Some Antineoplastic and Immunosuppressive Agents*, 26 (Lyon).

IARC (1982a) *IARC Monographs on the Evaluation of the Carcinogenic Risk of Chemical to Humans – Some Aromatic Amines, Anthraquinones and Nitroso Compounds, and Inorganic Fluorides Used in Drinking-water and Dental Preparations*, 27 (Lyon).

IARC (1982b) *IARC Monographs on the Evaluation of the Carcinogenic Risk of Chemical to Humans – Some Industrial Chemicals and Dyestuffs*, 29 (Lyon).

IARC (1983a) *IARC Monographs on the Evaluation of the Carcinogenic Risk of Chemical to Humans – Some Food Additives, Feed Additives and Naturally Occurring Substances*, 31 (Lyon)

IARC (1983b) *IARC Monographs on the Evaluation of the Carcinogenic Risk of Chemical to Humans – Polynuclear Aromatic Compounds, Part 1, Chemical, Environmental and Experimental Data*, 32 (Lyon).

IARC (1984) *IARC Monographs on the Evaluation of the Carcinogenic Risk of Chemical to Humans – Polynuclear Aromatic Compounds, Part 2, Carbon Blacks, MineraL Oils (Lubricant Base Oils, and Derived Products), and some Nitroarenes*, 33 (Lyon).

IARC (1985a) *IARC Monographs on the Evaluation of the Carcinogenic Risk of Chemical to Humans – Polynuclear Aromatic Compounds, Part 4, Bitumens, Coal-tars and Derived Products, State-oils and Doots*, 35 (Lyon).

IARC (1985b) *IARC Monographs on the Evaluation of the Carcinogenic Risk of Chemical to Humans – Allyl Compounds, Aldehydes, Epoxides and Peroxides*, 36 (Lyon).

IARC (1985c) *IARC Monographs on the Evaluation of the Carcinogenic Risk of Chemical to Humans – Tobacco Habits Other than Smoking; Betel-Quid and Areca-Nut Chewing; and Some Related Nitrosamines*, 37 (Lyon).

IARC (1985d) *IARC Monographs on the Evaluation of the Carcinogenic Risk of Chemical to Humans – Some Chemicals Used in Plastics and Elastomers*, 39 (Lyon).

IARC (1986a) *IARC Monographs on the Evaluation of the Carcinogenic Risk of Chemical to Humans – Some Naturally Occurring and Synthetic Food Components, Furocumarins and Ultraviolet Radiation*, 40 (Lyon).

IARC (1986b) *IARC Monographs on the Evaluation of the Carcinogenic Risk of Chemical to Humans – Some Halogenated Hydrocarbons and Pesticide Exposures*, 41 (Lyon).

IARC (1987a*) IARC Monographs on the Evaluation of the Carcinogenic Risk of Chemical to Humans – Silica and Some Silicates*, 42 (Lyon).

IARC (1987b) *IARC Monographs on the Evaluation of the Carcinogenic Risk of Chemical to Humans – Overall Evaluations of Carcinogenicty: An Updating of IARC Monographs Volume 1 to 42*, Supplement 7 (Lyon).

IARC (1989) *IARC Monographs on the Evaluation of the Carcinogenic Risk of Chemical to Humans – Diesel and Gasoline Engine Exhaust and Some Nitroarenes*, 46 (Lyon).

IARC (1990a) *IARC Monographs on the Evaluation of the Carcinogenic Risk of Chemical to Humans – Some Flame Retardants and Textile Chemicals, and Exposures in the Textile Manufacturing Industry*, 48 (Lyon).

IARC (1990b) *IARC Monographs on the Evaluation of the Carcinogenic Risk of Chemical to Humans – Pharmaceutical Drugs*, 50 (Lyon).

IARC (1991) *IARC Monographs on the Evaluation of the Carcinogenic Risk of Chemical to Humans – Chlorinated Drinking-water; Chlorination By-products; Some Other Halogenated Compounds; Cobalt and Cobalt Compounds*, 52 (Lyon).

IARC (1993a) *IARC Monographs on the Evaluation of the Carcinogenic Risk of Chemical to Humans – Some Naturally Occurring Substances: Food Items and Constituents, Heterocyclic Aromatic Amines and Mycotoxins*, 56 (Lyon).

IARC (1993b) *IARC Monographs on the Evaluation of the Carcinogenic Risk of Chemical to Humans – Occupational Exposures of Hairdressers and Barbers and Personal Use of Hair Colourants; Some Hair Dyes, Cosmetic Colourants, Industrial Dyestuffs and Aromatic Amines,* 57 (Lyon).

IARC (1994) *IARC Monographs on the Evaluation of the Carcinogenic Risk of Chemical to Humans – Some Industrial Chemical,* 60 (Lyon).

IARC (1995) *IARC Monographs on the Evaluation of the Carcinogenic Risk of Chemical to Humans – Dry Cleaning, Some Chlorinated Solvents and Other Industrial Chemicals,* 63 (Lyon).

IARC (1997) *IARC Monographs on the Evaluation of the Carcinogenic Risk of Chemical to Humans – Polychlorinated Dibenzo-para-dioxins and Polychlorinated Dibenzofurans,* 69 (Lyon).

IARC (1999a) *IARC Monographs on the Evaluation of the Carcinogenic Risk of Chemical to Humans – Re-evaluation of Some Organic Chemical, Hydrazine and Hydrogen Peroxide, Part One,* 71 (Lyon).

IARC (1999b) *IARC Monographs on the Evaluation of the Carcinogenic Risk of Chemical to Humans – Re-evaluation of Some Organic Chemical, Hydrazine and Hydrogen Peroxide, Part Two,* 71 (Lyon).

IARC (1999c) *IARC Monographs on the Evaluation of the Carcinogenic Risk of Chemical to Humans – Re-evaluation of Some Organic Chemical, Hydrazine and Hydrogen Peroxide, Part Three,* 71 (Lyon).

IARC (1999d) *IARC Monographs on the Evaluation of the Carcinogenic Risk of Chemical to Humans – Some Chemicals that Cause Tumors of the Kidney or Urinary Bladder in Rodents and Some Other Substances,* 73 (Lyon).

IARC (2000a) *IARC Monographs on the Evaluation of the Carcinogenic Risk of Chemical to Humans – Some Antiviral and Antineoplastic Drugs, and other Pharmaceutical Agents,* 76 (Lyon).

IARC (2000b) *IARC Monographs on the Evaluation of the Carcinogenic Risk of Chemical to Humans – Some Thyrotropic Agents,* 79 (Lyon).

IARC (2010) *IARC Monographs on the Evaluation of the Carcinogenic Risk of Chemical to Humans – Some Aromatic Amines, Organic Dyes, and Related Exposures,* 66 (Lyon).

ILO (1987) Internationl Labour Office. *Informe sobre la Utilización de Sustancias Químicas en el Trabajo.* Oficina Internacional del Trabajo (Ginebra).

INES (2007) "Another science, other technologies are possible: Meeting the challenges" – *Seminar organized by INES (International Network of Engineers and Scientists for global responsibilities) and WFSW (World Federation of Scientific Workers)* – Berlin, May 31st, June 1st.

INES (2011) "What's New in INES", 1. November 2011. <www.inesglobal.com>.

INESPE/Ethikschutzinitiative (2000) *Rundbrief an die Unterstuützer und Sympathisanten der Ethikschutz-Initiative*, 1-4.

Institute of Science in Society (2000) "Open Letter from World Scientists to All Governments Corcerning Genetically Modified Organisms (GMOs)".

International Conference on Cell Tower Sitting (2000) *Proceedings. International Conference on Cell Tower Siting*, Salzburg – June 7-8.

IPCS (1985a) International Programme on Chemcal Safety. *Environmental Health Criteria 47, Summary Report on the Evaluation of Short-Term Test for Carcinogens (Collaborative Study on In Vitro Tests)*, World Health Organization (Geneva).

IPCS (1985b) International Programme on Chemcal Safety. *Environmental Health Criteria 51, Guide to Short-Term Test for Detecting Mutagenic and Carcinogenic Chemicals*, World Health Organization (Geneva).

IPCS (1987) International Programme on Chemcal Safety. *Environmental Health Criteria 69, Magnetic Fields*, World Health Organization (Geneva).

IPCS (1990) International Programme on Chemcal Safety. *Environmental Health Criteria 109, Summary Report on the Evaluation of Short-Term Test for Carcinogens (Collaborative Study on In Vivo Tests)*, World Health Organization (Geneva).

IPCS (1993) International Programme on Chemcal Safety. *Environmental Health Criteria 155, Biomarkers and Risk Assessment: Concepts and Principles*, World Health Organization (Geneva).

IPCS (1999a) International Programme on Chemcal Safety. *Environmental Health Criteria 210, Principles for the Assessment of Risks to Human Health from Exposure to Chemicals*, World Health Organization (Geneva).

IPCS (1999b) International Programme on Chemcal Safety. *Environmental Health Criteria 214, Human Exposure Assessment*, World Health Organization (Geneva).

IPCS (2004) International Programme on Chemical Safety. *The WHO Recommended Classification of Pesticides by Hazards and Guidelines to Classification – 2004*, World Health Organization (Geneva).

IRPTC (1987a) International Register of Potentially Toxic Chemical. *IRPTC Datum Profile of 2,4,5-T*, United Nations Environment Programme (Geneva).

IRPTC (1987b) International Register of Potentially Toxic Chemical. *IRPTC Datum Profile of Aldrin*, United Nations Environment Programme (Geneva).

IRPTC (1987c) International Register of Potentially Toxic Chemical. *IRPTC Datum Profile of Chlordane.* United Nations Environment Programme (Geneva).

IRPTC (1987d) International Register of Potentially Toxic Chemical. *IRPTC Datum Profile of Chlorbenzilate,* United Nations Environment Programme (Geneva).

IRPTC (1987e) International Register of Potentially Toxic Chemical. *IRPTC Datum Profile of DDT*, United Nations Environment Programme (Geneva).

IRPTC (1987f) International Register of Potentially Toxic Chemical. *IRPTC Datum Profile of Dieldrin,* United Nations Environment Programme (Geneva).

IRPTC (1987g) International Register of Potentially Toxic Chemical. *IRPTC Datum Profile of Lindane*, United Nations Environment Programme (Geneva).

IRPTC (1987h) International Register of Potentially Toxic Chemical. *IRPTC Datum Profile of Maneb*, United Nations Environment Programme (Geneva).

IRPTC (1987i) International Register of Potentially Toxic Chemical. *IRPTC Datum Profile of Mirex*, United Nations Environment Programme (Geneva).

IRPTC (1987j) International Register of Potentially Toxic Chemical. *IRPTC Datum Profile of Parathion,* United Nations Environment Programme (Geneva).

IRPTC (1987k) International Register of Potentially Toxic Chemical. *IRPTC Datum Profile of Toxaphene, United* Nations Environment Programme (Geneva).

Ishikawa, K. (1985) *What is Total Quality Control? The Japanese Way* (New Jersey).

Jacobsson, P. (2004) Personal communication, Kungliga Teskniska Hogskolan, Stockholm.

Jenkinson, D. (1995) "Let science guide nitrate policy", *Farm Chemical International*, 9/1, 7.

Jerneloew, A. (1989) "Unido Environmental Programme". Draft UNIDO – Meeting 3 to 5 July 1989.

Johannes Paulus II (1990) "Mensaje de su Santidad JPII para la celebraciòn de la Jornada Mundial de la Paz", 1 Enero.

Jonas, H. (1984) *Das Prinzip Verantwortung* (Frankfurt am Main).

Jonas, H. (1987) „Ist erlaubt was machtbar ist?", *Universitas*, 42, 103-115.

Jones, L. (1999) "Science, medicine and the future: Genetically modified foods", *BMJ*, 318-581.

Jungen, B. (1985) "Integration of knowledge in human Ecology", *Humanekologiska skrifter*, 5, 27 (Göteborg).

Kafka, F. (2002) *El Proceso*, LIBROdot.com, <www.librosgratisweb. com/pdf/kafka-franz/el-proceso.pdf>.

Kafka, F. (2011) *El Castillo*, Wikipedia, <http://es.wikipedia.org /wiki/El_castillo_(novela)>.

Kant, E. (1921) *Fundamentación de la Metafísica de las costumbres,* trans. G. Morente, (Madrid).

Kapfelsperger, E. & U. Pollmer (1982) *Iss und stirb, Chemie in unserer Nahrung* (Köln).

Klug, A. (1999) "GM food debate", *The Lancet*, 354, 1729.

Knutti, E. & G.J. Kullman (1994) NIOSH *Health Hazard Evaluation Report – HETA 94-0033-2552*. CDC, NIOSH.

Kobila, E. de (2001) "Luces y sombras de la razón científica", *Cuadernos de la Diosa Episteme*, 2/2, 32-34.

König, W. (2006) „Die Lehre aus der Katastrophe von Tschernobyl", *Umwelt Medizin Gesellschaft*, 19/2, 87.

Kohn, A., et al. "Detection of Genotoxic Substances in Cancer Patients Reveiving Antineoplastic Drugs", *Annals of New York Academy of Sciences*, 776-791.

Korte F. (1988) Presentation, *Primer Congreso Internacional de Ecotoxicología*, 11 al. 15 de Abril, Buenos Aires, Argentina.

Kuhn, T. S. (1995) *La estructura de las Revoluciones Científicas*, Breviarios, Fondo de Cultura Económica.

Kurtzman, C.P., & A. Ciegler (1970) "Mycotoxin from a Blue-Eye Mold of Corn", *Applied Microbiology*, 20/2, 204-207.

Lachmann, P. (1999) "Health risks of genetically modified foods", *The lancet,* 354, 69.

Lakatos, I. (1982) *Die Methodologie der wissenschaftlichen For-schungsprogramme* (Wiesbaden).

Lambert, B., et al. (1986) "Report 7. Assays for Genetic Changes in Mammalian Cells", in: Montesano, R., H., et al., eds., *Long-Term and Short-Term Assays for Carcinogens: A Critical Appraisal, IARC Scientific Publication,* 83 (Lyon), 167-243.

Langbein, K., et al.. (1989) *Nutzen und Risiken der Arzneimitteln , EIM kritischer Ratgeber* (Germany).

Langfelder, E. & CH. Frentzel (2006) „20 Jahre nach Tschernobyl: Er-fahrungen und Lehren aus der Reaktorkatastrophe", *Umwelt Medizin Gesellschaft,* 19/2, 93-99.

Le Nouvel Observateur (2006) Entrevista de Marie-France Hirigoyen <http://librosyrecuerdos.blogspot.com/ 2009_07_01_archive.html>.

Leipert, C. (1986) „Ist humaner Wohlstand möglich?", *Universitas,* 6, 551-558.

Leloir, L.F. (1983) Comment in newspaper, *Diario La Nación* (Buenos Aires, 30 October).

Lenk, H. (1987) „Wirkungsforschung in vernetzen Systemen", *Universitas,* 6, 551-558.

LEY 11.723 (B.O. 30.9.33) Ley de Propiedad Intelectual – Artículo 17 – República Argentina.

Leymann, H. (1996) "Contenido y Desarrollo del Acoso Grupal/moral ("Mobbing") en el Trabajo", *European Journal of Work and Organiza-tional Psychology,* 5/2, 165-184, trans. F. Fuertes (Document in Inter-net) <http://www.anamib.com/debes_saber/mobbing.pdf>.

Liu, J., et al.. (1995) "Optimizing In Situ Hybridization of Lactoferrin mRNA in Mouse Uterine Tissue Using Digoxigenin-Labeled RNA Probes", *Cell Vison,* 2/5, 430-434.

Losey, J.E. (1999) *Polen tóxico de maíz Bt* (Ithaca).

Loukjanenko, V. (1990) "La Crisis del Agua en la URSS", *Salud* Mun-dial, Revista Ilustrada de la Organizazción Mundial de la Salud, Enero/Febrero.

Low, R. (1988) „Vom Prinzip Hoffnung zum Projekt Verantwortung", *Universitas,* 7, 727-731.

Lowe, X.R., et al.. (1995) "Aneuploidies and Micronuclei in the Germ Cells of Male Mice of Advanced Age", *Mutation Research,* 338, 59-76.

Lowe, X.R., et al.. (1998) "Epididymal Sperm Aneuploidies in Three Strain of Rats Detected by Multicolor Fluorescence In Situ Hybridization", *Environmental and Molecular Mutagenesis,* 31, 125-132.

Luke "Luke 5:36-39" <http://www.biblegateway. com/passage/?search=Luke%205:33-39;&version=NIV>.

Magge, B. (1973) *Popper* (Barcelona).

Margolin, B.H., et al. (1986) "Statistical Analyses for In Vitro Cytogenetic Assays Using Chinese Hamster Ovary Cells", *Environmental Mutagenesis,* 8, 183-204.

Marian (2003) *El Acoso Moral en el Lugar de Trabajo* (Document in Internet)<http://www.augcalicante.info/CartaNavegante/Opiniones/opiniones28.htm>.

Maritain, J. (1978) *Los Grados del Saber – Distinguir para unir* (Buenos Aires).

Mayer, S. & I. Meister (2000) *La liberación al. ambiente de organismos geneticamente modificados y su impacto potencial en países en desarrollo* (Manuscript).

McFee, A.F., et al. (1994) "Results of Mouse Bone Marrow Micronucleous Studies on 1,4-Dioxane", *Mutation Research,* 322, 141-150.

McLouglin, M. (2002) Personal communication.

Means, J.R., et al. (1988) "Acute, Subchronic, and Chronic Toxicity Studies of the Cardiotonic Isomazle (LY1753269 in Rats and Dogs (Abstract)", *The Toxicologist,* 8/1, 83.

Mercer, D.K., et al. (1999) "Fate of Free DNA and Transformation of the Oral Bacterium Streptococcus gordonii DL1 by plasmid DNA in Human Saliva", *Applied and Environmental Microbiology,* Jan, 6-10.

Mian, Z. & A. Glaser (2006) "Life in a nuclear powered crowd", *INES Newsletter,* 52, April, 9-13.

Michiels, F.M., et al. (1989) "Biological Effects of Asbestos Fibres on Rat Lung Maintained In Vitro", in: Bignon, J., et al., eds., *Non-Occupational Exposure to Mineral Fibres, IARC Scientific Publication,* 90 (Lyon), 156-160.

Mikkelsen, T. (1996) "The risk of crop transgene spread", *Nature,* 380, March.

Mira y López, E. (1950) *Cuatro gigantes del Alma* (Buenos Aires).

Mirsalis, J.C., et al. (1989) "Measurement of Unscheduled DNA Synthesis and S-Phase Synthesis in Rodent Hepatocytes Following In Vivo

Treatment: Testing of 24 Compounds", *Environmental and Molecular Mutagensis*, 14, 155-164.

Mitcham, C. (1989) *¿Qué es la filosofía de la tecnología?* (Barcelona).

Mitchell, P. (1999) "EU approves tighter regulations for genetically modified foods", *The Lancet*, 354.

Mitchell, P., & J. Bradbury (1999) "British Medical Association enters GM-crop affray", *The Lancet*, 353, 1769.

Mittelstrass, J. (1986a) „Interdisziplinarität – mehr als blosses Ritual", *Universitas*, 10, 203-208.

Mittelstrass, J. (1986b) „Interdisziplinarität – mehr als blosses Ritual", *Universitas*, 10, 1052-1055.

Molineux, R.J., et al. (2000) "Anti-Aflatoxicogenic Activity of Walnut Constituents" – *Aflatoxin/Fumonisin Workshop* – October 25-27, Yosemite, California, USA.

Montoya, V. Fragments from "La Envidia" <http://www.losnoveles.net/palabra2htm>.

Moore, K.G., et al. (1997) "Characterization of a Chitinase from TEX6 Inhibitory to Aspergillus flavus" – *Aflatoxin Elimination Workshop* – October 26-28, Memphis, TN, USA.

Morin, E. (1995) *Introducción al. pensamiento complejo* (Barcelona).

Morris, S.M., et al. (1995) "Programmed Cell Death and Mutation Induction in AHH-1 Human Lymphoblastoid Cells Exposed to m-amsa", *Mutation Research*, 329, 79-96.

Mott, L. & K. Snyder (1987) *Pesticide Alert – A Guide to Pesticides in Fruits and Vegetables,* Natural Resources Defense Council, (San Francisco).

Motta, A. (1985) *Profilaxis del Deterioro Fúngico y Formación de Micotoxinas en Base a la Medición de la Humedad Relativa Ambiente del Aire Intergranular.* Curso para Ingenieros Agrónomos. XII Jornadas Argentinas de Micología. San Luis. 9 al. 12 de Octubre, 95-109.

Motta, A. (1987) *Profilaxis del Deterioro Fúngico y Formación de Micotoxinass en Base a la Humedad Relativa Ambiente del Aire Intergranular.* Bolsa de Comercio de Rosario, (Rosario).

Motta, A. (1994) *Tecnogenologia: Verdad y Técnica – Actitudes y Consecuencias.* Colección Tecnogenia 6, (Rosario).

Motta, A. & G.M. Eguiazu (1989) "Fundamentos de una Ley de Tecnogenia" – Actas *Jornadas 2do Seminario Nacional Universidad y Medioambiente* – 25-27 October, Paraná/Entre Rios/Argentina.

Motta, A. & G.M. Eguiazu (1990) *Evaluación de Riesgo Ecotoxicológi-co Durante las Operaciones Normales de Uso, Almacenaje y Limpieza en el Laboratorio de una Casa de Altos Estudios.* Colección Tecnogenia 2, (Rosario).

Motta, A. & G.M. Eguiazu (1991a) "Variación de Parámetros de Calidad del Grano y Aceite de Girasol Almacenado a Diferentes a Humedades Relativas" – *Actas "Evolución". Primera Reunión Nacional de Oleaginosos* – Rosario 10 y 11 de Octubre, Bolsa de Comercio de Rosario, Rosario, Argentina, 434-441.

Motta, A. & G.M. Eguiazu (1991b) "La humedad relativa del aire inter-granular (HRAI) – Un nuevo parámetro para la comercialización de los granos" – *Actas "Evolución". Primera Reunión Nacional de Oleaginosos* – Rosario 10 y 11 de Octubre, Bolsa de Comercio de Rosario, Rosario, Argentina. 433.

Motta, A. & G.M. Eguiazu (1993) "Cinética de Rehidratación y Deterio-ro Biológico en Zea mays Almacenado a una Humedad Relativa del Aire Intergranular (HRAI) del 92 %", *Grasas y Aceites*, 6, 362-364.

Motta, A. & G.M. Eguiazu (2003) "El Desafío del Conocimiento de la Tecnogenia en la Enseñanza de la Tecnología", *UNR Ambiental*, 5, 49-58.

Motta, A. & G.M. Eguiazu (2004) "La Tecnopatogenología y su Contri-bución al. Manejo Poscosecha de Granos", *Aposgrán*, 85/1, 22-26.

Motta, A. & G.M. Eguiazu (2005) "Tecnopatogenología, Tecnopatogenia: La quinta aproximación". *Humanitas, Anuario del Centro de Estudios Humanísticos*, Universidad Autónoma de Nuevo León, 843-860.

Motta, A. & G.M. Eguiazu (2007) "La Tecnopatogenología y su carácter de ciencia. Propuesta metodológica, herramientas y otros aspectos. Refutación a algunas Objeciones". *Humanitas – Filosofía, Anuario del Centro de Estudios Humanísticos*, Universidad Autónoma de Nuevo León, 175-220.

Motta, E.J. (2011) Personal communication.

Mujeres en Red. "Violencia perversa", Extractos de Notas de la Conferencia de la Dra. M.F. Hirigoyen en Barcelona en Octubre 19, 2001 <www.acosomoral.org> and <http://www.nuestraedad.com.mx/violenciaperversa.htm>.

Neutra, R., et al. (1992) "Cluster Galore: Insights about Environmental Clusters from Probability Theory", *The Science of the Total Environment,* 127, 187-200.

NIEHS-DOE (1995) National Institute of Environmental Health Sciences and U. S. Department of Energy. *Question and Answers About E.M.F. Electric and Magnetic Fields Associated with the Use of Electric Power.* DOE/EE-0040.

Nietzsche, F.W. (1844-1900) Proverb <http://www.proverbia.net>.

NIH-NCI (1995) National Institute of Health – National Cancer Institute. *Understanding Gene Testing.* NIH Publication N° 96-3905.

NIH-NCI (2003) National Institute of Health – National Cancer Institute. *Cancer and the Environment - What You Need To Know - What You Can Do.* NIH Publication No. 03–2039.

NIOSH (1979) National Institute for Occupational Safety and Health. *A Guide to the Work-Relatedness of Disease.* Revised Edition, Kusnet, S. & M.K. Hutchinson, eds.

NIOSH-NIEHS-DOE (1996) National Institute for Occupational Safety and Health – National Institute of Environmental Health Sciences – U.S. Department of Energy. *Question and Answers EMF in the Workplace* – DOE/GO-10095-218.

Nuñez de Castro, I. (2000) "La Ética de la Investigación Científica", in: Cortina A. & J. Conill, eds., *Diez palabras clave en ética de las profesiones* (Navarra).

Nutzinger, H.G. (1986) „Das Konzept des qualitativen Wachstums und die Schwierigkeiten seiner Umsetzung", *Universitas*, 41, 1136-1148.

Olenchock, S.A., et al. (1989) "Effects of Different Extraction Protocols on Endotoxin Analyses of Airborne Grain Dust", *Scand. J. Environ. Health*, 15, 430-435.

Olenchock, S.A. (1990a) "Endotoxins – Biological Contaminants in Indoor Environments", in: Morey, P.R., et al., eds., *American Society for Testing and Materials*, ASTM STP 1071 (Philadelphia), 190-200.

Olenchock, S.A. (1990b) "Endotoxins in Various Work Environments in Agriculture – Development of Industrial Microbiology", *J. Of Ind. Microbiology*, 31/5, 193-197.

Olenchock, S.A. (1994) "Health Effects of Biological Agents: The Role of Endotoxins", *Appl. Occup. Environ. Hyg.*, 9/1, 62-64.

Paul *"First letter to Timothy"*, Christian Community Bible, 6,10, (Madrid).

Parr, D. (2000) *GM on trial: Scientific evidence presented in the defence of 28 Greenpeace volunteers on trial for their non-violent removal of a GM crop* (Greenpeace).

Pauling, L. (1965) „Die Wirklichkeit heutiger Gefährdung der Welt", *Universitas,* 43, 203-208.

Payne, G.A., et al. (2002) "Genetic Analysis of Inhibitory Proteins from Maize Seeds" – *Proceedings of the 2nd Fungal Genomics, 3rd Fumonisin Elimination and 15th Aflatoxin Elimination Workshops* – October 23-25, San Antonio, Texas, USA.

Payot, J. (1947) *El Trabajo Intelectual y la Voluntad* (Buenos Aires).

Peicovich, E. (2006) "Enfoques", *Diario La Nación* (Buenos Aires, 26 de Marzo).

Pengue, W. Personal communication.

Pérez Soliva, M. *El daño encubierto* <http://www.acosomoral.org/9Congreso7.htm>.

Petrosyan, V. (2005) Presentation – *INES Council Meeting 2005* – Vaquerias, Córdoba, Argentina.

Phillips, M.D., et al. (1991) "Induction of Micronuclei in Mouse Bone Marrow Cells: An Evaluation of Nucleoside Analogues Used in the Treatment of AIDS", *Environ. and Mol. Mutagens,* 18, 168-183.

Pirisi, A. (1998) "Genetically engineered foods debate sows seeds of discontent", *The Lancet*, 352, 382.

PNUMA (1982) Programa de las Naciones Unidas para el Medio Ambiente. "La Próxima Década", *Industria y Medioambiente*, N° 3.

PNUMA (1985a) Programa de las Naciones Unidas para el Medio Ambiente. *Registro Internacional De Productos Químicos Potencialmente Tóxicos*, Boletín, 7/1.

PNUMA (1985b) Programa de las Naciones Unidas para el Medio Ambiente. *Registro Internacional De Productos Químicos Potencialmente Tóxicos,* Boletín, 7/2.

PNUMA (1987) Programa de las Naciones Unidas para el Medio Ambiente. *Registro Internacional de Productos Químicos Potencialmente Tóxicos*, Boletín, 8/1.

PNUMA (1991) Programa de las Naciones Unidas para el Medio Ambiente. *Registro Internacional de Productos Químicos Potencialmente Tóxicos,* Boletín, 10/2.

Pompidou, A. (1997) "Research in Medical Ethics and Ethics of Research in the European Union", in: Gindro, et al., eds., *Research on Bioethics – Bioethics Research: Policy, M ethods and Strategies – Proceedings of a European Conference* – Roma, 23-25 November 1995, European Comission. Report EUR 17465 EN, 139-141.

Popper, K.R. (1973) *Conjectures and Refutations. The Growth of Scientific Knowledge* (London).

Preciado Patiño, J. "Resistencia a herbicidas: una amenaza latente", *Forrajes y Granos Agribusiness Journal.*

Preussmann, R. (1972) "On the Significance of N-Nitroso Compounds as Carcinogens and on Problems Related to their Chemical Analysis", in: Bogovski, P., et al., eds., *N-Nitroso Compounds – Analyasis and Formation, IARC Scientific Publication*, 3 (Lyon), 6-9.

Preussmann, R. (1976) "Chemical Carcinogens in the Human Environment – Problems and Quantitative Aspects", *Oncology,* 33, 51-57.

Preussmann, R. (1980) „Tumorbildung durch Schadstoffe: II Restrisiko", *Zeitschrift für Umweltpolitik,* 2, 649-659.

Pritchard, J.B. & J.R. Bend (1991) "Relative Roled of Metabolism and Renal Excretory Mechanisms in Xenobiotic Elimination by Fish", *Environmentla Health Perspectives*, 90, 85-92.

Purchase, I.F.H. (2004) "What determines the acceptability of genetically modified food?", *Toxicology and Applied Pharmacology* , Abstracts – ICTX Congress Special Issue, 197/3, 143.

Pusztai, A. (2000b) Presentation. *INES Conference: Challenges for Science and Engineering in the 21st Century* – Stockholm, Sweden – 14 to 18 June.

Quevedo, F. (1580-1645) Thought <http://despiertateya.blogspot.com/2008/03/donde-no-hay-justicia-es-peligroso.html>.

Rabovsky, J., et al. (1986) "In Vitro Effects of Straight-Chain Alkanes (n-Hexane through n-Decane) on Rat Liver and Lung Cytochrome P-450", *J. Of Toxicol. and Environ.Health*, 18, 409-421.

Rall, D.P. (1990) "Carcinogens in our Environment", in: Vainio, H., et al., eds., *Complex Mixtures and Cancer Risk, IARC Scientific Publication*, 104 (Lyon), 233-239.

Rammert, W. (1991) Personal communication. Freie Universität Berlin – Institut für Soziologie.

Rhodes, J. M. "Genetically modified foods and the Pusztai affair", *BMJ,* 318, 1284.

Ricco, R.R. (1993) *Calidad Estratégica Total: Total Quality Management* (Buenos Aires).

Ris, C.H. & P.W. Preuss (1988) "Risk Assessment and Risk Management: A Process", in: Cothern C.R., et al., eds., *Risk Assessment and*

Risk Management of Industrial and Environmental Chemical (Princeton, New Jersey), XV, 1-21.

Rohm & Haas (1986) "Listado de Hojas de Seguridad de Material – Maneb 80 R Y H", *Política sobre Seguridad, Salud y Medio Ambientel* (Buenos Aires).

Rolies, J.J. (1986) „Ist erlaubt , was möglich ist? Aufgaben einer Ethik der Medien", *Universitas*, 41, 135-141.

Ropohl, G. (1989) „An den Grenzen der Ingenieurethik", *Universitas*, 6, 561-568.

Rose, W.D. (1987) *Handbuch der krebsverursachenden Chemikalien, Kunststoffe und Strahlen* (München).

Saage, R. (1989) „Plädoyer für die Aufklärung wider die Vernunftkritik", *Universitas*, 3, 273-283.

Sachsse, H. (1985) „Die Krise der technischen Welt", *Universitas* 40, 407-414.

SAGUF (1983) *Praxisorientierte ökologische Forschung* (Bern).

Salvat (1978) *Enciclopedia Salvat* (Barcelona).

Samuel "Libro Segundo de Samuel", *Biblia de Jerusalén*, Capítulo 12, Versículo 3, (Bilbao).

San Martín, J. (1987) *Los Nuevos Redentores* (Barcelona).

San Martín, J. (1990) *Tecnología y Futuro Humano* (Barcelona).

San Pablo (a) "Primera Carta del Apóstol a Timoteo", *Biblia de Jerusalén*, Capítulo 6, Versículo 10, (Bilbao).

San Pablo (b) "Primera Epístola a los Corintios", *Biblia de Jerusalén*, Capítulo 6, Versículo 12, (Bilbao).

Sanders, T.A. (1999) "Food production and food safety", *BMJ*, 318, 1689-1693.

Sanguineti, J.J. (1977) *Augusto Comte: Curso de Filosofía Positiva*. Colección Crítica Filosófica, (Madrid).

Santurio, J. (2003) "Cuidado con la Calidad de los Cereales: Hongos y Micotoxinas". *Aposgrán*, 83/3, 49-52.

Scallet, A.C., et al. (2004) "Increased Volume of the Calindin D28k-Labeled Sexually Dimorphic Hypothalamus in Genistein and Nonynphenol-Treated Male Rats", *Toxicological Sciences*, 82, 570-576.

Schadel, E. (2005) "El dolor tantálico de Kant", *Cuadernos salmantinos de filosofía*, 32, 121-154.

Schaefer, O.F. (1989) „Reflexionen über ein holistisches Verständnis der Welt", *Universitas*, 8, 773-778.

Scheibe, E. (1987) „Gibt es eine Annäherung der Naturwissenschaften an den Geisteswissenschaften?", *Universitas*, 1, 5-17.

Schmähl, D., & H.R. Scherf (1984) "Carcinogenic Activity of N-Nitrosodimethylamine in Snakes (Python reticulatus, Scheider)", in: O'Neil, I.K., et al., eds., *Nitroso Compounds: Occurrence, Biological Effects and Relevance to Human Cancer, IARC Scientific Publication*, 57 (Lyon), 677-682.

Schmidt-Bleek, F. (2007) *Nutzen wir die Erde Richtig? – Die Leistungen der Natur und die Arbeit des Menschen* (Frankfurt am Main).

Schmitz-Feuerhake, I. (2006) „Anstiege bei Fehlbildungen, perinataler Sterblichkeit und kindlichen Erkrankungen nach vorgeburtlicher Exposition durch Tschernobylfallout", *Umwelt Medizin Gesellschaft*, 19/2, 100-108.

Schneider-Poetsch, H.J. (1987) „Technologiefeindlichkeit und die Verantwortung des Naturwissenschaftlers", *Universitas*, 11, 1158-1166.

Schuller, H.M., et al. (1987) "Cell Type-Specific Differences in Metabolic Activation of N-Nitrosodiethylamine by Human Lung Cancer Cell Lines", in: Bartsch, H., et al., eds., *Relevance of N-Nitroso Compounds to Human Cancer: Exposures and Mechanisms, IARC Scientific Publication*, 84 (Lyon), 138-140.

Scott, D., et al. (1991) "Genotoxicity under Extreme Culture Conditions – A Report from ICPEMC Task Group", *Mutation Research*, 257, 147-204.

Seemayer, N.H., et al. (1984) "Cell Cultures as a Tool for Detection of Cytotoxic, Mutagenic and Carcinogenic Activity of Airborne Particulate Mater", *J. Of Aerosol Science*, 15, 426-430.

Séneca, L.A. (61a.c.-31d.c.) Thought <www.rinconcastellano.com>.

Shakespeare, W. Act 1 Sc IV, Hamlet (Marcellus) "Something is rotten in the State of Denmark" <http://shakespeare.mit.edu/hamlet/ hamlet.1.4.html>.

Shi, X.Ch., et al. (1992) "Induction of micronuclei in rat bone marrow by four model compounds", *Teratogenesis, Carcinogenesis and Mutagenesis,* 11, 251-258.

Shiva Vandana (1995) *Monocultures of the Mind*, Third World Network.

Shotweel, O. (1983) "Aflatoxin detection and determination in corn", *Aflatoxin and Aspergillus Flavus in Corn,* Southern Cooperative Series Bulletin 279, 38-45.

Simonis, U. (1985) „Präventive Umweltpolitik", *Universitas*, 40, 121-130.

Simonis, U. (1989) „Entwicklung und Umwelt. Ein Plädoyer für mehr Harmonie", *Universitas*, 44, 1030-1039.

Sofuni, T., et al. (1990) "A comparison of chromosome aberration induction by 25 compounds tested by two chinese hamster cell (CHL and CHO) systems in culture", *Mutation Research*, 241, 175-213.

Sorenson, B., et al. (1995) *NIOSH Health Hazard Evaluation Report.* HETA 95-0160-257, CDC, NIOSH.

Standard Enciclopedic Dictionary, Funk & Wagnalls Publishing Company, Inc., The Clute International Institute, Los Angeles, 1971.

Strumpel, B. (1987) „Grüne Gefühle – Technokratische Argumente zum Wandel des Fortschrittsverständnisses", *Universitas*, 4, 341-348.

Stumpf, R. (2006) "El Mix energético del futuro – Parte II – Energía nuclear, adios a plazos", *Deutschland* 3, 11.

Swaminathan, S., et al. (1996) "Neoplastic transformation and DNA-binding of 4,4'-methylenebis(2-Chloroaniline) in SV40-immortalized human uroepitelial cell lines", *Carcinogenesis*, 17/4, 857-864.

Swartz, W.J. (1985) "Effects of carbaryl on gonadal development in the chick embryo". *Bull. Environ. Contam.. Toxicol*, 34, 481-485.

Swartz, W.J. & G.M. Mall (1989) "Chlordecone-Induced Follicular toxicity in mouse ovaries", *Reproductive Toxicology*, 3, 203-206.

Swartz, W.J. & R.L. Schutzman (1986) "Reaction of the mouse liver to kepone exposure", *Bull. Environ. Contam. Toxicol*, 37, 169-174.

Tacitus, P.C. (55 d.c.-120) Thought <www.rinconcastellano.com>.

Tecnogenia Ambiental: Resoluciones: Facultad de Ciencias Agrarias (CD) 152/88 – 110/89 – 045/95 – 090/95 – 143/95 – 117/91 – 145/95 – 042/98 – 132/99. Facultad de Ciencias Bioquímicas y Farmacéuticas (CD) 121/00 – Facultad de Humanidades y Artes (CD) 561/00.

Tengstrom, E. (1985) "Human Ecology: A new discipline", *Humanekologisks*, Skripen, 4. Göteborg.

Tenner, A (2004) "I + Dt info", *Revista de la Investigación europea*, 40, Febrero.

Teutsch, G.M. (1987) „Gerechtigkeit für Mensch und Tier", *Universitas*, 42, 835-847.

Thurau, M. (1989) *Gentechnik – Wer kontrolliert die Industrie?* (Frankfurt am Main).

Tirmenstein, M.A., et al. (1997) "Antimony-Induced Alterations in Thiol Homeostasis and Adenine Nucleotide Staus in Cultured Cardiac Myocytes", *Toxicology*, 119, 203-211.

Tolstoi, L.N. (1829-1910) Thought <www.rinconcastellano.com>.

Tomatis, L., et al. (2001) "Alleged 'misconceptions' distort perceptions of environmental cancer risks", *Environmental Cancer Risks,* The FASEB Journal, 15, 195-203.

Toynbee, A. "Is America neglecting her creative talents?", in: Taylor, C. W., ed., *Widening horizons and creativity.* (New York).

Treviño Ghioldi, S. (2005) "Guía práctica para casos de acoso psicológico: mobbing", *Diario Unión,* Año XVL, N° 214.

Tu, A.S., et al. (1992) "Morphological Transformation of Syrian Hamster Embryo Cells by Mezerein", *Cancer Letters,* 62, 159-165.

U.N.R. (1985) Resolución R.N. N° 1993/85 del 27/11/85 y C.S.P. N° 744/85 del 17/12/85 – Expediente N° 46200.

Ulmann, G. (1974) *Kreativitätsforschung* (Köln).

Universität Karlsruhe (2000) „Wissenschaftlichem Fehlverhalten entgegen treten", *UNIKATH* (Karlsruhe).

Universität Karlsruhe (2006) „CEDIM (Center for Disaster Management and Risk Reduktion Technology)", 24 (Abt. Forschung), (Karlsruhe).

US CPSC (1992) U.S Consumer Product Safety Commissión. *1992 – Annual Report to Congress.*

US DHEW-PHS (1979) *"National Toxicology Program – Fiscal Year 1980 – Annual Plan"*, U.S. Department of Health, Education and Welfare – Public Health Services. NTP 79-7.

US DHHS-PHS (1980) *"National Toxicology Program – Fiscal Year 1981 – Annual Plan"*, U.S. Department of Health and Human Services – Public Health Services.

US DHHS-PHS (1984) *"Report of the NTP Ad-Hoc Panel on Chemical Carcinogenesis Testing and Evaluation"*. Board of Scientific Councelors, U.S. Department of Health and Human Services – Public Health Services, National Toxicology Program.

US DHHS-PHS (1995) *"National Toxicology Program – Fiscal Year 1995 – Annual Plan"*, U.S. Department of Health and Human Services – Public Health Services.

US DHHS-PHS (2002) *"National Toxicology Program – Fiscal Year 2002 – Annual Plan"*, U.S. Department of Health and Human Services – Public Health Services, NIH Publication N° 03-5309.

US DHHS-PHS-FDA (1998). *Federal Food, Drug and Cosmetic Act – As Amended February 1998.* Sec. 409, 82. U.S. Department of

Health and Human Services – Public Health Services – Food and Drug Administration.

US DHHS-PHS-NIH-NTP (1992a) *"Toxicology and Carcinogenesis Studies of Monochloroacetic Acid (CAS Number 79-11-8) In F344/N Rats and B6C3F1 Mice (Gavage Studies)"*. U.S. Department of Health and Human Services – Public Health Services – National Institute of Health, National Toxicology Program, Technical Report Series N° 396.

US DHHS-PHS-NIH-NTP (1992b) *"Toxicology and Carcinogenesis Studies of 60-Hz Magnetic Fields in F344/N Rats and B6C3F1 Mice (Whole-Body Exposure Studies)"*, U.S. Department of Health and Human Services – Public Health Services – National Institute of Health, National Toxicology Program, Technical Report Series N° 488, NIH Publication N° 99-3978.

US DHHS-PHS-NIH-NTP (1992c). *"Toxicology and Carcinogenesis Studies of Magnetic Field Promotion (DMBA) Initiation in Female Sprague-Dawley Rats (Whole-Body Exposure/Gavage Studies)"*, U.S. Department of Health and Human Services – Public Health Services – National Institute of Health, National Toxicology Program, Technical Report Series N° 489, NIH Publication N° 99-3979.

US DHHS-PHS-NIH-NTP (2001) *Toxicology and Carcinogenesis Studies of p,p'-Dichorodiphenyl Sulfone (CAS N° 50-07-09) In F344/N Rats and B6C3F1 Mice (Feed Studies)*. T.R.S. 501. U.S. Department of Health and Human Services, Public Health Services, National Institutes of Health, NIH Publication N° 01-4435.

US DHHS-PHS-NTP (1985) *"Fourth Annual Report on Carcinogens"*, U.S. Department of Health and Human Services – Public Health Services – National Toxicology Program, National Institute for Environmental Health Sciences, PB 85-134633.

US DHHS-PHS-NTP (1991) *"Sixth Annual Report on Carcinogens"*. U.S. Department of Health and Human Services – Public Health Services – National Toxicology Program, National Institute for Environmental Health Sciences.

US DHHS-PHS-NTP (2002) *"10th Report on Carcinogens – 2002"*, U.S. Department of Health and Human Services – Public Health Services – National Toxicology Program.

US DHHS-PHS-NTP (2004) *"11th Report on Carcinogens – 2004"*, U.S. Department of Health and Human Services – Public Health Services – National Toxicology Program.

Vesonder, R.F. & W. Wu (1998) "Correlation of Moniliformin, but not Fumonisin B1 Levels, in Culture Materials of Fusarium Isolates to Acute Death in Ducklings Poultry", *Science*, 77, 67-72.

Volmar, R. (2002) „Schon Galilei schwindelte", *UNIKATH* , 3:2002 . Seite 20.

Voltaire, F.M. (1694-1778) Thought <www.rinconcastellano.com>.

von Uexkull, J. (1983) *Streifzüge durch die Umwelten von Tieren und Menschen* (Frankfurt am Main).

von Weizsäcker, E. (1986) „Fehlerfreundlichkeit als Evolutionsprinzip und Kritierium der Technikbewertung", *Universitas*, 41, 791-799.

von Wright, G.H. (1988) „Rationalität und Vernunft in der Wissenschaft", *Universitas*, 9, 1988-1945.

Walters, M., et al. (2003) "System Toxicology and the Chemical Effects in Biological Systems (CEBS) Knowledge Base", *EHP Toxicogenomics*, 111/1T, 15-28.

Wandscheider, D. (1989) „Gründe und Gegengründe. Der Streit der Experten in ethische Perspektive", *Universitas*, 41, 791-799.

Watson, R. (1999) "EU says growth hormones pose health risk", *BMJ*, 318, 1442.

Weinstein, I.B., et al. (1984) "Initial Cellular Target and Eventual Genomic Changes in Multistage Carcinogenesis", in: Börzsönyi, M., et al., eds., *Model, Mechanisms and Etiology of Tumour Promotion, IARC Scientific Publication*, 56 (Lyon), 159-184.

Westerholm, B. (1999) *God sed i forskningen* (Good Conduct in Research) (Stockholm).

Westerholm, B., et al. (2004) *Practical Ethics in Occupational Health* (Oxford).

Whitaker, T.B. (1993) *Testing Commodities for Aflatoxin in the International Market* (Leaflet).

Whitehead, A.J. & C. Orris (1995) "Food Safety through HACCP", *Food, Nutrition and Agriculture,* 15, 25-28.

WHO (1996) *Guidelines for drinking-water quality – Volume II – Health criteria and other supporting information*, Second Edition, World Health Organization.

WHO (1997) *Consecuencias sanitarias del accidente de Chernobyl – Resultados de los proyectos experimentales PIECCS y de los programas nacionales conexos – Informe recapitulativo,* World Health Organization.

WHO (1989) World Health Organization. "Environmental Epidemiology Network – List of Participants", *Environmental & Occupational Epidemiology*, PEP/89.16.

Whong, W.Z., et al. (1990) "Use of rat primary lung cells for studying genotoxicity with the sister Chromatid Exchange and micronucleus assays", *Mutation Research*, 241, 7-13.

Whong, W.Z., et al. (1992) "Comparison of DNA Adduct detection between two enhancement methods of the 32P-Postlabelling assay in rat lung cells", *Mutation Research*, 283, 1-6.

WHO-UNEP-FAO. *The Rotterdam Convention on the Prior Informed Consents Procedure for Certain Hazardous Chemicals and Pesticides in the International Trade*, World Health Organization, United Nations Environmental Programme, and Food and Agriculture Organization for the United Nations, Flyer.

Wild, W. (1984) „Vom Wahrheitsgehalt der Naturgesetze". *Universitas*, 39, 1067-1078.

Wishnok, J.S., et al. (1987) "The Ferret as a Model for Endogenous Synthesis and Metabolism of N-Nitrosamines", in: Bartsch, H., et al., eds., *Relevance of N-Nitroso Compounds to Human Cancer: Exposures and Mechanisms*, IARC Scientific Publication, 84 (Lyon), 135-137.

Witt, K.L., et al. (1992) "Induction of chromosomal damage in mammalian cells in vitro and in vivo by Sulfapyridine of 5-Aminosalicilic Acid", *Mutation Research,* 283, 59-64.

Witt, K.L., et al. (2000) "Micronucleated Erythrocyte Frequency in Peripheral Blood of B6C3F1 Mice from Short-Term, Prechronic, and Chronic Studies of the NTP Carcinogenesis Bioassay Program", *Environmental and Molecular Mutagenesis,* 36, 163-194.

Wyrobek, A., et al. (1995) "Aneuploidy on Late-Step spermatids of mice detected by two-chromosome fluorescence in sity hybridization", *Molecular Reproduction and Development,* 40, 259-266.

Yunus, M. (1999) *Hacia un Mundo Sin Pobreza* (Buenos Aires).

Zhu, S., et al. (1991) "Cytotoxicity, Genotoxicity, and Trasforming Activity of 4-(Methylnitrosoamino)-1-(3-pyridyl)-1-Butanone (NNK) in rat tracheal epithelial cells", *Mutation Research*, 261, 249-259.

Zinna G. (2004) Commentary in newspaper. *Diario La Capital* (Rosario 8 de Marzo).

Zip, M. (2001) „Kurswechsel im Verbraucherschutz", *Deutschland – Forum für Politik, Kultur, Wirtschaft und Wissenschaft*, 2, 7-10.